Diagnostic Reasoning

CASE ANALYSIS *in*
PRIMARY CARE
PRACTICE

Diagnostic Reasoning

CASE ANALYSIS *in* PRIMARY CARE PRACTICE

Jean Nagelkerk, PhD, RN, FNP-C

Professor and Director of Development and Grants
Grand Valley State University
Allendale, Michigan

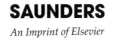

SAUNDERS

An Imprint of Elsevier

SAUNDERS
An Imprint of Elsevier
The Curtis Center
Independence Square West
Philadelphia, PA 19106

Editor-in-Chief: Sally Schrefer
Executive Editor: Barbara Nelson Cullen
Managing Editor: Sandra Clark Brown
Project Manager: Debbie Vogel
Production Editor: Ed Alderman
Design Manager: Bill Drone
Cover Designer: Teresa Breckwoldt

Library of Congress Cataloging-in-Publication Data

Nagelkerk, Jean M.
   Diagnostic reasoning: case analysis in primary care practice/Jean Nagelkerk.
   p.; cm.
   Includes bibliographical references and index.
   ISBN-13: 978-0-7216-8692-9   ISBN-10: 0-7216-8692-3
   1. Diagnosis—Case studies.   2. Nursing diagnosis—Case studies.   3. Clinical
medicine—Decision making—Case studies.   4. Nurse practitioners.   I. Title.
   [DNLM: 1. Nursing Diagnosis—Case Report.   2. Decision Making—Case Report.
3. Nurse Practitioners—Case Report.   4. Patient Care Planning—Case Report.   5. Primary
Health Care—Case Report.   6. Primary Nursing Care—Case Report. WY 100.4 N147d 2001]
RC71 .N24 2001
616.07'5—dc21

                                                                              00-045809

DIAGNOSTIC REASONING: CASE ANALYSIS IN PRIMARY CARE PRACTICE

Permissions may be sought directly from Elsevier's Health Sciences Rights
Department in Philadelphia, PA, USA: phone: (+1) 215 239 3804, fax: (+1) 215 239 3805,
e-mail: healthpermissions@elsevier.com. You may also complete your request on-line
via the Elsevier homepage (http://www.elsevier.com), by selecting 'Customer Support'
and then 'Obtaining Permissions'.

ISBN-13: 978-0-7216-8692-9
ISBN-10: 0-7216-8692-3

Printed in the United States of America

Last digit is the print number: 9   8   7   6   5   4   3

Contributors

Katherine Barbee, MSN, ANP
Adult Nurse Practitioner, Internal Medicine
Kaiser Permanente
Washington, DC
Chapter 12 Dermatological Disorders

Mary Moran Barr, RN, BSN, CCRN
Critical Care Nurse
St. Mary's Medical Center
Grand Rapids, Michigan
Appendix C Additional Case Study Exercise

Ruth Ann Brintnall, RN, MSN, AOCN, ANP
Assistant Professor
Grand Valley State University
Allendale, Michigan
Chapter 7 Cardiovascular Disorders
Chapter 9 Blood Dyscrasias
Chapter 16 Endocrine Disorders

Michelle Elmendorf, RN, BSN
Graduate Student
Grand Valley State University
Allendale, Michigan
Appendix C Additional Case Study Exercise

Kim Gillow, RN, MSN
Consultant
Cedar Springs, Michigan
Appendix C Additional Case Study Exercise

Penny Hinkle, RNC, MSN, NP, CS
Director of Partial Hospitalization
NW Center for Community Mental Health
Fairfax, Virginia
Chapter 15 Psychiatric Disorders

Roxana Huebscher, PhD, FNPC, CMT, HNC
Associate Professor
University of Wisconsin, Oshkosh College of
    Nursing
Oshkosh, Wisconsin
*Chapter 17 Integrating Complementary Therapies
    into Practice*

Wendy Muma, MSN, FNP
Family Nurse Practitioner
Spectrum Health
Grand Rapids, Michigan
Chapter 16 Endocrine Disorders

Jean Nagelkerk, PhD, RN, FNP-C
Professor and Director of Development and Grants
Grand Valley State University
Allendale, Michigan
*Chapter 1 Clinical Decision-Making in Primary
    Care*
*Chapter 2 Documenting the Health History and
    Physical Examination*
Chapter 5 Special Senses
Chapter 6 Respiratory Disorders
Chapter 8 Gastrointestinal Disorders
Chapter 10 Urogenital Disorders
Chapter 11 Women's Health
Chapter 13 Neurological Disorders
Chapter 14 Musculoskeletal Disorders
Chapter 16 Endocrine Disorders
Appendix B Assessment Aids
Appendix C Additional Case Studies
Appendix D Key to Abbreviations

Kathryn Niemeyer, MSN, RN, CCRN
Adjunct Faculty
Grand Valley State University
Allendale, Michigan
Cardiology Case Manager
Mercy General Health Partners
Muskegon, Michigan
Chapter 18 Common Herbal Therapies
Appendix A Common Supportive Herbs

Carol Patton, DRPh, MSN, CRNP
Assistant Professor of Nursing
Duquesne University
Pittsburgh, Pennsylvania
Chapter 3 Diagnostic Tests
Chapter 4 Diagnostic Imaging

Melanie Ranta, RN, BSN
Graduate Student
Grand Valley State University
Allendale, Michigan
Appendix C Additional Case Study Exercise

Christy Smolenski, MSN, RN, CEN, CS, FNP
Adjunct Clinical Faculty
Kirkhof School of Nursing
Grand Valley State University
Allendale, Michigan
Nurse Practitioner, Emergency Department
St. Mary's Medical Center
Grand Rapids, Michigan
Chapter 2 Documenting the Health History and
*   Physical Examination*

Reviewers

Patricia Diane Abbot, MSN, RN, ARNP
Lecturer, Family Nurse Practitioner Program
University of Washington School of Nursing
Lead Health Care Specialist, Urgent Care Services
University of Washington Medical Center
Seattle, Washington

Marilyn Alber, MSN, RN, CS, ARNP
University of Washington School of Nursing
Seattle, Washington

Thomas G. Bartol, MN, RN-C, FNP, CDE
Richmond Area Health Center
Richmond, Maine

Jennifer Elizabeth DiMedio, MSN, RN, FNP
West Chester Family Practice
West Chester, Pennsylvania

Marie Amos Dobyns, MD
Adjunct Clinical Professor of Medicine
George Washington University School of
　Medicine
Washington, DC

Sheila A. Dunn, MSN, RN, C-ANP
St. Louis Veteran's Affairs Hospital—Belleville
　Community-Based Clinic
Belleville, Illinois
St. Louis University
St. Louis, Missouri

Susan Flagler, DNS, RNC, WHCNP
University of Washington School of Nursing
Seattle, Washington

Janice A. Gagen, MSN, CANP, CDE
Georgetown University
Washington, DC

Carol Green-Hernandez, PhD, FNS, ANP/FNP-C
Project Director and Associate Professor, Primary
　Care Nurse Practitioner Program
The University of Vermont
Burlington, Vermont

ElDonna M. Hilde, MSN, RNC, WHNP
Assistant Professor
Georgia Southern University School of Nursing
Statesboro, Georgia

Nancy Mathes Horan, MSN, ANP
George Washington University College of Health
　Care Sciences
Washington, DC
George Mason University's Collaborative Nurse
　Practitioner Program
Fairfax, Virginia

Christine A. Hoyle, MN, ARNP
Lecturer, Primary Care Nurse Practitioner
　Program
University of Washington School of Nursing
Seattle, Washington

Joy Ann Laramie, MSN, CNP, ANP
George Washington University
Washington, DC
George Mason University
Fairfax, Virginia

Ann Maradiegue, MSN, CFNP
George Mason University
Fairfax, Virginia

Pamela Meredith, MSN, FNP
Adjunct Professor
George Washington University
Washington, DC

Terry L. Murray, RN, FNP
St. Joseph's Hospital
Savannah, Georgia

Christine Pintz, MSN, RNC, WHNP, FNP
Research Associate and Adjunct Faculty
George Washington University
Washington, DC

Jane Renfro, PhD, MS, BSN, ANPC
United States Department of Defense
Falls Church, Virginia

Cheryl Robertson, MSN, ANP-C, WHNP-C
Instructor, Nurse Practitioner Program
College of Nursing and Health Science
George Mason University
Fairfax, Virginia

Anne C. Thomas, PhD, RN, CS, ANP
Research Associate and Nurse Practitioner
Union Hospital
Terre Haute, Indiana
Adjunct Faculty, Family Nurse Practitioner
    Program
University of Southern Indiana School of Nursing
    and Health Professions
Evansville, Indiana

Margaret Venzke, RN, MS, CS, FNP
Instructor, Nurse Practitioner Program
College of Nursing and Health Science
George Mason University
Fairfax, Virginia

Preface

This text is designed to assist students and beginning advanced practice nurses to accurately diagnose common problems in primary care. The text provides a diagnostic framework for clinical decision-making using case study analysis. This text highlights those cases that clinicians will commonly diagnose and treat in practice. The focus is on managing common acute and chronic stable conditions across the life span in a culturally sensitive manner. The text provides a diagnostic framework from which practitioners can review and evaluate clinical data, postulate differential diagnoses, and formulate individualized treatment plans.

This case study text uses a holistic, patient-centered approach to diagnosing, treating, and delivering care. When an episodic treatment approach is used to deliver primary care services it often results in costly, fragmented care. This text presents a holistic framework to develop a comprehensive patient treatment plan to maximize the patient's resources, support systems, and community strengths and optimize quality of life. With this approach the practitioner and patient review the mutually agreed upon goals, evaluate progress, and establish new goals or reaffirm those that exist. Using this framework, the practitioner incorporates nursing, medicine, and complementary practices to address each patient's unique needs.

The use of case studies is a powerful learning tool. It is a teaching methodology that assists practitioners to apply information to practice in a controlled and supportive environment. Both novice and experienced practitioners find case study analysis a valuable asset in diagnostic reasoning. The case study methodology is one of the most effective teaching methods that I have used with nurse practitioners and medical students. By using real patient situations, students are able to work through each case systematically, assessing history and physical data, sorting cues and cue clusters, identifying appropriate differential diagnoses, selecting the single best diagnosis, and then formulating a detailed treatment plan. Experienced practitioners often use the case study format informally to discuss interesting cases, compare notes on how a patient problem was managed, and offer suggestions or alternatives to treatment plans. Using a case study approach provides an opportunity to work collaboratively, to share expertise, and to learn from one another in a structured environment.

The information presented in this text reflects the current recommendations for treatment approaches. Practitioners must continue to keep abreast of the changes that occur in the health-care field by reading journals, attending conferences, and consulting with peers when making choices about treatment plans. The aim of this text is to provide a method of examining common problems that practitioners treat on a daily basis, to assist them in diagnostic reasoning, and to assist in the development of holistic, comprehensive treatment plans.

The text is divided into three parts. Part One provides a review or overview of the diagnostic framework from which practitioners may choose to evaluate case studies. Often, beginning practitioners are challenged to efficiently and accurately collect and evaluate clinical data, develop diagnoses, and formulate a therapeutic plan of care. This unit provides a conceptual approach to diagnostic reasoning. Chapter 1 provides an introduction to primary care and case management of patients and describes the process of clinical decision making. Chapter 2 provides a review of the health history and physical examination. A functional health assessment approach is used and a family assessment is incorporated. The SOAP format is introduced and provides a systematic approach for practitioners to record the patient encounter. Documentation that is complete and accurate provides clear communication for interdisciplinary collaboration and provides the necessary documentation for reimbursement purposes. Chapters 3 and 4 review commonly ordered laboratory and imaging tests.

Part Two uses a systems approach to cover common problems that practitioners encounter in practice. The cases range from those that focus on health promotion and risk reduction to those that are emergent in nature. The most frequently encountered common problems and chronic conditions are examined with pharmacology integrated into each case analysis.

Chapters 5 through 16 present case studies using the conceptual framework provided in Part One. The final case study in each chapter presents the history and physical data and provides questions at the end of the case study to prompt individual analysis and group discussion. An instructor's manual is available for complete analysis of the final case study in each chapter as well as for the "optional" case studies in Appendix C. For each of the case studies, use the diagnostic reasoning process to review the history of present illness, functional health pattern assessment, and physical examination data. Use critical thinking to investigate potential diagnostic possibilities, evaluate cues and cue clusters, and to put the pieces of the diagnostic puzzle together. This text provides the opportunity to explore, analyze, and complete each case using a structured format. Before reviewing the discussion that is provided in each chapter, answer the following questions for each case study to guide your analysis.

- *What type of history data should be collected?*
- *What type of physical data should be collected?*
- *What are the differential diagnoses?*
- *What are the probable cause(s) of the presenting symptoms?*
- *What diagnostic tests should be ordered?*
- *What is your diagnostic impression?*
- *What is the therapeutic plan of care?*
- *What are the patient education and/or community resources?*
- *What is your follow-up plan?*

After answering the questions, read the answers and rationale for each of the sections. Then, in a group setting, alter the history of present illness to one of the alternative differential diagnoses and discuss the diagnostic reasoning process in relation to history, physical, and diagnostic data; differential diagnoses; diagnosis; and treatment plan. Discuss the diagnostic reasoning process employed in determining and the rationale for selecting the diagnosis.

The final unit focuses on integrating complementary therapies into practice and presents common herbal therapies. This text is intended to assist practitioners in becoming aware of the various complementary therapies that individuals are incorporating into their practices. It also identifies common herbs, their benefits and potential side effects, and herbal categories. Extensive references are included in these two chapters to encourage further exploration of complementary and herbal therapies.

This text is intended to provide a framework for diagnostic reasoning in case analysis and as such is not a comprehensive pathophysiological or medical text. The use of additional readings on select topics will enhance individual and class discussion. Suggested readings and when possible, Internet addresses have been included at the end of each chapter to encourage exploration and discussion of current trends and therapeutic plans of care.

ACKNOWLEDGMENTS

This book is dedicated to my husband, Tom Nagelkerk, and my children, Jonathon and Jennifer Nagelkerk, for their encouragement, love, and support.

To my friend and colleague, Beverly Henry, for her inspiration, guidance, and excellence in nursing.

To Christy Smolenski, who spent hours listening to ideas and reading manuscripts; to Andy Bostrom for assisting with editing the Psychiatric Disorders chapter; and to Mary Barr, who diligently worked with me to edit the Diagnostic Tests chapter.

And to my colleagues and students at the Kirkhof School of Nursing at Grand Valley State University.

Jean Nagelkerk

Contents

part one

1

CLINICAL DATA

CHAPTER 1

Clinical Decision-Making in Primary Care

Jean Nagelkerk

The recent debate over health care reform has made it clear that the challenge to improving the health of Americans lies in increasing access to primary care and the provision of services in a manner that reflects both quality and cost-effectiveness. Health goals for the nation have been delineated in the document *Healthy People 2010* (U.S. Department of Health and Human Services, 2000). The Healthy People 2010 document is a major initiative by the U.S. Public Health Service to improve the health of Americans. The central goals that were defined are: (1) to increase the quality and years of healthy life and (2) to eliminate health disparities. The nurse practitioner (NP) is well qualified to address the Healthy People 2010 goals at local, regional, and national levels by delivering quality, cost-effective primary care and by extending services to an increasing number of clients.

Primary care services are essential to meet the Healthy People 2000 objectives. Comparative data from states that participated in the Centers for Disease Control and Prevention's Behavioral Risk Factor Surveillance Survey showed an alarming trend toward unhealthy behaviors among citizens. The specific areas of concern are those that reflect access to timely health care, the lack of resources, and a need for lifestyle changes. There is a growing public awareness that many health care problems can be better managed through primary care services.

Primary care is a basic level of health care that focuses on an individual's total health needs and is typically provided in an outpatient setting. Primary health care providers such as NPs are essential to the provision of health promotion, risk reduction, and disease prevention services to people while keeping costs under control. Research shows that NPs provide holistic, high quality, cost-effective care to clients who present with common acute illnesses and stable chronic disorders (American Association of Colleges of Nursing, 1994). Research also indicates that clients who have an NP as their primary care provider are more knowledgeable about their health care problems and are better able to manage them (Brown and Grimes, 1992). NPs are needed to ensure access to primary health care for individuals, families, and groups. NPs are well positioned to encourage healthy lifestyles that reduce the risk of chronic illness such as heart disease, cancer, stroke, and lung disease; and to provide health promotion and preventative services that will lead to healthier lives for adults and children (AACN, 1994).

CASE MANAGEMENT

Primary care practice is central in health care. Primary care providers serve as the patient's gatekeepers to care. Gatekeeping requires careful coordination of primary, specialty, and in-patient care. It is the clinician who provides the gatekeeping function of organizing, coordinating, providing, and referring primary and acute care services for their patient population. Traditionally, case management has been used as a process of gatekeeping for those who are at high risk or those who are high-cost patients. "Case management is a collaborative process which assesses, plans, implements, coordinates, monitors, and evaluates options and services to meet an individual's health needs through communication and available resources to promote quality cost-effective outcomes" (Case Management Society of America, 1995).

Clinicians have tended to provide disease state management to their patients with chronic illnesses such as asthma, diabetes, and hypertension. Disease state management is the coordination of community-based care for chronically ill patients who may require intense use of resources (Ignatavicius, Workman, and Mishler, 1999). The goal of disease state management is to provide cost effective care with quality outcomes.

To provide holistic and humanistic primary care to patients, NPs must extend case management to all patients, not just to those who are high risk or high cost. The three essential functions of case management are coordination and facilitation, utilization management, and discharge planning (Cesta and Falter, 1999). Facilitation entails making sure that the patient receives the proper diagnostic tests, treatments, and consultation in a coordinated and expedient manner. The coordination function includes the review of services provided—to avoid redundancies and the possibility of overlooked and omitted diagnostics—as well as communication between interdisciplinary team members and coordination of efforts. The function of utilization managers is essential to juggle the patient services, diagnostic facilities, and the insurance resources to ensure that the patient receives essential services at a reasonable cost and acceptable quality. The discharge planning function includes the development of the therapeutic plan of care with the coordination of patient resources for optimal outcome and quality of life for both the patient and family or significant other. This is especially important for those experiencing chronic illnesses and those who require respite care.

According to Cesta and Falter (1999), community-based case management focuses on primary care and long-term, potentially lifetime, relationships. The NP possesses the prerequisite functions of case management and uses them to manage a caseload of patients. These case management functions will assist the NP's patients in navigating the health care system. Nurse practitioners who provide case management to their patients are able to assess the patient's health and functioning, interpret clinical and diagnostic data, develop detailed treatment plans, and access appropriate community and professional resources to improve healthy lifestyles, reduce risks, and prevent diseases.

CLINICAL JUDGMENT

Nurse practitioners who focus on their patients' needs and who assist communities in designing en-

vironments to humanize care are adept at making sound clinical judgments. Seasoned nurse practitioners engage in a holistic approach to the provision of health care. Their holistic framework encompasses the mind, body, and spiritual being of each patient. Routinely, they incorporate personalized factors that influence a patient's health and actively engage the patient in their plan of care. Not only do NPs diagnose and treat problems, they use preventative measures that incorporate the patient's social supports, nutrition, art, music, and relaxation to enhance a healthy lifestyle.

Nurse practitioners face both routine and complex decisions daily. Routine decisions are those that are well defined and have standardized treatments. They occur on a day-to-day basis and can be quickly managed with well-known treatment plans. Routine decisions encompass problems such as earaches, sore throats, and annual physical examinations. NPs regularly manage routine problems such as health promotion, risk prevention, and common acute problems. Complex problems, on the other hand, are those that are ambiguous and have no standardized treatments. These decisions require complex, abstract critical thinking and well-measured judgments. The NP must analyze more data that is loosely connected and develop a diagnostic plan in the face of uncertainty. An example of a complex decision is the differential diagnoses of abdominal or chest pain. The symptom of abdominal pain in a 21-year-old female requires complex decision-making. The clinician must piece together the data from the history, the physical examination (pelvic/rectal/abdominal), and laboratory data (possibly urine/quantitative HCG/urine dipstick/wet mount/gonorrhea and chlamydia cultures/CBC) to differentiate between the diagnostic possibilities and to determine whether emergency intervention is necessary.

Seasoned NPs are able to manage routine and complex decision-making efficiently. They have developed a process to make decisions and to weigh the uncertainty inherent in the clinical decision-making process. There are many uncertainties in making clinical decisions. The more common include errors in obtaining correct clinical data and interpreting it; uncertainty about treatment effects; variations in interpretation of clinic data; and the relation between clinical information and the absolute presence of disease (Weinstein et al, 1980). An example of an error in clinical data is a hemoglobin of 8.2 in a 5-year-old male presenting for a routine school physical, with no physical symptoms. A complete blood count was drawn showing a hemoglobin level of 12.5. If the practitioner had not ordered a complete blood count to further evaluate this disparity between the clinical presentation of the patient and the laboratory value, the child would have been treated based on inaccurate data.

DIAGNOSTIC REASONING

Diagnostic reasoning is a systematic approach to patient care. In this approach, the clinician moves from general data collection to specific data collection. Competing diagnoses are considered in the differential diagnosis, and clinical findings are compared to the potential diagnoses. A systematic approach to clinical decision-making provides a consistent structure from which clinicians can make optimal choices. The diagnostic reasoning process is multidirectional. Should the clinician need more data, he or she returns to an earlier stage in the diagnostic investigation.

It is important to use a comprehensive health assessment approach when engaging in diagnostic reasoning. A complete and accurate database (history and physical examination) is essential for each patient that enters a practice. In an ideal setting, all patients would have this database before the clinician would evaluate problem-focused concerns. In any situation, however, the NP can use a holistic approach when making clinical judgments. Table 1-1 shows the seven steps in the iterative process of diagnostic reasoning.

The first step in diagnostic reasoning is to promptly identify the presenting problem that caused the patient to seek care. The patient's concern should be documented and addressed completely. It is important to identify what the patient's concern(s) are, because often, the problem the clinician identifies as the priority is not the same problem that the patient feels is most pressing. For example, a patient may present for a sore throat and low-grade fever and incidentally be found to have high blood pressure. In order to have that patient hear about high blood pressure and be treated holistically, it may be necessary to discuss the treatment

Table 1-1
Steps in Diagnostic Reasoning

Steps	Process
Step One	Identifying the patient problem
Step Two	Assessing: collecting history and physical data
Step Three	Formulating competing diagnoses
Step Four	Ordering diagnostics
Step Five	Selecting a diagnoses
Step Six	Developing a treatment plan
Step Seven	Implementing and evaluating: follow-up

for the sore throat first. Otherwise, the patient may perceive that his or her concern is not being addressed and decide not to return for care of the hypertension.

The second step in the diagnostic process is assessing. In this step, the clinician systematically collects history and physical data. Data can be collected through interview, physical examination, record review, and by information (reports) from colleagues. The NP should be aware of the cultural, religious, and ethical components of the patient's care. The NP communicates effectively with the patient to collect accurate clinical data. Systematic observation while interviewing and conducting the physical examination provides a format for collection of pertinent data. In conducting the interview, the NP must be sure to collect data related to the problem as well as pertinent negatives—that is, those data that will help to strengthen or eliminate alternative diagnoses. Carpenito (1993) identifies the focuses of data collection as:

- Present and past health status
- Present and past coping patterns
- Present and past functional status
- Response to treatments
- Risk for potential problems
- Desire for a higher level of wellness

The focuses of data collection that Carpenito identifies are components of the database from which the NP manages the patient's care. The history and physical examination (H&P) provides the template for which a plan of care is developed and specific treatments are implemented. A comprehensive H&P is the backbone of the patient record. One of the NPs most useful tools is the history of the presenting illness. During the patient's description of the problem, the nature of the chief complaint is revealed. Therefore, an individual skilled in history taking can use focused questions to elicit rich data that will direct the physical examination. The NP who becomes proficient in history taking develops or uses a system to collect essential data on each patient problem. Table 1-2 lists seven history components that are addressed in order to get a complete picture of the patient problem or chief complaint.

A complete description of the patient problem is elicited by using the seven history components represented by the LCSTSAA format. The first component is the *location* (which may be focal or diffuse) of the discomfort or problem that the patient is experiencing. An example of the location of irritable bowel pain experienced by a patient may be generalized abdominal discomfort with palpation of the abdomen. A potential presentation for appendicitis might include localized pain in the right lower quadrant of the abdomen.

The second component is the *character or quality* of the patient problem. The clinician clearly identifies the intensity or type of pain or problem. For example, terms such as dull, aching, throbbing, stabbing, and band-like can be used to describe the type of pain. A patient who presents with a tension headache may describe a band-like pressure around the head, whereas a patient experiencing a migraine headache may describe the pain as sharp or stabbing.

The third component is the *severity* of the problem. Is it incapacitating? Can the patient work? Is the patient able to carry out activities of daily living and participate in family activities? Is the problem simply annoying? What is the severity of pain, based on a rating scale of 0 - 10 with 0 being no pain and 10 being the worst pain possible? Headaches are commonly scored on a rating scale to evaluate the success of the therapeutic plan of care.

Table 1-2
Seven History Components of a Patient Problem

Letter	History Component
L	Location
C	Character or quality
S	Severity
T	Timing: onset, frequency, duration
S	Sequence of the symptoms
A	Aggravating or alleviating factors
A	Associated factors and treatments

The fourth component is the *timing: onset, frequency, and duration* . When did the problem first begin? Has it occurred before? How frequently does the problem occur, and how long does it last? When evaluating the patient who presents with the chief complaint of headaches, it is important to have the patient keep a diary to determine what activities precede the headaches, what time of the day they occur, and how long they last. From the headache diary patterns can be discovered, triggers identified, and timing can be documented to determine the best treatment plan.

The fifth component is *sequence of the symptoms.* What is the order in which the pain or problem unfolds? If a patient complains of abdominal pain, nausea, and vomiting, it is important to find out which of these started first. Did the nausea and vomiting precede the abdominal pain, or did the pain cause the nausea and vomiting? In pregnancy, nausea and vomiting will often precede the abdominal discomfort, whereas with appendicitis, pain will often precede nausea and vomiting.

The sixth component is the *aggravating or alleviating factors* that increase or decrease the intensity of the patient problem. An example of this is illustrated in the patient who presents for low back pain. It is important to ask the patient if activity and/or sitting at rest affects the level of discomfort that is experienced. A patient with low back pain from a muscle strain will most likely experience pain with activity. A patient with a central cord dysfunction will experience pain with sitting or rest.

The seventh component is *associated factors and treatments*. Are there any other pertinent factors or symptoms influencing the patient's problem? Are there any pertinent data in the family history, past medical or surgical histories, or self-directed or provider-prescribed treatments that are associated with the patient problem? For example, a patient presents to the clinic with the chief complaint of a sore throat. Associated symptoms that the patient may report include swollen lymph nodes in the neck, high temperature, and fatigue. What prescription and nonprescription medications were used, and with what results? What herbal therapies or vitamin therapies were used, and with what results? Were any other treatments used? If so, what were the results? It is important to identify the herbal medications and alternative therapies that patients are using so that their effectiveness, potential side effects, and potential interactions with treatment plans can be determined. For example, should a patient need anticoagulation therapy, and warfarin (Coumadin) is prescribed, herbal products containing vitamins C or K may interfere with the efficacy of the prescribed medication.

Another example is the patient who presents with the chief complaint of abdominal pain. Using the seven history components of a patient problem the following data is elicited. The patient complains of 8-hour duration of knifelike, constant, unbearable pain in the right lower quadrant of the abdomen. Movement aggravates the pain. The patient vomited a small amount two times. The patient tried Tylenol Extra Strength and Alka Seltzer with no relief. The information contained in this description provides several cues as to potential differential diagnoses and clear direction for the physical examination and diagnostic testing this patient needs.

When interpreting data from the history and physical examination, the data are processed into cues and cue clusters. Cues may be primary or secondary data. Primary data include history information from the patient and physical examination data. Secondary data include information obtained from family and friends, health care providers, and diagnostic information. Cues are single pieces of information (for example, history data, signs, symptoms, and laboratory data) that may support or refute a specific diagnosis. Cue clusters are several pieces of data that, when linked together, are supportive of a specific diagnosis. Some cues are strongly linked to a problem, whereas others have only weak associations. For example, a patient who complains of a sore throat (symptom) may have malaise. This is a weak association because it is not specific for a single chief complaint. On the other hand, a red, beefy throat (sign) has a strong association for pharyngitis. Cues that have a strong association are clustered together to provide support for a specific diagnosis. Then these cues are weighed and attempts are made to fit them together like pieces of a puzzle to determine potential diagnostic possibilities.

Step three is the formulation of competing diagnostic alternatives. The goal in this step is to select the best diagnosis to assist the patient in achieving a high level of wellness. The process of formulating competing diagnoses is complicated and requires a broad knowledge base of nursing and medicine. Critical thinking about the nature of the cues and the cue clusters is used to generate possible diagnoses. Critical thinking is a self-questioning approach to making decisions. It requires careful and creative thinking. It involves asking, "How did this occur?" and "Why do we always manage a patient's care in this way?" Critical thinking is continual questioning of basic assumptions. It prompts clarity in the process of data collection, and encourages creativity and innovation with problem solving.

Many routine, straightforward decisions are made. At other times, decision-making will be uncertain and complex, requiring serious intellectual effort and well-developed critical thinking skills. Tanner et al (1987) found that nurses who limited their diagnostic options did not always include the correct diagnosis in their decision-making and overvalued the probability of a single diagnosis. Also, practitioners who did not systematically analyze decision options and consider competing differentials had a narrow focus to clinical decision-making and risked inaccuracies in diagnostic outcomes. Therefore, including a broad range of diagnoses in a differential and using a systematic approach to problem solving tends to generate more accurate diagnoses. The clinician needs to limit the number of diagnostic options to the top three to five to manage the diagnostic process effectively without excluding those diagnoses that should not be missed and that are potentially life threatening.

There are two types of problem-oriented clinical diagnostic reasoning: (1) focal, involving a single or limited number of body systems; and (2) constitutional, involving multiple systems requiring prompt treatment. The chief complaint of a severe sore throat is an example of focal, problem-oriented clinical diagnostic reasoning for a patient. The differential diagnoses include common causes such as group A beta-hemolytic streptococcal (GABHS) pharyngitis, viral pharyngitis, and infectious mononucleosis. Peritonsillar abscess is unlikely, but should never be missed due to potential airway compromise. An example of constitutional, problem-oriented clinical diagnostic reasoning is the patient who presents with fever. The differential diagnoses for fever are broad and involve many body systems to identify the etiology. Examples of possible differentials, which will depend on the patient's history and examination, include infections, malignancies, immune disorders, and metabolic disorders. The differential diagnoses engage the practitioner in a review of cue clusters for each diagnosis and ultimately, through decision-making, lead to the single best diagnostic possibility for the patient.

Step four is the ordering of laboratory or radiological tests to help support or refute the potential diagnoses. When ordering laboratory data, the practitioner must be aware of the degree of sensitivity and specificity of each test. The specificity of a diagnostic test is the proportion of patients who are free of a specific disease and are so identified by the test. The sensitivity of a diagnostic test is the proportion of the patients who have the specific disease and are so identified by the test. An example of sensitivity and specificity for a common laboratory test is the rapid test for detection of the streptococcal antigen. This test has a sensitivity of about 85% and a specificity of 98% (Goroll, May and Mulley, 1995).

Practitioners order many laboratory and radiological tests for patients. The NP must make the judgment as to whether the diagnostic value of the test outweighs its cost and the patient discomfort it may produce. Questions that need to be asked prior to ordering tests include the following:

- What data will the test provide?
- Would I treat the patient differently based on the test results?
- Is the test ordered diagnostic for the disease?

Diagnostic tests should be ordered prudently as they significantly increase the cost of health care and may cause unnecessary discomfort for the patient.

Step five is the selection of the single best diagnosis. By clustering the cues, it is easier to see patterns that point toward a specific diagnosis. For example, if the patient's cue cluster included abrupt onset of sore throat, fever, malaise, and red throat with gray exudate, you may suspect streptococcal pharyngitis. If the rapid test for detection of the streptococcal antigen were positive, it would further support your diagnosis. If it were not positive, you would reevaluate your differential diagnoses to determine the most likely diagnostic possibility. A pertinent negative in this case is the lack of an erythematous or fine red papular rash, refuting the diagnosis of scarlet fever. What is important is that the differential diagnoses are broad enough to include likely diagnostic probabilities so the correct diagnosis is not missed. As skill in the diagnostic process develops, a consistent structure to manage multiple problems is integrated into practice. For example, a male patient who presents with hypertension and benign prostatic hypertrophy could be given a variety of antihypertensive medications. But an alpha-blocker such as terazosin (Hytrin) could help both problems. The practitioner may also find that at times the exact diagnosis is uncertain until further testing is complete. Clear communication with the patient must be arranged to determine the next step in the treatment plan. An example of this is a patient presenting with heavy, irregular menses. A pelvic ultrasound may be necessary to confirm the physical examination of fibroids and enlarged ovary.

There may also be instances where the clinician, after making a diagnosis or evaluating the differential diagnostic possibilities, chooses to refer the patient to a specialist for further evaluation and treatment. The patient should be referred to the appropriate health care provider when the complexity or intensity of the patient problem is outside of the NP's scope of practice. Examples of problems that require a referral to a neurologist are new onset epilepsy and the inability to control seizures on the existing treatment regimen. Another example is the referral to an endocrinologist of a 32-year-old female who, on physical examination, is found to have a goiter. Often NPs co-manage the patient's care after the specialist has developed the therapeutic plan. The NP co-manages the patient's care by conducting follow-up on the specific problem as well as by providing preventive and ill care. The NP consults with the specialist as appropriate and establishes follow-up visits with the specialist on a semi-annual, annual, or as needed basis.

Practitioners often consult with peers or specialists to help evaluate patient problems. Patient outcomes often improve when the practitioner can work collaboratively with a network of individuals to manage patient problems. For example, the clinician may refer a pediatric diabetic patient to an endocrinologist for the development of a treatment plan and to co-manage the patient's care. The clinician may then call the endocrinologist for a consultation when the patient's blood sugar is high during an acute illness or when there are ketones in the patient's urine. The consultation may assist with managing the problem, or a visit to the endocrinologist may be scheduled. Another common practice of clinicians is to share information and confirm treatment plans when questions about patient care arise. For example, a clinician may call a gynecologist or a women's health nurse practitioner if there is a question on an abnormal Papanicolaou test or about dysfunctional bleeding on one of the patients under treatment.

Step six is the development of the best treatment plan for the patient. Development of the treatment plan commonly utilizes both nursing and medical knowledge. Patients appreciate a description of the malady, what can be done to prevent it in the future, and the likely trajectory or the course of their illness. Once the patient understand the prognosis or progression of the illness, the ability to cure or manage the problem, and the treatment options available, a specific treatment plan can be developed. For the treatment plan to be specific, it must include what is to be done, how it is to be done, what and who is to do it, when it is to be done, and for how long it is to be done (Carnevali, 1993; Weinstein et al, 1980). By using a specific treatment plan, the patient will better understand the directions and be able to carry them out accurately.

Here are two examples of specific treatments for a patient who is diagnosed with a urinary tract infection:

1. You (who is to do it) should drink at least two liters of water (what is to be done) each day (time it is to be done) for the next 2 weeks (how long it is to be done). In this example, orally (how it is to be done) is assumed.
2. You (who is to do it) should take one tablet of Bactrim DS (what is to be done) by mouth (how it is to be done) in the morning and one in the evening (time it is to be done) with fluids for a period of 10 days (how long it is to be done).

The interventions that clinicians order fall into three levels of prevention: primary, secondary, or tertiary care. When the clinician orders an intervention that is designed to prevent an illness, it is *primary prevention*. Examples of primary prevention include teaching nutrition to children to prevent obesity, encouraging the use of seat belts to minimize injuries, and providing adolescents with information about the hazards of smoking to prevent the use of cigarettes. *Secondary prevention* is the implementation of interventions to prevent illness or mortality by managing care during the asymptomatic period. Examples of secondary prevention include breast and testicular self-examination, treatment of an abnormal Papanicolaou test, and testing stools for occult blood. *Tertiary prevention* is the implementation of interventions to prevent complications or problems from established disease. Examples of tertiary prevention include rehabilitation programs for acute brain attacks; cardiac rehabilitation programs; and treating hyperlipidemia in a patient who has coronary heart disease to prevent the progression of atherosclerosis.

Summary

Practitioners who engage in careful analysis using critical thinking and diagnostic reasoning make sound clinical judgments. They use a comprehensive holistic health approach to analyze and cluster cues to make diagnoses. Expert practitioners creatively use data to piece together the diagnostic puzzle. There are many methods to analyze data and make decisions. Examples of methods of decision-making include pattern recognition, arborization, and exhaustive methods of data collection. This chapter presents one method of clinical decision-making that is a hypothesis generating approach. This method helps practitioners identify the essential elements in the diagnostic reasoning process. By using the steps in diagnostic reasoning and the seven history components of a patient problem, the practitioner has a framework to make clinical decisions. In Unit 2 of this text there are cases to analyze and use in making clinical judgments. Clinical decision-making is a careful, deliberate process that is at times fraught with uncertainty. These cases are designed to evaluate clinical problems using critical thinking skills and thereby arrive at diagnostic conclusions.

References

American Association of Colleges of Nursing: *Expanded roles for advanced practice nurses,* May 1994, Position Statement.

Brown S, Grimes D: *Meta-analysis of process of care, clinical outcomes, and cost-effectiveness of nurses in primary care,* Washington, DC, 1992, American Nurses Association.

Carnevali, D: *Diagnostic reasoning and treatment decision-making in nursing,* Philadelphia, 1993, J.B. Lippincott.

Carpenito, LJ: *Nursing diagnosis: application to clinical practice,* ed 5, Philadelphia, 1993, J.B. Lippincott.

Case Management Society of America: Standards of practice for case management, *J Case Manag* 1(3):6-16, 1995.

Cesta TG, Falter EJ: Case management. Its value for staff nurses, *Am J Nurs* 99(5):48-51, 1999.

Goroll A, May L, and Mulley A, editors: *Primary care medicine,* Philadelphia, 1995, Lippincott-Raven.

Ignatavicius DD, Workman ML, Mishler MA: *Medical-surgical nursing across the health care continuum,* ed 3, Philadelphia, 1999, WB Saunders.

Tanner CA, Padrick KP, Westfall UE, Putzier DJ: Diagnostic reasoning strategies of nurses and nursing students, *Nurs Res* 36(6):358-363, 1987.

United States Department of Health and Human Services: *Healthy People 2010: national health promotion and disease prevention objectives* (Conference edition in two volumes), Washington, DC, 2000, U.S. Government Printing Office.

Weinstein MC, Fineberg HV, Elstein AS et al: *Clinical decision analysis,* Philadelphia, 1980, WB Saunders.

Selected Readings

Eddy D: *Clinical decision-making,* Sudbury, Mass, 1996, Jones and Barlett.

Hamric AB, Spross JA, Hanson CM: *Advanced nursing practice: an integrative approach,* Philadelphia, 1996, WB Saunders.

Kassirer J, Kopelman R: *Learning clinical reasoning,* Baltimore, 1991, Williams and Wilkins.

Mengel MB: *Principles of clinical practice,* New York, 1991, Plenum Publishing.

Michigan Department of Public Health: *Behavioral risk factor surveillance survey,* Lansing, Mich, 1990, U.S. Centers for Disease Control and Prevention.

Oermann MH: Critical thinking, critical practice, *Nurs Manage* 30(4):40C-40F, 40H-40I, 1999. 175

CHAPTER 2

Documenting the Health History and Physical Examination

Jean Nagelkerk and Christy Smolenski

The health history is a key component of the patient's record and is often documented at the first visit. It provides an opportunity to develop a database, establish rapport, and build a strong patient-provider relationship. The purposes of the health history are to: (1) identify and document the patient's health problems, (2) identify the patient's health promotion needs, (3) identify potential health risks, and (4) describe the patient's personal and social lifestyle. During the health history, the subjective data is collected from the patient; if the patient is unable to provide complete information, data may be obtained from a knowledgeable significant other.

The complete history provides a comprehensive database that enables the practitioner to diagnose health status, begin to understand the context of the patient's environment, and to develop a patient-centered approach to care. Once a complete history database is collected, interval or focused histories are undertaken at subsequent visits. These histories are focused on the problem or problems that the patient is presenting at that visit, along with any new or pertinent data that may influence the patient's treatment plan.

CULTURAL CARE

America is becoming a more racially, ethnically diverse community (Dienemann, 1997). Health care providers must be culturally sensitive when delivering health care. During the process of collecting the initial or focused history, the NP must be sensitive to variations that may present due to cultural or ethnic origins. However, it is difficult for any single practitioner to know each cultural group's beliefs

and traditions. Many practitioners will provide care to multicultural groups, and often individuals within a cultural group may not hold the same beliefs (Geissler, 1994). Practitioners develop methods of communicating with patients that minimize demographic, social, and cultural biases. Table 2-1 provides information about dominant cultures in the United States. The information provided should be used as a guide or generalization about a specific dominant culture, but should not be used to stereotype individuals. The information provided in the table can assist health care providers to be more culturally sensitive in communication.

Since it is unrealistic to have an understanding of the culture for all ethnic or racial groups, health care providers can use the LEARN model to overcome barriers in cultural communication and to be sensitive to individual patient needs (Berlin and Fowkes, 1983). The LEARN model is applicable to all patient encounters, but is especially useful as a framework for facilitating communication between the NP and patients from different ethnic, racial, and cultural groups. The elements of the model are:

L — Listen to the patient describe the problem
E — Explain your understanding of the problem
A — Acknowledge and communicate the differences and similarities
R — Recommend a treatment plan
N — Negotiate the specifics of the patient's treatment

Practitioners who use the LEARN model elicit culturally sensitive histories. They listen more carefully while the patient describes the chief com-

Table 2-1
Dominant Cultures in the United States

Hispanic

Mexican-American

*Urban centers
  in the Southwest

Language: Spanish; 5.4% of American population
Religion: Predominantly Roman Catholic
Passive role in health care, visits only when acutely ill
Uses both traditional and folk medicine; *curandero* or folk healers view illness from religious and family context
Believe in external control over health and wellness
Family is important in health care decisions
Patriarchal, but mother is in charge of health care
Sustained eye contact is not polite
Focused on the present
Risk factors: Obesity, diabetes, and tuberculosis

Puerto Rican

*Urban centers
  in the Southwest

Language: Bilingual, speaking Spanish and English
Religion: Majority (85%) are Roman Catholic
Patriarchal, with women caring for the children and value placed on the extended family
Frequent use of folk healers, but will seek Western medicine
Believe in external control of health and illness, that illness may be a result of evil or a punishment for sin
Verbalize pain and discomfort loudly and openly
Classify foods and medicines as "hot" and "cold"
Strong stigma placed on mental illness
Risk factors: High prevalence of diabetes and hypertension

Cuban

*Florida
  and New York

Language: Bilingual, speaking Spanish and English
Religion: Roman Catholic
Strong family ties and values
Use Western medicine as well as healers called *santaria*
Decisions made by the family member that is most respected, most educated, or an elder
Male-dominated, with women as caregivers
Strong stigma placed on mental illness
Some believe in supernatural forces (e.g., "evil eye")
Risk factors: High prevalence of obesity

African-American

*Urban centers
  in the Southeast

Language: English; form 12.1% of American population
Highly heterogeneous group
Often, the female is the head of the household (2:1 ratio)
Mother typically has the role of making decisions for health care
Large network groups often provide support to one another
Health and illness are viewed as externally controlled
Folk medicine may be practiced, especially in the rural south
High mortality for African-American males from accidents and violence
Morbidity and mortality rates are high among African-Americans compared to the general population
Risk factors: Higher prevalence of heart disease, cancer, strokes, and lung disease

Modified from: Bowden VR, Dickey SB, Greenberg CS: *Children and their families,* Philadelphia, 1998, WB Saunders; Geissler EM: *Pocket guide to cultural assessment,* St Louis, 1994, Mosby; Giger JN, Davidhizar RE: *Transcultural nursing: assessment and intervention,* ed 2, St Louis, 1995, Mosby; Jarvis C: *Physical examination and health assessment,* ed 2, Philadelphia, 1996, WB Saunders; Lipson JG, Dibble SL, Minarik PA: *Culture and nursing care: a pocket guide,* San Francisco, 1996, University of California, San Francisco: Nursing Press; and Seidel H, Ball J, Dains J, Benedict G: *Mosby's guide to physical examination,* St Louis, 1995, Mosby.
*Locations with the highest population densities.

Table 2-1
Dominant Cultures in the United States—*cont'd*

Asian

Vietnamese-American

*Urban centers along the Pacific Coast

Language: Vietnamese; form 0.2% of American population
Major Religion: Buddhist
Herbal medicine is important
Illness is managed by self care and self medication
Seek care for acute illnesses only
Elders are respected and sought for wisdom and experience
Direct eye contact is considered impolite
Extended family is involved in health care; in traditional families, the oldest male makes health care decisions
May falsely answer "yes" or "no" to please the examiner rather than reflect a true answer
Risk factors: Tuberculosis

Japanese

*West Coast

Language: Bilingual, speaking Japanese and English
Religion: Shinto Buddhist, Christian
Use both Western and Oriental medicine
Nuclear and extended family is important
Approximately 50% marry outside of their ethnic group
Fathers are typically the head of the house and women are the primary care givers
The average consumption of soy is 40-120 mg daily, may contribute to lower incidences of hot flashes and cancers

Chinese

*West Coast:
California (40.1%);
also Hawaii (6.9%),
New York (18.1%),
Texas (3.3%),
and Illinois (3.6%)

Language: Cantonese, Mandarin, English (varies among individuals)
Religion: Taoism, Buddhist, Islam, Christian
Confucius's teachings are valued
Harmonious relationship with nature
Treatment is aimed at restoring the balance of *yin* and *yang*
Use Western medicine and medicinal herbs
Emphasis is on loyalty to family and tradition, individual needs deemphasized
Hierarchical leadership structure in families
Risk factors: High prevalence of hypertension, diabetes, and cancer

Caucasian

*Urban and rural areas throughout the United States

Language: English
Religion: Majority are either Protestant or Roman Catholic
Use Western medicine to treat illness, but there is growing use of complementary therapies for health and ill care
Internal or external control over health and ill care is influenced by educational level: those with more education tend to plan and make individual choices for health care
Nuclear families are central in individual's life
Usually patriarchal, with mothers caring and making decisions about health care; however, leadership structure in families varies
Risk factors: High incidence of obesity, breast cancer, and heart disease

*Locations with the highest population densities.

plaint in his or her own words. The practitioner describes what he or she heard the patient say, and checks for affirmation. If differences exist, they are then discussed to elicit the most accurate history, which provides focus for the physical examination and, ultimately, the formulation of the single best treatment plan. The treatment plan is presented, encouraging feedback about the patient's willingness and ability to implement the plan.

Various cultures have certain health beliefs that could affect a treatment plan. Actively listening to the patient's perceptions about the problem, the assessment of the available resources, and his or her own ability to carry out a specific treatment plan can strengthen the patient-provider relationship and assist the patient to optimal health. For example, Japanese women are more apt to consume soy products; these may interfere with supplemental thyroid and estrogen replacement therapy. If these women choose to continue taking large amounts of soy products, estrogen replacement therapy should not be instituted due to the mechanism by which soy acts upon the estrogen receptors (Glisson, Crawford, and Street, 1999). Willingness to work with the patient's personal lifestyle choices will strengthen the adherence to the collaborative treatment plan and the patient-provider relationship.

DEVELOPMENTAL STAGES ACROSS THE LIFESPAN

Listening carefully provides cues about the patient's level of development. Patient self-descriptions of occupation, relationships, and values and beliefs will also make the stage of development apparent. Researchers such as Erikson, Freud, Piaget, Maslow, and Kohlberg put forth several theoretical approaches to development that explain and predict human behavior (Freud, 1927; Power, Higgins, and Kohlberg, 1989; Thomas, 1985). Erikson (1963, 1986) clearly describes the process and stages of human psychological development. His work is based on the development of the self and the ego. The eight stages of human development, as identified by Erikson, are based on normative tasks that must be accomplished throughout the lifespan. These chronological stages, the corresponding developmental stages, and examples of tasks or activities that the individual must accomplish before moving to the next stage are shown in Table 2-2.

Table 2-2
Erikson's Developmental Stages

Chronological Stage	Developmental Stage	Tasks or Activities
Infants	Trust versus Mistrust	Attachment, investigates environment, adequate nutrition
Toddlers	Autonomy versus Shame and Doubt	Independence, playful, curious, improves physical skills
Preschool	Initiative versus Guilt	Independence, self-directed, even-tempered
School Age	Industry versus Inferiority	Peers important, independent decisions, enjoys school, self-confident
Adolescence	Identity versus Role Confusion	Independent, self-directed, even-tempered
Young Adulthood	Intimacy versus Isolation	Commitment, compromise
Middle Adulthood	Generativity versus Stagnation	Productivity, creativity, and nurturing
Older Adulthood	Ego Integrity versus Despair	Rearranging the past, reviewing accomplishments

Modified from: Erikson E: *Childhood and society,* 35th anniversary edition, New York, 1986, W.W. Norton.

Failure to meet a developmental task creates a situation in which the individual faces a crisis and is unable to reach a higher level of functioning. Once a developmental task is met, the individual is able to move on to the next developmental level. Individuals who have successfully moved to higher levels of development may have occasions where they relapse and must struggle with the conflict again for resolution. Conflicts are present at all stages of the life span and must be mastered again at higher levels for optimal functioning. For example, a toddler masters the core conflict of autonomy and advances to the next developmental stage. As an adolescent, he or she will again have to struggle with independence (autonomy) from parents when limitations are imposed. Erikson's theory is sensitive to the cultural, social, and historical context of human development (Bowden, Dickey, and Greenberg, 1998). Each individual will progress though the developmental stages at his or her own pace and achieve each developmental level through a range of socially acceptable methods.

By identifying the developmental stage of the patient, the practitioner may assess and discuss those activities that are pertinent to that individual. Anticipatory guidance that is culturally sensitive can be provided that parents and caregivers will find helpful as their children progress through the life cycle.

CHILDHOOD DEVELOPMENTAL MILESTONES

Discussing information about anticipated physical changes, developmental changes, and potential parenting strategies is useful for parents. Armed with knowledge of the typical physical activities and intellectual progressions, parents can work to assist their child in meeting developmental milestones (Boynton, Dunn, and Stephens, 1998). Table 2-3 lists the typical age that a child accomplishes specific activities or skills. Knowledge of normal skills in child development assists practitioners in assessing a child's developmental progression. Age-related normal skill acquisition in children does not occur at the same time for each child, but rather occurs within a range.

An excellent tool to use when assessing the developmental level of a young child is the Denver Developmental Screening Tool (Denver II, see Appendix B). The Denver II is a screening instrument developed to detect developmental delays in children ages 0 to 6 years old. The tool takes less than 25 minutes to complete and assesses four skill areas of children: gross motor, language, fine motor-adaptive, and personal-social. When questionable results are discovered, retesting should occur within 3 to 6 months. The Denver II is useful for screening infants, for performing longitudinal assessments of individuals, for following-up on children who have seen multiple providers, and for conducting pre-kindergarten screening (Jarvis, 1996). Many clinicians schedule the Denver II as part of every well child visit until the age of 6 years because developmental assessments are essential in early childhood. Any developmental lags or delays

Table 2-3
Normal Childhood Developmental Activities or Skills

Age	Activity or Skill
2 weeks	Coos
2 months	Turns head side to side when prone
4 months	Reaches for objects, rolls prone to supine
5 months	Rolls supine to prone, grasps objects
6 months	Sits unassisted, babbles, moves objects from one hand to the other
8 months	Crawls, begins pulling to stand
9 months	Drinks from a cup with help
1 year	Pincer grasp, says "mama" and "dada," stands alone, follows a single step command, begins to take steps
1 1/3 years	Walks
1 1/2 years	Drinks from cup independently, says two or three words together, scribbles
2 years	Feeds self
2 1/2 years	Dresses self, copies a circle, 75% of speech intelligible
3 years	Catches ball, rides tricycle, forms sentences, carries out a two- or three-step command
4 years	Uses pencil, copies a square
5 years	Copies a triangle
6 years	Ties shoes, copies a diamond

Modified from Bowden VR, Dickey SB, Greenberg CS: *Children and their families,* Philadelphia, 1998, WB Saunders; and Boynton RW, Dunn ES, Stephens GR: *Manual of ambulatory pediatrics,* ed 4, Philadelphia, 1998, JB Lippincott.

discovered during testing are referred for appropriate intervention. Early interventions assist the child to an optimal level of functioning. See Appendix B for an illustration of the Denver II and the directions for administration.

It is equally important for the practitioner to assess the developmental stage, activities, and tasks of adolescents and adults. A HEADS or PACES assessment should be conducted on each adolescent patient (Table 2-4). Topics that are often explored with adolescents include home life, school achievement, peer relationships, extracurricular activities, alcohol and drug use, sexual activity, smoking habits, ownership of weapons, and violence. Probing questions are often used to elicit information. The data that is gathered provides cues to developmental and other concerns of the adolescent. Once issues are identified, a treatment plan can be formulated and interventions implemented.

According to Erikson, adulthood is broken into three stages: young adulthood, middle adulthood, and older adulthood. Young adults are often working on beginning their careers, starting a family, and engaging in recreational activities. This is an exciting time, but the initiation of multiple roles can be confusing. The middle-aged adult is working at maximum capacity at work, at home, and in the community. At this point in life they are reflecting on priorities and creating schedules to manage their activities. The older adult has different needs and often is interested in community or volunteer activities. The practitioner can assist adult patients in reflecting upon their developmental tasks and providing resources, counseling, or referrals as needed.

FAMILY ASSESSMENT

Individual family members will present to your office for primary care. Family assessments are often completed on families that have special needs such as those with chronic illness, substance abuse, or dysfunctional family patterns. Many clinicians do not do family assessments as routine screenings, but conduct this assessment when problematic areas affect the individual. Other clinicians feel that health needs should always be addressed in the context of the family unit. Cultural sensitivity in assessing the context of the family enhances communication, goal setting, and accomplishment of treatment plans. "Family health is defined as a dynamic process that includes the activities a family uses to promote and protect the well-being of the family as a unit and the individual family members" (Bomar, 1996). Nurse practitioners who use a family nursing framework focus their interventions at the level of care that is needed for a particular patient or family. Each family member's behaviors and lifestyle influences the other family members' level of health.

Family nursing interventions occur at the individual level, family level, or family aggregates (groups). The level of nursing intervention depends on the problem or issues being addressed. Any level of intervention will ultimately affect the entire family because changes in financial resources, time, and lifestyle affect each family member. An example of an individual level of intervention is a patient that presents with an "itchy head" and is diagnosed with lice. Specific interventions, such as a prescription for medication and directions for removing the nits, need to be aimed at the individual. However, the entire family unit is affected because lice can be transmitted to other family members and precautions must be taken by the entire family to eradicate the problem. An example of a family level intervention would be counseling for a family unit where the child is being treated for behavioral problems at home and school. An example of a family aggregate intervention would be the organization and implementation of a community effort aimed to reduce violence in the neighborhood. As the nurse practitioner develops a solid provider-patient relationship, and begins to manage the care for each

Table 2-4 HEADS, PACES Assessments for Adolescents	
HEADS Questions*	**PACES Assessment†**
H=Home life	P=Parents, Peers
E=Extracurricular	A=Accidents (intentional and unintentional), Alcohol or other illicit drug activities
A=Alcohol	C=Cigarettes
D=Drugs	E=Emotional topics
S=Sexual activity, Smoking, and School	S=School, Sexual activity

*From Goldenring JM, Cohen G: Getting into adolescent heads, *Contemp Pediatr* 5:75, 1988.
†From DiFrancesco E: Getting teens to talk to you, *Pediatric News*, Aug. 19, 1992.

family member individually and as a group, it is possible to formulate interventions that improve the health of individual family members and the family unit as a whole. By taking into account the culture, social support structure, family resources, and physical environment of each patient, specific interventions can be developed and implemented.

Healthy family units interact openly and support one another by offering encouragement, helping with tasks, and sharing resources. There is a sense of trust and respect when the family engages in activities. The family pulls together in times of crisis and members assist one another. Family time is valued and activities are planned for relaxation, play, and work. Special times, such as meals, are reserved for the family and each member shares concerns, issues, and accomplishments. Healthy families share core values; some have a strong religious core, which further strengthens the family unit.

Families at risk for alteration in function often have difficulty managing major life stressors. Dysfunctional family patterns that create disharmony include poor communication, limited coping mechanisms, incongruity in power structure and family roles, and inadequate conflict resolution. Family members often escape the tense atmosphere in the home environment by working late, visiting friends, and pursuing recreational interests.

Nurse practitioners may wish to assess the level of family health functioning. The Family APGAR (Table 2-5) is a quick and easy-to-administer measure of family functioning (Smilkstein, 1978). This tool gives a general rating for the level of functioning of the family. Should problems be noted, further assessment of the family would be warranted. This tool is easy to administer and is a helpful tool when time is limited. It will help determine the type of assistance that may be needed by the family.

Should the Family APGAR Questionnaire reveal dysfunctional family patterns, a comprehensive family assessment may be conducted. Several different tools have been developed to evaluate family functioning. The administration and scoring, advantages and limitations of several other family assessment tools are described in Table 2-6.

For a comprehensive family assessment, tools like the Calgary family assessment model (Wright and Leahey, 1994) or Feetham family functioning survey (Roberts and Feetham, 1982; Feetham and Humenick, 1982) provide in-depth examination of family functioning.

Table 2-5
The Family APGAR Questionnaire

	Almost Always	Some of the Time	Hardly Ever
I am satisfied with the help that I receive from my family* when something is troubling me.			
I am satisfied with the way my family* discusses items of common interest and shares problem solving with me.			
I find that my family* accepts my wishes to take on new activities or make changes in my lifestyle.			
I am satisfied with the way my family* expresses affection and responds to my feelings such as anger, sorrow, and love.			
I am satisfied with the amount of time my family* and I spend together.			

Scoring: The patient checks one of three choices which are scored as follows: "Almost always" (2 points); "Some of the time" (1 point); or "Hardly ever," (0). The scores for each of the five questions are then totaled. A score of 7-10 suggests a highly functional family. A score of 4-6 suggests a moderately dysfunctional family. A score of 0-3 suggests a severely dysfunctional family.

From Smilkstein G: The family APGAR: a proposal for a family function test and its use by physicians, *J Fam Pract* 6(6):1231-1239, 1978.
*According to which member of the family is being interviewed, the provider may substitute for the word "family" either "spouse," "significant other," "parent," or "children."

Table 2-6
Family Assessment Tools

Tools	Supporting Theories or Models	Concepts Measured	Administration and Scoring	Advantages	Limitations
CFAM Calgary Family Assessment Model (Wright and Leahey, 1994)	Systems theory Cybernetics theory Communication theory Change Theory	Structural, developmental, and functional assessment of the family	An assessment and family intervention model; does not have a paper and pencil measure for families to complete Interview questions are suggested by Wright and Leahey (1994)	Comprehensive assessment model to evaluate multiple aspects of family life Data collected can be used directly to guide and support nursing interventions	Repeated contacts with family are necessary and optimal to obtain comprehensive assessment data
CHIP Coping Health Inventory for Parents (McCubbin, McCubbin, Cauble, and Nevin, 1979)	ABCX model Social support theory Family stress theory Theories of individual psychology of coping	Coping behaviors Coping patterns Coping strategies	45 self-report coping behaviors Hand scored	Each parent can complete the tool to get complete picture of family's overall coping strategy Can be used as pre- and post-test with intervention program aimed at strengthening coping	Not designed to evaluate child members of the family
CICI: PQ Chronicity Impact and Coping Instrument: Parent Questionnaire (Hymovich, 1983)	Crisis theory Coping theory	Impact of child's chronic illness Perceptions of stressors Coping strategies	48 items Scoring unknown	Identifies areas relevant for nursing interventions Can be used to measure outcome of intervention strategies	Only for families with chronically ill children
FACES III/ FACES IV Family Adaption and	Circumplex model	Cohesion Adaptability, flexibility Communication	30 items in four-point scale Likert-like scale Easy to administer	Measures relevant for nursing Measures real and ideal perceptions of	Family members may be unwilling to assess themselves

Name	Model	Subscales/Components	Administration	Uses	Limitations
Cohesion Scale (Olson, 1994 Olson, Portner, and LaVee, 1985; Olson and Wilson 1982)		Social desirability		the family	Assumes family has children
FAD Family Assessment Device (Epstein, Baldwin, and Bishop, 1983)	McMaster model of family functioning	Problem solving Communication Roles Affective responsiveness Behavior control General functioning	53 items Easy to administer	Measures area nurses could change through care plans	Requires individual to speak for family Not clear if useful with clients of different social and cultural backgrounds or in different life stages
Family APGAR Family Adaptability, Partnership, Growth, Affection and Resolve Test (Smilkstein, 1978)	Family structure, function, and social support	Adaptability Partnership Growth Affection Resolve	Five items Quick to administer	Measures relevant factors Can be completed by adults and children age 10 years and older	Not to be used to evaluate a family problem in depth
Family Satisfaction (Olson and Wilson, 1982)	Circumplex model	Family Satisfaction Cohesion Flexibility	14-Likert scale Easily administered Simple scoring procedures Norms obtained	Directly measures family satisfaction Takes into account normative backgrounds and cultural background	None identified

Continued

Modified from Bowden VR, Dickey SB, Greenberg CS: *Children and their families*, Philadelphia, 1998, WB Saunders.

Table 2-6
Family Assessment Tools—*cont'd*

Tools	Supporting Theories or Models	Concepts Measured	Administration and Scoring	Advantages	Limitations
F-Copes Family Crisis Oriented Personal Evaluation Scales (McCubbin, Larsen, and Olson, 1981)	Double ABCX model	Pile up family resources Meaning and/or perception of a crisis	30-item Likert scale Easily administered Three scales evaluate internal family coping patterns Five scales evaluate external family coping patterns	Identifies family with strong repertoire of coping behaviors	None identified
FES Family Environment Scale (Fuhr, Moos, and Dishotsky, 1981; Moos and Moos; 1976, 1984)	No theoretical position on the nature of families	Relationships Personal growth System maintenance Change	90 items—true-false Scoring is complex Standardized scores, two categories	Short form available Useful for measuring change after interventions Measures real and ideal	A research-oriented tool that does not have a clinical model associated with it; clinical utility is thus unclear
FFI Family Functioning Index (Pless and Satterwhite, 1973)	Family functioning	Communication Togetherness Closeness Decision-making Child orientation	15 items Quickly administered Complicated scoring	Identifies families at risk, not level of risk or distress	Not for families without children Not sensitive to short- or long-term change; thus does not measure change after a nursing intervention
FFFS Feetham Family Functioning Survey	Ecological systems approach	Three major areas of family relationships: between family and broader social units such as school and	Somewhat complicated scoring	Both parents complete the tool so that discrepant views of family life can be identified	Somewhat difficult to understand

Instrument (author)	Theoretical basis	Concepts measured	Items/Scoring	Clinical usefulness	Limitations
(Roberts and Feetham, 1982)		work; between family and subsystems within the family; and between family and individuals within the family		Measures factors nurses could change through care plans / Useful with middle-class families	
FILE Family Inventory of Life Events and Changes (McCubbin, Patterson, and Wilson, 1981)	Double ABCX Model	Pile up events, aA factor	Seven items / Can be hand scored / Evaluates life changes on 10 different scales	Can assess stress in a family at a single point in time / Examines the multiple stressors a family is experiencing	May be difficult for family members to remember events within the past year
IFF Inventory of Family Feelings (Lowman, 1980)	Families affective structure / Patterns of conflict relationships and alliances	Positive or negative feeling toward each member	38 items / Three point Likert-like scale / Easily scored	Focuses on a single dimension of interpersonal and family relationship	Limited clinical usefulness because of unidimensionality
SFIS Structural Family Interaction Scale (Perosa, Hansen, and Perosa, 1981)	Minuchin's family functioning theory	Enmeshment and disengagement / Neglect or overprotection / Rigidity or flexibility / Conflict or avoidance / Patient management / Triangulation of parent-child coalition / Detouring	85 items on four-point agreement scale / Easy to administer	Useful for family counseling and assessment	Length and complexity of tool make it difficult to use clinically

Taken from Bowden VR, Dickey SB, Greenberg CS: *Children and their families*, Philadelphia, 1998, WB Saunders.

THE HISTORY FORMAT

A holistic, patient-focused history format is presented to provide a foundation for case study analysis in Part Two. The history format is a systematic, organized tool designed to efficiently elicit a comprehensive database. In the nursing model, a comprehensive functional health assessment is obtained at the initial visit or at the time of the complete physical examination. The nursing model also includes health promotional activities in each category of the review of systems (ROS). For example, in the genitourinary ROS the use of Kegel exercises for stress incontinence would be noted. A functional health assessment may not be conducted using the medical model. Using the medical model, providers elicit a personal and social history instead of the functional health assessment. Table 2-7 lists the similarities and differences in the nursing and medical histories.

Due to time constraints and dictation costs, only positive history and pertinent negatives are documented on client records. A combination of closed and open questions yields useful, quality information. Closed questions are most useful when collecting factual, short, "yes or no" answers quickly. Open-ended questions elicit long, narrative answers that cue the interviewer into the patient's perceptions and needs.

The health history for a comprehensive database is presented in six sections. Each section is intended to provide prompts and should be expanded and altered throughout each patient visit. The sections include demographic data, past medical history, past surgical history, family health, functional health pattern, and a review of systems.

Table 2-7
Comparison of Nursing and Medical Histories

Medical History Components	Nursing History Components
Demographic data	Demographic data
Past medical history	Past medical history
Past surgical history	Past surgical history
Personal history	Functional health assessment
Social history	Health promotion activities
Review of systems	Review of systems

Family Health

Draw a family genogram or list the family health history. This should include information on the patient's grandparents, mother, father, siblings, and children, including ages (if deceased, add age and cause of death) and major illnesses for everyone listed.

Functional Health Patterns

The functional health patterns developed by Gordon (1992) are a holistic measure of the patient's cultural influences, biopsychosocial being, developmental stage, and environmental interactions. The functional health patterns provide a framework to ask questions about the patient's lifestyle. Patterns emerge from the patient's responses to questions posed about each functional pattern, and potential or actual diagnoses are generated. This holistic approach to patient assessment is presented in Table 2-8.

Review of Systems

In the review of systems, each body system is reviewed and assessed for symptoms or problems not previously discussed. A listing of systems and examples of system cues are contained in Table 2-9.

A sample health history of a 45-year-old African-American male who presents for a complete physical examination is presented in Figure 2-1. His last episodic visit was 6 months ago for acute bronchitis, and his last physical was 5 years ago.

Although all body systems will be assessed during a complete physical, the history data alerts the practitioner to specific body systems that require careful evaluation. In this sample history, J.R. has a positive family history for hypertension and diabetes. A careful review of his vital signs at this visit and over the past few years is important to analyze his blood pressure status. J.R. has smoked 1 pack per day for 10 years. The practitioner should pay particular attention to the heart, lung, and peripheral vasculature (extremities) assessment and look for any abnormalities secondary to this smoking history. J.R. also reports occasional itching of his hemorrhoids and an enlarged prostate. This information requires a careful review of any past PSA (prostate-specific antigen) lab data and a follow-up; or the drawing of an initial PSA at this visit for comparative purposes. A digital rectal examination should be performed to assess any progression of his prostate enlargement as well as an examination of his internal and external hemorrhoids. J.R. also reports occasional tension headaches, which should be evaluated by the physical examination of the HEENT and neurological system.

The Physical Examination The history or interview portion of the visit provides direction for the physical examination. The combination of the health history and physical examination database provides the necessary information for the skilled clinician to establish nursing and medical diagnoses, make clinical judgments, and evaluate the outcomes of the treatment plan.

In preparation for the physical examination, the environment should be arranged to be as private as possible. It should have adequate lighting, be at a comfortable temperature, and be equipped with an examination table. All equipment that is necessary for the examination should be arranged on a clean table. When examining the patient, expose only those areas that are being examined. The patient should be prepared for the physical examination with clear description of what will be done. Children should be called by their first names and parents or adults addressed as Mr., Ms., or Mrs. When examining a child, it is often important to have the patient or guardian present to obtain part of the history from them. Older children can answer many questions themselves, and they enjoy this interaction and participation in their health care. Observing the parent-child interaction during the visit can provide valuable information about relationships among family members. Adolescents should be asked questions directly, and time without parents in the examination area should be arranged. When examining older adults it is important to leave ample time for them to answer questions and change positions during the physical examination.

When applicable to the body system, the sequence of physical assessment techniques is inspection, palpation, percussion, and auscultation. An exception to this is the abdominal examination sequence. The abdomen is inspected first; auscultated second; percussed third; and palpated fourth. The practitioner inspects and auscultates the abdomen first because percussion and palpation can increase peristalsis and can give a false interpretation of bowel sounds (Jarvis, 1996).

THE PHYSICAL EXAMINATION

A focused physical examination is used by the clinician to investigate a specific body system related to the patient's chief complaint. A comprehensive, systematic, head-to-toe examination is conducted for a complete physical assessment. Table 2-10 details a physical examination format with examples of normal assessment data.

Table 2-11 lists specific information to assess when examining a neonate, infant or aging adult.

The cranial nerves are assessed under the neurological review of systems. Table 2-12 provides data to review the cranial nerves, their functions, and the methods of assessing them. The table shows the cranial nerves that are tested in-groups.

Table 2-13 presents information obtained in the physical examination of J.R.

Appendix B provides assessment aids to assist with the physical examination and documentation of findings.

DIAGNOSES AND THERAPEUTIC PLAN OF CARE

In summary, the following diagnoses can be made based on the history and physical data:

- Hypertension (Stage I): J.R. has documentation of an episode of high blood pressure 6 months ago and an elevation was seen on the visit today.
- Smoking Addiction: J.R. smokes 1 pack of cigarettes per day and has no plans to quit at this time.
- Benign prostatic hypertrophy (BPH)
- Tension headaches
- Cerumen impaction, left ear

J.R. has two cardiovascular risk factors. He has a family history of hypertension and he is a smoker. Using the criteria from the Sixth Report of the Joint National Committee on Prevention, Detection, Evaluation, and Treatment of High Blood Pressure (JNC VI, 1997), J.R. should institute lifestyle modifications. He should engage in a regular aerobic exercise program (35-40 minutes most days of the week); modify his diet by reducing sodium to 2 grams per day, limit red meats, and reduce the intake of dietary saturated fat and cholesterol; and he should actively pursue smoking cessation. A follow-up on the blood pressure should be performed in 1 or 2 months to assess the effectiveness of these lifestyle modifications.

For follow-up on the enlarged prostate, J.R. should continue with serial monitoring of his PSA levels annually. There is no need for medical treatment since he does not have disruptive urinary symptoms at this time.

J.R. has only occasional tension headaches that are responsive to Extra Strength Tylenol. This plan is working and should not be modified.

J.R. has an impaction of cerumen in his left ear. He should buy over-the-counter carbamide peroxide 6.5% (Debrox) otic drops, 5 drops to left ear qd times 5 days (12 ml) and be told to return for ear irrigation in one week.

DOCUMENTATION

Documentation is an integral component of the patient's medical record. Long ago, the medical record was the personal journal of the physician. Today, however, the medical record is a document used by multiple health-care providers to provide primary care. The purpose of the medical record has expanded to become pivotal in communicating the patient's current medical problems, health status, and past health-care practices. The medical record is also used for reimbursement; for diagnostic coding and classifying of levels of service (e.g., problem-focused, expanded, detailed, and comprehensive); for quality assurance and third party audits; and for coverage of medical legal issues (Edsall and Moore, 1995; Kettenbach, 1995; Larimore and Jordan, 1995; Owen and Moore, 1995). The use of multiple health care organizations, group and individual practices has made quality notes essential to communicate the health status of individuals across the life span.

Inadequate or limited documentation may bring the clinician monetary losses for reimbursable services provided or possibly result in legal liability. Continuity of patient care may suffer from inade-

quate documentation. Failure to document adequately may also result in the loss of credentialing by medical care organizations. Careful attention to accurate, concise documentation is therefore essential. Some health-care organizations have purchased or developed computerized patient records to gather, document, and analyze patient data. These state-of-the art health care tools offer a wide range of valuable services to the clinician. Effective information management systems assist the clinician in capturing and organizing essential elements for patient databases.

Various methods exist for documentation in the medical record. Lawrence Weed, M.D., developed the SOAP format to provide a systematic way for clinicians to document patient encounters. SOAP is a popular format for documenting simple episodic problems or follow-up visits. It assists health care providers to organize their cognitive process in clinical judgment to analyze patient information, make diagnostic decisions, and document the holistic patient encounter.

First, the health care provider enters the *chief complaint.* This entry consists of 2 to 7 words stated by the patient as the reason for seeking health-care services.

The *S* stands for *subjective data* that the patient or significant other describes as the pertinent information regarding the history of the present illness, significant past medical history (PMH), allergies, current treatments, and self-care measures. A detailed description of the patient problems may be elicited using the LCSTSAA format described in Chapter 1.

The *O* stands for *objective data.* This is measurable or observable data that the practitioner can gather by using the senses of sight, smell, hearing, and touch. Vital signs, height, weight, and systems that are examined in a head-to-toe fashion are documented. This section begins with a general survey and progresses systematically based on the body system and laboratory data related to the reason for the visit.

The *A* stands for *assessment* and includes the problem list or diagnoses elicited from the clinical evaluation. The diagnoses should include the status of the presenting problem (e.g., acute, stable, chronic, or resolving). If a diagnoses cannot be made for certain, then a symptom (e.g., vertigo, vomiting, or diarrhea) can be entered with potential rule out conditions if appropriate.

The *P* stands for *plan,* which identifies the outcomes for future evaluation. This is a detailed listing of diagnostic tests, therapeutic interventions, medications, and referrals. The follow-up plan is noted as to when the next visit should occur as well as the outcomes to measure. Detailed information should be included about the teaching completed during the patient visit. Counseling should include risk versus benefits of management options and procedures; and alternative risks discussed with the patient and significant other (if appropriate). Examples include teaching related to the illness or diagnoses, potential side effects of the medications, and therapies. Patient understanding of information given must also be documented.

The clinician must remember that if facts such as these are not documented, legally it is as if they never happened. Objective findings should be described. For example, the strength of the upper extremities should be documented as 4+/5 symmetric upper extremity strength rather than "normal." Pertinent negatives are important in making your clinical judgment with differential diagnoses. For example, documenting no headache, vomiting, or nuchal rigidity in a child who presents with fever demonstrates that common and potentially life-threatening conditions were considered and helps narrow the differential diagnoses.

The following SOAP example is from the history and physical data elicited from J.R.:

Chief Complaint: Headache

S: Occasional, throbbing, bandlike H/A for past 2 years; occurs once every 3 to 4 weeks when he works overtime in construction work; feels tightness in his neck and bilateral upper shoulders prior to the H/A onset; denies any fever, chills, dizziness, visual disturbance, N/V; H/A lasts for 5 to 6 hours if untreated, but resolves promptly with Extra Strength Tylenol; rates the pain as 5 on a 0-10 scale; usually does not interfere with ADLs; past medical history: smokes 1 pack per day for 10 years; HTN, +family history of HTN; no head injury or trauma

O: T: 98.4° F; P: 72; R: 16; BP 152/98; height, 6 feet even; weight, 212 pounds; BMI 29; alert and oriented ×4. Well-developed. Well-nourished. African-American male in NAD. Well-groomed. Speech clear. Smooth, independent gait. Head: normocephalic, without evidence of trauma, lesions, or tenderness. Face: symmetrical, expression appropriate. Eyes: sclera clear without lesions or exudate; PERRLA, optic discs sharp, well-defined, cream-colored, no exudates or hemorrhages, EOMs intact, visual acuity on Snellen chart 20/20 with glasses, 20/50 OU without glasses. Ears: pinna no lesions or scaling; L TM unable to visualize due to large amount of brown hard cerumen; R TM pearly gray, landmarks intact with distinct cone of light; Rinne, AC greater than BC au. Nose: patent bilaterally, septum midline, no discharge, polyps or sinus tenderness. Throat: oral mucosa pink, moist, no lesions, tonsils 0+, uvula midline, teeth with multiple fillings. Neck: supple without JVD, carotid bruits, thyromegaly, cervical lymphadenopathy, trachea is midline. Lungs: clear to auscultation and equal bilaterally, no adventitious breath sounds, resonant throughout lung fields. Cardiovascular: RRR without murmurs, no S3 or S4, PMI 5th ICS-LMCL, radial, pedal, and femoral pulses 2+ and equal bilaterally. Neuro: CN II-XII grossly intact, DTR 2+ bil symmetrical, muscular strength intact bil, no atrophy or tremors, Romberg neg, sensation intact to light touch and pinprick, able to heel-to-toe walk.

A: Tension H/A

P: Continue to use Extra Strength Tylenol prn; cold and heat therapy with mild neck and shoulder stretching BID, massage prn, imagery prn. Discussion on the cause and the treatment options for tension H/As. Instructions on heat and cold applications given and demonstration of neck and shoulder stretching done. Patient given a handout on massage therapy, reviewed with patient. Scheduled for classes on relaxation and imagery.

Table 2-8
Gordon's Functional Patterns

Examples of Activities/Behaviors

Health Perception-Health Management	**Health Promotion:** General health, mammogram, PAP, PSA, sigmoidoscopy, immunizations **Health Management:** Do you have a living will or advanced directive? (Management of overall health and well-being includes harmony of emotional, physical, and spiritual dimensions.) **Health Risks:** Tobacco use, alcohol use, recreational drug use, guns/other weapons in the home, family or environmental violence, smoke detectors, CO_2 monitor. Have you been physically or emotionally abused? **CAGE Questionnaire:** CAGE questions may be used to elicit drinking problems (Ewing, 1984): • Have you ever felt you ought to **C**ut down on drinking? • Have people **A**nnoyed you by criticizing your drinking? • Have you ever felt bad or **G**uilty about your drinking? • Have you ever had a drink first thing in the morning to steady your nerves or get rid of a hangover (**E**ye-opener)? **Infants:** For Infants use the SAFE questions: • S = Physical or environmental **S**afety concerns and **S**leep patterns • A = Appropriate **A**ctivity level • F = Adequate **F**ood and **F**luids • E = Adequate **E**limination. **Adolescents:** For Adolescent use the HEADS questions: • H = **H**ome life • E = **E**xtracurricular activities • A = **A**lcohol • D = **D**rugs • S = **S**exual activity, **S**moking, and **S**chool **Adult:** To conduct a general assessment and mental status, use the FROMAJE questions (Libow and Sherman, 1981): • F = **F**unction: the ability to perform self-care and an overall assessment of mental functioning • R = **R**easoning: the ability to think abstractly • O = **O**rientation: to time, person, place • M = **M**emory: assess immediate, short and long term • A = **A**rithmetic: assess intellectual ability • J = **J**udgment: able to select appropriate alternatives • E = **E**motional status: assess emotional well being and stability To conduct a detailed mental status examination, consider using the mini-mental status examination. See Appendix B for this tool and directions for its use
Nutrition/ Metabolic	Special diet or supplements, typical 24-hour food intake, appetite, weight loss or gain in past year, dentures, last dental appointment, swallowing problems, food restrictions
Activity/ Exercise	Self-care ability, exercise pattern, leisure activities, ability to perform activities of daily living
Sleep/Rest	Hours of sleep per night, insomnia, nightmares, snoring
Self Perception and Values/ Beliefs	Major loss, job change, or relationship change, body image, values, beliefs, goals
Coping-Stress	Source of support, stressful life events, coping mechanisms, recreation, hobbies, interests, spirituality
Role-Relationship	Support systems, living arrangements, social groups, working environment, marital or relationship status

Modified from Gordon M: *Manual of nursing diagnosis*, New York, 1992, McGraw-Hill.

Table 2-9
Review of Systems

System	Examples of System Cues
General	General health, unusual weight gain or loss; fatigue, weakness, fever, chills *Pediatrics:* Failure to gain weight appropriately for age, patterns of growth and development, activity/behavior, mother's health during pregnancy, labor and delivery, the perinatal period
Skin, Hair, Nails	Skin diseases, increased dryness or moisture, bruising, rashes, lesions, sun and wind exposure, color or texture change, abnormal hair or nail growth or loss, mole changes, jaundice *Pediatrics:* Jaundice as a newborn, cradle cap, eczema
HEENT	*Head:* Skull shape and size, any concussions or head injuries, history of headaches *Eye:* History of trauma or eye disease, visual disturbances (diplopia, photophobia, and scotoma), glaucoma or cataracts, eye drainage, itching or redness, blurred vision, glasses or contact lenses, last eye examination *Ear:* Ear infections, cerumen impactions, tubes in ears, hearing problems or deafness, occupational exposure to loud noises, tinnitus, vertigo *Nose:* Recurrent drainage, polyps, snoring, nasal stuffiness, nasal septum deviation, nosebleeds, sense of smell or loss of smell, frequency of colds, history of sinusitis *Throat:* Dental examination, dentures, bleeding gums, caries, lesions or soreness of lips, tongue, mouth, or throat; history of frequent tonsillitis or infections *Pediatrics:* Strabismus, difficulty seeing boards at school, multiple ear infections, ages at eruption of deciduous/permanent teeth, number of teeth at age 1 year, tubes in ears, braces or dental appliances
Neck	Vocal changes or hoarseness, goiter, lymph node enlargement *Pediatrics:* Neck control, webbing
Chest:	*Lungs:* History of emphysema, asthma, bronchitis, shortness of breath with or without exertion, number of pillows, number of stairs before SOB, cough, hemoptysis, exposure to environmental hazards, wheezing, exposure to tuberculosis (TB), dyspnea, TB test results, chest x-ray (CXR) results *Breasts:* Pain, lumps, dimpling, nipple discharge, scaling or cracks (fissures) around nipples, practice breast self-examination (BSE), last mammogram results *Pediatrics:* Exercise-induced asthma
Cardiovascular System	History of heart problems, heart murmurs, coronary artery disease, hypertension, congestive heart failure (CHF), chest pain, irregular heartbeat, palpitations, cyanosis, paroxysmal nocturnal dyspnea, exercise intolerance, edema, last ECG and results (if pertinent) *Pediatrics:* Change in skin color as a neonate

Continued

Table 2-9
Review of Systems—*cont'd*

System	Examples of System Cues
Gastrointestinal System	Bowel movement pattern and color, constipation, diarrhea, abdominal pain, flatulence, ulcers, gastroesophageal reflux disease, nausea and vomiting, rectal bleeding, hemorrhoids or fissures, heartburn, indigestion, rectal polyps, hepatitis, pancreatitis *Pediatrics:* Encopresis, pinworms
Genitourinary System	Urinary frequency, urgency, leakage, history of kidney infections, nocturia, hernia; sexually transmitted disease, sexual practices/orientation, history of abuse *Female:* Gravida, para, abortions, stillbirths, labor, delivery or post-delivery complications, method of birth control, pain or problems with sexual intercourse, vaginal discharge or dryness, pain with menses, intermenstrual/post coital bleeding, onset of menarche, last menstrual period, last Pap smear, any history of abnormal Pap smears *Male:* Circumcised, urethral discharge, penile lesions/sores, scrotal swelling, hernia or hydrocele, testicular pain or masses, change in libido, difficulty with erections or ejaculations, testicular self-examination, prostate problems, PSA test *Pediatrics*: Age toilet trained, bed-wetting, nocturnal emissions, Tanner's stages
Musculoskeletal System	Arthritis, full range of motion of joints, muscular disorders, pain, swelling of joints, stiffness, gait disturbances, history of back pain, kyphosis, lordosis, change in posture or height *Pediatrics:* Scoliosis, knee pain, hip pain
Endocrine System	History of diabetes, hypo/hyperthyroidism, skin striae, polydipsia, polyuria, weight changes, heat and cold intolerance, abnormal hair distribution, obesity *Pediatrics:* Early or late development of puberty, ambiguous genital development
Hematological System	Bleeding disorders, anemia, bruising, enlarged lymph nodes, blood transfusions, exposure to toxins or radiation *Pediatrics:* Sickle cell disease, blood cell disorder
Neurological System	Head injury, headaches, multiple sclerosis, seizures, strokes, tremors, tics, coordination problems, memory impairment, mental status, blackouts, depression, mood swings *Pediatrics:* Increased or small head size, bulging fontanels
Psychiatric System	Depression, suicidal/homicidal tendencies, mental health hospitalizations, drug/alcohol abuse, eating disorders, attention deficit disorder *Pediatrics:* Behavioral problems at school, peer relationships

Date of Assessment: October 2, 1998

Demographic Data:

Name: James Randolph   *Age:* 45   *Sex:* Male   *Ethnicity:* African-American

Date of Birth: 9/12/1953   *Occupation:* Construction Worker   *Religion:* Baptist

Historian: Self

Current Health Status: Patient ranks health as very good

Developmental Stage: Generativity versus Stagnation

Past Medical History:

Physical or Mental Illnesses/Injuries/Hospitalizations: Broken arm 1977

Past Surgical History: Appendectomy 1988; T&A 1964; Surgical repair GSW Right thigh 1972.

Childhood Illnesses: Measles, mumps, rubella, and chickenpox. Two episodes of severe strep throat 1969 and 1971.

Immunizations:

Immunization	Date(s)	Immunization	Date(s)
Diphtheria	7/10/98	HIB	
Pertussis		Measles	
Tetanus	7/10/98	Rubella	
Polio		Hepatitis B	4/94, 5/94, 9/94
Pneumovax		Varicella	

Allergies to Medications: Penicillin, breaks out in hives   *Other Allergies:* None

Transfusion History: # of Transfusions: None   *Year(s) of Transfusions:* None

Current Prescription or Over the Counter Medications/Herbs/Vitamins:

Medication/Herb/Vitamin	Dosage	Frequency
Multivitamin	1	qd
Vitamin E	200 mg	qd
Alka-Seltzer	1-2 tablets	prn indigestion
Tylenol ES	2 tablets	prn headaches

Family Health:

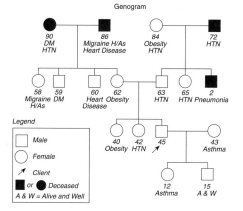

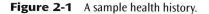

Figure 2-1   A sample health history.

Continued

Functional Health Patterns:

Health Perception-Health Management	Smokes 1 pack per day for 10 years. Drinks 2 glasses of red wine per week. Has experimented with marijuana, but does not use now. No current or past use of recreational drugs. Wears seatbelts, has a smoke detector and carbon monoxide detector at home. Has not completed advanced directives. Does not perform STE. Has not had a PSA test. Owns a handgun that he uses at a shooting range
Nutrition/Metabolic	Eats 3 meals per day with snacks. Eats 5 servings of fruits and vegetables, limits red meats, drinks 1 coffee and 1 coke per day, limits fat and salt intake, enjoys desserts
Activity/Exercise	Owns a treadmill, but rarely uses it, walks a little when the weather is nice, does wood cutting, shoveling snow, and cutting the grass. Plays basketball in the summer with his neighbors
Sleep/Rest	Sleeps 7 hours per day and is rested upon awakening, usually 11PM to 6AM, no difficulty falling asleep
Self Perception and Value–Beliefs	Enjoys helping others, attends church regularly
Coping–Stress	Enjoys outdoor activities. Talks with wife and friends when issues arise
Role-Relationship	Husband, father, son. Married

Review of Systems:

Skin, Hair, Nails	No dry skin, pruritis, bruising, sores, or lesions. No pigmentary or mole changes. Very slight hair thinning. Nails strong and intact
HEENT	Occasional throbbing, band like headache relieved with 2 Tylenol Extra Strength. No dizziness or syncope. Far-sighted with astigmatism. Wears bifocal glasses. Last eye exam May 1998 with Dr. Smith in Grand Rapids. No glaucoma, cataracts, pain, redness or infection. No blurred vision, flashes or spots, or changes in acuity. Hearing excellent. No tinnitus, pain, or infections as an adult. Gets frequent colds. No history of epistaxis, no sinus pain. Sense of smell good. Teeth in good condition. Several fillings. Regular dental checkups q 6 months with Dr. Radspa, Grand Rapids. No bleeding in gums, no pain, lesions, or sores in mouth. No hoarseness, pain or inflammation in throat
Neck	No changes in voice, hoarseness, goiter, or lymph node enlargement
Chest	No cough, dyspnea, pain, wheezing, hemoptysis, or pleurisy. No shortness of breath with exertion. No orthopnea or paroxysmal nocturnal dyspnea. No asthma or pneumonia. Environmental exposure to dusts
Cardiovascular System	No chest pain or pressure, palpitations, edema, leg cramps, varicosities, or claudication. No hypertension, anemia, bleeding tendency or blood transfusions. Blood type = O+. Negative sickle cell trait
Gastrointestinal System	Good appetite. Rare indigestion. No constipation, diarrhea, nausea or vomiting. No abdominal pain, jaundice, or bowel changes. Has daily bowel movement brown formed, no bloody or tarry stools. No excessive flatulence or belching. No history of hernia. Has hemorrhoids, which occasionally cause itching and mild discomfort, uses metamucil when this happens or increases vegetables in diet
Genitourinary System	No dysuria, pyuria, hematuria, polyuria, or urgency. No problems with urine stream. Wakes up once each night to void. Has enlarged prostate since 1995. Has no problem with sexual intercourse, no impotence, or unhappiness. No history of STDs. No scrotal or penile pain
Musculoskeletal System	No arthritis, muscular disorders, pains, swelling of joints, or stiffness. No gait disturbance or history of back pain. Full range of motion of all joints
Endocrine System	No history of diabetes, thyroid problems, hepatitis, pancreatitis, skin striae, polydypsia, polyuria, weight changes, or heat and cold intolerance
Hematological System	No bleeding disorders, anemia, bruising, enlarged lymph nodes, blood transfusions
Neurological System	No head injuries, rare tension headache relieved with Tylenol Extra Strength. No history of seizures, multiple sclerosis, strokes, tremors, tics, coordination problems, memory impairment, blackouts, mood swings. Rare situational depression – uses friends and partner to problem solve

Figure 2-1, *cont'd*   For legend see p. 29.

Table 2-10
Physical Examination Format

Parameter	Example of Normal
Vital Signs	BP R/L arm; pulse rhythm and strength; respiration rate, depth, strength; temperature and route; height; weight
General Appearance	Alert and oriented to time, place, person, and situation; well-nourished, well-groomed; speech clear; coordinated movements; in no apparent distress
Integument	
Skin	Smooth, moist, warm, good turgor, no edema, lesions, exudates
Hair	Color, smooth and evenly distributed, scalp pink without infestations
Nails	Pink and smooth, capillary refill less than 3 seconds, no clubbing
HEENT	
Head and face	Normocephalic, without evidence of trauma, lesions, or tenderness; symmetrical, expression appropriate
Eyes	PERRLA, optic discs sharp, well defined, cream color, no exudates or hemorrhages, EOMs intact, visual acuity, visual fields, cover/uncover tests
Ears	Pinna no lesions or scaling, External canal clear, TMs pearly gray, landmarks intact with distinct cone of light; able to hear whispered words; Rinne: AC greater than BC au, Weber without lateralization
Nose	Patent bilaterally, septum midline, no discharge, polyps or sinus tenderness
Throat	Oral mucosa pink, moist, no lesions, tonsils 2+, uvula midline
Neck	Supple without JVD, carotid bruits, thyromegaly, no cervical lymphadenopathy, trachea is midline
Lungs	Clear to auscultation and equal bilaterally, no adventitious breath sounds, resonant throughout lung fields, even respiratory effort
Cardiovascular	RRR without murmurs, no S3 or S4, PMI 5th ICS-LMCL, radial, pedal, and femoral pulses 2+ and equal bilaterally
Breast	Symmetrical, no tenderness, enlargement, dimpling, or masses, no nipple discharge, no axillary lymphadenopathy bilaterally
Abdomen	Flat, active bowel sounds, no abdominal bruits, soft, no masses or organomegaly, nontender, no inguinal lymphadenopathy, no CVA tenderness
Genital	
Female	External genitalia with no lesions, discharge, or rashes; vaginal mucosa pink and moist; cervix pink; parous os; no cervical motion tenderness; no adnexal masses, uterus not enlarged
Male	Penis circumcised (or not), no discharge or lesions, testes descended and without masses or tenderness
Rectal	No masses, lesions or hemorrhoids, hemoccult negative stool in anal vault, intact anal tone, prostate smooth with no nodules without evidence of hypertrophy
Extremities	Pink, warm, without edema, no varicosities, bilateral negative Homans' sign, joints without evidence of ligamentous laxity, effusions, erythema or swelling, full ROM of all joints, muscle strength 5+ and equal in upper and lower extremities
Neurological	CN II – XII grossly intact, DTR 2+ bilateral, symmetrical, muscular strength intact bilateral, no atrophy or tremors, Romberg neg, sensation intact to light touch and pinprick, able to heel-to-toe walk
Psychological	Mood and affect appropriate, smiling, emotive

Table 2-11
Specific Physical Examination Information for Neonates, Infants, and the Aging Adult

Neonate	APGAR at 1 and 5 minutes, lanugo, milia, cyanosis, jaundice, caput succedaneum, cephalhematoma, acrocyanosis, cutis marmorata, erythema toxicum, harlequin color change, Mongolian spots, telangiectatic nevi (stork bites)
Infant	Femoral pulses, cyanosis, venous hum, umbilical cord, descended testes, penis (circumcised or foreskin), head circumference, anterior and posterior fontanels, bossing, Barlow-Ortolani maneuver, Allis sign, language for age
Aging Adult	Senile purpura, arcus senilis, presbyopia, cherry angiomas, presbycusis, barrel chest, kyphosis, lordosis

Table 2-12
Cranial Nerves

Cranial Nerve	Function	Assessment
CN I: Olfactory	Sense of smell	Assess smell aromatic substance (e.g., vanilla extract)
CN II: Optic	Visual acuity and fields	Assess visual acuity and peripheral vision testing
CN III: Oculomotor	Pupillary constriction, extraocular movements, eyelid function, accommodation	Use penlight to check pupils, check for eyelid drooping, ability to follow moving objects, accommodation
CN IV: Trochlear		
CN VI: Abducens		
CN V: Trigeminal	Sensations of pain and touch, corneal reflex, open mouth and teeth clench, move jaw	Check the ability to clench teeth, corneal reflex intact, facial sensation bilaterally, check for atrophy
CNVII: Facial	Muscles of facial expression, taste buds of anterior 2/3 of tongue	Check the ability to smile, puff cheeks, wrinkle forehead; ability to identify sweet and salty tastes
CN VIII: Acoustic	Hearing	Check hearing; check air and bone conduction using a tuning fork
CN IX: Glossopharyngeal	Swallowing, gag reflex, taste on posterior 1/3 of tongue	Check ability to swallow, test gag reflex, ability to taste sour substances
CN X: Vagus	Uvula and soft palate rise, swallowing, speech quality	Check for swallowing, speech, and uvula rising
CN XI: Spinal Accessory	Trapezius and sternocleidomastoid muscle strength	Shrug shoulders and turn head side to side against resistance
CN XII: Hypoglossal	Tongue movement and quality of lingual speech sounds	Check for thickened speech and smooth symmetrical tongue movements

Table 2-13
Physical Examination of J.R.

Vital Signs	BP 152/98 L & R arms; apical pulse 72, regular; respirations 16, regular, nonlabored; temperature 98.4° F (ear); height, 6 feet 0 inches; weight, 212 pounds; BMI = 29
General Appearance	Alert and oriented X 4; well-nourished; well-groomed; speech clear; coordinated movements; in no apparent distress
Integument	
Skin	Dark complexion; skin moist, good turgor; no moles or bruising
Hair	Black, curly and evenly distributed; no dandruff, nits, or lice
Nails	Nail beds pink and smooth, capillary refill less than 3 seconds, no clubbing
HEENT	
Head	Normocephalic,
Face	Symmetrical, expression appropriate
Eyes	PERRLA; optic discs sharp, well defined, cream color; no exudates or hemorrhages; EOMs intact; visual acuity on Snellen chart 20/20 with glasses, 20/50 OU without glasses
Ears	Pinna no lesions or scaling; unable to visualize L TM due to large amount of brown, hard cerumen; R TM pearly gray, landmarks intact with distinct cone of light; Rinne: AC greater than BC au
Nose	Patent bilaterally, septum midline, no discharge, polyps, or sinus tenderness
Throat	Oral mucosa pink, moist, no lesions, tonsils +0, uvula midline, teeth with multiple fillings
Neck	Supple without JVD, carotid bruits, thyromegaly, no cervical lymphadenopathy, trachea is midline
Lungs	Clear to auscultation and equal bilaterally, no adventitious breath sounds, resonant throughout lung fields
Cardiovascular	RRR without murmurs, no S_3 or S_4, PMI 5th ICS-LMCL, radial, pedal, and femoral pulses 2+ and equal bilaterally
Breast	Symmetrical, no tenderness, enlargement, dimpling, or masses, no nipple discharge, no axillary lymphadenopathy
Abdomen	Well-healed slightly raised 6 cm scar RLQ; flat, active bowel sounds; no abdominal bruits or pulsatile masses; nontender, soft; no masses or organomegaly; no inguinal lymphadenopathy; no CVA tenderness
Genital	
Male	Penis uncircumcised, without lesions, no urethral discharge, testes descended without masses or tenderness, no hernias noted
Rectal	No masses, small external hemorrhoids, hemoccult negative stool in anal vault, intact anal tone, prostate smooth with no nodules, slightly enlarged
Extremities	Well-healed surgical scar on R posterior thigh; warm, without edema, no varicosities, joints without evidence of ligamentous laxity, effusions, erythema or edema, strength 5+
Neurological	CN II-XII grossly intact, DTR 2+ bilaterally symmetrical, Romberg neg, sensation intact to light touch and pinprick, sensory and motor function intact without deficits

References

Berlin EA, Fowkes WC Jr: A teaching framework for cross-cultural health care, *West J Med* 139(6):934-938, 1983.

Bomar PJ: *Nurses and family health promotion,* ed 2, Philadelphia, 1996, WB Saunders.

Bowden VR, Dickey SB, Greenberg CS: *Children and their families,* Philadelphia, 1998, WB Saunders.

Boynton RW, Dunn ES, Stephens GR: *Manual of ambulatory pediatrics,* ed 4, Philadelphia, 1998, JB Lippincott.

Dienemann JA: *Transcultural nursing: assessment and intervention,* ed 2, St Louis, 1997, Mosby.

Epstein N, Baldwin L, Bishop E: The McMaster Family Assessment Device, *J Marital Fam Ther* 9:171-180, 1983.

Edsall RL, Moore KJ: Exam documentation: charting within the guidelines, *Fam Pract Manag* 2(3):53-59, 1995.

Erikson E: *Youth: change and challenge,* New York, 1963, Basic Books.

Erikson E: *Childhood and society,* 35th anniversary edition, New York, 1986, W.W. Norton.

Ewing JA: Detecting alcoholism: The CAGE questionnaire. *JAMA* 252(14):1905-1907, 1984.

Feetham SL, Humenick SS: The Feetham family functioning survey. In Humenick SS, editor: *Analysis of current assessment strategies in the health care of young children and childbearing families,* Norwalk, CT, 1982, Appleton-Century-Crofts.

Freud S: Some psychological consequences of the anatomical distinction between the sexes, *International Journal of Psychoanalysis* 8:133-142, 1927.

Fuhr R, Moos R, Dishotsky N: The use of family assessment and feedback in ongoing family therapy, *American Journal of Family Therapy* 9(1):24-36, 1981.

Geissler EM: *Pocket guide to cultural assessment,* St Louis, 1994, Mosby.

Giger JN, Davidhizar RE: *Transcultural nursing: assessment and intervention,* ed 2, St Louis, 1995, Mosby.

Glisson J, Crawford R, Street S: The clinical applications of ginkgo biloba, St. John's wort, saw palmetto, and soy, *Nurse Pract* 24(6):28, 31, 35-36, 1999.

Gordon M: *Manual of nursing diagnosis,* New York, 1992, McGraw-Hill.

Jarvis C: *Physical examination and health assessment,* ed 2, Philadelphia, 1996, WB Saunders.

Joint National Committee on Prevention, Detection, Evaluation, and Treatment of High Blood Pressure: The sixth report, *Arch Intern Med* 157(21):2413-2446, 1997.

Hymovich DP: The Chronicity Impact and Coping Instrument: Parent Questionnaire, *Nurs Res* 32(5):275-281, 1983.

Kettenbach G: *Writing SOAP notes,* ed 2, Philadelphia, 1995, F.A. Davis Company.

Larimore WL, Jordan EV: SOAP to SNOCAMP: improving the medical record format, *J Fam Pract* 41(4):393-398, 1995.

Libow LS, Sherman F: *The core of geriatric medicine,* St Louis, 1981, Mosby.

Lipson JG, Dibble SL, Minarik PA: *Culture and nursing care: a pocket guide,* San Francisco, 1996, University of California, San Francisco: Nursing Press.

Lowman J: Measurement of family affective structure, *J Pers Assess* 44(2):130-141, 1980.

McCubbin H, Larson A, Olson D: *F-Copes,* Madison, WI, 1981, University of Wisconsin.

McCubbin H, McCubbin M, Cauble A et al: *Coping Health Inventory for Parents (CHIP),* St Paul, MN, 1979, University of Minnesota.

McCubbin H, Patterson J, Wilson L: *FILE,* St Paul, MN, 1981, University of Minnesota.

Moos RH, Moos BS: A typology of family social environments, *Fam Process* 15(4):357-371, 1976.

Moos RH, Moos BS: The process of recovery from alcoholism: III. Comparing functioning in families of alcoholics and matched control families *J Stud Alcohol* 45(2):111-118, 1984.

Olson D, Portner J, LaVee Y: *FACES III,* St Paul, MN, 1985, Family Social Science.

Olson D, Wilson M: *Family satisfaction,* Madison, WI, 1982, University of Wisconsin.

Owen A, Moore KJ: Don't read this article! *Fam Pract Manag* 2(2):47-53, 1995.

Perosa L, Hansen J, Perosa S: Development of the structural family interaction scale, *Family Therapy* 8(2):77-90, 1981.

Pless IB, Satterwhite B: A measure of family functioning and its application, *Soc Sci Med* 7(8):613-620, 1973.

Power CF, Higgins A, Kohlberg L: *Lawrence Kohlberg's approach to moral education,* New York, 1989, Columbia University Press.

Roberts CS, Feetham SL: Assessing family functioning across three areas of relationships, *Nurs Res* 31(4):231-235, 1982.

Seidel H, Ball J, Dains J, Benedict G: *Mosby's guide to physical examination* St Louis, 1995, Mosby.

Smilkstein G: The family APGAR: a proposal for a family function test and its use by physicians, *J Fam Pract* 6(6):1231-1239, 1978.

Thomas RM: *Comparing theories of child development,* ed 2, Belmont, CA, 1985, Wadsworth.

Wright LM, Leahey M: *Nurses and families: a guide to family assessment and intervention,* Philadelphia, 1994, F.A. Davis.

Selected Readings

Brennan PF, Daly BJ: Information requirements of advanced practice nurses, A*dv Pract Nurs* 2(3):54-57, 1996.

Olson D: Curvilinearity survives: The world is not flat, *Family Process* 33:471-478, 1994.

Taylor-Seehafer M: Nurse-physician collaboration, *J Am Acad Nurse Pract* 10(9):387-391, 1998.

Wells N, Johnson R, Salyer S: Interdisciplinary collaboration, *Clin Nurse Spec* 12(4):161-168, 1998.

CHAPTER 3

Diagnostic Tests

Carol Patton

KEY VARIABLES TO CONSIDER WHEN ORDERING DIAGNOSTIC TESTS

There are many factors that impact on decision-making and the ordering of diagnostic tests. The practitioner should order diagnostic tests in order to rule in or rule out a differential diagnosis. The diagnostic test should be client-centered with a clinical outcome that will provide benefit to the client. Many diagnostic tests ordered are unnecessary and provide little if any additional information to the treatment plan.

One of the most logical and succinct decision models for ordering diagnostic tests was developed by the American College of Physicians (ACP) (Taylor, 1998). According to ACP guidelines, there are five fundamental questions that should be asked when ordering any diagnostic test:

1. Why am I considering this test?
2. What question is this test supposed to answer?
3. Is the test capable of answering the question?
4. Do the benefits of testing outweigh the risks?
5. Does the benefit justify the test's cost?

The nurse practitioner must feel comfortable with the decision-making required to order diagnostic tests to rule in or rule out a given differential diagnosis. If the diagnostic finding will influence the treatment plan of the client, or affect client outcome in any way, the diagnostic test should be ordered. If the test result will not impact the decision-making and treatment plan, then one must question the cost/benefit ratio of the diagnostic component. The practitioner must consider whether or not there will be a clinical benefit in ordering the test.

Assessing the cost/benefit ratio is important when ordering diagnostic tests. Will the test yield a benefit to the patient? Benefit derived from a diagnostic test should equal or exceed the risk of performing the test. Benefit may be measured in a variety of ways. Cost/benefit analysis in ordering diagnostic tests should begin with a comprehensive assessment of the client. It is important for the practitioner to think in terms of a "stepped care approach" when ordering diagnostic tests. Many insurers will not approve or reimburse for a diagnostic test unless there is supporting rationale for ordering it. The stepped care approach is ordering the most cost-effective test that will yield useful diagnostic information. For example, ordering a plain film of a knee—instead of an MRI—is the first line diagnostic imaging study or primary diagnostic test. There are times when a more definitive diagnostic test should be ordered as the first line diagnostic test. The practitioner's documentation should reflect the rationale for the medical decision-making that occurred and how the decision was made. Documentation of decision-making is also essential in maintaining continuity of care in facilities where there may be multiple providers seeing a particular client.

The more accurate the practitioner's assessment and history-taking ability, the greater the yield in obtaining accurate, detailed information. Information gleaned from the client history and clinical examination provides a rich database and in most cases will be more helpful in making a diagnosis than a diagnostic test. For example, a client may provide a clinical history of acute cholecystitis, and clinically appear to have cholecystitis, but have normal laboratory data. It is over time and with clinical experience that the nurse practitioner develops keen, accurate assessment skills. There is a positive correlation between the novice practitioner and the number and sophistication of diagnostic tests ordered. Novice practitioners tend to over-order diagnostic tests, whereas the seasoned practitioner maximizes the use of history and physical data, ordering only essential tests in the work-up.

Ordering diagnostic tests also involves an ethical component. There are clients who need diagnostic tests to "rule in" or "rule out" a differential diagnosis and who may not receive them because they are uninsured or underinsured. When a client will benefit from a diagnostic test, the test should be ordered. In uninsured or underinsured cases it is critical to explore payment options and alternative resources. A client should never be deprived of a needed and justified diagnostic test due to lack of financial resources.

There are selected diagnostic screening tests that should be completed at specified intervals for specified vulnerable or high-risk populations. It is critical to keep accurate records of these screenings and outcomes. Examples include diabetics with HbA_{1C} and microalbumin of urine, and lipid profiles for those with hyperlipidemia. The practitioner should also be knowledgeable of drug levels that need to be monitored at specified intervals (e.g., Dilantin, lithium, and digoxin).

The ordering of unnecessary diagnostic tests may result in false-positive and false-negative results. When an unnecessary diagnostic test is ordered, there is an increase in health-care costs. Ordering unnecessary tests is an inappropriate use of health-care resources.

Sensitivity and specificity indicate the degree of accuracy of diagnostic tests. Sensitivity is the degree to which a specified diagnostic test is positive in a client with the disease. There is no diagnostic test that is 100% sensitive. This is because there will always be confounding variables that influence the test to have a false-positive or a false-negative. (A false-positive result indicates the person has the disease when this is not true. A false-negative result indicates the person to be free of the disease when this is not true.) The sensitivity of a diagnostic test indicates its ability to accurately determine the presence of disease. Specificity refers to the proportion of people who do not have the disease who test negative for the disease. There can be factors that influence false-positive and false-negatives in specificity as well as sensitivity (Table 3-1) (U.S. Preventive Services Task Force, 1996).

The results of diagnostic tests should be reported to the client in a timely, accountable manner. The practitioner should develop a notification system for diagnostic tests, and document this in the patient record. Notifying the client is always important, but is even more so when test results are abnormal. When test results are abnormal there is an increased chance of mortality and/or morbidity.

The client assessment should include a cultural assessment of the effect and/or potential impact of ordering diagnostic tests. For example, in some cultures women are not permitted to give permission to obtain their own diagnostic tests. Another person, perhaps the husband or a brother, is assigned to help the woman make these decisions or even to make them for her. This other person must be part of the decision-making process. Another example would be the patient in a third world country where health-care resources are scarce and treatment op-

Table 3-1
Factors that Affect Accuracy and Reliability of Diagnostic Tests

Sensitivity (True Positive)	Proportion of persons with the disease who test positive for the disease
Specificity (True Negative)	Proportion of persons without the disease who test negative for the disease
Positive Predictive Value	This is the proportion of persons who have tested positive who have the disease
Negative Predictive Value	This is the proportion of persons who tested negative and do not have the disease
Test Reliability	The ability for a diagnostic test to be reproducible. The ability to repeatedly obtain accurate results over time, reliability is positively correlated with positive predictive ability

Adapted from U.S. Preventive Services Task Force: *Report: guide to clinical preventive services*, ed 2, Media, Penn., 1996, Williams & Wilkins.

tions are limited. A diagnosis would do the person no good because the care needed, based on the diagnosis, is not available. A clinical example would be performing a test for detecting blood in the stool when there are no health-care resources available to treat a confirmed diagnosis of colorectal cancer.

The religious preference of the client is another variable to be considered when ordering diagnostic tests. Just as cultural variation needs to be considered in the decision-making process, so does the religious affiliation. One such example of religious influence on treatment would be the Jehovah's Witness prohibition on receiving blood or blood products. Such considerations are most important when deciding whether or not the outcome may lead to a conflict in treatment plans.

Genetics testing and its implications is an area of rapidly expanding importance. This is an area of tremendous technologic advance. For the most part, these test results are not unlike others in that they are often of a highly sensitive nature. Recognizing the need for genetics testing certainly falls under the purview of the practitioner. Results of genetic tests significantly impact the client and family as well as significant others. For example, a person known to carry the gene for Huntington's chorea might request genetic testing to see if he or she has the disease. But if the result is positive, the person has a 100% probability of getting the disease, as well as passing the gene on to offspring. This kind of case requires additional support services, such as a genetic counselor to help the client and family deal with the test results and their implications.

LABORATORY DATA

The decision to order laboratory data to "rule in" or "rule out" a specific diagnosis can be challenging from the perspective of what to order and what to do with the results that are obtained. Key variables to be factored into the equation of ordering laboratory tests include:

- Physical appearance of the client
- History of present illness and symptoms
- Chief complaint
- Vital signs
- Client age

- Clinical presentation of the client
- Associated clinical symptoms
- Existence of co-morbid conditions
- Current medications (including prescriptions, OTC, and botanicals-herbals)

The objectives when ordering diagnostic tests are to reduce morbidity and mortality, increase client well being, and achieve client satisfaction. The objectives for ordering diagnostic tests are listed in Box 3-1.

These objectives provide a guide for the laboratory work-up. One would always consider the sensitivity and specificity of each diagnostic test because these tests are not 100% accurate. Laboratory results must always be interpreted within the total clinical context, and we must recognize that diagnostic results may be fallible.

This chapter will present the most common laboratory tests used in primary care. For each diagnostic test there will be a brief discussion of basic pathophysiology, normal lab values, conditions that may cause abnormal lab values, and indications for use. A brief review of normal physiology is presented to help facilitate understanding of the significance of lab test results.

Box 3-1

Objectives for Ordering Diagnostic Tests

- To facilitate making a diagnosis in a client known to be sick
- To provide prognostic information for a person with a disease
- To identify an individual with sub-clinical disease or at risk for developing a disease
- To monitor ongoing therapy
- To reduce mortality and morbidity
- To improve client satisfaction
- To improve client sense of well-being

Adapted from Stoeckle JD: Principles of primary care. In Goroll A, May L, Mulley A, editors: *Primary care medicine: office evaluation and management of the adult patient*, ed 3, Philadelphia, 1995, JB Lippincott.

FLUID AND ELECTROLYTES

Description

In order to maintain homeostasis at the cellular level there must be balance in the structure and physiologic functioning of all body systems. Total body water consists of intracellular fluid (ICF) and extracellular fluid (ECF). Many processes at the cellular level influence the transport of water and nutrients between and within intracellular and extracellular fluid compartments. These processes involve passage of molecules through the cell membrane. This membrane is, by design, very discriminating about what it will allow to enter and exit the cell. This process is known as selective permeability. Selective permeability regulates the type and amount of fluid and solutes that will be allowed to enter and exit the cell membrane. This is a very dynamic operation, and balance between the intracellular and extracellular environments is critical in maintaining physiologic homeostasis.

SERUM OSMOLARITY

Serum osmolarity is the concentration of solute particles suspended in the plasma. There may be slight variations in plasma solute concentration without presenting an abnormal clinical picture. Serum osmolality is a measure of regulation of total body water and is normally 280 to 294 mOsm/kg. Serum osmolarity provides an assessment of hydration status and can be altered by a variety of disease states.

The balance between cellular intake and exchange of metabolic by-products occurs in a variety of ways. Some biological processes occur without energy expenditure, and others require energy sources to function at the cellular level. There are yet others that occur through voltage-gated channels that are highly specialized according to which ions need to enter or exit the cell. Chemical bonding of ions permits passage either directly or indirectly into voltage-gated channels, allowing balance to be maintained in the intracellular and extracellular environments. The major inorganic ions are Na^+, K^+, Ca^{++}, Cl^-, and HCO_3^-. In addition to the ions, there are uncharged organic compounds such as amino acids and sugars that require

specific transport mechanisms to move through the cell membrane. The movement of these solutes and fluids through the cell membrane requires energy sources.

Active mediated transport is one source of energy that facilitates movement of substances into and out of the cell. Active mediated transport provides a type of cellular communication involving movement of a protein transporter up a concentration gradient. This process requires energy. The energy source for active mediated transport comes primarily from cellular ATP (adenosine triphosphate). An example of this highly specialized transport would be the movement of Na^+ into the cell through voltage-gated sodium channels that are highly specialized for sodium transport only. Even a slight disruption in any component of this intricate process can lead to major electrolyte imbalances that manifest themselves in a variety of clinical presentations.

Passive mediated transport (also referred to in some texts as facilitated diffusion) is another mechanism of cellular communication important in maintaining balance of body fluids and solutes. Specific proteins passively carry the solute through the cell membrane without energy expenditure. An example of passive mediated transport is the movement of glucose molecules into red blood cells.

Some specialized receptors have a high affinity for the electrical charge of the substance to be transported. When there is alteration of either the receptor sites or the transport substances, there is a disruption of cellular balance that can result in abnormal physiologic conditions.

BLOOD COMPONENTS

Plasma, the liquid component of blood, consists of approximately 95% water. The solute portion of blood is made up of less than 1% solute. Solute is made up of 93% inorganic ions known as electrolytes, named so because of their electrical charges. The primary inorganic ions are Na^+, K^+, Cl^-, Ca^{++}, Mg^{++}, H^+, HCO_3^-, and phosphate.

Electrolytes have the ability to conduct electrical charges when dissolved in water. The positively charged ions are referred to as cations; negatively charged ions are called anions. It is the polarity of ions and their affinity for each other that allows passage and transport of nutrients and metabolic waste products into and out of the cell. The primary inorganic solutes help maintain homeostatic balance in the cellular environment. They keep water in the extracellular compartment, act as buffers, create membrane excitability in nerve and muscle cells, and participate in the coagulation process.

Proteins are another component of the blood plasma and constitute approximately 7% of total plasma weight. Serum proteins are albumins, globulins, and fibrinogen. The major function of plasma proteins is to provide nonpenetrating solutes that do not easily permeate cell membranes. Globulins act primarily as buffers and often bind through electrochemical affinity. They transport other plasma solutes such as hormones, lipids, vitamins, minerals, clotting factors, enzymes and their enzyme precursors, and antibodies across cell membranes. Globulins also play a key role in blood coagulation processes. Blood plasma also contains nutrients. These include glucose, carbohydrates, total amino acids, total lipids, cholesterol, individual vitamins, and individual trace elements.

Waste products are other solutes found in the serum plasma. These include: urea, obtained from protein metabolism; creatinine, from creatine metabolism; uric acid, from nucleic acid metabolism; and bilirubin, from hemoglobin breakdown.

PURPOSE OF OBTAINING SERUM OSMOLARITY AND ELECTROLYTES

Serum osmolarity and electrolyte tests are ordered to assess hydration status and to rule in/rule out a fluid or electrolyte imbalance. The practitioner should order serum osmolarity when there is severe disruption of body fluids resulting in cellular dehydration. Diabetic ketoacidosis is a classic instance in which it is important to evaluate serum osmolarity. Profuse diaphoresis may also potentiate the need for laboratory work-up in selected cases. Fluid losses are usually negligible, however, and not dramatic enough to warrant a laboratory work-up in a non-toxic, healthy appearing client. Table 3-2 lists the distribution of cations and anions in cellular compartments. Some common conditions that may warrant an electrolyte profile are listed on page 40.

Table 3-2
Distribution of Cations and Anions in Cellular Compartments

	Extracellular Fluid	Intracellular Fluid		Normal Range	
Cations			Adult	Newborn	Child
Na+	142 mEq/L	10 mEq/L	136-142 mEq/L	130-150 mEq/L	130-150 mEq/L
K+	5 mEq/L	156 mEq/L	3.8-5.0 mEq/L	<2 mos: 3.0-7.0	>12 mos: 3.5-5
Calcium	5 mEq/L	4 mEq/L	2.1-2.6 mEq/L	7d-2 yr: 1.6-2.6	2-14 yr: 1.5-2.3
Magnesium	2 mEq/L	26 mEq/L	1.25-1.75 mEq/L	1.5-1.8 mEq/L	1.5-1.8 mEq/L
Total	154 mEq/L	196 mEq/L			
Anions			Adults		
HCO_3^-	24 mEq/L	12 mEq/L	21-28 mEq/L		
HPO^2_4	2 mEq/L	40-95 mEq/L	0.5-1.25 mEq/L		
Proteins	16 mEq/L	54 mEq/L	64-83 mEq/L		
Total	42 mEq/L	106-161 mEq/L			
Other Negligible Anions	8 mEq/L	31 - 86 mEq/L			

Conditions indicating laboratory work-up for fluid and electrolyte disorders include the following:

- Suspected dehydration
- Prolonged vomiting or anorexia
- History of renal or electrolyte disorders
- Clients with cardiac history who are ill
- Suspected diabetes (particularly when acidosis is suspected)
- Intractable nausea, diarrhea, or vomiting in very young infants, children, diabetics, or the frail elderly
- Suspected differential diagnosis (possibly requiring a surgical intervention)
- Clients suspected of having acute bacterial illness
- Suspected heat exhaustion
- Clients suspected of having fluid volume overload
- Electrolyte profiles for baseline data during a routine physical examination
- Suspected drug toxicity
- Cardiac dysrhythmias
- Elderly presenting with history and symptoms indicating possible imbalance
- Very young children with acute severe illness

SODIUM

Sodium is the electrolyte that accounts for approximately 90% of extracellular cations. The normal range of extracellular Na^+ is approximately 14 times greater than the intracellular concentration. Na^+ moves in and out of the cell through highly specialized voltage-gated sodium channels via the process of active mediated transport. Any disruption in this transport process can result in a sodium imbalance.

Hyponatremia

Hyponatremia is a condition that results when serum sodium falls below 130 mEq/L. When this happens, in an effort to maintain serum osmolarity within normal limits, plasma water enters the cells. This produces cellular edema. Swelling of the cells of the central nervous system results in cerebral edema. Other clinical symptoms that can be evident are headache, peripheral edema, subnormal body temperature, tachycardia, hypotension, abdominal cramping, and nausea.

Depletion of serum sodium may be the result of a myriad of underlying causes. Possible causes of hyponatremia include the following:

- Renal disease
- Vomiting
- Diarrhea
- Cystic fibrosis
- Excessive diaphoresis
- Strenuous exercise
- Dilutional

Hypernatremia

Hypernatremia is the condition that results when serum sodium is greater than 150 mEq/L. Hypernatremia is most often the result of conditions that increase the loss of total body water, causing a hyperosmolar state. In an effort to maintain homeostasis, cells leak water into the plasma. This subsequently causes cells to shrink and can clinically present as irritability in the central nervous system, hypertension, temperature elevation, tachycardia, oliguria, anuria, and dry or flushed skin. Possible causes of hypernatremia include the following:

- Gastroenteritis
- Dehydration
- Decreased intake of free water
- Starvation
- Diabetes mellitus
- Coma
- Cirrhosis
- Cardiac failure
- Acute renal failure
- Chronic renal failure
- Nephrotic syndrome

POTASSIUM

K^+ is the major intracellular cation. The normal ranges for serum K^+ are 3.5 to 4.5 mEq/L. Potassium is essential for nerve excitability and the generation of action potentials. This activation allows for both cardiac and smooth muscle contractions. Potassium is primarily absorbed in the upper gastrointestinal tract and is exchanged for sodium in the lower bowel. Insulin and epinephrine increase cellular potassium uptake, and excretion is regulated primarily through the kidneys.

Hypokalemia

Hypokalemia results when the serum K^+ is less than 3.5 mEq/L. Most often a decreased potassium is the result of excessive loss through vomiting, gastric suction, or renal impairment. Very young children and the elderly are particularly vulnerable to potassium losses. Hypokalemia may be the result of a shift of extracellular potassium to the intracellular space in larger than normal amounts. Possible causes of hypokalemia include the following:

- Decreased intake
- Increased renal excretion
- Potassium-depleting diuretics
- Carbonic anhydrase inhibitors
- Defects in renal tubule
- Acid-base disorders
- Primary aldosteronism
- Thyrotoxicosis (rarely)
- Diabetic ketoacidosis
- Magnesium deficiency
- Mineralocorticoid excess
- Chronic metabolic alkalosis
- Antibiotics: gentamycin and amphotericin B
- Loss of potassium secondary to increased sodium conservation in the distal renal tubules

Clinical manifestations of hypokalemia can include changes in the electrocardiogram, particularly with respect to ventricular repolarization. Hypokalemia can result in many dysrhythmias, including but not limited to atrioventricular block, paroxysmal atrial tachycardia, and sinus bradycardia secondary to delays in ventricular repolarization. Other cardiac changes that can be seen on the ECG are a slightly peaked P wave, slightly prolonged P-R interval, S-T depression, a shallow T wave, and a prominent U wave. Alterations in myocardial conduction are related to the decreased action potential of myocardial cells and decreased myocardial membrane excitability. Other important clinical manifestations of hypokalemia may in-

clude weakness, particularly in large muscles of the extremities. In the extreme, hypokalemia could cause paralysis of the diaphragm with commensurate decrease in ventilatory effort. Hypokalemia can also result in loss of tone in smooth muscle throughout the body, including the gastrointestinal tract. This can be a cause of constipation, abdominal distention, or paralytic ileus. The hypokalemic client may also suffer from anorexia and nausea with or without emesis.

Hyperkalemia

A serum K^+ level greater than 5.5 mEq/L is considered hyperkalemia. Elevated serum potassium levels result primarily either from impaired renal excretion, excessive intake, or a shift of intracellular potassium to the extracellular space secondary to underlying pathology. Hyperkalemia can affect myocardial conduction. Examples of this effect on myocardial conduction can be evidenced by changes to the electrocardiogram. A wide, flat P wave; prolonged P-R interval; widened QRS; tall-peaked T waves; and a depressed S-T segment are all possible ECG abnormalities. Hyperkalemia can also present clinically as muscle cramping, diarrhea and abdominal cramping, and as generalized paresthesias. Possible causes of hyperkalemia include the following:

- Excess intake via parenteral routes
- Impaired renal function
- Acute or chronic renal failure
- Adrenal insufficiency
- Potassium-sparing diuretics
- Transcellular shifts
- Diabetic hyperglycemia
- Acidosis
- Beta-adrenergic blockade
- Digitalis toxicity
- Bactrim or ACE inhibitors

CHLORIDE

Chloride (Cl^-) is the most abundant extracellular anion. A normal range for serum chloride is 95 to 103 mmol/L. Chloride concentration is regulated secondary to sodium. When a sodium ion is reabsorbed in the renal tubules, either a chloride or a bicarbonate ion (HCO_3^-) is also reabsorbed. How much is absorbed is dependent on the acid/base balance of the extracellular fluid.

Chloride has four essential functions in the body: (1) to maintain osmolarity of the extracellular fluid; (2) to contribute to the acid/base balance; (3) to facilitate exchange of O_2 and CO_2 in red blood cells; and (4) as the major component of HCl in gastric juice.

Hypochloremia

Fluid volume depletion may result from several pathologic conditions and can cause hypochloremia. An example of this would be vomiting, because it decreases available chloride ions. This in turn produces an increased renal reabsorption of bicarbonate in the body's attempt to compensate and buffer the alkalotic state. The result is an increased excretion of hydrogen ions by the kidney and production of acidic urine (McCance, Huether 1998).

A low chloride can also result from use of diuretics such as thiazides, ethacrynic acid, and furosemide because these diuretics tend to produce a mildly alkalotic state in the body by increasing excretion of sodium, potassium, and chloride more than bicarbonate.

Hyperchloremia

An excess of chloride results in hyperchloremia. Hyperchloremia occurs most often with hypernatremia or with disease states that cause a metabolic acidosis. There are no specific symptoms that occur with excess chloride alone. High chloride levels are reflective of various underlying conditions that produce acidotic states.

MAGNESIUM

Magnesium is an important cofactor in many intracellular enzymatic reactions. Magnesium is particularly important in reactions involving protein synthesis, as a neurotransmitter, in myocardial conductivity, in muscle contractions, in receptor binding of neurohormones, in the functioning of voltage-gated channels, and in meeting energy demands at the cellular level (McCance and Huether, 1998).

Magnesium is located in bone and in intracellular spaces in the human body. Approximately 40% to 50% of magnesium is intracellular; the remaining portion is in bone storage. The normal serum magnesium level is 1.8 to 3.0 mg/dL. Between 1% and 2% of total body magnesium is present in extracellular fluid.

Hypomagnesemia

A serum magnesium less than 1.5 mEq/L results in hypomagnesemia. Hypomagnesemia manifests in symptoms including, but not limited to, neuromuscular irritability, tetany, tachycardia, seizures, and hypocalcemia and hypokalemia. The gastrointestinal tract and renal system help to maintain equilibrium in serum magnesium levels. Common causes of hypomagnesemia include the following:

- Alcoholism
- Renal tubular acidosis
- Diuretic therapy
- Hypercalcemia
- Hypoparathyroidism

Hypermagnesemia

Hypermagnesemia occurs when the serum level exceeds 2.5 mEq/L. Clinical manifestations of hypermagnesemia include, but are not limited to, depression of skeletal muscle activity, hypotension, bradycardia, palpitations, respiratory depression, and muscle weakness. Common causes of hypermagnesemia include the following:

- Phosphate-binding antacids (in persons with renal failure)
- Hypocalcemia
- Alcoholism
- Renal tubular acidosis

PHOSPHATE/PHOSPHORUS

Normal serum phosphate levels range from 2.5 to 4.5 mg/dl. Either phosphorus or phosphate levels may be reported by laboratories as phosphorus is one component of phosphate (Corbett, 2000). Phosphate is important in the formation and release of energy and is involved in enzymatic activities that occur at the cellular level. Phosphate is a primary inorganic solute dissolved in the plasma. Bone and intracellular fluid also contain phosphate. Serum phosphate is found as phospholipids, phosphate esters, and as the ionized form known as inorganic phosphate. Phosphate acts as a buffer in acid/base homeostasis in both intracellular and extracellular fluids. Phosphate transport is associated with glucose transport at the cellular level, and hyperglycemia will result in renal excretion of phosphorus in the urine. The kidneys are the primary regulators of serum phosphorus.

Phosphorus levels are closely aligned with serum calcium. The levels of calcium and phosphorus are carefully balanced by the interactions of parathormone (PTH), vitamin D, and calcitonin. These three hormones are responsible for the amount of phosphate and dietary calcium that are absorbed by the intestine. They also determine the absorption and deposition pattern of calcium and phosphate in bone, and regulate excretion of phosphate by the kidneys.

When conditions of hypercalcemia exist (i.e., levels above 10 mg/dL), patients will have low levels of serum phosphate (less than 2.5 mg/dL) or hypophosphatemia. Conversely, when hypocalcemia is present (less than 8.5 mg/dL), patients become hyperphosphatemic with levels of serum phosphate greater than 4.5 mg/dL.

Most phosphate is located intracellularly, and diseases that cause cellular destruction can result in a hyperphosphatemic state. A prime example of this is the excessive cell destruction that occurs as a result of systemic chemotherapy. When the cell membranes are disrupted by chemotaxis, an excessive amount of phosphate is released into the extracellular space.

Hypophosphatemia

A phosphorus level less than 2.5 mg/dl results in hypophosphatemia. Clients with low phosphate levels will develop signs and symptoms of hypercalcemia. Signs and symptoms of hypophosphatemia may include encephalopathy, irritability, confusion, paresthesias, seizures, coma, and electrocardiographic changes. Causes of hypophosphatemia include the following:

- Receiving total parenteral nutrition
- Prematurity in infants
- Low-birth-weight in babies
- Starvation syndromes
- Malabsorption syndromes
- Post-diabetic ketoacidosis
- Administration of corticosteroids
- Hyperparathyroidism
- Renal tubular defects
- Post-diuretic administration

Hyperphosphatemia

Normal phosphate levels can be as high as 6.0 to 7.0 mg/dl in infants and young children. Hyperphosphatemia occurs when serum phosphate levels exceed 4.5 mg/dl in adults. Possible causes of hyperphosphatemia include the following:

- Renal disease causing impaired excretion or glomerular filtration
- Bowel surgery with loss of jejunum
- Excess intake of aluminum hydroxide and carbonate in the bowel
- Hypoparathyroidism
- Excess administration of phosphate via oral or intravenous routes
- Administration of phosphate-containing enemas
- Administration of cytotoxic drugs

CALCIUM

The normal range for serum Ca^{++} is 8.6 to 10.5 mg/dl. Calcium is the major extracellular cation that helps promote and regulate neuromuscular and enzymatic activity, skeletal development, and blood coagulation processes. Primarily the bone, gastrointestinal tract, and kidneys regulate serum calcium levels. Calcium homeostasis occurs when there is a balance in the calcium absorbed via the gastrointestinal tract, the calcium excreted by the kidneys, and the distribution of calcium in bone and the extracellular compartments.

Hypocalcemia

Hypocalcemia results when the serum calcium level is less than 8.5 mg/dl. These clients can present with an increase in neuromuscular activity. Symptoms of hypocalcemia may include skeletal muscle cramping, hypocalcemic tetany, and laryngospasm (which can lead to asphyxiation and airway compromise). Electrocardiographic changes may include a prolonged Q-T interval secondary to prolonged ventricular repolarization and decreased myocardial contractility. The client may experience abdominal cramping and have hyperactive bowel sounds. Hypocalcemia may be a challenge to assess in the elderly who have an altered base line mental status, or in very young clients who cannot present an adequate history. This makes review of systems all the more important. Causes of hypocalcemia include the following:

- Insufficient dietary intake of vitamin D
- Decreased exposure to sunlight
- Removal of parathyroid glands, resulting in hypoparathyroidism
- Malabsorption of fat
- Low ionized calcium levels
- Abnormal metabolism of calcium
- Hyperphosphatemia
- Magnesium deficiency
- Acute pancreatitis

Hypocalcemia may result in severe gastrointestinal fluid losses. It can be very severe in the very young pediatric and frail elderly populations when individuals experience excessive diarrhea or vomiting. These patients may have decreased compensatory abilities and suffer extreme fluid and electrolyte loss in addition to calcium losses.

Hypercalcemia

An excess of calcium (greater than 12 mg/dL) results in hypercalcemia. Hypercalcemia is produced by an excess calcium influx into the extracellular fluid from the bone and a decrease efflux from the kidneys to the urine. Causes of hypercalcemia include the following:

- Parathyroid tumors
- Prostate cancer
- Breast cancer
- Cervical cancer
- Sarcoidosis

- Renal impairment
- Excess vitamin D intake
- Hyperparathyroidism
- Hyperthyroidism
- Immobilization
- Use of thiazide diuretics

Symptoms associated with serum hypercalcemia reflect the loss of cell membrane excitability. The cell membrane loses its ability to become refractory during depolarization, resulting in a hyperpolarized state and the decrease of cell membrane excitability. Commonly the symptoms will include lethargy, confusion, fatigue, nausea, constipation, anorexia, and generalized weakness. More specifically, clients with hypercalcemia can exhibit symptoms of decreased neuromuscular excitability (hyporeflexia), and in very young or elderly clients this may not be easily assessed. Clients with hypercalcemia may also exhibit signs of central nervous system depression; be at increased risk of spontaneous clinical bone fractures; experience vomiting, constipation, or renal calculi; and have high potential for cardiac dysrhythmias. These diagnoses are due primarily to the alteration in permeability of calcium ion channels in the cell membrane.

COMPLETE BLOOD COUNT (CBC)

Blood consists of plasma, blood cells, and platelets. The plasma is the liquid portion of the blood and is about 90% water. The solid constituents include white blood cells (WBCs), erythrocytes or red blood cells (RBCs), and platelets. Platelets are cell fragments that are derived from bone marrow-bound cells. At any given time, about a third of the body's platelets are in storage in the spleen, and are released into the blood as needed.

When Should a Complete Blood Count Be Ordered?

It is important to order a CBC when the client presents with acutely ill appearance. Client symptoms that warrant a CBC include a fever, intractable nausea or vomiting, abdominal pain, an infant less than 3 months with febrile state (in a very young infant this can be 100.5° F), a cough with febrile state, or a client of any age who appears to have either a viral or bacterial infection. Pneumonia is one of the most frequently occurring illnesses in the elderly and there may not be a high-grade fever associated with it.

In examining a client with acute abdominal pain and suspected appendicitis, there is the potential for a missed diagnosis if the clinician relies solely on the laboratory tests. Colucciello, Lukens, and Morgan (1999) reported that 10% to 60% of patients with appendicitis confirmed by surgery had a WBC that was within normal range. An elevated WBC, particularly with a left shift in neutrophils, is usually indicative of significant disease (Hamilton, Ruo, Wagner, 1998). In a client with abdominal pain, this is more than likely a perforated appendix or peritonitis. The WBC does provide useful information when surgical differential diagnoses are being considered in the client work-up; however it is equally important to note that the WBC should not be the critical piece of information in determining the client's plan of care. The WBCs are influenced by several factors including recent injections, seizures, and falls or other trauma. The WBC may lack sensitivity and specificity for abdominal presentations.

A CBC can be ordered with or without a differential and some laboratories will automatically perform the differential. Still other laboratories will perform a differential only if requested. When the white blood cell count is elevated, some laboratories will perform a manual differential.

Conditions warranting a complete blood count include the following:

- Unexplained, prolonged fatigue
- Hematochezia
- Hematemesis
- Hemoptysis
- Intractable abdominal pain
- Febrile state
- Fever or suspected septicemia in infant less than 3 months of age
- Suspected pneumonia in toxic-appearing client
- Acute abdominal pain
- Tachypnea
- Dyspnea
- Tachycardia
- Suspected cardiac disease
- Suspected anemia
- Suspected appendicitis

WHITE BLOOD CELLS (WBCS)

White blood cells are referred to as leukocytes and are divided into two groups, granulocytes and agranulocytes. Polymorphonuclear granulocytes include three types of leukocytes: neutrophils, eosinophils, and basophils. These cell types are named for their affinities for a particular color of laboratory dye. Eosinophils have an affinity for red dye; basophils have an affinity for blue dye; and neutrophils have little affinity for either dye. Leukocytes are located in the plasma but leave the blood stream to enter tissues. Neutrophils, basophils, and eosinophils are all phagocytes. Granulocytes contain many membrane-bound granules with enzymes that are capable of destroying microorganisms and digesting cellular debris. These same granules, located on the membranes, contain biochemical mediators that are important in immune and antiinflammatory responses. WBCs that do not contain granulocytes are called agranulocytes. These include monocytes and lymphocytes. Monocytes are transformed into macrophages and lymphocytes are transformed into plasma cells (B lymphocytes or T lymphocytes) that are responsible for cell-mediated immunity (McCance, Huether 1998).

Neutrophils

The most abundant type of granulocyte is the neutrophil. Neutrophils are also referred to as polymorphonuclear neutrophils (PMNs). They are the most numerous of white blood cells and make up approximately 55% of the WBC count in an adult. Most of the circulating neutrophils are of the mature form, having a segmented nucleus, and it is in this way that the laboratories identify them. Laboratories and clinicians sometimes refer to neutrophils as "segs" or segmented neutrophils. In contrast, the nucleus of the immature neutrophil does not appear in segments, but rather in bands. The term "bands" is derived from the microscopic appearance of the immature nucleus. (Some texts and references refer to the bands as "stabs," which is the German word for "rod.")

Neutrophils migrate from capillaries into tissue sites soon after an injury or invasion occurs. In the cellular space, neutrophils begin to phagocytize and digest microorganisms and other debris. After digesting microorganisms and debris, the neutrophils release potent digestive enzymes from the membranous granules. It is the release of these enzymes into the tissue that prepares the tissue for healing. Neutrophils only live 1 to 2 days.

Eosinophils Eosinophils make up only 1% to 4% of the total WBC count. Eosinophils are instrumental in control of inflammatory responses and in the response to invasive parasites. Eosinophils ingest antigen-antibody complexes in inflammatory responses. Clinical conditions in which the eosinophil counts would be higher than normal include an allergic response to an allergen and an intestinal parasite manifestation.

Basophils

Basophils make up 0.75% or less of the total leukocytes in an adult. Basophils are segmented polymorphonuclear granulocytes. Basophilia is associated with allergic reactions and mechanical irritations. The lifespan of basophils is not known. Basophils have cytoplasmic granules that contain histamine, bradykinin, serotonin, and heparin. The exact mechanisms of basophilic action are still not completely understood.

Agranulocytes

Agranulocyte is the name given to monocytes, macrophages, and lymphocytes. Unlike granulocytes, agranulocytes do not contain lysosomal enzymes for breaking down and digesting cellular invaders. These lymphocytes aid in bodily defense through activity at the cellular level. Monocytes are a type of leukocyte that is larger than a granulocyte, with a "horseshoe-shaped" nucleus and few cytoplasmic granules. Monocytes are immature macrophages. Formed in the bone marrow, monocytes circulate in the blood stream for approximately 36 hours. After this initial circulation, the monocytes mature into macrophages. Macrophages migrate predominantly to lymphoid tissues in the liver, spleen, lymph nodes, peritoneum, and gastrointestinal tract. In these specific body tissues, macrophages remain in an active state for months or years. Monocytes and macrophages contain large vacuoles that are used to ingest cellular invaders. Monocytes and macrophages are responsible for aiding in immune and inflammatory responses through a process known as phagocytosis.

Lymphocytes

The final type of leukocyte is the lymphocyte. Lymphocytes account for about 36% of the total leukocytes. Leukocytes are primarily responsible for the body's immune response. Lymphocytes are a type of leukocyte that contains a large nucleus and a scant amount of cytoplasm. Lymphocytes are the cells that create cellular immunity. There are many types of lymphocytes present in the body. The major ones are the T cells, B cells, and mature B cells (otherwise referred to as plasma cells). The lifespan of lymphocytes is quite varied. Lymphocytes may live for days, months, or years, depending on the specific cell type and function.

WBC Count: Normal Lab Values

When a white blood cell count is requested, it is important to note that the report includes the total number of cells and the percentage of each type of WBC. The total WBC is usually 5,000 to 10,000 leukocytes/mm^3 of blood. The differential (percentage of each of the cell types) consists of the proportion of the five types of leukocytes in a sample of 100 white blood cells. Absolute numbers of cell types may change, but the total number in the differential must always equal 100%. An elevation of immature neutrophils is referred to as "a left shift," and usually indicates a bacterial infectious process. A WBC count greater than 10,000 with a left shift (neutrophil percentage greater than 75% of the differential) is usually considered abnormal (Table 3-3, Box 3-2).

Erythrocytes

The main function of erythrocytes is to transport oxygen in the blood. The bi-concave shape of this cell allows it great flexibility to move through macrocirculation and allows maximum diffusion of

Table 3-3
Normal Ranges for WBC Differential

	Total (WBC/mm^3)	Percentage
Adult Male/Female	4300 – 10,000	
Bands/Stabs (Immature Neutrophils)		3%-5%
Granulocytes (Polymorphonuclears)		
Neutrophils (Segs)		51%-67%
Eosinophils		1%-4%
Basophils		0%-1%
Agranular Leukocytes		
Lymphocytes		25%-33%
Monocytes		2%-6%
Total Percentage of Differential		100%

Box 3-2

Normal Variants for WBC Differential

Smokers tend to have higher total WBCs.

Pregnancy tends to produce leukocytosis and counts may be up to 16,000/mm^3. This is mostly due to an increase in neutrophils with a slight increase in lymphocytes.

Newborns on the day of birth can have WBC counts of 18,000 to 40,000/mm^3, but these counts will drop to the adult levels in approximately 14 days. Wider ranges in differential values will decrease and move toward normal adult levels as time passes after birth.

Children will have more lymphocytes than neutrophils until age 5 to 8 years. A normal WBC count can be 14,500/mm^3, depending on age. Laboratories will have relative values for the differential at various ages.

Elderly persons may have decreased WBC counts due to the aging process.

gases into and out of the cells. The most important feature of an erythrocyte is that it contains hemoglobin. Hemoglobin has an affinity for oxygen, acts as a buffer, and helps transport carbon dioxide. Erythrocytes only survive about 120 days and require replacement. The generation of new RBCs is called erythropoiesis. Normal erythrocyte values are calculated as the number of red blood cells/mm^3 (Table 3-4).

Hemoglobin and Hematocrit

Hemoglobin is the most important feature of the erythrocyte or RBC. To maximize its hemoglobin content, a single erythrocyte contains several hundred million hemoglobin molecules to the exclusion of almost everything else. Normal adult hemoglobin levels are 16 g/dL for men and 14 g/dL for women (Table 3-5). The percentage of erythrocytes in a specified volume of blood is called the hematocrit. The hematocrit is obtained after centrifuging the blood. The hematocrit of "packed cell volume" essentially represents the percentage of total blood volume occupied by erythrocytes. The normal hematocrit is about 45% for men and about 42% for women (Table 3-6). (These figures are calculated based on a person with a weight of 70 kilograms and approximately 5.5 liters of circulating blood volume.)

Reticulocytes

Reticulocytes are produced in the bone marrow and have a web-like appearance for which they were named (from the Latin *re' te*, meaning "net"). Reticulocytes are immature red blood cells and their count helps in the differential diagnosis of anemia. A normal reticulocyte count (percentage of the total RBC count) is 0.5% to 1.5% for adults (Table 3-7). The reticulocyte count will have normal variations in certain clients. For example, there is a slight increase during pregnancy, and the count will be increased 3% to 5% in newborns during the first week of life. The reticulocyte count also increases in hemolytic anemia, hemoglobinopathies, sickle cell anemia, 3 to 4 days after a hemorrhage,

Table 3-4
Normal Erythrocyte Values

Red Blood Cells (RBC)		SI Units
Adult females	4.0–5.5 million/μl	$4.0–5.5 \times 10^{12}$/L
Pregnant		
Trimester 1	4.0–5.0 million/μl	$4.0–5.0 \times 10^{12}$/L
Trimester 2	3.2–4.5 million /μl	$3.2–4.5 \times 10^{12}$/L
Trimester 3	3.0–4.9 million/μl	$3.0–4.9 \times 10^{12}$/L
Postpartum	3.2–5.0 million/μl	$3.2–5.0 \times 10^{12}$/L
Adult males	4.5–6.2 million/μl	$4.5–6.2 \times 10^{12}$/L
Children		
Newborn		
Day 1	4.1–6.1 million/μl	$4.1–6.1 \times 10^{12}$/L
Days 2–8	5.1 million/μl	5.1×10^{12}/L
Days 9–13	5.0 million/μl	5.0×10^{12}/L
2–8 weeks	3.8–5.6 million/μl	$3.8–5.6 \times 10^{12}$/L
3–5 months	3.8–5.2 million/μl	$3.8–5.2 \times 10^{12}$/L
6–11 months	4.6 million/μl	4.6×10^{12}/L
1–2 years	3.6–5.5 million/μl	$3.6–5.5 \times 10^{12}$/L
3 years	4.5 million/μl	4.5×10^{12}/L
4 years	4.0–5.2 million/μl	$4.0–5.2 \times 10^{12}$/L

Taken from Chernecky CC, Berger BJ: *Laboratory tests and diagnostic procedures,* ed 2, Philadelphia, 1997, WB Saunders.

Table 3-5
Hemoglobin (Hb, Hgb), Blood

		SI Units
Females	12–15 g/dl	7.1–9.9 mmol/L
Pregnant	10–15 g/dl	6.3–9.3 mmol/L
Males	14–16.5 g/dl	8.7–11.2 mmol/L
Children		
Neonates	14–27 g/dl	9.6–15.5 mmol/L
3 months	10–17 g/dl	6.1–9.6 mmol/L
1–2 years	9–15 g/dl	5.6–9.0 mmol/L
6–10 years	11–16g/dl	5.8–9.6 mmol/L
Panic levels	<5 g/dl	<3.1 mmol/L
	>20 g/dl	>11.2 mmol/L

Taken from Chernecky CC, Berger BJ: *Laboratory tests and diagnostic procedures,* ed 2, Philadelphia, 1997, WB Saunders.

Table 3-6
Hematocrit (HCT), Blood

		SI Units
Females		
Adult	35%–47%	0.35–0.47
Pregnant	30%–46%	0.30–0.46
Adult males	42%–52%	0.42–0.52
Neonates	42%–68%	0.42–0.68
3 months	29%–54%	0.29–0.54
Children		
1–2 years	35%–44%	0.35–0.44
6–10 years	31%–43%	0.31–0.43
Panic levels	<15% or >60%	<0.15 or >0.60

Taken from Chernecky CC, Berger BJ: *Laboratory tests and diagnostic procedures,* ed 2, Philadelphia, 1997, WB Saunders.

after increased RBC destruction, and after treatment of anemias. The reticulocyte count decreases in cases of iron deficiency, aplastic and untreated pernicious anemias, chronic infection, radiation therapy and exposure, marrow tumors, endocrine disorders and myelodysplastic syndromes.

Immature reticulocytes are found in the bone marrow until they become mature erythrocytes. The reticulocyte count is of clinical significance in conditions that may involve impairment of red blood cell production. Conditions that indicate a need for the reticulocyte count include:

Table 3-7
Reticulocyte Count, Blood

Norm: Comprises 1%–2% of the total RBC count		SI Units
Adult females	0.5%–2.5%	$0.005–0.025 \times 10^{-3}$
Adult males	0.5%–1.5%	$0.005–0.015 \times 10^{-3}$
Cord blood	3.0%–7.0%	$0.030–0.070 \times 10^{-3}$
Newborn	1.1%–4.5%	$0.011–0.045 \times 10^{-3}$
Neonates	0.1%–1.5%	$0.010–0.015 \times 10^{-3}$
Infants	0.5%–3.1%	$0.005–0.031 \times 10^{-3}$
Children >6 months	0.5%–4.0%	$0.005–0.040 \times 10^{-3}$

Taken from Chernecky CC, Berger BJ: *Laboratory tests and diagnostic procedures,* ed 2, Philadelphia, 1997, WB Saunders.

- Clients undergoing chemotherapy who have suppression of all blood cell lines including erythrocytes
- Differential diagnosis of anemia
- Impaired renal function producing a decrease in RBCs

Disorders of RBCs

An elevated RBC count is called polycythemia or erythrocytosis. Polycythemia vera (PV) is a myeloproliferative disorder in which there are excessive numbers of erythrocytes. Not only are there abnormal numbers of circulating erythrocytes, but it also appears that there is myeloproliferation of all cells including RBCs, WBCs, and platelets. There can be increases in RBCs that are not pathologic, such as that which occurs at higher altitudes or with rigorous physical training. Bone marrow will increase production of RBCs to accommodate the demands for increased need for oxygenation under these circumstances. This is a nonpathologic state and requires no treatment.

Decreased numbers of erythrocytes result in anemia. The actual term "anemia" can mean either a decrease in the number of RBCs, a decrease in the hemoglobin level of RBCs, or a decrease in both. A decrease in RBCs can result from abnormal loss of blood, from atypical destruction of RBCs, from impairment or deficiency in the critical elements needed to produce erythrocytes, or due to the suppression of bone marrow.

The diagnosis of anemia is based on the hemoglobin and hematocrit values. The evaluation of a client suspected to have anemia would include a thorough client history, physical assessment, CBC, and peripheral blood smear (to determine the size of the RBCs), and a reticulocyte count. Also useful in diagnosis are tests to determine the client's iron, ferritin, vitamin B_{12}, and folate values.

Erythrocyte size and shape are important in making the diagnosis of anemia. Erythrocyte size, shape, and hemoglobin-carrying capacity are determined by the hemoglobin, hematocrit, erythrocyte count, mean corpuscular volume (MCV), mean corpuscular hemoglobin (MCH), and mean corpuscular hemoglobin concentration (MCHC). In most laboratory settings these values are integral to the CBC.

Mean Corpuscular Volume (MCV)   The mean corpuscular volume is the arithmetic mean or average of an individual red blood cell denoted in cubic microns (μm^3). The normal MCV is 86 to 98 μm^3.

When the MCV is less than 86 μm^3, the erythrocytes are considered to be microcytic. Microcytic erythrocytes are present in iron deficiency anemia, lead intoxication, and chronic inflammation. Thalassemia major and thalassemia minor are also conditions that result in microcytic anemia and that affect the hemoglobin concentration of the RBCs.

An MCV that exceeds 98 μm^3 results in a macrocytic erythrocyte. Clinical examples of macrocytic anemias are seen in pernicious and folic acid deficiency anemias, anemia of pregnancy, hemolytic and aplastic anemias, inflammation, liver disease, alcohol intoxication, and following a total gastrectomy. An anemia that occurs with an erythrocyte of normocytic shape is blood loss anemia. In blood loss, the erythrocytes are of normal shape and hemoglobin-carrying capacity, but the number of them has decreased.

Mean Corpuscular Hemoglobin (MCH)   MCH is the amount of hemoglobin present in one erythrocyte. This weight is recorded in picograms (pg). The normal MCH ranges from 27 to 32 pg per single erythrocyte. Hyperlipidemia and high heparin concentrations falsely elevate MCH. WBC counts of greater than 50,000 falsely elevate Hgb values and also falsely elevate MCH values.

Mean Corpuscular Hemoglobin Concentration (MCHC)

The MCHC represents the percentage of hemoglobin that occupies one erythrocyte. The normal range of MCHC is 31% to 38%. An MCHC less than 30% indicates that the erythrocytes have a decreased hemoglobin concentration and are "hypochromic." An example of the most common type of hypochromic anemia is iron deficiency anemia. Chronic blood loss anemia and thalassemia also result in low MCHC values. Hyperchromic refers to erythrocytes that have excessive coloration. Usually erythrocytes can hold a limited capacity of hemoglobin, so MCHC levels that are high indicate spherocytosis. MCHC is usually decreased in pernicious anemia (Tierney, McPhee, and Papadakis, 2000) (Table 3-8).

Red Blood Cell Distribution Width (RDW)

The RDW is a useful laboratory parameter that assists in determining variation in the actual width of one erythrocyte. It also helps to determine the differential diagnosis of anemia. For example, in anemia of chronic disease, there is low-normal MCV with a normal RDW, whereas in early iron deficiency anemia, there is low-normal MCV and elevated RDW (Fischbach, 2000). The normal range for the RDW is 11.5% to 14.5%.

Vitamin B_{12} and Folate

The measurement of vitamin B_{12} and folate in the serum is important information to obtain if initial laboratory tests reveal an elevated MCV and a low reticulocyte count. Vitamin B_{12} and folate levels are used to make the definitive diagnosis of macrocytic anemia due to dietary deficiency or with malabsorption. The normal vitamin B_{12} level is 205 to 876 pg/ml. A value from 140 to 204 pg/ml is a borderline result. Results can also vary in the elderly, who may have lower values due to less absorption in the aging gut.

Normal folic acid levels should be greater than 3.3 ng/ml. A value between 2.5 and 3.2 ng/ml is borderline. Again, aged persons may have lower folic acid levels due to decreased gastric absorption.

Serum Iron

The serum iron level (Fe) is a direct reflection of the amount of serum iron present in the body (Table 3-9). The client should not take any iron supplements for 24 hours preceding the test. There is also a diurnal variation in serum iron levels, which may be as much as 10 times higher in the evening (Fischbach, 2000). Serum iron levels should therefore be drawn in the morning.

Serum Ferritin

Serum ferritin levels reflect the amount of iron stored in the body and is a reliable indicator of total body iron (Fischbach, 2000). A decreased ferritin of less than 10 ng/ml is associated with iron-deficiency anemia. Elevated levels of ferritin that are greater than 400 ng/ml indicate iron excess and may be due to hemochromatosis, hemosiderosis, iron administration, liver disease, malignancies,

Table 3-8
Classification of Anemias

Cell Classification	Type of Anemia	Laboratory Findings
Normochromic, normocytic	Acute blood loss	Normal MCV, MCH, MCHC
Microcytic, hypochromic	Iron deficiency	Decreased MCV, MCH, MCHC
Macrocytic	Vitamin B_{12} deficiency	Increased MCV, variable MCH
	Folic acid deficiency	and MCHC

Table 3-9
Normal Values of Serum Iron, Ferritin, TIBC, and Transferrin Saturation

Test	Normal Range
Serum iron	50-150 µg/dl
Serum ferritin	20-400 ng/ml
Total iron-binding capacity (TIBC)	250-410 µg/dl
Transferrin saturation	20%-50%

hyperthyroidism, or thalassemia. A serum ferritin level is a very inexpensive diagnostic test used in detecting iron deficiency anemia and is excellent in distinguishing between simple iron dficiency anemia and anemia of chronic disease (Barkin, Green, Johnson et al, 1998).

Total Iron-Binding Capacity

Total iron-binding capacity (TIBC) is the availability of iron to bind with erythrocytes. It increases in iron deficiency anemia, with use of oral contraceptives, during pregnancy, with blood loss, and in acute liver damage.

Transferrin

Transferrin saturation is an indirect calculation of serum iron. It is derived from mathematical calculation of the total iron binding capacity and serum iron levels. The formula is

$$\frac{Serum\ iron}{TIBC} \times 100\% = \%\ transferrin\ saturation$$

Platelets

Platelets are a blood component comprised of cell fragments from larger cells known as megakaryocytes. Platelets do not have a cell nucleus, do not contain DNA, and therefore cannot replicate. Platelets do contain cytoplasmic granules, which carry biochemical mediators that assist in hemostasis. A normal circulating platelet volume is 140,000 to 340,000 platelets/mm^3. Normal variants in platelet counts are seen under the following conditions:

- In females during the first few days of menses (increased)
- Immediately after labor and delivery (usually increased)
- In newborns (decreased)

Thrombocytopenia

Low platelet counts (below 100,000 platelets/mm^3) are termed thrombocytopenia. Clients with platelet counts of 50,000 platelets/mm^3 or less are at increased risk of bleeding from minor trauma. Those at greatest risk of spontaneous hemorrhage—such as petechiae, frank spontaneous bleeding from gums, ecchymotic areas on the skin, purpura, ecchymosis or spontaneous bleeding from mucous membranes—are those whose platelet counts are between 10,000 and 15,000 platelets/mm^3. These clients require emergency attention and usually in-patient admission. A platelet count of less than 10,000/mm^3 indicates the presence of a life-threatening condition.

Platelets are formed in the bone marrow and removed from the body by the spleen. Platelets aggregate in the vessel on the wall and begin the coagulation process. Among the causes of thrombocytopenia are medications that interfere with platelets and impede the coagulation process. One such medication that is commonly prescribed is Bactrim, a sulfa preparation.

Thrombocytosis

Thrombocytosis results when platelet counts are greater than 400,000 platelets/mm^3. In this instance, the client is at increased risk of excessive blood coagulation. A person with a high platelet count usually is asymptomatic until values reach 400,000 platelets/mm^3. Situations that produce transient thrombocythemia include but are not limited to infectious processes, trauma, stress, exercise, and ovulation. There are two types of abnormal thrombocythemia referred to in some texts: (1) primary thrombocythemia and (2) secondary thrombocythemia (also referred to as reactive thrombocythemia). Primary thrombocythemia is the result of a myeloproliferative disorder in which platelet production exceeds 600,000 platelets/mm^3. These individuals have hyperplasia of megakaryocytes and often clinically manifest with hypersplenism and/or episodes of hemorrhage or thrombosis. There has to date been no clear identification of the exact cause of primary thrombocythemia. Clients with primary thrombocythemia can be asymptomatic, and the finding may be incidentally noted on a routine CBC. Secondary (or reactive) thrombocythemia is often caused by malignancy of the lung, stomach, and colon, and it can also manifest in clients who have undergone splenectomy.

The lifespan of platelets is approximately 10 days. There are many variables that can influence production of platelets. Pathological conditions underlying severe platelet dysfunction include but are not limited to myeloproliferative disorders, leukemias, dysproteinemias, and myelodysplastic pathology.

RENAL FUNCTION: BUN AND CREATININE

The measurement of serum blood urea nitrogen (BUN) and creatinine levels is an assessment of renal function. Urea is the end product of the body's protein metabolism. It is formed in the liver and is circulated to the kidneys for excretion in the urine. The serum BUN provides a value that indicates glomerular function. The kidney excretes approximately 50% of urea, and the remaining 50% is recycled. The normal adult BUN is 8 to 25 mg/dl. There may be a slight variance in serum BUN levels between the sexes, with men having slightly higher levels than women. Other factors that can cause normal increases in BUN are late pregnancy, advanced age (elderly clients may have a decrease in their glomerular filtration rate), and many drugs. Decreases in BUN occur in low-protein, high-carbohydrate diets; persons with smaller muscle mass; early pregnancy; and with many drugs. It is essential to know whether or not a client has a history of elevated BUN and creatinine or if this is a new finding. This data will have a significant impact on the treatment plan, and the importance of renal function cannot be overestimated.

A baseline BUN and creatinine should be documented so that therapies that may have an impact on renal functioning can be accurately assessed. For example, a baseline BUN and creatinine level should be obtained prior to administering an aminoglycoside, or prior to intravenous injection of contrast media (given in certain imaging studies, such as the intravenous pyelogram). Diabetic clients are more prone to renal impairment and are at higher risk of developing renal failure. Renal function may need to be monitored more closely in high-risk client populations. Impaired functioning may delay renal excretion of commonly prescribed medications (including but not limited to Demerol, phenothiazines, and digoxin). BUN and creatinine also can be elevated with prolonged use of lipid-lowering drugs. Clinical indicators of an elevated BUN include the following:

- Dehydration
- Decreased renal blood flow
- Clients receiving tube feedings
- Gastrointestinal bleeding

The level of serum creatinine is changed only by alterations in renal functioning. Renal function is reflected by the BUN/creatinine ratio. In the case of gastrointestinal bleeding, the BUN will reflect a marked elevation, whereas the creatinine will remain within normal limits. This is because the kidneys are functioning normally, but there is an elevated level of protein being filtered through the kidneys. Clinical examples of a decrease in the BUN/creatinine ratio would include decreased protein intake, overhydration, and clients experiencing liver failure. In these persons the BUN is decreased but not the creatinine. An elevated creatinine level occurs when there is damage to a large number of nephrons in the kidney.

BUN/creatinine ratios range from $1:6$ to $1:20$ with the mean usually $1:10$. In renal failure both BUN and creatinine will be elevated. Clients with renal insufficiency, such as those with diabetes mellitus, will often have mildly elevated BUN on baseline.

URINALYSIS

A routine urinalysis (UA) is one of the most frequently ordered laboratory tests in both routine physical examinations as well as in establishing differential diagnoses. It is a good screening test that is indicative of a person's overall state of health, as well as the health of the urinary tract. A dip urinalysis is very easily performed in the office and can reveal a wealth of information. A typical urinalysis looks for color, clarity, pH, specific gravity, odor, glucose, ketones, protein, nitrates, bacteria, and leukocytes.

Normal urine pH is 4.5 to 8.0 (the average person's urine has a pH of 5 to 6). A low urine pH can be caused by certain foods, emphysema, pyrexia, and starvation. A high urine pH could indicate bacteriuria, chronic renal failure, respiratory disease with loss of CO_2, or salicylate intoxication. Some antibiotics cause elevated urine pH. Dark yellow to amber urine could indicate bilirubin, could be caused by drugs such as chlorpromazine (Thorazine) and nitrofurantoin (Macrobid, Macrodantin), by excess riboflavin, or by eating too many carrots. Orange urine can be caused by bile pigment, rifampin, some oral anticoagulants, or the drugs phenazopyridine (Pyridium) and sulfasalazine (Azulfidine). Cloudy urine may indicate the presence of pus, red blood cells, or bacteria, or may be normal. Urine glucose is usually negative, as are ketones, proteins, and nitrates. False negative results can be obtained when patients have been taking vitamin C, levodopa, or salicylates. Positive urine glucose usually occurs in patients who do not have their diabetes under good control and "spill" sugar into the urine. Ketones may be present in alcoholism, diabetes mellitus, eclampsia, and ketoacidosis. Transient proteinuria can occur with dehydration, with excessive protein in the diet, emotional stress, exposure to cold, strenuous exercise, fever, post-hemorrhage, and with sodium depletion. Proteinuria may have more serious implications and requires a full urine work-up. However, it might be wise to repeat the dip UA before incurring the expense of a 24-hour urine collection. There are other categories of disease that can be prerenal, renal, glomerular, interstitial, tubular, and postrenal; and a number of drugs that cause proteinuria. Nitrates in the urine are indicative of bacteriuria. A routine urinalysis should be obtained on any client who complains of pain or burning with urination, flank pain, abdominal pain, fever, chills, nausea, vomiting, diarrhea, or visible blood in the urine. Elderly clients who have a history of chronic urinary tract infections should have a urinalysis when they are symptomatic and at the completion of antibiotic therapy for a urinary tract infection. In the case of a bacterial urinary tract infection, as evidence in the microscopic report, a urine culture should be obtained. It is preferable to obtain the culture and sensitivity prior to the initiation of antibiotic therapy, but the client's presentation may warrant starting therapy before the C&S results are obtained.

RBCs in the Urine

A microscopic examination of the urine should be requested if any of the routine values are elevated. For example, hematuria is the presence of blood in the urine. If the urinalysis is positive for blood in a non-menstruating female, a microscopic examination should be performed to determine how many RBCs are present. Urine becomes pink in color when there are approximately 20 to 30 RBCs per high power field. It becomes red at approximately 100 RBCs per high power field (Gleich, 1999). If the microscopic examination reveals RBCs too numerous to count, this will most certainly influence the treatment. Common causes of hematuria include the following:

- Renal calculi
- Sloughing of urethral cells after chemotherapy
- Malignancy
- Urinary tract infection
- Menstruation
- Vaginal bleeding

Hematuria is not normal, and there should be an extensive work-up of these clients. Hematuria can indicate serious pathology and the patient can be asymptomatic. According to Gleich (1999), it is normal to have 0 to 3 RBCs in high-powered microscope field. The complete diagnostic work-up for a client with hematuria—to rule out malignancy—would consist of assessment and clinical evaluation, creatinine level, urinalysis, urine culture, urine cytology, intravenous pyelogram, and cystoscopy; then advance to ultrasound and CT scan of kidneys to rule out renal mass, obstruction, and renal calculi (Box 3-3).

WBCs in the Urine

When the urinalysis is positive for WBCs the microscope may reveal 30 to 50 WBCs, which is indicative of a serious urinary tract infection and may be a precursor to urosepsis. This can result in death if not aggressively managed. A repeat urinalysis should be performed on any client who has been treated for a urinary tract infection to be certain the microorganisms have been eradicated. The urine should have had a culture analysis in order to determine the effectiveness of the antibiotic therapy chosen.

A urinalysis positive for leukocyte esterase and nitrites is indicative of a urinary tract infection and

Adapted from Gleich P: Hematuria: just UTI – or something more ominous, *Consultations in Primary Care: Consultant* 39(8):2235-2242, 1999.

> ## Box 3-3
>
> ## Significant Findings Related to Hematuria
>
> Urine should not contain more than 0-3 RBCs. Greater than 3 RBCs per high-power field is probably not innocent.
>
> There is a 1 in 4 chance that gross hematuria is a transitional cell neoplasm.
>
> Dysmorphic RBCs, RBC casts, or protein may indicate glomerular damage and increased risk of renal parenchymal disease.
>
> Patients with microhematuria should have twice-yearly urinalysis and cytologic examination for approximately 3 years after initial evaluation or until the hematuria resolves.

urine cultures should follow. Ideally, the specimen should be the first voided in the morning after the urine has incubated in the bladder for 4 hours or more. Bacteria produce nitrites by converting metabolites from food nutrients to nitrites. The leukocytosis esterase test identifies enzymes found in granulocytes, histocytes, and trichomonas. A positive leukocyte esterase, combined with a positive nitrite, is highly sensitive (95%) and specific (85%) for a urinary tract infection. Clients who present with fever, costovertebral angle (CVA) tenderness on palpation, and nausea or vomiting should be suspected of having pyelonephritis, and there is clear indication for obtaining urine cultures.

A 24-hour urine collection should be done on clients who are hypertensive and when adrenal gland pheochromocytoma is being ruled out. It is critical that this test should be done on the workup of any unexplained hypertension before proceeding with further diagnostic work-up (Isselbacher, 1994).

Human Chorionic Gonadotropin (HCG)

A fertilized ovum secretes human chorionic gonadotropin (HCG) 8 to 10 days after conception.

The urine test can accurately be performed 2 days after missed menses. The serum test can detect pregnancy in as little as 1 week postconception. An HCG level should be obtained either by urine or serum sample in any female of childbearing years who has the potential to be pregnant. This should be done prior to some diagnostic work-ups, particularly those involving risk of exposure to the fetus. Such risk would be associated with x-rays, CT scans, and many drug therapies. There are very few medications that are not potentially teratogenic, particularly in the first trimester of pregnancy. It is critical for the nurse practitioner to know when to order a qualitative HCG versus a quantitative HCG. The qualitative HCG indicates that the client is either pregnant or not. The quantitative value indicates an actual level of hormone consistent with the gestational age of the fetus. It is important to obtain the quantitative test in the case of threatened abortion or after spontaneous abortion to determine if the levels are decreasing and if further treatment is indicated. Serial monitoring of quantitative HCG may be conducted to evaluate gestational age. The normal HCG levels for a nonpregnant female and for a pregnant female through 12 weeks gestation are shown in Table 3-10.

THYROID PROFILE

The tests most widely used in clinical practice are serum immunoassays for thyroid-stimulating hormone (TSH) and free thyroxine (FT$_4$). Table 3-11 lists the results of a normal thyroid profile. TSH levels are decreased and FT$_4$ is elevated in patients with primary hyperthyroidism. TSH can also be suppressed by thyroid hormone administration in either excessive or replacement amounts. Other conditions associated with low TSH may include pregnancy, HCG-secreting trophoblastic tumors, acute psychiatric illness, and administration of glucocorticoids. Some drugs can cause mild suppression of TSH without clinical hyperthyroidism. Theses include NSAIDs, amphetamines, octreotide, opioids, and certain calcium channel blockers.

A client with hypothyroidism will have an elevated TSH level and a decreased free thyroxin index (FTI) or FT$_4$ level. Autoimmune disease may

Table 3-10
Normal HCG Levels

HCG		SI Units
Males	<5.0 mIU/ml	<5.0 IU/L
Females		
Nonpregnant	<5.0 mIU/ml	<5.0 IU/L
≤1 week gestation	5–50 mIU/ml	5–50 IU/L
2 weeks gestation	50–500 mIU/ml	50–500 IU/L
3 weeks gestation	100–10,000 mIU/ml	100–10,000 IU/L
4 weeks gestation	1000–30,000 mIU/ml	1000–30,000 IU/L
5 weeks gestation	3500–115,000 mIU/ml	3500–115,000 IU/L
6–8 weeks gestation	12,000–270,000 mIU/ml	12,000–270,000 IU/L
12 weeks gestation	15,000–220,000 mIU/ml	15,000–220,000 IU/L

Taken from: Chernecky CC, Berger BJ: *Laboratory tests and diagnostic procedures,* ed 2, Philadelphia, 1997, WB Saunders.

Table 3-11
Normal Thyroid Profile

Test	Normal Range
Thyroxine (T_4)	4-11 μg/dl
T_4 (expressed as iodine)	3.2-7.2 μg/dl
T_3 resin uptake	25%-38% relative uptake
TSH	10μU/ml

also falsely elevate serum TSH levels by interfering with the assays. TSH levels may also be increased by dopamine antagonists, phenothiazines, and atypical antipsychotics.

A thyroid profile is essential in any client who reports heart palpitations or irregular heart beat; a client diagnosed with new onset atrial fibrillation; or in clients experiencing rapid unexplained weight loss, nervousness, or insomnia. Clients who have unexplained menstrual disorders, myalgias, fatigue, weakness, constipation, weight change, hyperlipidemia, and anemia also need to be thoroughly assessed.

Clients at risk for developing thyroid disorders include but are not limited to those with a family history of thyroid problems, those with diabetes, persons with elevated triglycerides, persons with autoimmune disorders, and persons taking lithium and amiodarone.

FASTING BLOOD GLUCOSE

A fasting blood glucose (FBS) should be ordered when the client history or clinical presentation indicates that diabetes mellitus is a differential diagnosis. The diagnosis of diabetes can be made by a fasting blood glucose higher than 126 mg/dl on more than one occasion (Tierney, McPhee, and Papadakis, 2000). For an accurate test to be done, clients should be normally active and free from any acute illness. The client should have no food intake for at least 4 hours prior to the test, but water intake is permissible. Persons with diabetes should withhold insulin for at least 4 hours prior to the test. Since fasting plasma glucose is known to increase with age, providers should be more tolerant of slight abnormalities in people over 70. It should be noted that a random blood glucose over 200 mg/dl with a standard glucose intake prior to the sample can also be used to make the diagnosis of diabetes mellitus. Repeat fasting blood glucose levels should be done in 2 to 3 months to monitor patient compliance and efficacy of various antidiabetic agents.

HEMOGLOBIN A_{1c}

Hemoglobin A_{1c} (HbA$_{1c}$) is used to monitor changes in blood sugar over time, and is perhaps the single most important tool in accurately measuring the degree of diabetic control. By measuring glycosylated hemoglobin (the binding of glucose to the hemoglobin molecule), the HbA_{1c} reflects glycemic control. Since glycohemoglobins circulate within red blood cells—whose life span is approximately 120 days—they generally reflect the state of glycemic control over the preceding 8 to 12 weeks. HbA_{1c} is expressed as a percentage. Normal values of HbA_{1c} are approximately 4% to 6% of the total hemoglobin. The desired level is a glycosylated HbA_{1c} less than 7% with a fasting glucose of less than 140 mg/dl. The HbA_{1c} is reliable and provides a valid index of what glucose control has been over time. This test needs to be done every 6 months to 1 year for maintenance and assessment of control in diabetes, and perhaps more frequently in those who have difficulty with control or who present more difficult compliance issues. The American Diabetic Association endorses biannual HbA_{1c} levels.

MICRO-ALBUMINURIA

Protein is almost always completely reabsorbed by the kidneys and is undetectable in the urine.

Clients with type 2 diabetes mellitus should have a micro-albuminuria level at the time of diagnosis and annually thereafter. Urine protein (in the absence of blood) is significant in the development of diabetic nephropathy. The microvasculature of the kidneys becomes damaged and can no longer filter proteins. Diabetic nephropathy is usually evidenced by the presence of protein in the urine.

ERYTHROCYTE SEDIMENTATION RATE (ESR)

When a sample of well-mixed venous blood is allowed to stand, all of the red cells settle to the bottom of the tube. The rate at which they fall is called the erythrocyte sedimentation rate (ESR). There are several methods used to measure the sed rate, with the Westergren method being the most commonly used. Table 3-12 lists normal values for the sed rate.

An elevated erythrocyte sedimentation rate is indicative of an inflammatory process somewhere in the body. The ESR is a nonspecific test, however, because there are many differential diagnoses and clinical conditions that can affect it. The sed rate can be affected by any condition that would cause

Table 3-12
Normal Values for Erythrocyte Sedimentation Rate

Adult male	1-13 mm/hr
Adult female	1-20 mm/hr
Pregnant female	44-114 mm/hr
Male >50 years	1-20 mm/hr
Female >50 years	1-30 mm/hr
Child	1-13 mm/hr

cells to clump or by conditions that produce an increase in globulins or fibrinogen. While the sed rate may confirm that an inflammatory condition does exist, it does not identify the source of the inflammation. Moreover, the sed rate is normally elevated in pregnancy.

The conditions most likely to cause an elevated ESR are inflammation and tissue insult. In a nonpregnant client, the most likely cause of an elevated ESR greater than 100 mm/hr is an inflammatory process or disease, a malignancy, or a collagen vascular disease such as arthritis. A sed rate should be ordered in clients suspected of having rheumatoid arthritis or inflammation of joints. It is also the number one diagnostic tool in diagnosing temporal arteritis (giant cell arteritis). A diagnosis of temporal arteritis can be made on clinical examination, sed rate, and a temporal artery biopsy.

LIPID PROFILE

All patients with known cardiovascular disease should be screened for elevated lipids. The only exceptions are patients in whom lipid lowering is not indicated or desirable for other reasons (Tierney, McPhee, and Papadakis, 2000). A complete lipid profile includes examination of total cholesterol, high-density lipoprotein (HDL) cholesterol, triglyceride levels, and low-density lipoprotein (LDL) cholesterol. Table 3-13 lists the normal values for an adult lipid profile, which usually includes total cholesterol, triglycerides, HDLs and LDLs. The U.S. Preventative Services Task Force (1996) recommends lipid screening in men age 35 and older and women age 45 and older, unless there is significant family history or other risk factors present to warrant testing sooner.

Table 3-13
Normal Levels for the Adult Lipid Profile

Total cholesterol	140-199 mg/dl
Triglycerides (VLDL)	35-160 mg/dl
High-density lipoproteins (HDL)	32-85 mg/dl (more than 35 mg/dl is desirable)
Low-density lipoproteins (LDL)	Less than 130 mg/dl

Hyperlipidemia is considered to be present when a client has elevated serum cholesterol or triglycerides significant enough to produce symptoms of coronary heart disease or pancreatitis. Some of the most common secondary causes include but are not limited to diabetes; excessive alcohol ingestion; hypothyroidism; renal nephrosis; liver disease; and use of certain medications, particularly corticosteroids, diuretics, and beta-blockers.

The desirable total cholesterol level should be less than 200 mg/dl and the HDL should be greater than 35 mg/dl. Borderline high cholesterol is 200 to 239 mg/dl, and a value greater than 240 mg/dl is considered high. The ideal LDL cholesterol would be less than 130 mg/dl. Borderline high-risk is considered 130 to 159 mg/dl, with high risk any level greater than 160 mg/dl. Triglycerides are also low-density lipoproteins, less dense than LDLs, and are also referred to as VLDLs (very–low-density lipoproteins).

It is important to obtain a lipid panel on clients who have a known familial history of hypercholesterolemia, significant coronary heart disease, peripheral vascular disease, or carotid disease. It is important to obtain the total cholesterol, HDL and LDL levels for these clients at least annually. Once again, it is important to document the significant risk factors, and to use these values to determine the best course of treatment. Diet and exercise treatment may not be enough if lipids are elevated and there are more than two additional risk factors present. It is also important to keep in mind the need to evaluate serum levels of children who have a significant family history in order to intervene early in the process.

LIVER PROFILE

The liver profile measures the activity of enzymes that help reflect hepatic function. Enzymes that assess hepatic functioning are alkaline phosphatase (AP), aspartate aminotransferase (AST), alanine aminotransferase (ALT), bilirubin, and lactate dehydrogenase (LDH). A liver profile usually includes albumin, total bilirubin, direct bilirubin, alkaline phosphatase, AST, and ALT. Liver function tests are helpful in making the differential diagnosis involving hepatic functioning. Liver functions only need to be obtained once and are usually not repeated unless there is risk of hepatic disorder or the client develops symptoms. AST and ALT should be monitored, however, in patients taking drugs that have the potential for causing hepatocellular dysfunction. Persons at risk for altered hepatic functioning include those with the following conditions:

• History of alcohol abuse
• History of intravenous drug abuse
• Viral hepatitis
• Nasal cocaine use
• History of hepatitis B
• History of hepatitis C
• History of blood transfusion
• At-risk sexual behavior
• Tattoos
• Body piercing
• History of family death due to liver disease
• Hemachromatosis
• Clients on statin medications to lower cholesterol

ALBUMIN

Albumin is a protein produced by the liver and released into the plasma. Albumin is a very large protein molecule and is essential for maintaining oncotic and osmotic pressure gradients in the body. The usual production of albumin in an adult is approximately 12 to 14 grams per day. Normal serum albumin in an adult is 3.8 to 5.6 g/dL. Under normal conditions, a small amount of albumin is lost through the mucosa of the gastrointestinal tract. Aging and conditions of malnutrition can contribute to the loss of albumin. Serum albumin levels should be obtained in clients with edema (both peripheral and ascites), liver disease, or suspected malnutrition. An elevated serum albumin level is rarely of any consequence and is a rather benign finding. A low serum albumin, however, creates fluid balance problems and can be indicative of a number of disease states. Low serum albumin can be present in malnutrition, congestive heart failure, hyperthyroidism, lymphatic leukemia, stress, burns, collagen diseases, and diabetes. Liver damage can lead to a decrease in albumin synthesis, but serum albumin is not a reliable indicator of liver disease alone. Many other non-hepatic factors contribute to decreased albumin levels.

ALKALINE PHOSPHATASE (AP)

Total serum alkaline phosphatase (AP) is a reflection of several isoenzymes found in hepatoparenchymal osteoblasts, the renal epithelium, the intestinal mucosa, bones, and the placenta. High concentrations of alkaline phosphatase are present during periods of rapid growth or cellular injury. Table 3-14 lists the normal levels of alkaline phosphatase, which is measured in units per liter. Indications for concern about alkaline phosphatase levels include the following:

- Skeletal diseases characterized by marked osteoblastic activity
- Local hepatic lesions (e.g., tumor, abscess) causing biliary obstruction
- Supplement other liver enzymes and gastrointestinal enzyme tests

Approximately 50% of the measured enzyme is produced in the bone and approximately 50% by the liver. Because children are growing rapidly, they will have higher alkaline phosphatase levels due to increases in osteoblastic activity—approximately 2 to 4 times that of an average adult. Serum AP levels are lower in women than men during the middle years; then the value tends to rise in women. Normal levels also tend to be higher in older women secondary to bone reabsorption. It is important to indicate the client's age on the laboratory requisition in order to reliably interpret values.

A serum AP greater 142 units/L is considered elevated. The AP level is elevated 3 to 10 times nor-

Table 3-14 Normal Alkaline Phosphatase Levels	
Adults	17-142 units/L
Children	70-530 units/L
Pregnant women	30-200 units/L

mal in hepatobiliary disease that impairs hepatic excretory function. It is also elevated in parenchymal disorders such as hepatitis and cirrhosis and in metastatic disease. Other conditions causing elevated serum alkaline phosphatase levels include the following:

- Bone disease
- Liver disease or dysfunction
- Drug effects
- Heart failure
- Hyperthyroidism
- Lymphoma
- Leukemia
- Primary biliary cirrhosis
- Primary sclerosing cholangitis
- Drug-induced hepatotoxicity
- Cholelithiasis

BILIRUBIN

Bilirubin is a by-product of the destruction of aged red blood cells. Bilirubin is transported from the blood after it attaches to the large albumin molecules. In the liver, the bilirubin and the albumin become conjugated and are then excreted as bile. Laboratory tests are available to measure both direct and indirect bilirubin. Table 3-15 lists normal bilirubin levels for different client populations. Clients should fast at least 8 hours before bilirubin levels are tested. Fat intake, particularly if it has been large, will interfere with test results. Bilirubin levels should also not be drawn for 24 hours after a client has had a dye injected for other radiological or diagnostic studies. In neonates, the blood sample for bilirubin is taken from the heel.

Total bilirubin levels can be separated into direct and indirect bilirubin. The unconjugated bilirubin is also known as indirect bilirubin, and the con-

Table 3-15
Normal Bilirubin Levels

Adults and children (not newborns)	Indirect (unconjugated)	0.1-1.0 mg/dl
	Direct (conjugated)	0-0.4 mg/dl
	Total (includes both)	0.1-1.0 mg/dl
Newborn		
Term Infant	Total bilirubin first 24 hours	<6 mg
	Up to 48 hours	<8 mg
	2-5 days	<12 mg
Premature Infant	Total bilirubin first 24 hours	<8 mg
	Up to 48 hours	<12 mg
	2-5 days	<16 mg
Pregnancy	May be slightly elevated: usually normal	

jugated bilirubin is known as direct bilirubin. Usually, a diagnosis is made based on whether the problem is primarily hepatic or cholecystic. The type and amount of bilirubin levels can determine this. Indirect bilirubin levels can be calculated by subtracting the direct levels from the total. A direct bilirubin should only be done if the total is greater than 1.0 mg/dl.

HYPERBILIRUBINEMIA

In the client with elevated levels of unconjugated (lipid soluble or indirect) bilirubin, a mild jaundice is expected. This is usually due to cholestasis, which can be benign; or it can occur in the third trimester of pregnancy. Splenomegaly occurs in hemolytic disorders (except sickle cell disease) with an elevated indirect bilirubin. When there is an elevation of total bilirubin greater than 1.0 mg/dl, and conjugated (water soluble or direct) bilirubin is also elevated, biliary obstruction, hepatocellular disease, or intrahepatic cholestasis can be suspected.

SERUM AMINOTRANSFERASES

The aminotransferases, referred to in most literature as transferases, are enzymes located predominantly in the liver hepatocytes. Aspartate aminotransferase (AST or SGOT) and alanine aminotransferase (ALT or SGPT) are sensitive indicators of liver abnormalities. These aminotransferases are indicative of hepatocellular injury. AST

Table 3-16
Normal Values for Liver Enzymes

	ALT	AST
Adults	0-35 U/L	0-35 U/L
Elderly	Slight increase	Slight increase
Newborn	Higher	2-3 times higher

Levels for the normal female are slightly lower than males on the AST. There are no gender differences seen in ALT levels.

and ALT elevations are the accepted markers of hepatitis A (Table 3-16).

Alanine Aminotransferase

The normal levels of ALT differ in men, women, and children. There can be a great deal of variation in values obtained according to the lab method used.

The transaminases are found in large quantities in liver tissue, but are also present in myocardial tissue, skeletal muscle tissue, and renal cells. ALT levels will increase with various types of tissue trauma but it is not specific to the tissue type. ALT levels will be increased in liver diseases including, but not limited to, hepatitis, mononucleosis, and cirrhosis. There will also be elevation of ALT levels in hydatidiform mole, Reye's syndrome, congestive heart failure, and eclampsia. The greatest levels of

ALT are found in the liver; therefore, elevations are often indicative of liver pathology.

Aspartate Aminotransferase

AST is found in myocardial cells, hepatocytes, and skeletal muscle. AST levels will be elevated in liver disease. Serum levels may reach significantly high levels before jaundice is physiologically evident. Under normal conditions, the levels of AST are low. These levels might be lower in very extensive liver disease when the liver is no longer functioning. Conditions that warrant liver function testing include the following:

- History of high-risk sexual behavior
- History of intravenous drug abuse
- Alcohol abuse
- Hepatitis or exposure to hepatitis
- Mononucleosis with jaundice
- Excessive nausea and vomiting with jaundice
- Abdominal pain with focal tenderness over the right upper quadrant
- Clay-colored stools
- Clients who are being treated with medications for hypercholesterolemia, especially the somatostatin drugs
- Jaundice of the skin or sclera

Liver function tests may not include prothrombin time, partial thromboplastin time, and international normalized ratio, and these may need to be requested separately. Some laboratories also require amylase and lipase to be requested separately.

PT, PTT, INR, AND PLATELETS

Blood coagulation is the process by which blood forms a gelatinous substance otherwise known as a clot. The clotting process is dependent on many factors and consists of several steps. There are two clotting pathways, the intrinsic and extrinsic, which merge to form one clotting cascade. The common link between the intrinsic and extrinsic pathways is a substance called thrombin.

All substances in the intrinsic pathway required for coagulation to occur are from the blood. The components necessary for the extrinsic pathway are from substances external to the blood. The intrinsic

and extrinsic pathways converge at factor Xa. Xa catalyzes and assists in conversion of prothrombin to thrombin. In turn, this catalyzes the formation of fibrin, which is necessary for the platelet plug, the first step in coagulation. There can be many differential diagnoses as well as specified pharmacological agents that interfere with either the intrinsic or extrinsic pathways or the resulting clotting cascade.

Routine tests used to determine clotting ability of the blood are prothrombin time (PT), partial thromboplastin time (PTT), international normalized ratio (INR), and platelets (Table 3-17).

Prothromin Time

The PT indicates the effectiveness of prothrombin, as well as fibrinogen and clotting factors V, VII, and X. Prothrombin (factor II) is a plasma protein. Factor II is produced by the liver and is the test used to measure clotting effects of anticoagulant medications such as Coumadin. The PT reports the time in seconds that it takes the blood to clot when certain chemicals are added. The client's PT value/second will be greater than the control value when anticoagulation is desired.

A decreased PT of 8 or 9 seconds (with a control of 11 or 12 seconds) may indicate malignancy or thrombophlebitis. It should be noted, however,

Table 3-17
Normal PT and PTT

Normal PT	
Adult	Control 11-16 seconds (±2 seconds)
Newborn	May be higher in premature infants
	Reference values may be 12-21 seconds

Normal PTT	
Adult	25-38 seconds or 60-90 seconds if not activated
Newborn	Levels higher than adults until age 3 months
Pregnancy	Normally decreased
Women	Levels may be decreased with use of oral contraceptives

that a decreased PT alone is not a clinically significant diagnostic tool.

Partial Thromboplastin Time

The PTT is useful in detecting various abnormalities in the intrinsic clotting cascade. The PTT reflects the activities of fibrinogen; prothrombin; and factors V, VIII, IX, X, XI, and XII. If an abnormal PTT is reported, further specific testing is needed to determine if there is a specific clotting defect. The PTT is used to monitor heparin therapy. Because specific chemicals are added to the sample, the test is reported as *activated PTT*. Just as with the prothrombin time, the patient's PTT is compared to a control value. No percentage is reported in the PTT. For a client on heparin therapy, the desired PTT would be 1.5 to 2.5 times the control value.

International Normalized Ratio

When values are reported in seconds or percentages, it can be a problem because the results will vary depending on the reagent used. The INR ensures a standardized reporting by accounting for variation in the test results. Laboratory reports include both the PT ratio and the INR for decision-making in coagulation testing.

Platelets

Platelets are an extremely critical element in the coagulation process. Without them, the platelet plug—the critical first step in clotting—will not occur. When the platelet count falls below 50,000/μL, the client is at risk of a clotting deficiency. There are many medications that have the inherent ability to interfere with platelet aggregation. These include, but are not limited to, aspirin and aspirin-containing products, nonsteroidal antiinflammatory medications, tricyclic antidepressants, alcohol, and beta-blockers. Preoperatively, the preferred platelet count is 100,000 /μL (Patton, 1999).

RHEUMATOID PANEL

When immune complexes are formed (for example, as in the case of rheumatoid arthritis), polymorphonuclear neutrophils (PMNs) are stimulated.

PMNs, in turn, secrete enzymes into the collagen in joint spaces. These enzymes eventually destroy healthy structures. Peck (1998) reports that many patients with either rheumatoid arthritis or an inflammatory arthritis will have normal rheumatoid factors and erythrocyte sedimentation rates. The diagnostic tests most useful in confirming the clinical suspicion of rheumatoid arthritis are rheumatoid factor (IgM), antinuclear antibody (ANA) and variants, and the ESR.

Rheumatoid factor is common in approximately 70% of the clients with rheumatoid arthritis; however, in terms of sensitivity and specificity of the test, it is important to know that a negative value does not necessarily mean that the disease is not present. The ESR and C-reactive protein (CRP) levels may also be elevated, but the same holds true in other diseases of a rheumatologic nature.

A positive CRP, like the ESR, can indicate an inflammatory process or tissue destruction but it does not provide any degree of specificity as to the nature of the infectious process. CRP is not normally present in the blood of healthy individuals. CRP is a highly nonspecific test. ESR is still the preferred test in the diagnosis and monitoring of rheumatoid arthritis. Other lab studies that are particularly helpful in the diagnosis of arthritis are the rheumatoid factor (RF), antinuclear antibody (ANA), and antistreptolysin O titer (ASO) (Baum, 1999).

The RF detects abnormal proteins in clients with rheumatoid arthritis. The normal rheumatoid factor should be less than 60 IU/ml. The RF test actually tests for different types of IgM antibodies. RF can be present in clients with other diagnoses; however, it is present in higher levels in persons with rheumatoid arthritis. It should be noted that the assay level does not correlate with severity of the disease. Other patient populations testing positive for RF include, but are not limited to, those testing positive for tuberculosis, bacterial endocarditis, syphilis, and those with collagen or connective tissue diseases.

Antinuclear antibodies are gamma globulins that are present in clients with selected autoimmune disorders. ANA are highly specialized and directed against components of the cell nucleus. Most of these antibodies are of the IgA class, and ANA is primarily used to assist in the diagnosis of systemic lupus erythematosus (SLE). Most clients with SLE will have elevated ANA titers. The ANA titer can also be elevated in rheumatoid arthritis, scleroderma, carcinomas, TB, as well as in hepatitis.

There is some variation in ANA titers in the elderly; the titers tend to be increased in the elderly despite the absence of immune disorders. The ANA titer is positive if it is greater than 40 or if the diluted serum ratio is 1 : 8.

The antistreptolysin O titer is used to detect recent infection with group A beta-hemolytic streptococcus. Infection involving group A beta strep leaves antigens in the form of measurable antibodies in the serum. Serum antibodies to streptolysin O are present and detectable approximately 7 to 10 days after an acute infection with streptococcus. These antibody levels will peak at approximately 2 to 4 weeks and can remain elevated for weeks or months, indicating the previous strep exposure. There are cases where a false positive can occur, such as in other pathologies including liver disease. Table 3-18 lists normal ASO levels.

H-PYLORI *(HELICOBACTER PYLORI)*

In 1985 the American College of Physicians (ACP) prepared a policy statement in response to what was perceived as an overuse of diagnostic testing in dyspepsia syndromes. The ACP statement emphasized the need to utilize clinical judgment; exercise technologic restraint; and, when possible, treat the client with dyspepsia provisionally. Clients with a suspected diagnosis of peptic ulcer disease (PUD) should be treated empirically, and evaluation of that treatment should precede laboratory testing.

The empiric treatment protocols for PUD should be a minimum of 3 weeks if the client remains stable and is progressing positively with the therapy. After 6 to 8 weeks of empiric therapy, the client should then undergo laboratory and diagnostic testing. The criteria for determining need for further testing should include the criteria that the client's symptoms are improved but not resolved.

H-pylori can be detected in several ways. These include a breath analysis with nonradioactive ^{13}C urea; serum levels; and biopsy specimens, usually obtained during an endoscopic examination. The serum test for H-pylori is limited and tests primarily for IgG antibodies to H-pylori. There is also the consideration that there is a high prevalence of H-pylori in asymptomatic clients. These clients will test positive even in the absence of symptoms. Some practitioners also use Campylobacter-like organism testing (CLO) because it is relatively inexpensive to perform, is highly accurate, and is available in most laboratories.

LIPASE

Lipase is a highly sensitive and highly specific test for assessing the function of the pancreas. The pancreas is located rather retroperitoneally in the body and the symptoms associated with pancreatitis can be varied. Serum lipase is the test of choice in diagnosing pancreatitis. The pancreas is the major source of lipase, a coenzyme specific to pathologies involving the pancreas. Serum lipase levels have a wide degree of sensitivity and specificity ranging from 70% to 80%. Pancreatic carcinoma or trauma may result in elevated serum lipase. The normal lipase level should be 23 to 300 U/L.

AMYLASE

Amylase is an enzyme that functions in the breakdown of starch in the body. The serum amylase range is 25 to 130 IU/L and is designated in Somogyi units/dl. Amylase is produced in the pancreas; in the salivary glands; and, in some cases, by tumors in the lung. After it is produced, the largest amount of amylase travels to the intestine to begin the breakdown of starch. Normally there is a very small amount of amylase present in the serum. The kidneys usually excrete amylase, hence amylase will be mildly elevated in clients with renal failure. A low serum amylase level is usually of no consequence and is a benign finding.

Amylase levels are helpful in the differential di-

Table 3-18 Normal ASO Titers	
Preschool	1:85
Ages 5-18 years	1:170
Adults	1:85

agnosis of parotiditis (mumps). Serum amylase is an important diagnostic test when ruling out a surgical abdomen, or in abdominal pain where there is a high index of suspicion for pancreatitis. Serum amylase can begin to rise 3 to 6 hours after the onset of pancreatitis. Not all patients with pancreatitis will have a high serum amylase.

There is no clinical correlation between the degree of elevation of amylase levels and disease prognosis. Sensitivity for diagnosing pancreatitis based on serum amylase levels varies from 45% to 95%. Amylase is considered elevated when it is greater than 150 Somogyi units/dl. Conditions that may result in elevated amylase levels include the following:

- Perforated ulcer
- Mesenteric infarction
- Salivary gland disease (commonly, parotiditis)
- Chronic renal failure
- Amylase-secreting cancer
- Pancreatitis
- Ovarian tumor
- Lung tumor
- Salivary gland tumor
- Peritonitis
- Acute appendicitis
- Peptic ulcer disease
- Intestinal obstruction
- Ruptured ectopic pregnancy
- Diabetic ketoacidosis

References

Barkin JS, Green R, Johnson B et al: A practical work-up for the patient with anemia, *Patient Care for the Nurse Practitioner* April:30-42, 1998.

Baum J: Rheumatoid arthritis: how to make the most of laboratory tests in the work-up, *Consultations in Primary Care: Consultant* 38(5):1341-1348, 1999.

Chernecky CC, Berger BJ: *Laboratory tests and diagnostic procedures,* ed 2, Philadelphia, 1997, WB Saunders.

Colucciello SA, Lukens TW, Morgan DL: Assessing abdominal pain in adults: a rational, cost-effective, and evidence-based strategy. In *Emergency medicine practice,* vol. 1, Marietta, Ga., 1999, Pinnacle Publishing.

Corbett JV: *Laboratory tests and diagnostic procedures with nursing diagnoses,* ed 5, Upper Saddle River, N.J., 2000, Prentice Hall.

Fischbach F: *A manual of laboratory diagnostic tests,* ed 6, Philadelphia, 2000, JB Lippincott.

Gleich P: Hematuria: just UTI – or something more ominous, *Consultations in Primary Care: Consultant* 39(8):2235-2242, 1999.

Goroll A, May L, Mulley A, editors: *Primary care medicine: office evaluation and management of the adult patient,* ed 3, Philadelphia, 1995, JB Lippincott.

Hamilton J, Ruo P, Wagner J: Appendicitis: unmasking the great masquerader, *Patient Care for the Nurse Practitioner,* July:11-27, 1998.

Isselbacher KJ et al: *Harrison's principles of internal medicine,* ed 13, New York, 1994, McGraw-Hill.

McCance KL, Huether SE: *Pathophysiology: The biologic basis for disease in adults and children,* ed 3, St Louis, 1998, Mosby.

Patton CM: Preoperative nursing assessment of the adult patient, *Semin Perioper Nurs* 8(1):42-47, 1999.

Peck B: Rheumatoid arthritis. Early intervention can change outcomes, *Adv Nurse Pract* 6(7):34-38, 41, 1998.

Stoeckle JD: Principles of primary care. In Goroll A, May L, Mulley A, editors: *Primary care medicine: office evaluation and management of the adult patient,* ed 3, Philadelphia, 1995, JB Lippincott.

Taylor RB, editor: *Family medicine: principles and practice,* New York, 1998, Springer-Verlag.

Tierney LM Jr, McPhee SJ, Papadakis MA, editors: *Current medical diagnosis and treatment,* ed 39, New York, 2000, Lange Medical Books/ McGraw-Hill.

U. S. Preventive Services Task Force: *Report: guide to clinical preventive services,* ed 2, Media, PA, 1996, Williams & Wilkins.

Suggested Readings

Adelman AM, Richardson JP: Gastritis, esophagitis, and peptic ulcer disease. In Taylor RB, editor: *Family medicine: principles and practice,* New York, 1998, Springer-Verlag.

Bouska Lee CA, Barret CA, Ignativicus DD: *Fluids and electrolytes: a practical approach,* ed 4, Philadelphia, 1996, F.A. Davis.

Chernecky CC, Krech RL, Berger BJ, editors: *Laboratory tests and diagnostic procedures,* Philadelphia, 1993, WB Saunders.

Goldman L, Bennet JC, editors: *Cecil textbook of medicine,* ed 21, Philadelphia, 2000, WB Saunders.

Vander A, Sherman J, Luciano D: *Human physiology: the mechanisms of body function,* ed 7, Boston, 1998, McGraw-Hill.

Williamson KM, Thrasher KA, Fulton KB et al: Digoxin toxicity: an evaluation in current clinical practice, *Arch Intern Med* 158(22):2444-2449, 1998.

CHAPTER 4

Diagnostic Imaging

Carol Patton

IMAGING STUDIES

There are many different imaging techniques available to assist the practitioner, including sophisticated imaging techniques that may or may not employ the use of radiation. Imaging techniques that provide enhanced diagnostic capability include computed tomography scanning (CT scan), magnetic resonance imaging (MRI), radionuclide bone scanning, ultrasound, radioisotope scanning, angiography, and fluoroscopy.

Plain Radiographs (Plain Films)

Plain radiographs employ radiation and are usually the first line imaging technique utilized in most acute extremity symptoms (Simon and Koenigsknecht, 1996).

General Radiographic Concepts Plain x-rays are also referred to as plain radiographs (Mettler, 1996). Plain x-rays account for the majority of radiological images. When a plain film is taken, an x-ray beam is passed through the client's body. The x-ray is absorbed differently by the various types of tissue or structures that the beam must pass through.

Four densities in the human body influence penetration of x-ray beams: these are air, fat, water, and bone (Mettler, 1996). The lungs appear darker on a plain film because the air in them is less dense than fluid, allowing the radiation beams to pass through more readily. Bones appear white on plain films because their thickness and calcium content absorbs the x-ray beam (Mettler, 1996). Plain films are not particularly diagnostic with regard to soft tissue and vasculature.

A thorough and accurate assessment of the client must occur prior to ordering any diagnostic radiological procedures. It is of particular importance to consider the client's age when ordering x-rays. Every attempt should be made to protect the client from excessive or unnecessary radiation exposure. There are standards for shielding clients and for determining amounts of radiation exposure. In the practice of evidence-based medicine, the history and mechanism of injury may not justify an x-ray, and the benefit of obtaining the film may not outweigh the risks involved. For example, a female client who is 6 weeks pregnant tells you that she twisted her ankle 2 weeks ago. She has been able to bear weight, but wonders if she may need an x-ray because the pain has persisted. The practitioner needs to weigh the benefit of obtaining the film against the teratogenic risk to the fetus during the first trimester. Other questions to consider include: Will obtaining the film change the treatment plan and influence client outcome? Can the client be effectively shielded to protect the fetus from exposure to radiation?

Careful thought and attention must be paid when ordering an emergent or diagnostic x-ray on any female of childbearing age. Women in this age group often deny the chance of pregnancy when the possibility exists. The teratogenic effect of radiation on a fetus exposed in utero has been documented, especially during the first trimester of pregnancy (Mettler, 1996, Taylor, 1998). Guidelines for irradiating the pregnant or potentially pregnant patient are listed in Box 4-1.

Consumer Demands for Imaging Studies The client and/or significant others may present to the practitioner demanding an x-ray. In such cases, the consumer has an expectation and will not be satisfied with less. Health-care providers can educate and explain the risk/benefit ratio, but in some instances the

Box 4-1

Guidelines for Irradiating the Pregnant or Potentially Pregnant Patient

1. Do not irradiate the abdomen, pelvis, lumbar spine, or hips of a woman in the first trimester of pregnancy unless it is clearly medically indicated.
2. Whenever possible, defer the examination or choose an alternative imaging modality (for example, ultrasound).
3. When evaluating a pregnant woman with modalities that use ionizing radiation, limit the number of images or views obtained; take only those required to ensure adequate care.
4. If the abdomen or pelvis of a pregnant patient is accidentally irradiated, the radiology department needs to be notified. A radiation safety officer can estimate the radiation dose to the fetus. This calculation can be used to determine the potential effect to the fetus.

From Wiest PW, Roth PB, editors: *Fundamentals of emergency radiology,* Philadelphia, 1996, WB Saunders.

consumer can be insistent and will not be satisfied even after a careful explanation. These challenging cases must be handled on an individual basis. For example, a parent might demand a skull film on a 6-month-old infant who has fallen from a low dressing table onto a carpeted floor. The infant may have hit his head, but had no loss of consciousness or behavioral changes. The parent may insist on a skull x-ray, though the test of choice in head trauma would be a CT scan of the brain if there was an index of suspicion of skull fracture or if the infant's behavior was abnormal after the fall. If there was no history of loss of consciousness, normal clinical examination, and no behavioral changes, the CT scan would not be indicated.

There have been many strategies and models, both formal and informal, for decision-making about which radiological studies to order. To date there has been no model that documents a consensus on ordering diagnostic imaging tests. In 1995, the American College of Radiology sparked an initiative to identify decision-making criteria that would assist health-care providers when some method of diagnostic imaging, if any, is appropriate (American College of Radiology, 1995). These concepts are integrated throughout the chapter.

Tomography

There are two types of tomography, conventional and computed. Computed tomography (CT) is also referred to in some texts and by the lay public as a CAT scan (computed axial tomography). The CT image is generated by passing a rotating beam of x-rays through the affected body part. The CT scan is a more sophisticated diagnostic imaging modality, but it delivers 10 to 100 times more exposure to radiation than do plain films (Mettler, 1996). A CT scan should be ordered only in specific circumstances, and is used predominantly for processes involving the brain and abdomen.

The CT scan may involve the use of a contrast medium, given to the client either by oral or intravenous method. The decision regarding the use of contrast should be discussed with the radiologist as to when this media is appropriate. For example, it is the standard of care to give the client oral contrast prior to a CT of the abdomen and pelvis in order to fully visualize structures. From a legal perspective, there is risk of liability if a client suspected of having liver or splenic injury is given a CT of the abdomen without oral contrast and a splenic or liver injury is missed based on decreased test sensitivity and specificity. In the case of suspected appendicitis, a CT scan without IV contrast is 96% sensitive, 99% specific, and has a 90% accuracy rate in supporting the differential diagnosis (Mountz and Hetherington, 2000).

The conventional CT scan is useful in evaluating an extremity when plain films are inconclusive or difficult to evaluate. CT scans provide visualization of radiographic cross sectional slices. CT scans provide density readings via a two dimensional image of bone and soft tissue. CT scans are more specific and detailed in depicting soft tissue injuries, and frequently are utilized in injuries or diagnoses involving the brain and abdomen (Simon and Koenigsknecht, 1996).

The use of contrast media is contraindicated in some client populations. For example, persons allergic to shellfish are at risk of untoward outcomes with the use of intravenous iodine contrast. Another key consideration regarding contrast with CT scan is the assessment of renal functioning. It is critical to have baseline lab data on the client's renal function, such as a blood urea nitrogen (BUN) and creatinine (Cr), prior to giving contrast. Persons with a known history of renal impairment may have difficulty clearing the contrast from their bodies. The potential for renal compromise is compounded in diabetic clients who are on Glucophage. Glucophage may be discontinued prior to intravenous contrast and 48 hours after receipt of the contrast media. There will be institutional variation on acceptable levels of renal functioning. This is an issue usually discussed in collaboration with the radiologist.

Another key consideration regarding the use of contrast involves the CT scan of the brain. This should be ordered without intravenous contrast when a bleed is suspected. If a cerebral bleed is present, contrast media will expand it. A cerebral bleed should be suspected when the client says "this is the worst headache I have ever had."

Other indications for a CT include suspected CVA, new onset seizure disorder with no prior history, new onset confusion, behavior changes after head trauma, head trauma with questionable or witnessed loss of consciousness, head trauma without loss of consciousness if the client is taking Coumadin or other anticoagulants, visible or palpable deformity of the skull, raccoon's eyes, Battle's sign, large hematoma of the scalp, head injury with altered mentation, excessive vomiting, or lethargy associated with head trauma. In non-trauma cases, the majority of CT scans can be ordered on an outpatient basis.

Magnetic Resonance Imaging

Magnetic resonance imaging is a technique that allows body structures to be visualized through application of varying magnetic fields. The alignment of atoms in the body generates radio waves that can be graphically depicted. MRIs have excellent contrast resolution and allow visualization of soft tissue, anatomic structure, and vasculature with extreme clarity. The relationship of tissue properties and the magnetic fields results in a tomographic

image. The key points of plain films, CT scans, and MRI are summarized in Table 4-1.

The advantages of MRI, in addition to the excellent resolution, include the lack of ionizing radiation and no requirement for any contrast media injection (Novelline, 1997). MRI has a very high sensitivity to neoplastic areas and vasculature abnormality, as well as to areas of inflammation. MRI is the diagnostic test of choice when there is suspicion of brain tumor, multiple sclerosis, or other central nervous system pathologies and all other diagnostic workups have failed to be conclusive. MRI is the most sensitive imaging technique in diagnosing a necrotic hip, and the test of choice in distinguishing between benign and malignant tumors (Simon and Koenigsknecht, 1996). The MRI is also a valuable diagnostic tool for clients with musculoskeletal symptoms who have normal plain films but who continue to have persistent pain or loss of functional ability (Novelline, 1997).

Client preparation for an MRI consists of assessment for any metal implants or a history of claustrophobia, and a current weight. Persons weighing more than 300 pounds will not fit in some scanning units and must be referred to a facility that has an "open" unit that can accommodate exceptional weight. These open MRI units also work well for clients who suffer from claustrophobia. These clients may be prescribed a low dose anxiolytic such as Ativan or Valium prior to the scan. Clients with metal implants cannot be scanned because ferrous metal in the body may cause critical injury to the client. For example, an intraocular metal foreign body may cause retinal hemorrhage, and intracranial aneurism clips may cause intracranial hemorrhage. Middle ear prosthetics and nerve stimulation devices may be contraindicated. Although rarely a contraindication, inform the radiologist about cardiac pacemakers and implanted venous acces devices. Many stainless steel orthopedic implants are not ferromagnetic and therefore are not affected by the MRI (Chernecky and Berger, 1997).

Ultrasound

In ultrasound imaging, a narrow beam of sound wave is directed at a particular part of the body, then translated by a transducer into an electrical

Table 4-1
Key Points of Plain Films, the CT Scan, and MRI

Imaging Study	Benefits	Potential Limitations
Plain Films	Good for extremity injuries. Less costly than more advanced imaging modalities	Do not provide detailed information on soft tissues Have to remain in position until film is obtained, making it difficult if client is in pain or in very young
CT Scan	Provides a clearer image of soft tissue and other structure	10 to 100 times increased absorption of radiation over plain films Increased cost May require oral/IV contrast; renal impairment may limit use of contrast media Client needs to be calm and still during imaging. This may require sedation in young children or combative elderly clients
MRI	Excellent visualization of soft tissue, anatomic structure, and vasculature No ionizing radiation No need for contrast media Diagnostic test of choice in suspected brain tumor, multiple sclerosis, central nervous system pathologies	Expensive, ranging from $100-$1000 Slower, and unless scanner is "open" client may require sedation due to claustrophobia

signal. This signal specifies the physical density of tissue as well as sound velocity (Novelline, 1997).

Ultrasound is attractive to clients because it is painless, safe, and noninvasive. It is useful in diagnostic evaluation for obstetrics, pediatric, gynecologic, and testicular studies.

Ultrasound as a diagnostic imaging technique has an overall high sensitivity and specificity. Lowe et al (1998) report a sensitivity rate of 55% and a specificity rate of 99%, indicating that ultrasound as a diagnostic test is both sensitive and specific. Client preparation for ultrasonography is an important consideration. It is essential for the client to have a full bladder and an empty bowel prior to ultrasound. This preparation is particularly important for pelvic ultrasounds because bowel loops are filled with stool and can appear on ultrasound as cysts, masses, or as a cul-de-sac mass. The client may be required to have a Foley catheter inserted to ensure a full bladder before the pelvic ultrasound. Inadequate client preparation could result in a false-negative test result or lead to an inconclusive study and un-

warranted further diagnostic studies. Adequate and complete client preparation can avoid delays and provide more accurate diagnostic data.

Several other factors can result in inconclusive ultrasound results. It is more difficult to obtain an accurate abdominal ultrasound in an obese client because of sound wave transmission and interpretation. In early pregnancy, to rule out an ectopic pregnancy or a spontaneous abortion, the preferred test is a transvaginal ultrasound. This provides a much more definitive visualization of the uterus, ovaries, and fallopian tubes. The practitioner must explain the necessity of the procedure to the client and significant others. Without this explanation, the client may refuse. This often happens in the case of threatened spontaneous abortion and the client thinks the transvaginal probe will cause her to abort. She and the significant other must be told this will not harm the fetus but that the test results will be quite helpful in making the diagnosis.

A distinct advantage of ultrasound is that it can differentiate between solid and fluid-filled masses by measuring the absorption of sound waves. Ultrasound can distinguish between cystic masses and solid masses. The cystic, fluid-filled mass produces sound waves with an echo, whereas the solid mass absorbs sound waves. The disadvantage of ultrasound is that although it can distinguish between fluid-filled and solid masses, it does not differentiate between benign and malignant tissues.

Novelline (1997) describes five major advantages that make ultrasound very attractive for diagnostic testing:

1. Ultrasound does not utilize ionizing radiation; this results in decreased exposure to biological injury.
2. Ultrasound is less expensive than CT or MRI.
3. Ultrasound can be performed at the bedside (cardiology, OB, ED).
4. The "real-time" ultrasound can provide moving images such as motion of the heart wall and the opening and closing of valves.
5. Ultrasound can be performed from several different planes, enabling views of greater anatomic regions.

Ultrasound should be the first line diagnostic in cases of suspected cholecystitis, ectopic pregnancy or tubo-ovarian abscess, appendicitis, testicular torsion, hydrocele, threatened abortion, or deep vein thrombosis, as well as in pregnancy. Ultrasound is usually performed in the second trimester (12 to 16 weeks) according to the American College of Radiology (1995). Transvaginal ultrasound is used to determine gestational age, as well as to diagnose selected anomalies of the fetus. In the event of threatened abortion, the transvaginal ultrasound can provide information about an intrauterine pregnancy, whether or not the fetus is viable, if the ovaries are within normal limits, and if there is a fluid in the cul de sac.

Nuclear Imaging

Nuclear imaging consists of intravenous injection of a radioactive isotope, usually Technetium-99m (^{99}Tc). Though it has a relatively short half-life in the body, this isotope has an affinity to certain physiologic substances in the body. Once ^{99}Tc has been

administered intravenously, the client must wait a designated time (usually 1 to 2 hours) and then have the scan. The scan will determine uptake of the isotope in a particular area. Other common isotopes are thallium-201 (used in cardiac stress tests); technetium Tc 99m-pertechnetate (used in thyroid scans); technetium Tc 99m-macroaggregated albumin (used in lung scans); and technetium 99m-methylene diphosphonate (used in bone scans).

Nuclear scans utilizing radioisotopes provide a pictorial record of "hot spots" in an area, and the graphic display reflects increased areas of metabolic activity. Single photon emission computed tomography (SPECT) is another nuclear diagnostic method, as is positron emission tomography (PET) scans. PET scans are utilized most often in oncology clients to track disorders such as colorectal carcinomas; soft tissues cancers; lung, head, and neck cancers; primary carcinomas; and breast and metastatic brain tumors (Mountz and Hetherington, 2000).

Most nuclear scans are performed on an outpatient basis with the exception of the ventilation perfusion (V/Q) scan in suspected pulmonary embolism. Indications for a nuclear scan include the following:

- When there is an index of suspicion for osteomyelitis
- In a lung scan when pulmonary embolism is being ruled out
- For a thyroid scan when ultrasound has proven inconclusive
- In a thallium stress test when the client has chest pain of unknown etiology

DECISION-MAKING FOR PLAIN FILMS

According to the American College of Radiology (ACR, 1995), the usual starting point for diagnostic imaging is the plain x-ray. Plain films enable examination of anatomic structures. If these findings are normal, and client symptoms persist, a more sophisticated diagnostic imaging study may be warranted.

The ACR attempted to determine when it is appropriate to order diagnostic x-rays. Extensive input from physicians and numerous health-care providers was elicited in order to develop practical and credible clinical decision-making criteria for ordering these tests. It was decided that the practitioner ordering the radiological test must understand the rationale for ordering the test, as well as the specified and predicted limitations of the specified tests.

Another set of decision-making criteria for ordering plain x-rays was developed in Canada and is known as the Ottawa Rules (Box 4-2). The Ottawa Rules were developed to determine which clients have indications for x-rays based on clinical examination. These rules were designed for clinical examination of extremities and are not limited to injuries. These are specific, detailed clinical indicators for extremity x-rays including, but not limited to, injuries of the knee, ankle, wrist, elbow, and hand.

The Ottawa Rules provide clear, concise indicators for ordering x-rays. Clinical research reports a positive correlation between better decision-making and implementation of the Ottawa Rules. The sections that follow will describe the most commonly ordered diagnostic radiological tests.

GENERAL CONCEPTS RELATED TO RADIOLOGIC IMAGING

Plain films (referred to in some texts as standard films) provide a two-dimensional view of three-dimensional information. In order to obtain accuracy, x-rays will be ordered to be taken from different views.

X-rays usually consist of anterior-posterior (front to back) views, posterior-anterior (back to front) views, lateral (side to side) views, or oblique (at an angle) views. These views are necessary to provide accurate detail in a specific area. For example, if the practitioner orders only an anterior-posterior film when a fracture is suspected there will be no data to determine if there is angulation. Angulation indicates the degree of displacement in the bone and is essential information in order for the orthopedist to decide the treatment plan. The client will have to to be moved into different positions to maximize radiologic technique. This is extremely difficult, if not impossible, if the client cannot cooperate or lie quietly. Adequate pain control will facilitate imaging and maximize efficiency.

X-rays are indicated when there is known or suspected trauma or injury. Information about the

---

Box 4-2

Ottawa Rules for Obtaining X-rays of Knee, Ankle, Wrist, Elbow, Foot, and Hand

Knee
- Only if client is older than 55
- Isolated tenderness of the patella
- Tenderness at the head of the fibula
- Inability to flex the knee 90 degrees
- Inability to bear weight at the time of trauma or presently

Ankle
- Only if there is pain in the malleolar zone and any of the following:
- Focal tenderness at posterior edge or tip of the lateral malleolus
- Bone tenderness posterior edge or tip of medial malleolus
- Inability to bear weight at the time of trauma or presently

Wrist
- If there is discrete tenderness or obvious deformity
- Localized pain
- There is no tenderness above (do wrist film only)
- Focal tenderness on radial and ulnar sides
- No tenderness beyond the wrist joint (do wrist film only)

Elbow
- When the client reports a "dull" ache
- If there is difficulty localizing the pain

Foot
- Only if there is pain in the midfoot zone and any of the following:
- Bone tenderness at the base of 5th metatarsal
- Bone tenderness at the navicular
- Inability to bear weight at the time of trauma or presently

Hand
- Required only if there is focal tenderness or obvious deformity.

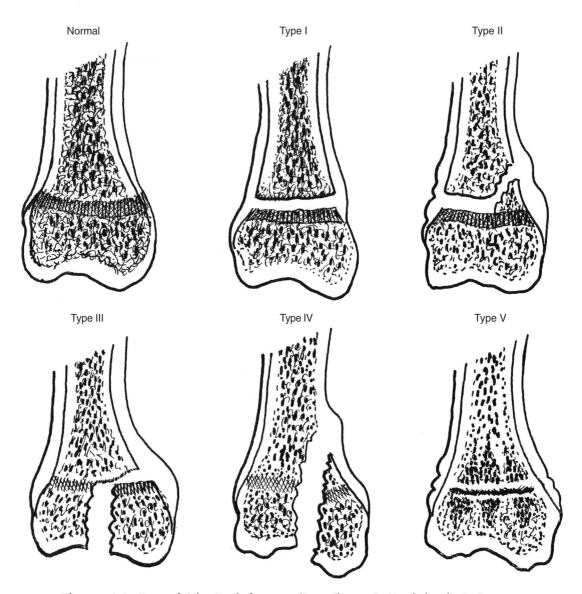

Figure 4-1   Types of Salter-Harris fractures. (From Simone R, Koenigsknecht S: *Emergency orthopedics,* ed 3, Stamford, Conn., 1996, Appleton & Lange.)

mechanics of the injury will help determine the diagnostic test as well as the views that should be ordered. A work-related injury may be a potential for a disability claim. X-rays are also important to obtain when there is a history of trauma in the pediatric and adolescent population. There is great potential liability for a missed epiphyseal fracture in pediatric clients. An injury to the growth plate otherwise referred to as the epiphysis will result in delayed growth of the bone in the affected extremity.

Epiphyseal fractures are also known as Salter-Harris fractures. The five classifications of Salter-Harris fractures are illustrated in Figure 4-1. The epiphyseal fracture may be missed on film readings; therefore it is important that there be clinical correlation with the affected extremity. It is extremely helpful when the person who examines the client also reviews the films for clinical correlation. An epiphyseal fracture may not be radiologically visible, and treatment must be based on clinical examination. Epiphyseal fractures that are not readily seen are referred to as occult fractures. Children often have occult fractures in joints. These are commonly the result of a fracture through the epiphyseal plate. The epiphyseal plate is also known as the "growth plate."

Only 6% of all epiphyseal fractures are type I Salter fractures; however it is important that the practitioner be aware of them because clients usually present as normal on plain films. Clinically, these clients will have focal tenderness, limited or decreased range of motion, and swelling over the epiphyseal plate.

In the adult population, the scaphoid bone in the hand is a common place for an occult fracture. A client with a scaphoid fracture also referred to as navicular fracture will present with tenderness in the hand over the anatomic area known as the snuffbox (Figure 4-2). This anatomic area is located near the wrist, a space that once was used to place smokeless tobacco or snuff. A scaphoid fracture in this area can be present without obvious alteration of bone integrity on a plain film. Clinical examination of a person with a scaphoid fracture will reveal tenderness over the area. Trauma to this area can also disrupt the arterial blood supply, leading to necrosis of the scaphoid bone in the hand.

Missed scaphoid fractures are highly litigious, as are missed epiphyseal fractures. Clients who are at risk of having an occult fracture should be properly splinted and referred to an orthopedist for evaluation. Clients should be advised that some fractures may not be seen on the initial x-ray, and if pain persists and they are not pain free in 7 to 10 days, they may need a repeat film. The rationale for this is that some fractures do not show up readily but will show up on repeat films obtained 7 to 10 days after the injury. The diagnosis should be "rule out occult fracture" or "possible epiphyseal fracture." The documentation by the practitioner in the medical record should include data that the patient and the significant other (in the case of children,

the parents) are informed of the potential of an occult fracture and the necessity for reevaluation and/or follow-up by an orthopedist.

Head

Plain films of the skull do not usually provide benefit to the client. Skull films are not particularly helpful; some texts refer to skull films as "useless" (Mettler, 1996). If the client history reveals head trauma without loss of consciousness, a plain film will yield little benefit. If the client reports a significant head trauma with loss of consciousness, however, a CT scan of the head without intravenous contrast would be the diagnostic test of choice. The CT scan will be used to rule out hematoma or obvious bleeding. If the clinical examination reveals palpable or visible evidence of crepitus or obvious skull deformity, the test of choice would be either a CT scan of the brain without intravenous contrast or, in tertiary care centers, an MRI.

A CT scan may be indicated in some children with headaches. The decision for enhanced diagnostic imaging should be based on the clinical examination and neurological assessment of the child (Diamond, 1999). Neuroimaging is indicated if there are clinical indicators for significant intracranial pathology. According to Diamond and Moore (1999), neuroimaging is indicated in clients with headaches when certain high-risk clinical features are noted. These features are listed in Table 4-2.

In cases where head trauma has been significant enough to produce loss of consciousness, a CT scan will provide a higher yield and may rule out a cerebral bleed. These scans should only be done without intravenous contrast because the contrast media can extend a bleed. Cerebrovascular accidents (CVAs) can be hemorrhagic or ischemic (Mettler, 1996). In the event of an acute hemorrhagic stroke, the bleed can be visualized as very dense on the CT scan. A negative CT scan result does not rule out a stroke if the CT is obtained within 12 hours of the onset of symptoms. The client must be treated clinically because the CT scan can produce a false-negative result.

It is difficult to detect an ischemic stroke on CT scan unless there is some mass effect, whereas an MRI in this situation would have a high yield because edema can be detected (Mettler, 1996).

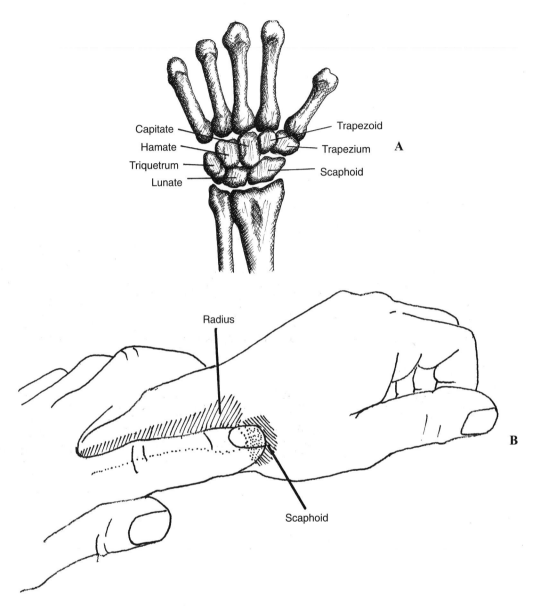

Capitate
Hamate
Triquetrum
Lunate
Trapezoid
Trapezium
Scaphoid

A

Radius

Scaphoid

B

Figure 4-2 **A,** The scaphoid bone in the hand is a common place for an occult fracture. **B,** A client with a scaphoid fracture will present with tenderness in the hand over the anatomic area near the wrist known as the "snuffbox." (From Simone R, Koenigsknecht S: *Emergency orthopedics,* ed 3, Stamford, Conn., 1996, Appleton & Lange.)

Indications for CT scan of the brain with intravenous contrast include, but are not limited to, metastasis or dementia (which is usually not very helpful, showing atrophy with or without chronic changes; see Box 4-3). Multiple sclerosis can usu-

ally only be effectively imaged by the MRI (Mettler, 1996).

CT scans should be done in clients of any age, if indicated. It is important to note that some clients will need to be sedated in order to have

Table 4-2
Incidence of Clinically Significant
Intracranial Disease

Symptom/Population	Incidence
Sudden severe headache	1 in 3
Acute unexplained headache	About 1 in 16
Recent onset headaches (weeks to months)	About 1 in 300
Chronic daily headaches	1 in 1000
Typical migraine	1 in 3000
General population	1 in 3000

Adapted from Diamond S, Moore KL: When is MRI or CT warranted?, *Consultations in Primary Care: Consultant* 39(9):2529-2532, 1999.

Box 4-3

Indications for Ordering a CT Scan of the Head

- History of head trauma with unknown loss of consciousness but change in behavior
- History of head trauma with known loss of consciousness
- Head trauma in client on anticoagulant therapy
- Head trauma in client with known bleeding dyscrasia
- New onset seizure disorder
- Unexplained new onset neurologic changes
- Unexplained new onset confusion

---

them remain quiet during the scanning. For example, a young child or an elderly patient with dementia might have to be sedated in order to lie quietly enough to obtain an accurate diagnostic CT scan.

Sinus Films

The Waters' view provides the best view of sinuses. In this view, the head is tilted back, providing optimal visualization of the maxillary sinuses. A lateral view increases visualization of the sphenoid sinuses. It is inappropriate to order sinus films for young children to rule out sinusitis. Children do not have well-developed sinuses until about 5 to 6

years of age. Most often the diagnosis of sinusitis can be made based on clinical examination of the client and palpation of the maxillary and frontal sinuses.

A client with sinusitis would have air-fluid levels in the sinus. Trauma to the sinuses may also produce air-fluid levels. Clients with chronic sinusitis will have a thickening of the sinuses as well as an indistinct appearance on plain films (Mettler, 1996).

Facial Fractures

When a client reports facial trauma, diagnostic imaging may be needed to rule out facial fractures. The imaging study should be a CT of the facial bones. Plain films are often used to detect a facial fracture, but serious fractures can be missed. The decision to order facial films really lies in the urgency of the results and how this will affect client outcome. For example, a client who has been in an altercation and is clinically suspected of having a fracture of the orbit should have a CT of facial bones.

Mandible Films

A fall or trauma to the chin can produce a fracture in the mandible. Most often these mandibular fractures occur in the temporomandibular joint (TMJ). A TMJ fracture will induce pain when the client attempts to open the mouth. Range of motion of the jaw will be impaired. The clinical examination may reveal focal tenderness over the TMJ region, or there may be crepitus. A mandibular fracture is a certainty if there is malocclusion after the injury. The clearest visualization of this anatomic area is with a Panorex view of the mandible. The Panorex provides a view as though the mandible were flattened out and is the image of choice. A plain film, usually a standard oblique view of the mandible, can be obtained but it is more difficult to interpret and should only be done if Panorex is not available. Mandibular fractures are common in persons who have had direct trauma such as a fist to the chin or falling and hitting chin on a hard surface. Many toddlers fall while learning to walk and suffer a laceration to the chin. In these cases, a mandibular fracture should be ruled out.

Nasal Bones

Nasal bone films are useful in determining depression or lateral deviation after nasal trauma. Parents bring their children to have nasal films after sports injuries or other facial trauma. The customary expectation is that a bone that could be fractured should be filmed regardless of the yield or cost benefit. In other words, health-care consumers may demand a film that essentially has little or no benefit. Nasal fractures are often the result of sports-related injuries such as a player's arm striking another player in the nose or a blow to the nasal area from a ball, bat, or hockey stick.

Orbital Fractures

An orbital fracture may result when there has been direct trauma to the globe of the eye. An orbital fracture is a significant injury and, more often than not, is due to direct trauma from a small object. The mechanism of action is through the pressure created on the eyeball that actually fractures the medial or inferior orbit walls. The Waters' view of the sinuses is the best film for determining this type of fracture (Novelline, 1997). A missed orbital fracture can result in meningitis because of its anatomic proximity to the meninges.

Le Fort Fracture

A Le Fort fracture is most often the result of substantial facial trauma. Le Fort fractures are referred to in some texts as blow-out fractures (Novelline, 1997). A Le Fort fracture is most commonly seen in sports-related injuries where there is a blow to the face with a baseball or a baseball bat (Novelline, 1997). In these types of blunt trauma to the face, it is critical to order a CT of facial bones to rule out a Le Fort fracture.

These fractures are classified as Le Fort I, II, and III. A Le Fort I is a fracture through the maxilla and can be the result of direct trauma to the upper mouth with an object. The Le Fort II is more extensive, resulting in injury to the maxilla, nose, and the inferior and medial orbital walls. A Le Fort III is even more extensive and results in a separation of the face and the skull. The Le Fort III is associated with a high mortality rate and intense facial and head trauma.

A CT of facial bone would provide a higher yield of accurate findings than plain films. It is easier to miss a Le Fort I fracture on a plain film than with CT of facial bones.

Zygoma Films

At the zygomatic process, the zygomatic arch and the skull form a bony ring. This area has been described as "pretzel-like" (Mettler, 1996). When a pretzel breaks, it does not break in one place, but rather in multiple places. For this reason if a fracture of the zygoma is suspected, a "jug handle" view should be ordered. This view allows a look at the zygomatic arch.

In a fracture of the zygoma, if the mechanism of injury is forceful or traumatic enough, the provider needs to rule out a tripod fracture. The tripod fracture actually includes breaks in four structures: the zygomatic arch, lateral orbital rim, inferior orbital rim, and the lateral wall of the maxillary sinus (Mettler, 1996). These fractures occur most commonly in children and the elderly when the person has fallen and landed with full force on the chin. This type of fracture should be ruled out in any client who has a chin laceration or history of jaw trauma, particularly if there is malocclusion of the teeth.

Soft Tissue of the Neck

Films for soft tissue of the neck should be ordered when there is any suspicion of interference with the client's airway (Novelline, 1997). This means that soft tissue of the neck films should be ordered whenever there is suspicion of foreign body, retropharyngeal abscess, tonsillar abscess, croup, suspected obstruction, epiglottitis, thyroid mass, history of direct trauma, or subcutaneous emphysema.

Soft Tissue Mass

A routine radiograph should be ordered first on any soft tissue mass. If the plain film is negative, then MRI should be done. A plain film is necessary because a view of the bones and soft tissue will be helpful in selecting the second study (ACR, 1995). The MRI will help evaluate soft tissue masses.

Spinal Column

Cervical Spine Plain cervical spine films should be ordered when there has been a history of cervical spine trauma. These films should include an open mouth view to visualize the odontoid, and AP and lateral views as well as good visualization of C7 and T1. These views are the minimal standard for cervical spine trauma. In patients who present complaining of lateral neck pain following a history of trauma, but who have normal plain films, flexion and extension views are warranted. These are common in injuries related to sports such as wrestling, and after automobile trauma in which the person was seatbelted and jolted forward.

In cervical spine injuries, when plain films are normal, yet there is persistent pain or neurological indications, an MRI of the cervical spine should be ordered. It is important to note that a CT scan should not be a first line diagnostic method in evaluation of a cervical spine injury. Prior to the CT, there should always be a plain film of the complete cervical spine. The plain film is essential to evaluate stability and integrity of the cervical spine prior to obtaining the CT scan. It is important to understand that a CT scan of the cervical spine will not give a true picture of the alignment of the vertebral bodies.

An MRI of the cervical spine is the diagnostic test of choice in evaluation of the cervical spine if plain films are normal and neurologic signs or symptoms are present. If there is contraindication for MRI, or there is no MRI capability, then it would be appropriate to order a CT myelography. CT myelography is the standard of care if and only if MRI is not available or the client cannot tolerate having an MRI.

If there is suspected damage to the C2 vertebra based on plain films, conventional tomography or CT with reformatting should be done.

Thoracic Spine A thoracic spine film should be ordered when there is a history of trauma or when the client complains of symptoms. Plain thoracic films of the thoracic spine are taken in the AP and the lateral views (Mettler, 1996). The AP view provides an assessment of the alignment of the vertebra as well as the integrity of the bone mass, vertebral pedicles, and the paraspinous ligaments. Children have a normal variant that could be misinterpreted as a fracture in thoracic spine films. This is an apophysis that is seen on the lateral view and could be mistaken for a fracture. Another common variant found in older persons, particularly women with osteoporosis, are compression fractures of the mid- to lower thoracic spine. The challenge in these clients is not whether or not these are new or old fractures, but rather if they could be indicative of metastatic disease.

There are clients who have felt a "pull" or "tearing" at work while lifting an object. In these cases, the yield from a plain film will not be much; however, the plain film does have benefit in allowing a look at the baseline integrity of the structure and composition of the bones. This is particularly helpful and important in cases involving Workman's Compensation, and when injuries have the potential to result in lost time or work-related claims. For example, when a person with chronic back problems gets injured at work, a plain thoracic film could allow visualization of degenerative joint disease. This kind of disease increases the likelihood of chronic pain and further exacerbates symptoms. This official radiological report then becomes a permanent part of the health care record.

A client experiencing pain in the thoracic spine unrelated to trauma could have a thoracic spine tumor, although this is a very rare presentation. Elderly women with osteoporosis typically will present with acute pain for compression fracture of the thoracic spine.

Lumbar Spine X-rays of the lumbosacral spine are indicated for low back pain in the following circumstances: a recent significant trauma; evidence of malignancy in the body; age less than 18 or more than 50 years; unresolved back pain for longer than 10 days; prior to specialist referral; in cases of fever, weight loss, adenopathy, or other signs of systemic illness; with a history of alcoholism or IV drug use; with a history of tuberculosis; in the presence of neurological deficits; and when litigation or compensation is intended.

The lumbar portion of the spine is a common site for injury. The majority of persons who present with chronic back pain or acute injury to the spine, present with lumbar region symptomatology. The lumbar views which should be ordered are AP, lateral, another lateral of L5-S1, and oblique views

(Mettler, 1996). The additional view of L5-S1 is necessary because of the increased soft tissue and the need for increased penetration of these areas to adequately visualize the bones.

As with any spine film, the AP view allows visualization of alignment, in this case of the sacroiliac (SI) joint and sacrum. This is important because the SI joint can be narrowed in some pathologies (particularly with ankylosing spondylitis) or it can be widened (in the event of a pelvic fracture). The LS spine area is another very common site for vertebral subluxation. An oblique view of the LS spine provides information regarding the facets, which are typically referred to as the "Scottie dog."

The fractures occurring most frequently in the lumbar spine area are wedge compression fractures and burst fractures. Degenerative changes can be visualized on plain radiographs; however, a CT or MRI could be used as a second level of diagnostic testing. The anatomic area for the CT scan should be specified because the CT is made up of many cuts through each plane of the disk spaces. The MRI is used most often as a second diagnostic test. The MRI is particularly helpful in diagnosing a protruding disk or extreme degenerative changes. The MRI is the standard of care in diagnostic imaging to rule out neuronal impingement.

Upper Extremity Films

Shoulder and Humerus Symptomatology of the shoulder usually requires a plain AP or PA view of the shoulder in which the arm is internally and externally rotated. These views help to visualize the humeral head and are particularly helpful in diagnostics related to symptomatology or posttraumatic events. An AP view was determined by the American College of Radiology to be the standard to rule out a fracture or dislocation following acute shoulder trauma. There has been controversy among experts about whether or not to obtain axillary lateral or transcapular "Y" radiological views of the shoulder when a fracture or dislocation is suspected. The Y view or the axillary view aids in assessing the humeral head in reference to the glenoid fossa. Posterior dislocations of the shoulder are rare; anterior dislocations account for over 95% of all shoulder dislocations. Most practitioners will order these views based on the clinical

criteria of whether or not the client can move the shoulder.

AP and lateral views of the shoulder should be obtained if it appears dislocated or if the client reports a decreased range of motion. It is very important to order the AP and lateral views in order to assess the degree of angulation in the event of a dislocation.

Persistent shoulder pain lasting 2 weeks posttrauma, with initial normal radiographic findings, should have plain films repeated prior to ordering any additional tests such as CT scan or MRI. If there is an index of suspicion for a rotator cuff tear in the shoulder, and plain films are normal, the client should have an MRI of the shoulder. These clients typically present with a history of dull, aching pain that has been persistent; with or without a history of prior injury or trauma; and a limited ability to abduct the arm higher than 25 to 45 degrees. If there is no history of known trauma, these clients will usually report a chronic aching pain in the shoulder that has persisted for quite some time. Rotator cuff injuries often result from a jolting or shearing force to the shoulder.

A shoulder film will allow visualization of the acromioclavicular (AC) area as well as the scapula. A view of the AC space can be obtained by having the client hold weights in both hands. This weight helps to extend the acromioclavicular space and determine an AC separation. The acromioclavicular separation can also be suspected on clinical examination of the client without this special view.

While it is highly irregular and very difficult to fracture a scapula, a scapular film can be ordered. A scapular fracture would usually be trauma-related, such as after a fall or significant blunt injury. Scapular fractures are quite rare.

Elbow Many falls in persons of all ages will result in a trauma to the elbow, particularly the olecranon area. These clients present with an inability to fully flex or extend the arm. This clinical finding is common in radial head fractures. The primary bony injury is difficult to detect by x-ray. In the adult, the lateral view will usually have a bulging of the anterior fat pad known as "sail sign" (because it takes on the appearance of a boat sail) or the presence of a posterior fat pad. Even if the bones appear normal these positive fat pad signs are indicative of an occult or hidden radial head fracture and should be referred for orthopedic evaluation.

The common elbow injury in children is a radial head dislocation often referred to as nursemaid's elbow. This injury is often the result of trauma, particularly when someone attempts to pull or raise the child by the hand with elbow full extended. Often this dislocation will be reduced while attempting to get plain films of the child's elbow.

A plain film should be ordered if there is a history of trauma to the patient. For example, a parent might report that the child fell while running and has not used the arm since the fall. In this case there is a high index of suspicion for a fracture, and the practitioner would not want to reduce the dislocation until a fracture is ruled out. This is very important, particularly in the child who may have an epiphyseal fracture. Supracondylar fractures in children are very serious due to neurovascular compromise, and these injuries warrant emergency orthopedic evaluation and treatment.

Wrist   Plain films of the wrist include the AP, lateral, and oblique views. Children up to the age of 12 years usually warrant a comparison view of the opposite extremity. It is important for the practitioner to explain this necessity to the parents, who often perceive that the radiology technician is making a mistake or that the child is receiving too much radiation exposure. Comparison views enable comparison of areas difficult to assess. This is particularly true in cases such as a suspected epiphyseal fracture in the wrist.

A majority of falls in all age groups result in fractures to the hand or wrist area. This is true in osteoporotic women, who have markedly decreased bone density secondary to severe bone demineralization. Any time there is a history of fall or trauma, and complaint of pain in the wrist, a plain film consisting of AP, lateral, and oblique views is indicated.

The most common fractures in the wrist area are Colle's fractures, involving a fracture of the distal radius; and a fracture of the ulnar styloid. There are 8 carpal bones in the hand: the trapezoid (lesser multangular), trapezium (greater multangular), capitate, hamate, triquetrum, pisiform, lunate, and scaphoid or navicular.

In the event of a suspected navicular fracture, a special navicular view may be ordered. Navicular fractures are one of the most commonly missed fractures. In the event of tenderness in the wrist area known as the snuffbox, this must be treated aggressively as an occult navicular fracture. A navicular fracture is critical to assess for because there is a unique arterial blood supply in this area. An undiagnosed or missed navicular fracture can result in aseptic necrosis to the hand. It is for this reason that the practitioner must be aware of the liability involved in any missed fracture. A missed navicular fracture carries an increased liability.

Hand   Hand films should include the AP, lateral, and oblique views. Hand films should be ordered when there is a history of trauma or when the client reports pain that is unexplained. Even in the event that a client presents with an injury of the hand (including digits) that may be as much as 7 days prior, it is important to obtain plain films of the area. Many clients will have what they believe to be a minor trauma to the hand and treat it conservatively. They present to the practitioner because the pain has persisted. Persistent pain after an injury is important because sometimes, early in a fracture, there is hyperemia of the fracture with accompanying reabsorption of calcium.

A client can have a very small avulsion fracture in the joint space of the fingers. In orthopedic literature, these are classified as orthopedic emergencies. Failure to identify an avulsion fracture of the joint can result in a frozen joint. This is particularly important in younger clients. In children, this type of avulsion can involve the epiphysis and result not only in a frozen joint but also in retarded growth because of the epiphyseal involvement. There may be no definite observable fracture in these cases, and the official radiology report may be somewhat noncommittal in stating that there is no definite fracture observed. It may, however, suggest repeat films in 7 to 10 days (Mettler, 1996) or recommend clinical correlation. Clinical correlation means that the area of question in the x-ray correlates to the client's area of pain. If the client is focally tender or point tender in the area of question on the x-ray, this indicates a fracture.

Practitioners may be questioned about the rationale for repeat films. Once again, this information should be included in the client's medical record to justify the treatment plan and rationale for care. This is a litigious area, and the practitioner must take care to be fully aware and knowledgeable about the pitfalls and hazards involved with missed fractures.

Plain films of the hand should also be done when there is any index of suspicion of foreign body. Often a client will deny any recollection of a foreign body; however, this is an important diagnostic "rule out." A missed foreign body carries a very high price tag in terms of liability. Clients must always be advised of the potential of a missed foreign body, and documentation of this conversation should be placed in the client's medical record. There should also be an entry that the client and/or significant other verbalize knowledge and understanding of the potential for a missed foreign body and implications of the same.

Common foreign bodies in the hand are metallic fragments, glass, lead, and fragments of wood. Metallic foreign bodies are easy to spot on x-ray, but lead and wood usually are not. There is controversy over films when glass is a suspected potential foreign body. Glass is usually radiopaque and not clearly visible; however it is usually recognized because of its shape or distinct sharpness. Some practitioners will only get a plain film to rule out glass as a foreign body if there is a potential that the glass contained lead.

There are two very common fractures of the hand: the boxer's fracture and the Bennett and Rolando fracture. A boxer's fracture usually occurs when the client strikes an object with a clenched fist, resulting in a fracture at the base of the fifth metacarpal. There is usually a high index of suspicion of this fracture based on clinical examination, and the films confirm it as well as being helpful in noting whether or not there is any degree of angulation or displacement of the bones. The Bennett and Rolando fracture is a triangular fracture at the base of the first metacarpal.

Lower Extremity Films

Pelvis   When there is a history of fall or trauma, AP and oblique views should be obtained on the plain film. The AP pelvis will provide views of the iliac wings, ischium, pubis, bilateral hips, and the LS spine. Client history is very important,

and the decision to order pelvic films is not always clear-cut. For example, an elderly person may forget that he or she had a fall prior to the onset of discomfort, and there may be no other clinical indicators of prior trauma (such as bruising). An elderly woman with significant osteoporosis who sustains a fall may report no immediate loss of functional status; but over time she may develop an inability to ambulate or to move from lying to sitting or sitting to standing positions because of extreme pain in the hips or pelvic areas. In this population, pubic rami fractures can often be missed. In some cases the pubic rami fracture may not be seen but the client has agonizing pain and cannot ambulate.

Clients with pubic rami fractures will often complain of groin pain. Clients with pubic rami fractures sometimes must be admitted secondary to inability to ambulate and intractable acute pain. They will often require pain control in the form of either intramuscular or intravenous analgesia.

A coccyx film is a commonly ordered film that is not really helpful or contributory in any way to the treatment plan. It does appear in Western cultures that people demand to know if there is a fracture even if this information does not change the decision-making and treatment plan. A film showing a fractured coccyx will not alter client care at all. To say that a coccyx film is never useful would be inaccurate: the film may be of some value in documenting baseline if there is potential liability or suspected abuse. The rationale for a coccyx film should be carefully documented in the client medical record in the event the decision is called into question at some future time.

Some pelvic traumas may warrant a CT scan. If trauma was sufficient to cause a pelvic fracture, there indeed may be surrounding soft tissue injury or a hematoma within the pelvis (Mettler, 1996). There may be serious or life-threatening injuries, such as renal damage, even when plain films are negative. Suspicion is based on the client's clinical examination. This is particularly important when there is a potential for a fragment in the SI joint. This is a common problem in elderly osteoporotic women who have had a fall or other trauma and ambulate with severe pain or not at all.

Hip   Plain films of the hip should consist of an AP view; "frog leg" view, if possible; and a lateral view. In the event of a hip fracture, this is essential in determining the degree of angulation, if any. The frog leg view allows abduction of the hip. The goal in plain films of the hip is to determine the relationship of the acetabulum and the head of the femur (Mettler, 1996).

The most common fractures in the hip are of the acetabulum or the intertrochanteric region (Novelline, 1997). Hip fractures may be missed in the elderly client because there may be extensive osteoporosis.

Some clients cannot provide an adequate history, and may have experienced trauma that was neither witnessed nor known. It is critical to assess whether or not there has been any recent injury, no matter how slight or insignificant it may have seemed to the client or the significant other. For example, a nursing assistant helping place a client in bed slips and loses her balance, falling across the side of the bed. The assistant presents for examination 10 days later, complaining of extreme left hip pain, but reports that she had ambulated on the extremity for 10 days and never suspected a fracture. Some practitioners erroneously believe that if the client can ambulate, then the extremity is not fractured. This is certainly not the case and there are many exceptions to this way of thinking.

An AP pelvis film should be ordered when there is an index of suspicion for avascular necrosis in the hip. The frog leg view is a necessity in suspicion of avascular necrosis in order to evaluate the femoral head from an anterosuperior perspective (Novelline, 1997). If the plain film reflects a mottled femoral head, and there is suspicion for avascular necrosis in a painful hip, an MRI is the next step. The MRI would provide a definitive diagnosis in this case. The MRI is the most sensitive and highly specified modality in determining avascular necrosis if plain films are negative and pain persists.

Femur Femur films should be taken from AP and lateral views. It is important to ascertain whether or not there is angulation or dislocation of the femur. On occasion, the x-ray technician may report difficulty in obtaining quality or provide limited films because of the client's acute pain, particularly if there has been a traumatic event or there is acute exacerbation of chronic pain. The client should be medicated to a level of comfort in order to obtain the best views.

Knee A child or adolescent who presents with nontraumatic knee pain should have an AP standing or supine knee film. The same films are deemed to be the minimal mandatory films on a child or adult who presents with patellofemoral (anterior) knee pain. Lateral and axial views are also indicated in patellofemoral (anterior) knee joints as the mandatory minimal views.

The American College of Radiology (ACR, 1995) recommends as the mandatory minimal standard that an adult with nontraumatic, nonlocalized pain have an AP, lateral view of the knee. The ACR also recommends that an MRI is indicated in a child or adolescent with non-patellofemoral symptomatology if the initial plain AP and lateral views were not diagnostic or significant. An MRI is indicated in a child with a suspected joint effusion.

Lateral knee films would be taken with the client's knee in partial flexion. This view is important in determining whether or not there is a joint effusion as well as integrity of the patella (Mettler, 1996). AP and lateral views of the knee are useful in determining fractures, degenerative joint disease, and integrity of the proximal tibia and distal femur.

There are two additional views of the knee that the practitioner should be familiar with. These are the sunrise view and the tunnel view. The sunrise is a view looking from the top down and it helps to determine the relationship of the patella to the anterior femur. In the tunnel view, the knee is more flexed and the x-ray captures more of the tunnel that is created by the femoral condyles.

MRI of the knee is much more definitive for diagnosing more subtle ligamentous injuries, including anterior cruciate ligament as well as medial and lateral meniscus pathologies. MRIs are commonly done in sports-related knee injuries.

Tibia/Fibula Tibia films should include both AP and lateral views. It is crucial that films include the entire length of the bone and go from the tibial plateau to the ankle joint (Mettler, 1996). Tibia fractures are not always discrete, and a client can complain of knee or tibial plateau pain for several weeks or months after an injury in which the ankle or knee was slightly twisted. Once again, the practitioner should be cautious not to focus on recent traumatic events, but rather to query the client about previous injuries that may have seemed slight at the time.

Another commonly missed injury to the tibia occurs when a force causes the client to twist while keeping the feet planted in place. This can produce enough torque to twist the tibial plateau and cause an avulsion fracture in this area. Again, there will be no obvious findings on clinical examination and the fracture can be missed.

Ankle   Ankle films should be obtained in AP, lateral, and oblique views because there are a number of fractures which can only be visualized in the oblique view and not in AP or lateral views. The oblique view provides a detailed view of the mortise (Mettler, 1996). The most common ankle injuries occur in either the lateral or medial malleolar areas.

The lateral injury commonly occurs when the mechanics of the reported injury involved an outward rolling of the ankle (inversion), or that the client came down on the outside of the ankle. These clients often say they have not been able to bear weight on the extremity since the event.

Medial malleolar injuries occur with trauma the client reports as a twisting inward (eversion) of the ankle. Sometimes the trauma is so great or conditions are such that the client will have a break in both the lateral and medial malleolus. This is referred to as a bimalleolar fracture. In other situations the client literally shatters the medial and lateral malleolar areas as well as the distal tibia. This fracture is referred to a trimalleolar.

Clients who have sustained significant ankle trauma and have no fractures, but may have joint laxity or extreme ligamentous tenderness, should be reevaluated by the orthopedic surgeon. They may, in fact, be candidates for an MRI to determine the extent of the ligamentous injury.

Foot   When a foot film is clinically indicated, films should be obtained in the AP, lateral, and oblique views. As in the hand, the dorsum of the foot contains many smaller, more well-rounded bones that can suffer occult fractures. These commonly occur when a person jambs a foot into the brake while attempting to stop quickly to avoid an accident. This type of fracture was seen so often in pilots who pushed their feet into the cockpit that it was named "aviator's fracture" (Mettler, 1996). It is important to tell the client about this, and also to document the potential of a missed fracture in the foot or in any part of the body that is not pain free and functioning normally within a reasonable time. As previously mentioned, clients should always be advised to have the extremity reevaluated in 7 to 10 days if the pain persists. Another fracture that can be missed in foot trauma is the calcaneal or talus fracture. This can occur when a client falls, landing on the feet on a hard surface.

A client may also deny having any fall or trauma in the foot but actually have a stress fracture from repetitive or strenuous activity. Stress fractures usually can be seen distally in the second, third, or fourth metatarsal.

Chest Films   Chest x-rays are usually done in a healthy client in the PA (posterior/anterior) view. In this view, the x-ray beam is shot from behind the standing client toward the anterior side. A lateral chest film should also be ordered unless the client is not able to stand or to tolerate this. The upright position allows for greater visualization of vessels. This is important because airways can demonstrate poor inspiratory effort and appear as an abnormal chest if the client does not stand and take a deep breath in and hold it during the film.

In a frail, debilitated, or emergent client, the film of choice will be an AP view, usually a portable film or one taken while the client is in a lying or semi-Fowler's position. In this case, a lateral view is not usually obtained for obvious reasons.

The major difference between the PA and AP views is the degree of penetration. The heart will appear larger on the AP than on the PA view. The best chest film is the PA, lateral and upright position, to maximize inspiration and visualization of the tissue with increased and maximum spreading of the pulmonary vasculature.

Chest films should typically be performed in the client who presents with a febrile illness and there is no apparent source; in clients who are dyspneic, debilitated, or febrile; and in those clients who cannot verbally communicate their symptoms. It is critical to obtain a chest film in any infant less than 6 months of age who presents with a febrile illness. An infant or toddler greater than 3 months of age is considered to be febrile with a temperature of 100.4° F (38° C) or higher. A significant fever is reported to be 101.3° F. (38.5° C). Fever may have differing interpretations, and the age of the child and the source of the fever are the significant considerations. If there is no visible source for the fever (for example, otitis media or acute pharyngitis), a chest film to rule out pneumonia is essential. A chest film is also essential in a febrile elderly client, particularly those who cannot provide a history or review of systems.

In cases where the clinical examination is unimpressive, and the client is taking and retaining fluids without nausea or vomiting and there are no co-morbid pathologies, a chest film to rule in or rule out pneumonia may not be necessary.

Some clients believe they should have a chest x-ray and be hospitalized if they are diagnosed with pneumonia. Community-acquired pneumonias are often treated on an outpatient basis, and the client is admitted only when this outpatient therapy fails. Approximately 4 million adults are diagnosed each year with community-acquired pneumonia (Meehan et al, 1997). From this total, there will be approximately 600,000 hospital admissions for pneumonia. The elderly population is at high risk for developing community-acquired pneumonia.

A chest film should be obtained when there is any obvious airway compromise. For example, a client who has any clinical indicators of respiratory compromise such as a low pulse oximetry value (less than 90% on oxygen or room air) should have a chest film. Preferably, this would include PA, lateral, and upright views if the client can tolerate this without further compromise to rule out underlying pathology. When there is limited movement of air on auscultation, and airway impairment is present, a chest film is needed. This would be the case in a spontaneous pneumothorax, when a client reports the sudden onset of a sharp, knifelike pain followed by difficulty in breathing. A higher incidence of spontaneous pneumothorax is seen in thin, young men (Mettler, 1996). There may be a need for an additional end-expiratory view (which accentuates the abnormality) to visualize a small, apical pneumothorax.

A chest film should also be obtained in a client with a history of choking or emesis while lying supine. A clinical example would be the client residing in a long-term care facility who has had choking episodes. Examples of those at high risk for aspiration pneumonia or airway compromise would be debilitated elderly clients who have decreased mobility and altered mentation.

Any client suspected of having a pulmonary embolus should have a chest film prior to any more definitive diagnostic tests such as a ventilation perfusion (V-Q) scan. Clients with chest pain should always have a plain film. Plain films are helpful in identifying infiltrates, effusion, or a widened mediastinum (as would be present in aortic aneurysm). If plain films raise an index of further suspicion, the client should have more definitive diagnostics such as a V-Q scan of the lungs or a chest CT on an emergent basis. In the event of pulmonary nodules or index of suspicion of metastasis of a carcinoma, a chest CT could be ordered on an outpatient basis, as could a bronchoscopy with biopsy.

Another time a chest film should be ordered is when there is a history of chest wall trauma or shortness of breath or when rib fractures are suspected. However, it is usually unnecessary and practically useless to obtain rib films in these clients. Once again, the Western culture leads clients to want to have their diagnosis supported with proof. They may appear dissatisfied when informed by the practitioner that rib films are not helpful or necessary. They should be informed that the film of choice is a chest PA and lateral to rule out a pneumothorax. A plain x-ray that reveals a rib fracture will not in any way change the treatment plan.

Abdominal Films The most common abdominal film will be of the kidney, ureters, and bladder (KUB). These films help determine mechanical ileus or intestinal obstruction due to foreign body (FB), neoplasm, gallstones eroding into the gut, meconium bezoars, enteroliths, worms, adhesions, stenosis, hernias, volvulus, and intussusception. They also help determine distended bowel, in the flat plate; and stepladder pattern of air-fluid levels, in the upright or decubitus films. They may also be helpful in renal or biliary tract disease when looking for abnormal calcifications. These films are taken with the client lying in a supine position. Mettler (1996) points out that the term KUB is somewhat misleading since the kidneys, ureter, and bladder are usually not seen on a plain film of the abdomen. Despite this fact, KUB is still a widely used term.

An abdominal film allows a visualization of the bowel gas patterns, the anatomical bony structure, soft tissue, and also the bases of the lungs. Abdominal films are very important in determining any "free air" in the peritoneum, a significant finding. Normally the stomach will have some air in it, and when a client is lying on his/her back, this bubble will move to the anterior portion of the stomach. This would be a normal finding on abdominal films.

Abdominal films include an upright abdomen and an upright PA chest (or left lateral decubitus if the client is unable to stand), providing a 3-dimensional view of the abdomen. This is an absolutely necessary view of the abdomen because it helps to visualize whether or not there is any free air in the peritoneum under the diaphragm, which would be a significant finding and could indicate a rupture of the intestinal viscus.

A client who reports a history of intractable vomiting or abdominal pain should have an abdominal series to rule out obstructive patterns and underlying pathologies. Usual signs and symptoms may be absent or altered in children, the elderly, or immunosuppressed individuals. Further studies such as IV pyelography, unltrasound, or abdominal CT may be indicated in certain patient presentations.

References

American College of Radiology: *Appropriateness criteria for imaging and treatment decisions,* Restin, Va., 1995, ACR Publications.

Chernecky CC, Berger BJ: *Laboratory tests and diagnostic procedures,* ed 2, Philadelphia, 1997, WB Saunders.

Diamond S: *Migraine in children: how to recognize, how to treat,* Consultations in Primary Care: Consultant 39(7):2045-2054, 1999.

Diamond S, Moore KL: When is MRI or CT warranted?, *Consultations in Primary Care: Consultant* 39(9):2529-2532, 1999.

Lowe SW, Pruitt RH, Smart PT, Dooley RL: Routine use of ultrasound during pregnancy, *Nurse Pract* 23(10):60, 63-6, 71, 1998.

Meehan TP et al: Quality of care, process, and outcomes in elderly patients with pneumonia, *JAMA* 278(23):2080-2084, 1997.

Mettler FAJr: *Essentials of radiology,* Philadelphia, 1996, WB Saunders.

Mountz J, Hetherington HP

Novelline RA: *Squire's fundamentals of radiology,* ed 5, Boston, 1997, Harvard Publishing.

Simon KR, Koenigsknecht SJ: The Extremities. In *Emergency orthopedics,* ed 3, Stamford, Conn. 1996, Appleton & Lange.

Taylor RB, editor: *Family medicine: principles and practice,* New York, 1998, Springer-Verlag.

Supplemental Readings

Felson B, Weinstein AS, Spitz HB: *Principles of chest roentgenology,* Philadelphia, 1965, WB Saunders.

McBride PE, Underbakke G: Dyslipidemias. In Taylor RB, editor: *Family medicine: principles and practice,* New York, 1998, Springer-Verlag.

Scheffleer KJ, Tobin RS: *Better x-ray interpretation,* Springhouse, Penn., 1997, Springhouse Publishing.

Washington LJ, Holder MS, Kirksey OW et al: Fever in infants: appropriate management strategies, *Clin Rev* 9(2): 51-64.

part 2 two

CASE ANALYSIS

CHAPTER 5

Special Senses

Jean Nagelkerk

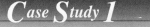

Case Study 1

CHIEF COMPLAINT: Ear Pain

History of Present Illness M.J., a 3-year-old Caucasian male, presents with his father and four siblings, complaining of a sore ear. The patient has a 2-day history of low-grade fever, right ear pain, and crying more than usual. The father has not noticed any drainage from either ear. M.J. has had cold symptoms for a week consisting of a runny nose with thick yellow discharge, cough that occurs mainly at night, and a mild sore throat. He does not have a rash, N/V, H/A, or diarrhea. Negative history of sinusitis and environmental allergies. No history of ventilating tubes. Mother and father smoke in the home and car. Appetite is OK, but he is taking less overall. Elimination is fine. Activity is slightly decreased. Motrin has been given for fever and pain with some relief.

Past Medical History Two visits for ear infections over the past year

Past Surgical History Unremarkable

Family History Mother, father, three brothers and one sister, A&W

Developmental Stage Autonomy versus Shame and Doubt

Role-Relationship Lives with mother, father, three brothers, and one sister in a three-bedroom ranch in the country. Father works second shift in a local factory and mother works day shift at a fast-food restaurant. M.J. and his siblings stay with a neighbor who has five children for 1 hour every day while they wait for their mother to get home from work.

Sleep/Rest M.J. goes to bed at 8:30 PM and sleeps until 9 AM. He takes one nap in the afternoon for 2 to 3 hours.

Nutrition/Metabolic Breakfast, cold or warm cereal; lunch, sandwich or macaroni and cheese; dinner, vegetables, pasta, and meat. Snacks on fruits, crackers, and cookies

Activity/Exercise Is very active playing with his brothers and sister. Enjoys the neighbor children and plays outdoors when supervised

Coping/Stress Enjoys mom and dad reading to him. Watches television whenever he can. Likes to play at the park

Health Management Immunizations up to 6 months

Medications Poly-Vi-Flor drops 1 ml (0.25 mg) qd

Allergies PCN

Pertinent Physical Findings

Vital Signs Height 38 inches; weight 35 pounds; temperature 101.2° F; heart rate 96; respirations 22

HEENT External canals clear. Right TM erythemic with distorted cone of light and indistinct landmarks. Right TM erythemic without bulging or retraction, no drainage noted, and decreasing mobility on insufflation. Left TM pink with distinct cone of light; mobility intact on insufflation. Sinuses: No frontal or maxillary sinus tenderness. Nose: Pink nasal mucosa with yellow drainage. Pharynx: Pink with tonsils 2+ bilaterally. Uvula midline. No cervical lymphadenopathy

Heart Regular rate and rhythm, no murmurs, no S_3 or S_4

Lungs Lungs clear to auscultation

History Data Questions specific to the chief complaint of ear pain include the following:

- For how long and where are you having pain (inside the ear or outside the ear)?
- Are you having itching or drainage from your ear?
- Do you have a runny nose, nasal congestion, headache, sore throat, cough, nausea or vomiting, diarrhea, rashes, or fever?
- Do you have hearing loss, tinnitus, or dizziness?
- Did your symptoms start with an upper respiratory infection?
- Do you have a history of ear infections, sinusitis, or environmental allergies?
- How many ear infections have you had in the past year?
- Have you ever had ventilating tubes placed in your ears?
- Does anyone smoke in the house or car?
- Do you go to daycare?

Physical Examination Data   The focused examination for the chief complaint of ear pain includes vital signs, HEENT (may need to assess conductive hearing loss in adult patients or children who have repeated ear infections; evaluate for tragus, mastoid, and frontal and maxillary sinus tenderness; document assessment findings for the external auditory canal), neck (evaluate lymph node involvement and nuchal rigidity), heart, and lungs.

Differential Diagnoses*   Acute otitis media, serous otitis media, chronic otitis media, otitis externa, mastoiditis, foreign body, TMJ (in an adult patient) (Table 5-1)

Probable Causes of the Presenting Symptoms
Acute otitis media in children under the age of 2 years accounts for 26% of all visits (Rubin et al, 1996). A viral infection typically precedes acute otitis media, causing eustachian tube swelling. The swelling results in accumulation of fluids, which then become infected by bacteria. The three most common organisms causing acute otitis media are *Streptococcus pneumoniae* (40% to 50%),

Haemophilus influenzae (20% to 30%), and *Moraxella catarrhalis* (10% to 15%) (Barnett and Klein, 1995; Jacobs, 1996). Patients are more likely to have spontaneous resolution of acute otitis media if the causative organism is *H. influenza* or *M. catarrhalis* than if it is *S. pneumoniae*. If bullae are noted on the tympanic membrane, an organism that must be considered is *Mycoplasma pneumoniae*. For chronic otitis media, the most common organisms are *P. aeruginosa*, *Proteus* sp., *Staphylococcus aureus*, and mixed anaerobes.

Risk factors for acute otitis media include a history of an upper respiratory infection, allergies, sinusitis, barotrauma, age (higher in infants and children), gender (males more at risk than females), race (Caucasians and Native Americans have a greater incidence), and smoking or exposure to second-hand smoke. Group daycare also increases the exposure to multiple pathogens and puts the child at high risk for acute otitis media.

Diagnostic Tests   Other than tympanometry, no diagnostic tests would be considered for acute otitis media. Tympanometry is the evaluation of the patency and mobility of the tympanic membrane. In otitis media with effusion there is decreased mobility of the tympanic membrane. When tympanostomy tubes are present there is not an airtight seal so the tympanometric reading will be flat. If the patient has frequent episodes of acute otitis media, and there is hearing impairment or speech problems, then audiometry should be done. Rarely will tympanocentesis be performed, and then usually only when the child is less than 2 months old, the patient is critically ill, or for those who do not respond to several antibiotic courses.

Diagnostic Impression   The patient presents with complaint of sore ear. He is running a low-grade fever and crying more than usual. The physical examination reveals R TM erythemic with decreased mobility. M.J.'s diagnosis is acute otitis media (AOM), most likely a result of his upper respiratory infection.

Therapeutic Plan of Care   Amoxicillin is the drug of choice for simple uncomplicated AOM. The standard recommended dosage of amoxicillin is 40 to 50 mg/kg/day bid or tid for 10 days (Dow-

---

*Acute sinusitis and viral pharyngitis may also cause eustachian tube dysfunction. See page 106 for a discussion of viral pharyngitis and page 110 for a discussion of acute sinusitis.

Table 5-1
Ear Pain Differential Diagnostic Cues

Diagnosis	Signs and Symptoms	Lab Data	Treatment
Acute Otitis Media	Otalgia, irritability, fever, erythemic TM, decreased movement of TM	None	Amoxicillin, amoxicillin clavulanate, cefuroxime axetil, ceftriaxone (IM) (see pages 86-87 for antibiotic doses); antihistamines (e.g., loratadine [Claritin] 10 mg QD, cetirizine [Zyrtec] l0 mg qd); or decongestants (e.g., pseudoephedrine HCl [Sudafed] 120 mg bid prn, or phenylpropanolamine HCl 75 mg/guaifenesin 400 mg [Entex LA] bid prn may be used for symptom relief, especially if allergies are possible contributing factor), analgesics, antipyretic, topical Auralgan, otic drops prn
Serous Otitis Media	TM dull and hypomobile, may have conductive hearing loss, air bubbles behind TM	None	For children, oral antibiotics as for acute otitis media; if no resolution after several months, then ventilating tubes. For adults, try decongestant and check for sinusitis and allergies
Otitis Externa (Swimmer's Ear) Preventative measures include using ear plugs when swimming and using 2-3 drops of 1:1:1 solution of vinegar/isopropyl alcohol/water after each water exposure	Otalgia, pruritus, purulent discharge, Hx of water exposure or mechanical trauma, erythema and edema of ear canal, movement of auricle elicits pain	None	Protect from moisture and further trauma; otic drops containing aminoglycoside and antiinflammatory corticosteroid (e.g., neomycin sulfate, polymyxin B sulfate, and hydrocortisone [Cortisporin Otic Suspension]), instill 4 gtts in ear canal qid × 7 days; remove purulent discharge and use wick if ear canal is swollen
Mastoiditis	Postauricular pain, erythema, spiking fever	Radiography shows coalescence of the mastoid air cells	ENT referral, intravenous antibiotics, and myringotomy for C&S. Mastoidectomy if medical therapy fails
Foreign Body	Otalgia, pruritus	None	Removal—do not use aqueous irrigations with items such as insects and beans because they swell
Chronic Otitis Media	Perforation of TM, purulent aural discharge, pain only with acute exacerbation, conductive hearing loss	None	Regular removal of debris; use ear plugs to protect from water exposure, topical antibiotic drops for exacerbation; definitive treatment is surgical
TMJ	Otalgia made worse by chewing or bruxism	None	Soft diet, local heat to masticatory muscles, massage, analgesics, dental referral, stop gum chewing

ell et al, 1999). However, there is evidence supporting a 5 to 7 day course of antibiotics for children older than 2 years of age with uncomplicated AOM (Dowell et al, 1998; Kozyrskyi et al, 1998). For those who are at high risk (that is, younger than 2 years old, with chronic or recurrent otitis media, or with a ruptured tympanic membrane), 10 days of antibiotic therapy is recommended.

For patients who are at high risk for drug-resistant *Streptococcus pneumoniae* (DRSP), the new recommended dosage of amoxicillin is 80 to 90 mg/kg/day (Dowell et al, 1999). High risk factors for DRSP include antimicrobial exposure within the past 3 months, age under 2 years, and attendance at daycare. An alternative therapy to amoxicillin is the use of amoxicillin-clavulanate (Augmentin) 80 to 90 mg/kg/day in two divided doses with the clavulanate dosage remaining at about 10 mg/kg/day to help decrease the incidence of diarrhea.

However, M.J. is allergic to penicillin, so we must use another agent that will cover the most common organisms that cause acute otitis media. Alternative agents are cefuroxime axetil (Ceftin) 30 mg/kg/day in two divided doses; and intramuscular ceftriaxone (Rocephin) in a single injection of 50 mg/kg. (In children who have experienced a treatment failure on another antibiotic, a three-dose regimen of ceftriaxone may be superior.)

Alternative therapies to amoxicillin were recommended by the Centers for Disease Control and Prevention's DRSP Working Group if they met the criteria of effectiveness against beta-lactamase–producing *H. influenzae* and *M. catarrhalis* and against *S. pneumoniae* and most DRSP strains (Dowell et al, 1999). The alternative therapeutic agents include cefuroxime axetil (Ceftin), amoxicillin-clavulanate (Augmentin), and ceftriaxone (Rocephin).

Trimethoprim-sulfamethoxazole (very inexpensive and effective) could be used with this patient, but its reported DRSP effectiveness is about 25%. Erythromycin, a macrolide, has been reported to have DRSP effectiveness of about 10%. Prophylaxis is used when a patient has recurrent ear infections that involve three episodes in 6 months or six episodes in a year. Generally, a low dose of amoxicillin or sulfisoxazole is given daily for several months.

M.J. needs to have his immunizations updated. At his visit today he will need to receive a dose of DTaP (diptheria and tetanus toxoid and acellular pertussis vaccine); MMR (measles, mumps, and rubella vaccine); and Hib (*H. influenzae* type b conjugated vaccine). Also at this visit, a discussion should be held with his father to review the effects of second-hand smoke on increased susceptibility of his children, his wife, and himself to upper respiratory infections. Preventative strategies such as smoking outdoors and not in enclosed areas (e.g., automobiles) would be one option if he and/or his wife are unable or not ready to quit smoking.

Patient Education and/or Community Resources   Preventative measures include no smoking around the children, limit or eliminate daycare, and no bottle propping.

Follow-Up Plan   If there is no improvement in 2 or 3 days, the patient should return for a reevaluation and the antibiotic should be switched to a different classification. Treatment failure with the therapeutic plan occurs when there is no improvement of ear pain, fever, otorrhea, and redness or bulging of the tympanic membrane. Patients who have been on an antibiotic recently have an increased risk of carrying an infection with a resistant strain of pathogen. Otherwise, schedule a visit in 2 to 3 weeks for a recheck. If the patient has recurrent ear infections, refer to an ENT specialist for evaluation of tympanoplasty with ventilating tubes or antibiotic prophylaxis. Children who are placed on prophylactic antibiotics should be evaluated every 4 weeks.

Case Study 2

CHIEF COMPLAINT: Red Eye

History of Present Illness   R.K. is a 29-year-old African-American female who presents with a chief complaint of gradual onset of left red eye of 2 days duration. She noticed the redness in her eye when she was applying make-up yesterday morning. She denies eye or head trauma. When she awakens in the morning her left eye is matted shut with yellow drainage. R.K. has soft contact lenses, but she has not worn them to the office today. She visits Dr. Kemp, an ophthalmologist, annually. Her last appointment was 9 months ago. Her left eye feels gritty and she feels like rubbing it all the time. She has no visual disturbance, photophobia, eye pain, or N/V. R.K. had "red eye" several years ago and was given eye drops with success. R.K. works as a nurse's aide in a nursing home and her employer has insisted that she see a health care provider. She reports that she has been providing care for an elderly lady who also has eye drainage. R.K. denies allergies, herpes simplex infection, and sexually transmitted diseases. She reports that she does have a new sexual partner. R.K. has been putting Visine in her left eye to keep it clean.

Past Medical History Abnormal Pap × 2, is seeing a gynecologist for follow-up; acute bronchitis every fall and winter; broken right arm in 1996

Past Surgical History T&A, 1975; Right breast mass, which was benign, in 1998

Family History Mother age 49, breast cancer; father age 51, HTN; sisters aged 31, 33, and 34, A&W; brother age 32, deceased; two children A&W

Developmental Stage Intimacy versus Isolation

Role-Relationship R.K. is single and lives with her mother, her three sisters and their five children, and her two children in a small house in the city. She has been dating a man for the past 3 months. Her mother and sisters help care for her children when she works. The biological father does not assist with childcare or financial support.

Sleep/Rest Falls to sleep anywhere from 11 PM to 2 AM and awakens about 8 hours later feeling rested. Works second shift at the nursing home. Uses OTC sleeping pills when she has a problem falling to sleep. Takes the sleeping pills about once per week.

Nutrition/Metabolic Breakfast, donuts and coffee; lunch, fast food or will make pasta dishes; dinner, eats a hot meal at work. Snacks on cookies and candy, popcorn, chips, and soda

Activity/Exercise Does not engage in any formal exercise programs

Coping/Stress Her mother and sisters offer her a great deal of support. Attends a Baptist church every Sunday

Health Management Drinks a glass of wine socially. Smokes marijuana about once a week with her friends. Nonsmoker. Td: 3/27/98. Has a smoke detector and carbon monoxide detector in her house. States her boyfriend has slapped her on three occasions. Her sister has a gun in the house for protection.

Self-Perception and Values/Beliefs R.K.'s goal is to save enough money to return to school to become a teacher. She has a strong work ethic and enjoys her job. R.K. enjoys her children and spends time with them in community activities. She feels she is heavy and would like to lose weight.

Medications Triphasil one pill every day
Allergies NKMA

Pertinent Physical Findings
Vital Signs Height 5 feet 6 inches; weight 135 pounds; BMI 30; temperature 97.6° F; heart rate 82; respirations 16; blood pressure 132/80

EENT Visual Acuity per Snellen Chart 20/20 OU without correction, PERRLA, EOMs intact. Left Eye: No corneal abrasions or dendritic lesions noted with the application of fluorescein dye to the left eye. No foreign bodies noted with eversion of the eyelid. Cornea clear, pink palpebral conjunctiva, mild injection of the conjunctival vessels in the bulbar conjunctiva. No ciliary flush. Purulent yellow discharge on lower lid. Right eye: cornea clear, palpebral and bulbar conjunctiva clear. No discharge on lower lid. Funduscopic: optic discs sharp, well defined, cream color, no exudates or hemorrhages. Ears: TMs gray, distinct cone of light. Nose: clear. Pharynx: pink, uvula midline, tonsils surgically absent, no lesions. No preauricular or cervical lymphadenopathy

Heart Apical pulse 82, regular rate and rhythm; no murmurs, S_3 or S_4

Lungs Lungs clear.

Diagnostics
Diagnostic Tests None

History Data Questions specific to the chief complaint of red eye include the following:

- How long have you had the redness in your eye(s) and did it begin abruptly or gradually?
- What were you doing when you noticed the redness in your eye (determine if recent eye trauma)?

- Are the symptoms confined to just one eye or do you experience symptoms in both eyes?
- Are the symptoms constant or intermittent?
- Do you have visual disturbances? Do you wear glasses or contact lenses?
- How often do you see an ophthalmologist, for what condition(s), and what medications do you use?
- Do you have eye pain? If so, describe the intensity and frequency.
- Do you have light sensitivity (photophobia)?
- Do you have itching, tearing, crusting, or discharge (determine if mucoid or purulent)?
- Has anyone around you had similar symptoms of red eye?
- Have you had red eye before? If so, how frequently?
- Do you have a history of allergies, herpes simplex infection (past or recent outbreak), or sexually transmitted diseases?
- Do you have a new sexual partner (assess the possibility of chlamydial or herpes simplex conjunctivitis)?
- Have you had a recent upper respiratory infection?
- Do you have nausea or vomiting (may be from increased intraocular pressure or acute glaucoma)?

Physical Examination Data   The focused examination for the chief complaint of red eye includes vital signs, EENT, neck, heart, and lungs.

Differential Diagnoses   Bacterial conjunctivitis, viral conjunctivitis, chlamydial conjunctivitis, allergic conjunctivitis, chemical burns, subconjunctival hemorrhage, corneal abrasion, acute iritis, acute angle-closure glaucoma (Table 5-2)

Probable Causes of the Presenting Symptoms
In a primary care office, the most common eye complaint is "red eye." A red eye is due to hyperemia of the conjunctival, episcleral, or ciliary vessels (Morrow and Abbott, 1998; Tierney, McPhee, and Papadakis, 1999). An inflammatory, infectious process, or trauma (Kelley, 1997) can cause the hyperemia.

It is important to elicit a thorough history and detailed eye examination because the causes of red eye may be minor to severe with loss of vision. Examination of the conjunctiva may provide a clue to the cause of the problem. Diffuse redness from vessel engorgement on both the palpebral and bulbar conjunctiva is usually a result of conjunctivitis. A ciliary flush (also called circumcorneal injection or perilimbal flush) is created by intraocular or corneal inflammation and requires emergency care. A ciliary flush is a pinkish or red defined area around the corneal border.

The most common cause of red eye is conjunctivitis. In bacterial conjunctivitis, the patients experience mucopurulent discharge, typically starting in one eye, and have no visual disturbance or photophobia. The most common organism in temperate zones is *Pneumococcus*. In tropical zones, *Haemophilus aegyptius* is most prevalent. In chronic conjunctivitis, either *Staphylococcus aureus* or *Moraxella lacunata* is most often the causative organism. *Neisseria* infection may also cause a very purulent discharge, and without treatment can lead to visual loss and systemic disease.

Diagnostic Tests   Culture and smears of the drainage are not required unless there is treatment failure or a gonococcal infection is suspected (Uphold and Graham, 1998). If gonococcal infection is suspected, a stained smear and culture should be obtained. Conjunctival smears are rarely necessary or done. In bacterial conjunctivitis, a conjunctival smear will have polymorphonuclear leukocytes, whereas with viral conjunctivitis there will be eosinophils. When an infected corneal ulcer is present, refer to an ophthalmologist; do not scrape and obtain a sample. Clotting studies may be considered if a coagulopathy is suspected. With cellulitis, a CBC with differential and blood cultures may be ordered.

The use of fluorescein stain with a blue filter is helpful in assessing corneal infection or abrasion. A slit-lamp is a microscopic instrument with specialized lighting system that enables the visualization of the anterior chamber of the eye. This instrument is useful in finding infection of conjunctiva, iris, opacity, and corneal abrasions. A Hruby lens may be used to visualize the posterior vitreous and retina.

Table 5-2
Red Eye Differential Diagnostic Cues

Diagnosis	Signs and Symptoms	Lab Data	Treatment
Bacterial Conjunctivitis	Diffuse conjunctival injection, purulent discharge, gritty feeling in affected eye(s), matted lids in morning	Cultures and smears of discharge not necessary unless treatment fails or gonoccal infection is being considered	Sodium sulfacetamide (Sulamyd) ophthalmic ointment, 10% 0.5-1.0 cm in conjunctival sac bid for 7-14 days *OR* 10% solution 2 gtts q4 hours for 7-14 days; *OR* bacitracin/ polymyxin (Polysporin) ointment 0.5-1.0 cm in conjunctival sac bid for 7-14 days. If accompanied by OM, treat with oral agent such as amoxicillin-clavulanate (Augmentin) or trimethoprim-ulfamethoxazole (Septra). Warm compresses prn
Viral Conjunctivitis	Diffuse conjunctival injection, watery discharge, scratchy feeling in affected eye(s)	None	Topical antibiotics as in bacterial conjunctivitis to prevent secondary infection. Warm compresses
Chlamydial Conjunctivitis	Diffuse conjunctival injection, purulent discharge, gritty feeling in affected eye(s), STD, preauricular lymphnodes, cobblestone appearance on palpebral conjunctiva	Culture and smears	Doxycycline (Vibramycin) 100 mg bid × 10 days and topical erythromycin (Ilotycin) ophthalmic ointment qd
Allergic Conjunctivitis	Diffuse conjunctival injection, mucoid discharge, scratched feeling in affected eye(s), tearing, puffy lids	None	Cromolyn sodium (Opticrom) ophthalmic solution 4% 1-2 gtts qid × 4 days and systemic antihistamines
Chemical Burn Alkali injuries have a poor prognosis because there may may be rapid corneal penetration	Diffuse conjunctival injection, tearing, pain in affected eye(s), may have corneal abrasions	pH testing – use pH 6.0-8.0 test paper – pH should be near 7.0	Removal of the irritant by irrigating the affected eye(s) with saline solution or plain water as soon as possible after exposure. Emergent referral. Do not neutralize alkali or acid solution. Check pH after irrigation (should be neutral)
Subconjunctival Hemorrhage	Sudden, unilateral bright red eye, may cause elevated cornea	None	No treatment; will spontaneously resolve over a 2-week period

Continued

	Table 5-2
	Red Eye Differential Diagnostic Cues—cont'd

Diagnosis	Signs and Symptoms	Lab Data	Treatment
Corneal Abrasion	Circumcorneal conjunctival injection, blurred vision, pain, photophobia, watery discharge, corneal epithelial defects	None	Consider use of cycloplegic agent at the office to dilate pupil and relieve ciliary muscle spasms, which cause pain. Prescribe a topical antibiotic. May patch affected eye and recheck the next day. If suspect infection of of cornea immediately send to ophthalmologist
Acute Iritis	Circumcorneal conjunctival injection, may have blurred vision, aching pain with eye movement, photophobia, constricted or irregular pupil, ciliary flush	None	Immediate referral to ophthalmologist
Angle-Closure Glaucoma	Circumcorneal conjunctival injection, blurred vision, severe pain, mild photophobia, cloudy cornea, moderately dilated and sluggish or fixed pupil, N/V, H/A, halos, increased intraocular pressure	Tonometry	Immediate referral to ophthalmologist

Diagnostic Impression This patient presents with purulent discharge, injected bulbar conjunctiva, and a gritty feeling in the affected eye. These symptoms are characteristic of bacterial conjunctivitis.

Therapeutic Plan of Care Prescribe a topical antibiotic such as sodium sulfacetamide (Sulamyd) ophthalmic solution 2 gtts q 4 hours for 7 days. Many patients prefer ophthalmic solution to the ointment. Ointment can cause a film that creates blurred vision. Either solution or ointment is effective for treatment. Update the adult tetanus for this patient since it is more than 10 years since her last immunization.

Neomycin causes an allergic response (keratitis) in 5% of patients who use it topically. Erythromycin ophthalmic ointment (Ilotycin) may be used 0.5 to 1 cm qid if allergic to other categories of topical preparations. Topical ophthalmologic steroids should not be prescribed by a primary care practitioner because they can make the infection worse and a corneal ulcer could form quickly, causing a perforation (Goroll, May, and Mulley, 1995).

Encourage R.K. to discontinue the Visine eye drops and discard them to prevent reinfection. She should be instructed not to wear her contact lenses until after the medication is complete and the infection is resolved. R.K. should thoroughly clean the contact lenses before wearing them to prevent reintroduction of the infection.

R.K. has verbalized that her boyfriend has slapped her on three occasions. The practitioner should assess the frequency, duration, and nature of the injuries at this visit. The most common locations of injuries include the head, neck, and torso. Being of female gender is the major risk factor for being a victim of abuse. R.K. should be asked if anyone (e.g., family or friends) knows of the abuse (Ashur, 1993). She should be queried to see if she knows how to get help and if she feels in danger. Offer to establish an appointment with a counselor or to provide her with access to community resources. It is important to listen to R.K. in a nonjudgmental manner and support her in making her decisions. Describe the cycle of violence where the abuser inflicts injury, asks for forgiveness, and then repeats the cycle over again. Provide time for R.K. to verbalize and develop a plan. State laws require health care providers to report suspected abuse of children, elderly, and disabled adults. There are no laws that require reporting of suspected abuse for competent adults who choose to stay in abusive relationships. It is required that injuries caused by violent weapons such as guns or knives be reported to law enforcement agencies (Uphold and Graham, 1998).

Patient Education and/or Community Resources Patients should be instructed to notify you immediately if there are visual problems or increased pain. Instruct on the use of warm moist compresses as needed. Discuss the infectious nature of the condition and encourage good handwashing and the use of separate towels and washcloths. Certain cosmetic products, such as mascara and eyeliners, may need to be discarded to prevent reinfection. Discuss the contagious nature of bacterial conjunctivitis. Point out the importance of proper handwashing to prevent the spread of infection from one individual to another. Instruct patients to refrain from rubbing eyes to prevent the spread of infection to the unaffected eye. Inform the patient that the eye secretions are infectious for a minimum of 24 hours after antibiotic use. Teach the patient to instill the topical ophthalmic medication in the inner aspect of the lower eyelid.

Follow-Up Plan The patient should return to the office in 2 days if there is no improvement or if symptoms increase. R.K. should schedule a routine follow-up visit in 2 to 3 weeks to review her concerns about being overweight, discuss partner abuse, and address sleep hygiene. At the follow-up visit information can be provided about weight management, discussion of the use

of marijuana, and the use of over-the-counter sleeping pills. Providing useful information on sleep hygiene, activity, and diet management will be useful to R.K. She should be encouraged to continue her follow-up of the abnormal Pap smears.

Case Study 3

CHIEF COMPLAINT: Blurred Vision

History of Present Illness B.N. is a 69-year-old Caucasian male who complains of sudden onset of left eye pain and blurred vision while raking leaves in his yard 4 hours ago. He reports seeing a halo around lights, and his left eye is red. B.N. states that he rapidly developed severe pain in his left eye and he is light sensitive. He is also having problems focusing with his left eye and he feels his vision is poor. He is nauseated and has vomited × 1. He does not have a family history of glaucoma. B.N. denies the use of anticholinergic medications and steroids.

Past Medical History HTN, hyperlipidemia, and osteoarthritis

Past Surgical History Left inguinal hernia repair in 1982

Family History Mother died of a stroke at age 60; father died at age 72, HTN; brother 65, HTN and hyperlipidemia; sister age 72, osteoarthritis and hypothyroidism; sister age 71, breast cancer

Developmental Stage Ego Integrity versus Despair

Role-Relationship Lives alone in a small house in the suburbs. Wife died 2 years ago from colon cancer. Has three children and eight grandchildren who visit regularly. Frequently dines out and travels with a lady friend

Sleep/Rest Routinely goes to bed at 11 PM and arises at 7 or 8 AM. Uses Ambien for sleep difficulties. Usually only needs the sleeping pills when he feels stressed, which occurs about once every 3 to 4 weeks. States he worries about his children and grandchildren if he perceives they have any problems.

Nutrition/Metabolic Breakfast, hot cereal or a donut; lunch, sandwich, soup, or a salad with fruit; dinner, dines out at a local restaurant with friends often. Usually orders a complete meal that includes a meat, potato dish, vegetable, bread, dessert, and coffee. Does not usually have a snack.

Activity/Exercise   Walks at least 1 mile every day. In addition, he walks his dog twice a day.

Coping/Stress   Is very close to his children and talks with them almost daily. He also shares concerns with his lady friend. He is very active at church and helps organize social events.

Health Management   B.N. does not smoke or drink alcohol. He wears glasses. Td: 1/9/97. He does not have an advanced directive or living will. B.N. has a smoke detector in his house. He does not own a firearm.

Medications   Moexipril HCl (Univasc) 15 mg qd; atorvastatin (Lipitor) 10 mg qd; and zolpidem tartrate (Ambien) 5 mg at HS prn

Allergies   NKMA

Pertinent Physical Findings

Vital Signs   Height 5 feet 8 inches; weight 164 pounds; BMI 25; temperature 98.2° F; heart rate 88; respirations l6; blood pressure 144/88

Eyes   Visual acuity per Snellen chart, 20/30 OD, 20/50 OS with corrective lenses; 20/50 OD, 20/70 OS without corrective lenses; EOMs intact. Upper lids have loose skin but do not droop. Right eye, PERRLA. Funduscopic: Optic disc sharp, well-defined, cream color, no exudates or hemorrhages. Cornea clear. Conjunctiva without erythema. Left eye: Pupil moderately dilated and nonreactive to light. Cornea steamy. Eye erythemic. Funduscopic: Nasal displacement of the vessels and enlargement of the cup. Pallor of the disc

Heart   Apical pulse 88, regular rate and rhythm; no murmurs, S_3 or S_4

Lungs   Clear to auscultation

Diagnostics

Diagnostic Tests   Tonometry shows elevated intraocular pressure in the left eye of 60 mm Hg (normal intraocular pressure is 10 to 22 mm Hg); right eye, 20 mm Hg

History Data   Questions specific to the chief complaint of blurred vision include the following:

- Is one eye affected, or both eyes?
- When did the blurred vision first occur and is it intermittent or constant?

- Do you have any pain, visual loss, or headaches?
- Did the pain and visual loss (central or peripheral) occur suddenly or gradually?
- Do you have light sensitivity (photophobia)?
- Do you have a family history of glaucoma or eye disorders?
- What medications are you on (check for anticholinergic medications or steroids)?

Physical Examination Data   The focused examination for the chief complaint of blurred vision includes vital signs and an eye examination.

Differential Diagnoses   Open-angle glaucoma, angle-closure glaucoma, macular degeneration, temporal arteritis, diabetic retinopathy, cataract (Table 5-3).

Probable Causes of the Presenting Symptoms Risk factors for acute angle-closure glaucoma include being elderly, being farsighted, and being Asian. Acute onset of angle-closure glaucoma results from blockage of aqueous humor outflow by closure of a preexisting narrow anterior chamber angle (Greene et al, 1996). This occurs more often in the elderly because they have physiologic enlargement of the lens. Pupil dilation by pharmacological mechanisms such as anticholinergic agents or sitting in a darkened environment (movie theater) may precipitate angle-closure glaucoma (Tierney, McPhee, and Papadakis, 1999).

Diagnostic Tests   Tonometry to assess intraocular pressures. Often, in primary care settings, the Schiötz tonometer is used: it is small, easy to operate, and can be performed quickly. The tonometer is covered with a disposable casing and placed on the anesthetized eye to measure intraocular pressure.

Diagnostic Impression   This patient has a tonometry measurement of 60 mm Hg and symptoms that are indicative of angle-closure glaucoma. The patient is also experiencing sudden onset of pain and blurred vision in his left eye with halos around lights. With angle-closure glaucoma, intraocular pressures may be 50 to 90 mm Hg. With chronic open-angle glaucoma, pressures rise gradually to 30 to 50 mm Hg.

Table 5-3
Blurred Vision Differential Diagnostic Cues

Diagnosis	Signs and Symptoms	Lab Data	Treatment
Open Angle Glaucoma	Insidious onset, gradual loss of peripheral vision, tunnel vision, elevation of intraocular pressure, cupping of the optic disc, halos around lights	Tonometry	Ophthalmologic referral. Topical treatment is usually initiated. B-adrenergic blocking agent (e.g., timolol [Betimol], 1 gtt of 0.25% or 0.5% solution q 12 hours; **OR** levobunolol [Betagan] 0.5%; **OR** metipranolol [OptiPranolol] 0.1-0.6% bid). Epinephrine eye drops 0.5%-1% may be used alone or with betaxolol (Betoptic). Carbonic anhydrase inhibitors (e.g., acetazolamide [Diamox]) are used until surgery or laser treatment when topical therapy is inadequate. Laser trabeculoplasty is used in addition to topical therapy to postpone surgery. Surgical trabeculectomy is done when medical and laser therapy is ineffective
Angle-Closure Glaucoma	Circumcorneal conjunctival injection, blurred vision, severe pain, mild photophobia, cloudy cornea, moderately dilated and sluggish or fixed pupil, N/V, H/A, halos, increased intraocular pressure	Tonometry	Immediate referral to ophthalmologist. Laser peripheral iridectomy is usually done. Pilocarpine (Pilopine) 4% 1 gtt qid may be used to treat the underlying angle closure
Macular Degeneration Atrophic (dry) Exudative (wet)	Typically progressive bilateral vision loss (central vision), although rarely may be sudden	None	Ophthalmologic referral. If severe loss may do laser photocoagulation of subretinal neovascular membranes (if membrane is far enough away from the fovea). Vision aids, oral vitamins and minerals (specifically zinc) may have beneficial effects
Temporal Arteritis	H/A, eye pain, may or may not have visual distubance (loss), tenderness over the temporal artery, fever, sweats	Erythrocyte sedimentation rate (ESR). If ruling out infection, do WBC	Immediate referral to ophthalmologist. Start on high dose prednisone 60 mg/d for at least 1-2 months before tapering. Monitor ESR. Biopsy of temporal artery

Note: Consider the possibility of trauma or a foreign body in the eye. When the patient often feels like something is in the eye, perform a complete eye assessment and evaluate for a foreign body. When the patient presents with a history of trauma, assess for a hyphema (blood in the anterior chamber of the eye). When a hyphema is present there is usually significant eye injury such as retinal detachment, ruptured globe, or lens dislocation, any of which requires emergent intervention.

Continued

Table 5-3 Blurred Vision Differential Diagnostic Cues—cont'd			
Diagnosis	**Signs and Symptoms**	**Lab Data**	**Treatment**
Diabetic Retinopathy	Blurred or diplopia or asymptomatic, no redness or pain, proliferative or nonproliferative retinopathy	FBS, Hgb A1C	Ophthalmologic referral. Annual ophthalmoscopic examinations through dilated pupils. Laser photocoagulation may be needed
Cataract	Progressive blurred vision, lens opacities, no redness or pain	None	Ophthalmologic referral. Surgical correction by removal of cataract and implantation of an intraocular lens

Therapeutic Plan of Care Immediate ophthalmologic referral is indicated for this ocular emergency.

Patient Education and/or Community Resources Routine follow-up visits should be scheduled with an ophthalmologist.

Follow-Up Plan Follow-up with the ophthalmologist. Schedule a routine physical, assess patient's sleep habits. Ambien is a hypnotic and can be habit-forming. Discuss natural methods of sleep management. Review information with the patient on advanced directives and living wills.

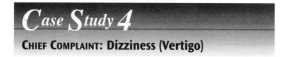

Case Study 4

CHIEF COMPLAINT: Dizziness (Vertigo)

History of Present Illness C.S. is a patient new to your practice. She is a 42-year-old Caucasian female who presents with chief complaint of dizziness and nausea for 2 days. The dizziness and nausea lasts from 1 to 3 minutes and has occurred three to nine times per day, requiring her to lie down. When she is lying down, she must keep her eyes open or she feels as though she is spinning around the room. If she walks during a "spell" she feels like she is a "drunken sailor" and fears that she will fall. C.S. has not been able to work since the symptoms started. C.S. reports that she had a bad cold 2 weeks ago. She is currently taking no medications for her dizziness.

Past Medical History Menses, menstrual cramps seem to be increasing; her flow is heavier (changes super absorbent tampons every 2 hours days 1 through 4, every 4 hours days 5 and 6, and then uses a pad days 7 through 9) and lasts longer (8 or 9 days)

Past Surgical History T&A 1965; D&C (8 years ago after miscarriage)

Family History Mother age 65, hypothyroidism; father age 68, HTN; brother age 44 and sister age 40, A&W

Developmental Stage Generativity versus Stagnation

Role-Relationship Has been married for 19 years and has two children, a son age 10 and a daughter age 8. C.S. works as a press operator in a local factory on the first shift. The family frequently entertains and enjoys outdoor activities. C.S. has not felt up to camping, biking, and swimming because of her tiredness and her husband has urged her to inform her care provider of this problem.

Sleep/Rest Falls to sleep at 11 PM and awakens at 6 AM. States she feels tired more often than not and just doesn't have much energy. At least once a week will lay down when she gets home from work and nap from 30 minutes to 1 hour.

Nutrition/Metabolic Breakfast, peanut butter on toast and a glass of orange juice or milk; lunch, sandwich, chips, and cookie or cake; dinner, meat, potatoes or pasta, vegetable, and bread. The family eats together for dinner and everyone helps cook and clean up the dishes. Snacks occasionally on fruit, sweets, or chips

Activity/Exercise Until 6 months ago had been exercising twice a week with her girlfriend at the YMCA. She quit because she felt too tired.

Coping/Stress Her husband and her girlfriend are very supportive of her, and she talks with them when she has problems. Attends a Lutheran church on holidays. Does not feel she has too much stress in her life at this time.

Health Management Td: 1/12/96. Nonsmoker. Alcohol, glass of white wine for dinner. C.S. has a smoke detector and carbon monoxide detector in her home. They do not have weapons in the home. Last Pap smear was 3 years ago (normal) and she has never had a mammogram. C.S. and her husband use condoms for birth control.

Self-Perception and Values/Beliefs C.S. is very happy with her life and enjoys her husband and children.

Medications Motrin 800 mg every 8 hours prn with food for menstrual cramps

Allergies PCN, Keflex

Pertinent Physical Findings

Vital Signs Height 5 feet 2 inches; weight 136 pounds; BMI 25; temperature 98.2° F; heart rate 76; respirations 12; blood pressure 130/80

HEENT PERRLA. Funduscopic: Optic discs sharp, well-defined, cream color, no exudates or hemorrhages, EOMs intact without nystagmus. Rinne, AC>BC bilateral; Weber, nonlateralizing. Ears: TMs gray, distinct cone of light. Sinuses: Nontender; Nose: Clear. Pharynx: Pink, tonsils surgically absent. Cervical lymphadenopathy: None. Neck: No carotid bruits

Heart Apical pulse 72, regular rate and rhythm; no murmur, S_3, or S_4

Lungs Clear to auscultation

Abdomen Soft, nontender, no masses or organomegaly, active bowel sounds

Neurological CN II-XII grossly intact. DTRs 2+ upper and lower bilaterally. Babinski: Negative. Romberg: Negative. Tandem gait test: WNL. Hallpike maneuver: + Vertigo for 1-minute duration. Slight lateral nystagmus resolving within 5 seconds

Diagnostics

Diagnostic Tests + Hallpike maneuver

History Data Questions specific to the chief complaint of dizziness include the following:

- How often do you experience dizziness, and for how long?
- What precipitates or causes and relieves the dizziness?
- Describe the feeling of dizziness.
- Have you or do you feel like fainting (syncope)?
- Do you feel like you or the room is spinning around (vertigo)?
- Do you feel unsteady or have a sense of imbalance (may indicate a sensory deficit, cerebellar dysfunction, Parkinson's, vertebrobasilar insufficiency, or anxiety)?
- Have you had a recent upper respiratory infection?
- What medications are you taking? (Aminoglycosides, cancer chemotherapeutic drugs, and loop diuretics may cause ototoxicity; drugs that suppress the central nervous system may cause dizziness; and drugs that affect the circulatory system can cause postural hypotension and create a feeling of fainting or syncope.)
- Do you use herbal therapies and vitamins (megavitamin doses may be neurotoxic)?
- Do you have diabetes mellitus, thyroid dysfunction, heart problems, cataracts, or a psychiatric condition?
- Have you noticed any changes or difficulty in walking?

During the history, try to differentiate between organic disease and a nonorganic disease such as anxiety. If it is organic, differentiate between vestibular (spinning sensation) and nonvestibular (syncope or fainting sensation). Finally, if it is vestibular, determine if it is peripheral (ear) or central (brain) (Kelley, 1997).

Physical Examination Data The focused examination for the chief complaint of dizziness includes vital signs, HEENT, neck, heart, lungs, abdomen, and neurological. Make sure to include the Hallpike (Nylen-Barany) test.

Differential Diagnoses Labyrinthitis, Meniere's disease, vestibular neuronitis, positional vertigo, posttraumatic vertigo, acoustic neuroma, vertebrobasilar artery disease, central lesions (tumors of the brainstem or cerebellum), anxiety, drug toxicity, cardiovascular problems, metabolic conditions, multiple sclerosis (Table 5-4).

Probable Causes of the Presenting Symptoms The patient who presents with dizziness challenges the practitioner to determine the specific cause of the presenting complaint. The differential for dizziness is broad, and it is often compounded by a vague history. It is essential to determine whether the patient is experiencing fainting episodes or syncope (which are often from a cardiovascular cause) as opposed to vertigo or a feeling of the room spinning. C.S. recently recovered from an upper respiratory infection. There is inflammation of the labyrinth, creating vertigo and disequilibrium. The vestibular end organ is composed of the three semicircular canals, a utricle, and a saccule (Greene et al, 1996). With inflammation of the vestibular end organ there is disruption of the orientation of the body in space, creating a sense of disequilibrium, vertigo, and often nausea and vomiting.

Diagnostic Tests C.S. had a + Hallpike maneuver. To perform the Hallpike maneuver, have the patient sit with the head turned to the right side then quickly position the patient in the supine position with the head hanging over the edge of the table and check for nystagmus. Repeat on the opposite side (Uphold and Graham, 1998). The Hallpike maneuver is depicted in Figure 5-1.

C.S. does not require any further diagnostic tests for the symptoms of dizziness at this time. Should C.S.'s symptoms persist, further testing would be indicated.

C.S. also complains of fatigue, tiredness, and lack of energy. She has not had a physical examination in 3 years. A physical examination with laboratory testing should be scheduled. Laboratory tests to consider include a CBC with differential (assess anemia), TSH (assess thyroid function, mother has hypothyroidism), and BS (assess for diabetes). In addition, she needs a Pap smear (last Pap 3 years ago) and a mammogram (C.S. has not had a mammogram).

Diagnostic Impression C.S. presents with recent history of an URI, vertigo, and nausea of 2 days duration, and a + Hallpike maneuver. These symptoms are most likely from acute labyrinthitis. C.S. also presents with fatigue, which must be evaluated further. Potential causes of the fatigue include heavy menstrual flow, hypothyroidism, diabetes, and gastrointestinal bleeding.

Therapeutic Plan of Care C.S. should begin taking an antihistamine medication such as meclizine (Antivert) 25 mg tid for 5 to 7 days (depending on the persistence of symptoms) and then taper the medication. C.S. should not go to work for 1 or 2 days until symptoms resolve because she is a press operator. She should have bed rest for a day.

Patient Education and/or Community Resources Discuss the nature of the problem with C.S. Describe the usual course of symptoms and complete resolution. Instruct her to return if the symptoms do not resolve, if they continue to progressively worsen, or if they reoccur.

Follow-Up Plan C.S. should return to your office in 2 to 4 weeks for a reevaluation of the dizziness and a complete physical examination and evaluation of fatigue. She should return sooner if there is no improvement, if the condition worsens, or if symptoms return.

Table 5-4
Dizziness Differential Diagnostic Cues

Diagnosis	Signs and Symptoms	Lab Data	Treatment
Labyrinthitis	Severe vertigo that lasts days to a week, tinnitus, hearing loss (usually temporary)	None unless symptoms persists	Antihistamines (e.g., meclizine [Antivert] 25 mg tid and taper; or dimenhydrinate 25-50 mg po q6 hours). Scopolamine low-dose transdermal 0.5 mg/day. Bed rest and exercise program
Meniere's Disease (Endolymphatic Hydrops)	Episodic vertigo for 1-8 hours at a time, low-frequency sensorineural hearing loss, nausea, tinnitus, ear fullness. Common in young adults	Audiometry Brainstem Auditory Evoked Responses to distinguish between cochlear and retrocochlear lesions Caloric testing demonstrates impairment of thermally induced nystagmus on the involved side	Low-salt diet (<2 gm per day) Diuretic (e.g., hydrochlorothiazide [Dyazide] 50-100 mg qd). Possibly intratympanic gentamicin to the abnormal side. Rarely, surgical decompression of the endolymphatic sac if medical failure
Vestibular Neuronitis	Frequently occurs in spring and summer following a viral infection. Vertigo, emesis, disequilibrium lasts several days to weeks. No hearing loss	None	Antihistamines (e.g., meclizine [Antivert] 25 mg tid and taper; or dimenhydrinate 25-50 mg po q6 hours). Scopolamine low-dose transdermal 0.5 mg/day. Bed rest and exercise program
Positional Vertigo Benign positional vertigo is common in the elderly	Vertigo occurring in clusters that lasts several days caused by changes in head position, lasting 10-60 seconds	None	Physical therapy to teach customized habituation protocols
Posttraumatic Vertigo	Vertigo that usually subsides after several days. If basilar skull fracture, may have deafness	CT scan of head for head	Treat underlying condition
Acoustic Neuroma (Vestibular Schwannoma)	Unilateral hearing loss (may be sudden), vertigo, dysequilibrium	Audiometry Auditory evoked responses Enhanced MRI	Microsurgical excision

Continued

Table 5-4
Dizziness Differential Diagnostic Cues—cont'd

Diagnosis	Signs and Symptoms	Lab Data	Treatment
Vertebrobasilar Artery Disease	Common in the elderly. Vertigo caused by changes in posture or extension of the neck	Magnetic resonance angiography	Vasodilators and aspirin
Central Lesions	Gradual onset of vertigo progressively worse and constant. Vertical nystagmus without latency. Unstable gait. Positive Romberg	Electronystagmorgraph MRI for suspected parenchymal lesions of the brain stem or cerebellum CT if suspect abnormality of the bony labyrinth	Treat underlying condition
Anxiety	Intermittent dizziness or lightheadedness, hyperventilation, tingling of digits of the extremities	None or labs to rule out underlying abnormality (e.g., FBS, TSH, CBC)	Treat underlying conditions Counseling Anxiolytics or antidepressants
Drug Toxicity	Depending on the drug can cause tinnitus and vertigo	None	Discontinue medication
Cardiovascular Problems (e.g., cardiac dysrhythmias, orthostatic hypotension)	Dizziness or lightheadedness (syncope versus vertigo), a fainting sensation as opposed to vertigo (spinning). May have faint, irregular or fast heart rate	ECG CBC	Treat underlying condition
Metabolic Conditions (e.g., anemia, thyroid dysfunction, diabetes mellitus)	Dizziness or lightheadedness as TSH, FT_4	CBC FBS, HgB, A_1C	Treat underlying condition
Multiple Sclerosis	Occasionally presents with vertigo, weakness, numbness, and diplopia Symptoms may initially disappear and then reoccur	MRI may show periventricular plaques	Refer to neurologist for treatment plan Burst of steroids May try beta interferon or Copolymer 1

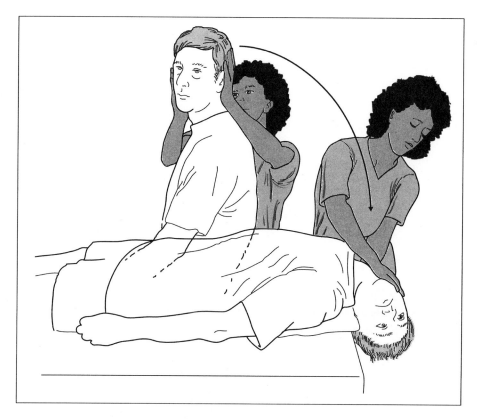

Figure 5-1   Demonstration of the Hallpike maneuver to elicit vertigo. (Rubin RH et al: *Medicine: a primary care approach*, Philadelphia, 1996, WB Saunders.)

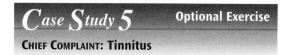

Case Study 5

Optional Exercise

CHIEF COMPLAINT: Tinnitus

History of Present Illness: K.R., a 36-year-old Hispanic male, presents with chief complaint of ringing in his ears while he is awake. He has noticed this for the past 4 months, but thought it would go away. The ringing is continuous, and the only thing that helps is to drown out the ringing with a radio or television. He describes it as irritating, but not pulsatile. He works at the airport loading and unloading luggage from planes. K.R. reports that the ringing seems worse after working all day at the airport. He denies head trauma, ear surgery, recent air flight or diving, H/A, dizziness, or ear drainage. Denies a recent upper respiratory infection. Negative past medical history for DM, HTN, or thyroid disorders. He sought advice from a *curandero* who provided him with herbs, but the ringing persisted.

Past Medical History   Unremarkable

Past Surgical History   Unremarkable

Family History   Mother age 62, DM; father age 65, HTN; sister age 41, DM; sister age 42 and brother age 44, A&W

Developmental Stage   Intimacy versus Isolation

Role-Relationship   Lives in the suburbs with his wife and their three daughters ages 5, 7, and 9. Their extended families are close and visit often. K.R. has worked at the airport for 10 years loading and unloading baggage.

Sleep/Rest Goes to bed at 11:30 PM and awakens at 6:30 AM rested.

Nutrition/Metabolic Breakfast, cereal and toast; lunch, rice, soup, and sandwiches; dinner, beans, rice, vegetables, and bread. Snacks on fruit, vegetables, and sweets

Activity/Exercise Does not engage in planned exercise. Feels he is busy enough with working at the airport carrying luggage, caring for his yard, and playing with his children

Coping/Stress Talks with his father, his brother, and wife if he has concerns. Attends a Catholic church every Sunday

Health Management Td: 1/12/96. Smokes 1 pack of cigarettes per day for 20 years. Drinks 1 or 2 beers in the evening

Medications None

Allergies NKMA

Pertinent Physical Findings

Vital Signs Height 5 feet 11 inches; weight 207 pounds; BMI 29; temperature 98.2° F; heart rate 88; respirations 16; blood pressure 148/92

HEENT Eyes: PERRLA, EOMs intact. Ears: TMs gray bilaterally. Nose: Clear. Pharynx: Pink, tonsils +0, no cervical lymphadenopathy. Rinne: AC>BC. Weber: Tone lateralizes to the left ear

Heart Apical pulse 88, regular rate and rhythm; no murmurs, S_3, or S_4

Lungs Lungs clear to auscultation, slightly diminished breath sounds in the bases

Neurological CN II-XII grossly intact. DTR 2+ bil symmetrical; muscular strength intact bil, no atrophy or tremors; Romberg and Babinski, negative; sensation intact to light touch and pinprick; able to heel-to-toe walk; gait stable

Diagnostics

Diagnostic Tests Audiometry: Bone and air conduction are equally diminished. Right ear 20 dB at 250 and 500 Hz, 30 dB at 1000 Hz, 40 dB at 2000, 4000, and 8000 Hz. Left ear 20 dB at 250, 500, 1000, 2000, 4000, and 8000 Hz. (Testing indicates mild hearing loss in the right ear [e.g., trouble hearing the soft-spoken voice].)

Discussion Questions

What type of history data should be collected?

What type of physical data should be collected?

What are the differential diagnoses?

What are the probable causes of the presenting symptoms?

What is your diagnostic impression?

What is the therapeutic plan of care?

What are the patient education and/or community resources?

What is your follow-up plan?

Discussions for optional case study exercises can be found in the accompanying Instructor's Manual.

References

Ashur ML: Asking about domestic violence: SAFE questions (letter to the editor), *JAMA* 269(18):2367, 1993.

Barnett ED, Klein JO: The problem of resistant bacteria for the management of acute otitis media, *Pediatr Clin North Am* 42(3):509-517, 1995.

Dowell SF, Butler JC, Giebink GS, Jacobs MR, Jernigan D, Musher DM, Rakowsky A, Schwartz B: Acute otitis media: management and surveillance in an era of pneumococcal resistance-a report from the drug-resistant *Streptococcus pneumoniae* therapeutic working group, *Pediatr Infect Dis J* 18(1):1-9, 1999.

Dowell SF, Marcy SM, Phillips WR, Gerber MA, Schwartz B: Otitis media: principles of judicious use of antimicrobial agents, *Pediatrics* 101:165-171, 1998.

Goroll, May, and Mulley: *Primary care medicine*, ed 3, Philadelphia, 1995, Lippincott-Raven.

Greene H, Fincher RM, Johnson W et al: *Clinical medicine*, St Louis, 1996, Mosby.

Jacobs MR: Increasing importance of antibiotic-resistant *Streptococcus* pneumoniae in acute otitis media, *Pediatr Infect Dis J* 15(10):940-943, 1996.

Kelley W: *Textbook of internal medicine*, ed 3, Philadelphia, 1997, Lippincott-Raven.

Kozyrskyi AL, Hildes-Ripstein GE, Llongstaffe SEA et al: Treatment of acute otitis media with a shortened course of antibiotics: a meta-analysis, *JAMA* 279:1736-1742, 1998.

Morrow GL, Abbott R: Conjunctivitis, *Am Fam Physician* 57(4):735-746, 1998.

Rubin H, Voss C, Derksen DJ, Gateley A, Quener RW: *Medicine: a primary care approach*, Philadelphia, 1996, WB Saunders.

Tierney L, McPhee SJ, Papadakis MA: *Current medical diagnosis and treatment*, Stamford, Conn., 1999, Appleton & Lange.

Uphold C, Graham M: *Clinical guidelines in family practice*, Gainesville, Fla., 1998, Barmarrae Books.

Selected Readings

Feder HM, Gerber MA, Randolph MF, Stelmach PS, Kaplan EL: Once-daily therapy for streptococcal pharyngitis with amoxicillin, *Pediatrics* 103(1):47-51, 1999.

Kendrick R: Gradual painless visual loss: glaucoma, *Clin Geriatr Med* 15(1):95-101, 1999.

CHAPTER 6

Respiratory Disorders

Jean Nagelkerk

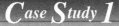

CHIEF COMPLAINT: Sore Throat

History of Present Illness A.T., a 4-year-old Native American female accompanied by her mom and 2-year-old sister, is complaining of a sore throat. Upon further questioning you learn that she has a 3-day history of a sore throat, low-grade fever, and that mom feels she has been "cranky." A.T. does not have a runny nose, cough, or rash. She does not have a history of ear infections, ventilating tubes, or sinusitis. She has not been eating solid foods, but is drinking well. She is eliminating with no problems. She has been waking up at least once a night with a fever. She is active during the day, but lays around more than usual. Mother has been giving her Tylenol every 4 to 6 hours for her fever while she is awake. Mom states that she has been in daycare with her sister and that one of the other children in the daycare had strep throat.

Past Medical History Chickenpox age 2; negative prior history of streptococcal pharyngitis

Past Surgical History None

Family History Mother, A&W; father, history of alcoholism; sister, A&W

Developmental Stage Initiative versus Guilt

Role-Relationship Lives in a small apartment in the city with her mother, father, and sister. Plays with children at the park in the neighborhood. Father smokes in the house

Sleep/Rest Typically will go to bed at 8 PM and sleep until 8 AM. Will take a nap in the afternoon

Nutrition/Metabolic Breakfast, toast or oatmeal with skim milk; lunch, macaroni with cheese or sandwich and fruit; dinner, pasta, rice, or potatoes, meat, and vegetables. Snacks on cookies, fruit, and crackers

Activity/Exercise Plays with her sister and is very active throughout the day. Enjoys the park and playing on the playground equipment

Coping/Stress Enjoys playing with her friends and sister and having mom read to her. Enjoys watching television, which mom limits to 1 hour per day. Attends a nondenominational church about once a month with her parents

Health Management Immunizations are up-to-date. Family combines Western medicine with a healer who gives them herbs and roots for different ailments. Mom is unsure of the names of the herbs she is given from the healer. There are no guns in the apartment. There is a smoke detector in the apartment.

Medications None

Allergies NKMA

Pertinent Physical Findings

Vital Signs Height 40½ inches; weight 35 pounds; temperature 100.2° F with antipyretic; heart rate 98; respirations 20

Skin Brown, moist; no sores, lesions, or rashes

HEENT Ears, TMs gray. Nose, clear. Red, beefy throat with a fetid smell. No palatine petechiae present. Uvula midline. Tonsils 2+ with white-gray exudate bilaterally. Tender, slightly enlarged submandibular lymph nodes palpable bilaterally

Heart Heart rate regular; no murmurs, S_3, or S_4

Lungs: Lungs clear to auscultation

Abdomen Soft, nontender, no masses or organomegaly

Diagnostics
Diagnostic Tests   + rapid strep test

History Data   Questions specific to the chief complaint of sore throat include the following:

- Where is the discomfort located?
- When did the symptoms begin?
- What is the severity of the sore throat?
- Have you had a fever? (If so, what is the temperature range?)
- Do you have a runny nose (rhinorrhea), cough, or postnasal drip?
- Do you have any swallowing problems or drooling (may indicate peritonsillar abscess)?
- How much fluid are you drinking?
- Do you have any lesions in your mouth (consider hand-foot-mouth disease, herpes simplex)?
- Do you have nausea or vomiting, abdominal pain, headache, or rashes (a rash may be symptomatic of scarlet fever)?
- Do you have a history of allergies, sinusitis, or bronchitis?
- Is anyone that you have close contact with sick with similar symptoms (to determine if the patient has had an exposure to a streptococcal or other infection)?
- What medications, herbs, or treatments have you used to alleviate the symptoms?

Inquire about the patient's smoking history. Inquire about sexual practices in an adult or a sexually active individual in whom a STD is suspected.

Physical Examination Data   The focused examination for the chief complaint of a sore throat includes: Vital signs, skin, HEENT, neck, heart, lungs, and abdomen. (**Note:** Be cautious with examination of the pharynx in a young child who is drooling or has a stridor. The child may have epiglottitis and an examination can initiate airway compromise.)

Differential Diagnoses   Group A beta-hemolytic streptococci (GABHS) pharyngitis, peritonsillar abscess, viral pharyngitis, infectious mononucleosis, epiglottitis, *Neisseria gonorrhea* pharyngitis (sexual history), *Mycoplasma* or *Chlamydia* pharyngitis, and sinusitis (see page 110 for discussion of sinusitis). Table 6-1 lists the differential diagnoses for a sore throat with signs and symptoms, laboratory data, and treatment.

Probable Causes of the Presenting Symptoms
The sore throat results from streptococcal organisms causing severe mucosal inflammation from bacterial extracellular factors (Rubin et al, 1996). If treatment is not instituted, the following sequelae may result: rheumatic valvular disease, scarlet fever, local abscess formation, and acute poststreptococcal glomerulonephritis.

Table 6-1
Sore Throat Differential Diagnostic Cues

Diagnosis	Signs and Symptoms	Lab Data	Treatment
Group A Beta-Hemolytic Streptocci (GABHS) Pharyngitis	Sudden onset of fever, anterior cervical adenopathy, posterior pharynx, erythematous, with pharyngotonsillar exudate, H/A, mild odynophagia	Rapid test for group A streptococcal antigen, throat cultures	Pen-Vee K, penicillin G benzathine, amoxicillin, or may use a macrolide (e.g., erythromycin [E-Mycin]) if PCN allergic; or a cephalosporin (e.g., cephalexin [Keflex] 500 mg bid × 10 days, or cefadroxil monohydrate [Duricef] 500 mg bid × 10 days)
Peritonsillar Abscess	Severe sore throat, odynophagia, trismus, medial deviation of the soft palate, scratchy voice/muffled, or shift of uvula to opposite side	Culture drainage from abscess	Emergent ENT referral for an incision and drainage of abscess, antibiotic therapy, and tonsillectomy if reoccurrence

Continued

Table 6-1
Sore Throat Differential Diagnostic Cues—cont'd

Diagnosis	Signs and Symptoms	Lab Data	Treatment
Viral Pharyngitis (Most common)	Scratchy throat, clear nasal drainage, cough; no or minimal lymphadenopathy and erythema of pharynx; no exudate	None or rapid test for group A streptococcal antigen; or throat culture	Supportive care with increased rest and fluids, adequate nutrition, warm salt gargles and throat lozenges prn (caution with young children—may be a choking hazard), acetaminophen (Tylenol) or ibuprofen (Motrin); NSAIDs decrease inflammation and provide analgesia
Infectious Mononucleosis	Marked lymphadenopathy (posterior cervical chain), temperature elevation (may be as high as 102°-104° F), and whitish tonsillar exudate; gradual onset of pharyngitis, soft palate palatine petechiae, fatigue, H/A, malaise, hepatosplenomegaly	Heterophil agglutination test or anti-EBV titer; may exhibit lymphocytosis indicates with atypical lymphocytes May order liver enzymes if assessment hepatomegaly	No contact sports for at least 1 month, and if patient has splenomegaly, this must be resolved; rest, adequate nutrition/fluids, supportive care; take measures to avoid transmission (e.g., handwashing, no sharing glasses, avoid kissing)
***Neisseria Gonorrhea* Pharyngitis**	Sore throat, exudate on tonsils, low grade fevers; consider vaginitis/urethritis in sexually active patients	Throat cultures, Gram stain smears; possible DNA probe and wet mount	Ceftriaxone, cefixime, ciprofloxacin, ofloxacin, erythromycin (if allergic); co-treat for chlamydia
Mycoplasma Pharyngitis	Gradual onset of low grade fever, sore throat, H/A	Throat C&S	Macrolide and supportive care as with viral pharyngitis
Epiglottitis	Odynophagia, drooling, swollen, erythematous epiglottis, toxic appearance Compromised airway leading to respiratory distress (stridor)	Lateral x-ray of the neck (soft tissue) may show a large, swollen epiglottis, which may resemble an upward pointing thumb (Wiest and Roth, 1996) Direct visualization only in adult patients Blood cultures	Emergency referral for hospitalization for intravenous antibiotics and dexamethasone May require intubation

The most common symptoms associated with streptococcal pharyngitis include tonsillar exudate, fever, anterior cervical adenopathy, and absence of cough. Of those patients presenting with three of the four most common symptoms, 21% will test positive for streptococcal pharyngitis. Of those who have four of the four most common symptoms, 43% will test positive (Ruppert, 1996).

Diagnostic Tests Many clinicians order rapid test for group A streptococcal antigen, which is approximately 85% sensitive and 95% specific (Goroll, May, and Mulley, 1995). Throat cultures are the gold standard, with a sensitivity of 90% and specificity of 99%.

Diagnostic Impression The patient presents with recent onset of a red, beefy throat with a fetid smell; tonsils +2 with white exudate; and a + rapid strep test. This presentation is most likely group A beta-hemolytic streptococci (GABHS) pharyngitis. Should the patient return with repeated episodes of streptococcal pharyngitis, consider a viral pharyngitis with streptococcal colonization.

Therapeutic Plan of Care Penicillin is the medication of choice to prevent further complications. Penicillin V potassium (Pen-Vee K) tid × 10 days is the most inexpensive and specific for the streptococcal organism. Penicillin G benzathine may be administered intramuscularly in those who are on vacation, those who have no place to store medications, or those patients who may not comply with the daily medication regimen. Amoxicillin provides a broader coverage and is also inexpensive. Amoxicillin should not be administered if infectious mononucleosis is suspected because many patients develop a rash. GABHS and infectious mononucleosis co-occur in approximately one third of patients (Tierney, McPhee, and Papadakis, 1999). If the patient is allergic to penicillins, then a macrolide such as erythromycin may be used. If the patient is allergic to both penicillins and macrolides, then a cephalosporin may be used.

Antibiotics approved for once-a-day dosing for the treatment of streptococcal pharyngitis include cefixime (Suprax), azithromycin (Zithromax), ceftibuten (Cedax), and cefadroxil (Duricef). The antibiotics given once a day are more expensive than penicillin V potassium or amoxicillin and have a broader spectrum of antimicrobial activity (Prescriber's Newsletter, March 1999).

Patient Education and/or Community Resources The patient should be instructed to increase her rest and to increase the amount of fluids she is taking. Warm saltwater gargles as needed will help with the discomfort of the sore throat, as will Popsicles. Over-the-counter lozenges such as Cepacol lozenges, cough drops, or analgesic lozenges such as Cepastat may be helpful. NSAIDs may be used as needed to decrease inflammation, to provide analgesia, and for the antipyretic effects. Patients who have streptococcal pharyngitis should not return to school or work until they have been on antibiotics for 24 hours. In order to prevent a reinfection of streptococcal pharyngitis, encourage the patient to get a new toothbrush. For older children or adults with orthodontic appliances such as a retainer, encourage disinfection of the appliance (Prescriber's Newsletter, March 1999). Watch for signs and symptoms of acute pharyngitis in other family members. Counseling and information about the effects of second-hand smoke on the children's health should be reviewed.

Follow-Up Plan If no improvement is seen in 48 hours, or if symptoms persist or worsen, schedule an appointment; otherwise, return for routine well and ill visits.

Case Study 2

Chief Complaint: Sinus Congestion and Pressure

History of Present Illness A.N. is a 32-year-old Asian-American female who presents with a 10-day history of pressure over her cheeks that is worse when bending forward. A.N. describes a thick, yellow nasal discharge; low-grade fever; intermittent cough; and a generalized headache. She reports having a cold 2 weeks ago, at which time she experienced clear nasal discharge, intermittent cough, and a mild sore throat. She denies having a toothache, recent dental work, or asthma. A.N. uses Afrin nasal spray two squirts qid since the onset of her cold 2 weeks ago. She reports that she is allergic to cats, and that her cousin who moved in 1 month ago brought a longhaired brown cat to live with them.

Past Medical History   Has episodes of "gastritis" that she was treated for, but now uses TUMS about once a month with relief. Had hepatitis A 5 years ago

Past Surgical History   Unremarkable

Family History   Mother age 50, GERD; father age 54, A&W; three sisters, ages 24, 26, and 28, A&W; brother age 30, A&W

Developmental Stage   Intimacy versus Isolation

Role-Relationship   Single, works as a seamstress in a sewing factory. Lives with her family in a one-story home in the inner city. Her family works together to care for one another. Family members share resources, and frequently invite extended family members, friends, or other individuals without a place to live to stay with them.

Sleep/Rest   Sleeps from 8:30 AM to 3:30 PM. Adjusts her sleeping patterns on her days off to be awake a few hours during daytime. Does not have trouble falling to sleep.

Nutrition/Metabolic   Breakfast, cold cereal and milk; lunch, packs a box lunch for work and usually has a sandwich, raw vegetables, and chips; dinner, eats with her family and they usually have a rice dish with vegetables. Snacks on vegetables and fruit

Activity/Exercise   Does not engage in planned exercise

Coping/Stress   Her family supports one another and she can count on them in times of need. Her father takes the lead in problem solving and decision-making. She enjoys swimming and reading. Does not attend church regularly

Health Management   Immunizations are up to date. Nonsmoker. Alcohol, none. Has a smoke detector and carbon monoxide detector. States she lives in an old neighborhood that is unsafe at night because of drug sales, prostitution, and alcohol use. Several individuals in the neighborhood own weapons such as knives or guns. She keeps to herself and stays in at night except when she works.

The family is trying to save enough money to move to a safer area.

Medications   Tums, prn; Q10 (a herbal supplement) 1 qd; garlic tablets 2 qd

Allergies   NKMA

Pertinent Clinical Findings

Vital Signs: Height 5 feet 0 inches; weight, 128 pounds; BMI 25; temperature 99.2° F (ear) without antipyretics; heart rate 68; respirations 16; blood pressure 130/82

HEENT   Eyes: no periorbital swelling or allergic shiners; conjunctiva clear, sclera white, iris intact. Ears: external canals clear; TMs gray intact with dull cone of light bilaterally. Sinus: + maxillary sinus tenderness bilaterally, − frontal sinus tenderness, tragus, and mastoid nontenderness. Clouded transillumination of maxillary sinuses bilaterally. Nose: congested with swollen red mucosa bilaterally, purulent, yellow drainage, no polyps. Pharynx: buccal mucosa pink and moist, no lesions, tonsils 1+; posterior pharynx erythremic with cobblestone appearance, no exudate, no cervical lymphadenopathy

Heart   Apical pulse 68, regular rate and rhythm, no murmurs, S_3 or S_4

Lungs   Clear to auscultation, no adventitious breath sounds, resonant throughout lung fields

Diagnostics

Diagnostic Tests   None

History Data   Questions specific to the chief complaint of sinus pressure include the following:

- Where is the pressure located (localize what sinus is involved)?
- How severe is the discomfort? Does the pressure increase with bending (pressure typically increases with sinusitis)?
- How long have you had these symptoms?
- Do you have nasal discharge? If so, what is the amount, consistency, and color (purulent, yellow may indicate sinusitis; clear may indicate allergic rhinitis)?
- Have you had an upper respiratory infection, dental abscess, or have you used nasal sprays recently (predisposing factors to sinusitis)?

- Do you have a toothache, fever, fatigue, headaches, or puffiness around the eyes or on the forehead?
- Do you have a history of allergies, asthma, immunodeficiency, diabetes, or leukemia?
- Do you smoke or use recreational drugs (snorting cocaine may damage the nasal mucosa and septum)?

Physical Examination Data The focused examination for the chief complaint of sinus pressure includes vital signs, HEENT (may need to assess conductive hearing loss in adult patients or in children who have repeated otitis media; evaluate for tragus, mastoid, and frontal and maxillary sinus tenderness), neck (evaluate lymph node involvement), heart, lungs, and neurological (if suspect intracranial suppuration).

Differential Diagnoses Acute or chronic sinusitis, uncomplicated upper respiratory infection (see pages 104-112 for presentation of upper respiratory infections), allergic rhinitis, vasomotor rhinitis, dental abscesses, migraine or cluster headaches (see pages 233-241 for presentation of headaches), nasal polyps, tumors (Table 6-2)

Probable Causes of the Presenting Symptoms
Sinusitis is a common medical disorder; in fact, it is the fifth most common reason that antibiotics are prescribed (Williams, 1995). According to Williams et al (1992), the best clinical predictors of sinusitis include the following: (1) a history of no improvement while on a nasal decongestant, (2) colored nasal drainage, (3) maxillary toothache, and the physical examination findings of (4) abnormal transillumination and (5) purulent nasal drainage. Results from that study indicate that there is a 92% probability of sinusitis with all five positive clinical predictors. Predisposing factors to sinusitis include a history of an upper respiratory infection, a dental abscess, a history of allergies, and the use of vasoconstrictor nasal sprays (Black et al, 1999). The sequela of sinusitis with a URI occurs in 0.5% to 5.0% of the population. The most common sinuses involved are the maxillary (87%), ethmoidal (65%), sphenoidal (39%), and the frontal (32%) (Goroll, May, and Mulley, 1995).

In sinusitis, fluids and pus collect in the sinuses. Either a virus, allergy, or obstruction in the nasal mucous membrane produces edema and blockage of normal drainage. The accumulated fluid becomes secondarily infected by microorganisms. The most common organisms in acute sinusitis include *Streptococcus pneumoniae, Haemophilus influenzae, Moraxella catarrhalis,* and other streptococci. In chronic sinusitis, the most common organisms include *H. influenzae, S. pneumoniae,* anaerobic organisms (aerobic streptococci and bacteroides species), *Staphylococcus aureus* (20% of cases), and other streptococci. Though rare, sinusitis caused by fungi is extremely difficult to treat effectively and requires emergent care. Those at risk for rhinocerebral fungal infection include patients with poorly controlled diabetes or those with leukemia. Patients who have a toxic appearance with sinusitis or who have central nervous system involvement should have an emergent referral.

Patients who have frontal sinusitis are at risk for osteomyelitis of the frontal bones. Symptoms include fever, H/A, and edema over the involved bone (Pott's puff tumor). A complication of ethmoidal sinusitis includes orbital infection, which begins with edema of the eyelids. Other complications of sinusitis include septic cavernous sinus thrombophlebitis and intracranial suppuration, which require emergent care.

Diagnostic Tests A.N. should not have any diagnostic tests unless her symptoms become recurrent or unless there is a treatment failure. The gold standard for the diagnosis of sinusitis is sinus puncture, lavage, and aspiration of secretions from the antrum (Black et al, 1999). However, this test is rarely performed because of the invasive nature of the diagnostic procedure. A computed tomography (CT) is the *noninvasive* gold standard for sinusitis and is ordered when surgery is considered or for recalcitrant cases (sensitivity is about 100%; specificity 65%). Sinus films are often the first diagnostic test to be ordered for those who fail treatment or who have complicating factors (sensitivity 70%; specificity nearly 100%). If a maxillary sinusitis is suspected, then a single Water's view is almost as reliable as a complete sinus series (Black et al, 1999).

Table 6-2
Sinus Pressure Differential Diagnostic Cues

Diagnosis	Signs and Symptoms	Lab Data	Treatment
Sinusitis Acute (<3 weeks duration) Chronic (>3 months duration)	Nasal congestion, fever, purulent nasal discharge, facial pain worse with bending over, intermittent sore throat, tooth pain, H/A *Maxillary sinus symptoms:* Pain and pressure over the cheeks, may be referred to the teeth and hard palate via branches of the trigeminal nerve *Frontal sinus symptoms:* Pain and tenderness over the forehead *Ethmoid sinus symptoms:* pain over the retro-orbital area and lateral wall of the nose *Sphenoid sinus symptoms:* Pain in the retro-orbital, frontal, and facial areas In *chronic sinusitis* nasal discharge and congestion are prominent Fever, H/A, and pain are mild or absent	In most cases the clinical findings are adequate to diagnose sinusitis. In patients with recurrent, persistent sinusitis despite antibiotic therapy, or with atypical presentations, consider ordering sinus films. Sinus films include the Caldwell (frontal), Waters (maxillary), lateral (sphenoid), and submentovertical (ethmoid) views. Presence of sinus opacification, air-fluid levels, or mucosal thickening is indicative of sinusitis. CT of sinuses is reserved for those who have negative x-rays and are symptomatic and for those with complicated disease. MRI is useful in differentiating mucosal inflammation from tumor. Nasal cultures are not useful as they do not correlate with sinus fluid and there are many false-positive isolates of staphylococcal species.	Treatments of uncomplicated acute sinusitis include decongestants (e.g., pseudoephedrine [Sudafed] 60-120 mg tid-qid), nasal decongestant sprays (e.g., oxymetazoline [Afrin], one or two sprays in each nostril every 6-8 hours for 1-3 days—do not administer longer or may have rebound nasal congestion [rhinitis medicamentosa]) Antibiotics effective in uncomplicated acute sinusitis include amoxicillin or trimethoprim-sulfamethoxazole, often used for 14 days or 7 days after symptoms subside When beta-lactamase–producing *H. influenza* and *Moraxella* are of concern, consider using amoxicillin-clavulanate (Augmentin), cefaclor (Ceclor), loracarbef (Lorabid), azithromycin (Zithromax), or clarithromycin (Biaxin) Other treatments include increasing fluids, local application of heat, and inhalation of steam With chronic sinusitis cover beta-lactamase–producing organisms with antibiotics and use for longer time frame (21-30 days). Refer if recurrent or if emergent condition arises
Rhinitis *Allergic Rhinitis* Due to allergen exposure Symptoms become more intense	Sneezing, nasal congestion and watery discharge; itching of the eyes, nose, and throat; tearing and postnasal drip; allergic shiners, conjunctiva has	Allergy testing may help determine allergens Skin testing is often used by preparing allergens (e.g., dusts, molds) and using a needle to introduce them	Avoid allergens. For perennial allergic rhinitis, dust with damp cloth, use a dehumidifier, use a pillow encased in an allergen-impermeable cover, cover

Table 6-2
Sinus Pressure Differential Diagnostic Cues—cont'd

Diagnosis	Signs and Symptoms	Lab Data	Treatment
Rhinitis—cont'd			
with subsequent exposure Seasonal allergies (e.g., pollen) Perennial allergies (e.g., animal dander, dust, and mold)	cobblestone look, nasal salute. Nasal mucosa may appear pale and edematous Symptoms are usually worse in the AM and PM.	under the skin; if a wheal and flare occurs within 20 minutes, it is a positive test Sinus films if sinusitis is suspected	the mattresses with an elastic fabric casing, avoid fur-bearing animals, toss old newspapers to prevent mold growth Trial topical corticosteroids such as flunisolide (Flonase), two sprays in each nostril qd; or beclomethasone dipropionate (Beconase), two inhalations in each nostril bid May use oral antihistamine (e.g., loratadine [Claritin], fexofenadine [Allegra], and cetirizine [Zyrtec]). Other treatment options include oral decongestants, intranasal decongestants (use cautiously due to rebound phenomena), anticholinergics (e.g., ipratropium nasal spray), intranasal cromolyn, oral corticosteroids (for short periods)
Vasomotor rhinitis Abnormal autonomic responsiveness that results in vascular dilation dilation of the vessels No correlation to allergens Typically adult onset Negative family history of allergies	Abrupt onset of congestion and nasal discharge are most common symptoms Emotional upset, sexual arousal, and extreme temperatures can often trigger symptoms Itching is absent	Smears of nasal secretions for eosinophils have limited specificity; if infection is present, a large number of neutrophils will be observed Radioallergosorbent testing (RAST) has modest sensitivity, high specificity, and high cost—usually only done for equivocal or special cases Most often diagnosis is made on clinical data Skin testing is negative Nasal smear is negative	No definitive treatment Avoid triggers such as temperature changes, strong perfumes or odors, tobacco smoke, and emotional upsets Try humidification of the home in the winter Do not use decongestant nasal sprays May use physiological nasal saline solution such as Ocean or Salinex or make saline nasal drops by putting 1/4 tsp salt in 8 oz of water and boiling; may use when cool May try topical ipratropium (an antihistamine) or a mild adrenergic agent (e.g., pseudoephedrine [Sudafed])

Continued

Table 6-2
Sinus Pressure Differential Diagnostic Cues—cont'd

Diagnosis	Signs and Symptoms	Lab Data	Treatment
Dental Abscess	Swelling (may be fluctuant) in the mucosa adjacent to the tooth involved Severe pain May have difficulty opening mouth May experience a low-grade fever	Specialist may order x-rays to evaluate dental caries and confirm abscess	Referral to a dentist or oral surgeon Strong analgesia for the discomfort and antibiotic such as Pen-Vee K or amoxicillin Drainage of the abscess
Nasal Polyps Asthma and aspirin sensitivity increases the likelihood of nasal polyps	Sense of blockage of a nostril, diminished sense of smell, possible nose bleeds. Polyps are pale, edematous and covered with mucosa	None	For small polyps may try a topical nasal steroid spray (e.g., beclomethasone 42 ug/spray) May need referral to ENT Often will require surgical removal
Tumor	Symptoms of sinusitis (see above) Also, may experience CNS disturbances, epistaxis, persistent pain, cranial neuropathies	Sinus films may show destruction of the bone MRI would identify tumor	Refer to specialist for evaluation and treatment

Diagnostic Impression   A.N. presents to your office with the following: pressure over her cheeks that is worse with bending, purulent nasal discharge, and generalized headache. The upper respiratory infection, use of Afrin nasal spray (3 weeks duration), and the presence of a cat in her home environment were predisposing factors to the acute sinusitis.

Therapeutic Plan of Care   A.N. should be prescribed an antibiotic (amoxicillin 500 mg tid × 14 days) and a combination decongestant and antihistamine (because of the allergen exposure). A.N. could use loratadine 10 mg/pseudoephedrine sulfate 240 mg (Claritin-D 24-hour) 1 qd for 7 to 14 days. Antihistamines should be avoided in patients who do not have an allergic component because they cause thickening of the secretions and decrease the outflow of sinus secretions. A.N. should

discontinue use of the Afrin nasal spray and be instructed on the proper use of a nasal decongestant and the side effect of rebound congestion. A.N. should help her cousin find a new home for the cat to remove the allergen in her environment. She should increase fluid intake to 2 liters per day.

Patient Education and/or Community Resources   The patient should be instructed to return if there is no improvement or if the severity of the symptoms increases. Instruct the patient to return immediately if there is periorbital swelling, ptosis, diminished extraocular movements, high fever, or alteration in consciousness. Patients should increase their intake of fluids and humidify the air. Local warmth to the affected sinuses as needed and steam inhalation may decrease congestion. Patients should not swim, scuba dive, or fly during the acute phase of their sinusitis. Those who smoke should be encouraged to quit. A discussion of the impact of smoking on the respiratory tract and the options available for smoking cessation may be beneficial. For those who have an allergic component to the sinusitis, avoidance of the allergens will help decrease the frequency of infections.

Provide instruction on intranasal medications for patients who need to use them. Instruct the patient to clear the nasal passages prior to using the medication. While in an upright position, the patient should spray the medication into each nostril, but away from the nasal septum. The medication should be administered rapidly and the patient should retain the medicine for 5 to 10 minutes. The patient should cleanse the intranasal canister after each use.

Follow-Up Plan   The patient should be reevaluated in 48 to 72 hours if there is no improvement. Depending on the severity of the patient's symptoms, either switch to a different antibiotic or refer to a specialist. Otherwise, the patient should be reevaluated in 14 days.

Case Study 3

CHIEF COMPLAINT: Cough and Chest Congestion

History of Present Illness   N.T., a 48-year-old Caucasian male, presents complaining of sudden onset (2-day history) of a bad, nagging cough with an occasional expectoration of a small amount of thick, rust-colored sputum; slight shortness of breath; low-grade fever; chills; and malaise. He denies weight loss and diaphoresis. He has a history of a cold with symptoms 1 week ago. He took some Tylenol Extra Strength and some Robitussin DM with minimal relief. He is taking fluids, but eating less and sleeping poorly because of the cough and chills. He denies a history of asthma, COPD, TB, and acquired immunodeficiency. He has not had an exposure to anyone with an infectious disease.

Past Medical History   HTN

Past Surgical History   None

Family History   Father, 70, HTN; mother, 68, arthritis; one sister, 46, and one brother, 44, A&W

Developmental Stage   Generativity versus Stagnation

Role-Relationship   N.T. has been married to his second wife for 5 years. With his first wife, N.T. has twin boys who are 24 years old. Both of his sons are on their own, have finished college, and have jobs. N.T. feels he has a good relationship with his current wife. They talk over major decisions and discuss problems until they agree upon a resolution. He lives with his wife in a ranch house in the suburbs and works in construction, repairing roads. N.T. is looking forward to retirement because the job is becoming more physically demanding.

Sleep/Rest   Falls asleep at 10 PM and awakens rested at 5 AM. Does not use sleep aids

Nutrition/Metabolic   Breakfast, donut and coffee; lunch, eats either at fast food restaurants or takes a bag lunch with a sandwich, chips, Coke, and piece of fruit; dinner, wife cooks a meal from various Mexican, Italian, and American menus. Usually snacks on sweets

Activity/Exercise   Does not have a planned exercise program. Feels he gets enough exercise at work with his construction job

Health Management   Smokes one pack per day for 15 years; alcohol, one beer twice a week in the evening; recreational drug use, none

Self-Perception and Values/Beliefs   Is content with his life, but is considering changing jobs because the construction work is very physically demanding. Enjoys the time he has with his wife

Medications   Moexipril (Univasc) 15 mg qd for hypertension

Allergies   NKMA

Pertinent Physical Findings

Vital Signs   Height 6 feet 1 inch; weight 205 pounds; BMI 27; temperature 101.4° F; heart rate 92; respirations 24; blood pressure 132/86

HEENT   Ears: TMs gray. Sinuses: No frontal or maxillary tenderness. Nose: Pink nasal mucosa. Throat: Pink, uvula midline, tonsils 1+. Nodes: No cervical lymphadenopathy

Heart   Apical pulse 92 regular rhythm; no murmurs, S_3, or S_4

Lung   Fine rales in the RLL, whispered pectoriloquy and vocal fremitus present, dullness to percussion in RLL, no rubs, lung expansion equal, O_2 Saturation 96%, PEFR 500

Diagnostics

Diagnostic Tests   Chest x-ray shows infiltrates in the right lower lobe

History Data   Questions specific to the chief complaint of cough and chest congestion include the following:

- How long have you had your symptoms of cough and chest congestion?
- Did your symptoms begin gradually or did they occur suddenly?
- Is your cough occasional or constant?
- Do you have any expectoration when you cough? If so, how often, what color, what is the consistency, and the amount of expectoration?
- Do you have a fever, rhinorrhea, chills, sore throat, or headache?
- Do you have chest pain, shortness of breath with exertion or dyspnea, fatigue, malaise, blood in your sputum, night sweats, nausea, or diarrhea?
- What is your alcohol intake?
- Do you use or have you used recreational drugs?
- Do you smoke? If so, how many packs per day and for how many years?
- What is your occupation?
- Are you up to date on your immunizations?
- Do you have a history of bronchitis, pneumonia, or sinusitis?
- Do you have asthma, chronic obstructive pulmonary disease, acquired immunodeficiency, a history of tuberculosis, hypertension, or congestive heart failure?
- Have you recently been exposed to anyone who has an infectious illness?

Physical Examination Data   The focused examination for the chief complaint of chest congestion includes vital signs, HEENT, heart, and lungs.

Differential Diagnoses   Acute bronchitis, pneumonia, congestive heart failure, asthma, acute exacerbation of chronic bronchitis, bronchiolitis, pulmonary embolism, lung abscess, tuberculosis, bronchogenic carcinoma (Table 6-3)

Probable Causes of the Presenting Symptoms
Acute pneumonia is usually caused by infection of the lower respiratory tract. Infectious particles invade the alveolar surfaces and create an inflammatory response through activation of the cytokines. Inflammatory exudate is produced and causes the systemic symptoms of chills, fever, and fatigue (Bartlett et al, 1998; Kelley, 1997). There is considerable overlap between the presentation of "typical" and "atypical" pneumonias, which may not be distinguished reliably on clinical grounds. The most common organisms for the differential diagnosis of chest congestion are listed in Table 6-4.

Diagnostic Tests   Consider ordering a CXR (PA and lateral) when clinical signs and symptoms are suggestive of pneumonia. When a patient has pneumonia, the chest x-ray will show infiltrates (Figure 6-1).

The CBC will show WBCs in the range of 15,000 to 30,000/ml in bacterial pneumonia (with shift to the left), WBC greater than 10,000/ml in 20% of cases in atypical pneumonia, and WBC greater than 10,000 count in anaerobic pneumonia. Patients who have viral infections may exhibit a higher proportion of lymphocytes in their CBC. Consider a chemistry profile to assess liver and renal function; Gram stain and culture of sputum to evaluate microorganisms; blood cultures, if bacteremia is suspected, to evaluate microorganisms; and oxygen saturation and peak expiratory flow rate to quickly assess respiratory status. Arterial blood gases may be ordered in the emergency room or hospital to assess respiratory exchange.

Diagnostic Impression   N.T. presents with sudden onset of cough with rust-colored sputum production, low-grade fever, chills, and shortness of breath. These clinical symptoms are likely caused from a community-acquired pneumonia (bacterial).

Therapeutic Plan of Care   This patient is 48 years old, in no acute distress, with stable hypertension treated with a single agent. His history, physical, and diagnostic data indicate a bacterial

Text continued on page 119.

Table 6-3
Chest Congestion Differential Diagnostic Cues

Diagnosis	Signs and Symptoms	Lab Data	Treatment
Acute **Bronchitis**	Acute cough, low-grade fever, coarse rhonchi may clear with cough, fatigue, wheeze	None or CXR	Supportive, antibiotics seldom indicated; if elect antibiotics, give erythromycin, tetracycline, amoxicillin, or trimethoprim-sulfamethoxazole
Acute Exacerbation of Chronic Bronchitis	Increased sputum with color change, low-grade fever, dyspnea, increased cough, coarse rhonchi and moist crackles	None or CXR	Aerosolized bronchodilators, systemic corticosteroids, antibiotics such as amoxicillin, trimethoprim-sulfamethoxazole, tetracycline, or erythromycin (macrolide)
Bronchiolitis (Pediatric occurs in those less than 2 years of age)	Fever, coryza, cough, tachypnea, wheezing, suprasternal and intercostal retractions	None or CXR	Oxygen or mist therapy, antibiotics only if bacterial infection is suspected; ribavirin aerosol for those seriously ill with RSV, those with co-morbid conditions, or those with immunodeficiency
Pneumonia		Lab data for all categories of pneumonia:	Determine if hospitalization is needed (see page 119)
Bacterial	Abrupt onset, shaking chills, pleuritic chest pain, fever, tachycardia, tachypnea, rales	Chest x-ray, CBC if considering hospitalization, Gram stain and C&S of sputum if important to isolate pathogens, blood cultures if hospitalized, oxygen saturation to assess respiratory status	Outpatient therapy: If less than 60 years old and without co-morbidity, use a macrolide (e.g., erythromycin [Ery-Tab] 500 mg bid × 10 days) or
Atypical	3-4 day onset, severe nonproductive cough, fever, fatigue, chills, rales		tetracycline (e.g., doxycycline 100 mg bid × 10 days); if suspect *H. influenza* (with risk factors like smokers or COPD), use clarithromycin (Biaxin)
Anaerobic	Symptoms present for 3-5 weeks, chronic productive cough fever (102° F)		250-500 mg bid × 7-14 days or azithromycin (Zithromax) 500 mg qd for day 1 then 250 mg qd days 2-5. If over 60 years of age or have a co-morbid condition, use a second generation cephalosporin (e.g., cefuroxime [Ceftin] 250-500 mg bid × 10 days), trimethoprim-sulfamethoxazole (Bactrim

Continued

	Table 6-3		
	Chest Congestion Differential Diagnostic Cues—cont'd		
Diagnosis	**Signs and Symptoms**	**Lab Data**	**Treatment**
Pneumonia —cont'd			DS) bid × 14 days, or a beta-lactamase inhibitor or the newer fluoroquinolones (e.g., levofloxacin [Levaquin] 500 mg qd × 7-14 days [under age 18 not recommended])
Lung Abscess	Insidious onset of fever, weight loss, cough, poor dental hygiene, foul smelling sputum, malaise	Chest x-ray shows thick-walled solitary cavity surrounded by consolidation	Penicillin G intravenously then penicillin V orally until CXR shows stabilization (usually takes a month or more); use clindamycin if PCN allergy
Pulmonary Tuberculosis	Unexplained mild to marked cough lasting more than 3 weeks, fatigue, weight loss, fever, night sweats, hemoptysis	Sputum specimens for stain and culture × 3 morning specimens The tuberculin skin test is used as a screening tool to identify individuals who have been exposed to tuberculosis CXR	The Centers for Disease Control and Prevention (1993) has published three treatment options for patients without HIV infection. The first involves a four-drug regimen with isoniazid, rifampin, pyrazinamide, and either ethambutol or streptomycin. The total duration of therapy should be at least 6 months and at least 3 months after sputum cultures convert to convert to negative All cases of tuberculosis should be reported to the local and state public health department Tuberculosis should be managed by a skilled clinician that routinely manages patients who have tuberculosis
Bronchogenic Carcinoma	Cough, dyspnea, anorexia, weight loss, hemoptysis	Sputum for cytology CXR Bronchoscopy may be indicated	Refer to a specialist for evaluation and treatment: surgery, chemotherapy, radiation therapy

Table 6-3
Chest Congestion Differential Diagnostic Cues—cont'd

Diagnosis	Signs and Symptoms	Lab Data	Treatment
Pulmonary Embolism	Sudden onset of dyspnea, chest pain, apprehension, tachypnea, syncope, hemoptysis, diaphoresis, tachycardia, pleuritic pain, pleural friction rub	CXR ABG ECG Ventilation-perfusion lung scan Doppler ultrasound	Emergent refer for immediate treatment Anticoagulation therapy Thrombolysis in select cases Select patients may undergo percutaneous low-resistance venous filters or embolectomy
CHF	Shortness of breath, orthopnea, cough, dyspnea on exertion, paroxysmal nocturnal dyspnea, lower extremity edema, tachycardia, third heart sound, elevated venous pressure, rales, cardiac enlargement	ECG to assess myocardial ischemia, MI, LVH, or dysrhythmia CXR to evaluate gross cardiac size and pulmonary pathology (may show Kerley B sign: thin, parallel lines that extend from the pleural surface into the subpleural lung [Wiest, 1996]; or effusion) Echocardiogram to assess anatomical structures (ejection fraction, wall motion, and valve function) Cardiac catheterization if valvular or coronary artery disease must be assessed Other tests based on diagnostic cues (e.g., CBC if suspect anemia, blood cultures if suspect endocarditis, digoxin level if suspect toxicity)	Treat underlying problem; if no specific cause is identified, medical management is indicated Moderate salt restriction (2 grams of sodium) Gradual exercise program Diuretic therapy for relief of symptoms ACE Inhibitors are standard treatment for CHF Digitalis is reserved for those who are symptomatic on diuretics and ACEs *Calcium channel blockers tend to aggravate CHF In select cases, hydralazine, alpha-adrenergic blockers, and beta-blockers may be evaluated for use Other treatment options include: Coronary revascularization for those with CAD For severe cases, cardiac transplantation, cardiomyoplasty, ventricular reduction may be considered

*CHF differential is presented in Chapter 7 on page 138.

Table 6-4
Common Microorganisms

Diagnosis	Microorganisms
Acute Bronchitis	Usually a virus: Influenza A and B virus, adenovirus for adults; respiratory syncytial virus (RSV) for children. Infrequent bacteria are *Streptococcus pneumoniae, Haemophilus influenzae,* and *Moraxella catarrhalis; Mycoplasma pneumoniae* and *Chlamydia pneumoniae* in older children and young adults
Acute Exacerbation of Chronic Bronchitis	*S. pneumoniae, H. influenzae, M. catarrhalis,* and respiratory viruses
Bronchiolitis	*M. pneumoniae* is most common, may have co-infection with other bacteria, RSV or *H. influenzae*
Pneumonia	*S. pneumoniae, H. influenzae, M. pneumoniae, C. pneumoniae; S. aureus, H. influenza, Klebsiella pneumoniae, Enterobacter aerogenes* are more common in the elderly, those who are immunocompromised, and alcoholics. *S. pneumonia* and *S. aureus* are common with patients with splenectomy or spleen problems

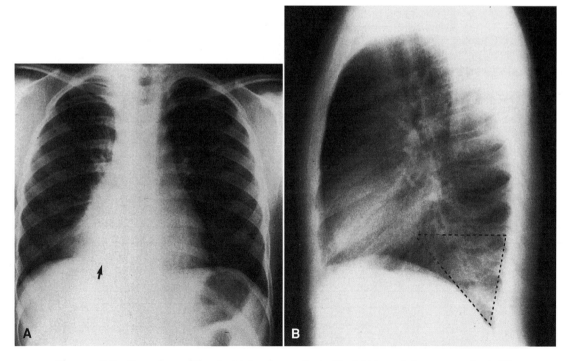

Figure 6-1   X-ray views of the chest taken in a patient with right lower lobe pneumonia. **A,** PA view demonstrates consolidation obscuring the right medial hemidiaphragm *(arrow).* **B,** Lateral view reveals retrocardiac opacification *(dashed triangle).* It is an important diagnostic key to remember that the spine becomes more radiolucent as one proceeds from cephalad to caudal on the lateral projection. Any opacity in this area, however subtle, requires careful consideration. (From Wiest P, Roth P: *Fundamentals of emergency radiology,* Philadelphia, 1996, WB Saunders.)

Text continued from page 114.

pneumonia. He can be treated on an outpatient basis with an oral agent. A macrolide such as clarithromycin for 10 to 14 days would be appropriate as he is a smoker and he is less than 60 years of age.

The following clinical findings indicate a need for hospitalization for pneumonia: age 65 or older, coexisting conditions, temperature higher than 101° F, respiratory rate greater than 30, systolic BP less than 90 or diastolic BP less than 60 mm Hg, multilobular involvement on CXR or other abnormal CXR findings, and noncompliance with the treatment plan. Other clinical symptoms that require hospitalization include heart rate >125, altered mental status, and respiratory hypoxia or acidosis (PO_2 <60; pH <7.35). Hospitalization may also have to be considered for patients who lack home support or who fail to respond to antibiotics after 48 to 72 hours.

A discussion of the impact of smoking on the respiratory system and the predisposition to upper and lower respiratory tract infections and the risk for lung cancer should be reviewed. Encourage N.T. to have an annual flu vaccination.

Patient Education and/or Community Resources Discuss smoking cessation. Increase fluids to a minimum of 2 liters per day and ensure adequate rest. Encourage the patient to complete the full course of antibiotics—even if feeling better—to prevent reoccurrence.

Follow-Up Plan If symptoms show no improvement in 48 hours, or are worsening, the patient should return immediately. Otherwise, schedule an office visit in 1 to 2 weeks to reevaluate the clinical symptoms. If the patient is a smoker, age 65 or older, or immunologically compromised, order CXR in 6 weeks to assess resolution of infiltrates.

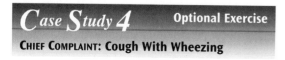

Case Study 4 **Optional Exercise**

CHIEF COMPLAINT: Cough With Wheezing

History of Present Illness S.K., a 64-year-old Caucasian female, presents complaining of insidious onset of a dry cough with wheezing and occasional chest tightness for 7 weeks duration. She has been told she has a breathing condition and was given a Ventolin inhaler and 10 refills and instructed to use it qid prn. She has been using it four times a day for the past 5 days with minimal relief of the wheezing and chest tightness. She is sleeping poorly because she wakes up with some chest tightness. Her appetite is good. She thinks she has allergies because in the fall and spring she has more problems with wheezing than normal.

Past Medical History HTN

Past Surgical History Vaginal hysterectomy with bilateral salpingo-oophorectomy at age 49

Family History Mother age 90, hypothyroidism; father age 88, HTN; sister age 69, hypothyroidism; sister age 67, A&W

Developmental Stage Ego Integrity versus Despair

Role-Relationship S.K. has been divorced for 15 years. She has one son who is married and lives 25 miles away. She lives alone in a small condominium. Is retired from her job as a fourth grade teacher. Has a female friend (Harriet, age 72) with whom she travels on vacations and dines out twice a week at local restaurants. Her son visits every other month, and she talks with her daughter-in-law or son once a month.

Sleep/Rest Falls to sleep at 11 PM and awakens at 7 AM.

Nutrition/Metabolic States she eats three meals per day and feels they are nutritious. Snacks on healthy foods such as fruits, raw vegetables, and crackers

Activity/Exercise Does not engage in planned exercise. Feels she walks about ½ mile per day with her normal daily activities.

Coping/Stress Harriet is her main source of support for decision-making. S.K.'s son is also important in her life, but he is busy with his career, his wife, and two young sons. Attends church every Sunday

Health Management S.K. is a ½ pack-per-day smoker for 15 years. Immunization status: Last Td 1986. Enjoys a glass of red wine in the evening. Has a smoke detector and carbon monoxide detector. Has completed a living will. Last mammogram was 5 years ago

Self-Perception and Values/Beliefs States she is happy with her accomplishments and does volunteer once per month at a local shelter for the homeless. Admits to often feeling lonely

Medications   Propranolol HCl (Inderal) 40 mg bid; ASA 325 mg qam because her neighbor told her it prevented heart disease
Allergies   NKMA

Pertinent Physical Findings
Vital Signs   Height 5 feet 2 inches; weight 136 pounds; BMI 25; temperature 98.6° F; heart rate 72; respirations 20; BP 136/86; O_2 saturation 94%; PEFR 350

HEENT   Ears: TMs gray with distinct cone of light. Nose: pink nasal mucosa. Throat: pink, uvula midline, tonsils 1+; nodes, no cervical lymphadenopathy

Heart   Apical pulse 72, regular rhythm, no murmurs, S_3 or S_4

Lung   Scattered wheezes throughout lung fields and diminished breath sounds in the bases

Diagnostics
Diagnostic Tests   Spirometry + for moderate obstruction

Discussion Questions

What type of history data should be collected?

What type of physical data should be collected?

What are the differential diagnoses?

What are the probable causes of the presenting symptoms?

What is your diagnostic impression?

What is the therapeutic plan of care?

What are the patient education and/or community resources?

What is your follow-up plan?

Discussions for optional case study exercises can be found in the accompanying Instructor's Manual.

References

Bartlett JG, Breiman RF, Mandell LA, File TM: Community-acquired pneumonia in adults: guidelines for management, *Clin Infect Dis* 26(4):811-838, 1998.

Black ER, Bordley DR, Tape TG, Panzer RJ: *Diagnostic strategies for common medical problems,* ed 2, 1999, American College of Physicians.

Centers for Disease Control and Prevention: Initial therapy for tuberculosis in the era of multidrug resistance. Recommendations of the Advisory Council for the Elimination of Tuberculosis, *MMWR* 42(RR-7):1-8, 1993.

Chernecky CC, Berger BJ: *Laboratory tests and diagnostic procedures,* ed 2, Philadelphia, 1997, WB Saunders.

Goroll AH, May LA, Mulley AG: *Primary care medicine,* ed 3, Philadelphia, 1995, Lippincott-Raven.

Kelley W: *Textbook of internal medicine,* ed 3, Philadelphia, 1997, Lippincott-Raven.

Prescriber's Letter: *Pediatrics* March 1999 (ISSN No. 1073-7219):14.

Prescriber's Letter: *Pediatrics* June 1999 (ISSN No. 1073-7219):33.

Rubin H, Voss C, Derksen DJ, Gateley A, Quenzer RW: *Medicine: a primary care approach,* Philadelphia, 1996, WB Saunders.

Ruppert SD: Differential diagnosis of common causes of pediatric pharyngitis, *Nurse Pract* 21(4):38-42, 44, 47-8, 1996.

Tierney L, McPhee SJ, Papadakis MA: *Current medical diagnosis and treatment,* Stamford, Conn., 1999, Appleton & Lange.

Wiest P, Roth P: *Fundamentals of emergency radiology,* Philadelphia, 1996, WB Saunders.

Williams JW Jr: Sinusitis: beginning a new age of enlightenment, *West J Med* 163(1):80-82, 1995.

Williams JW Jr, Simel DL, Roberts L, Samsa GP: Clinical evaluation for sinusitis: making the diagnosis by history and physical examination, *Ann Intern Med* 117(9):705-710, 117, 1992.

Selected Readings

Armitage KB, Gross P, Yamauchi T: Respiratory infections: which antibiotics for empiric therapy? *Patient Care for the Nurse Practitioner* 2(1):30-34, 39-45, 1999.

Cozad J: Infectious mononucleosis, *Nurse Pract* 21(3):14, 16, 23, 27, 1996.

Fine MJ, Auble TE, Yealy DM, Hanusa BH, Weissfeld LA, Singer DE, Coley CM, Marrie TJ, Kapoor WN: A prediction rule to identify low-risk patients with community-acquired pneumonia, *N Engl J Med* 336(4):243-250, 1997.

Hanson MJS: Acute otitis media in children, *Nurse Pract* 21(5):72, 74, 80, 1996.

Kennedy MM: Influenza viral infections: presentation, prevention, and treatment, *Nurse Pract* 23(9):17, 21-22, 25-28, 1998.

King DE, Pippin HJ Jr: Community-acquired pneumonia in adults: initial antibiotic therapy, *Am Fam Physician* 56(2):544-550, 1997.

Madison JM, Irwin RS: Chronic obstructive pulmonary disease, *Lancet,* 352:467-473, 1998.

Poe RH, Israel RH: Chronic cough: a strategy for work-up and therapy, *J Respiratory Diseases* 18(6):629-641, 1997.

CHAPTER 7

Cardiovascular Disorders

Ruth Ann Brintnall

Case Study 1

CHIEF COMPLAINT: Physical Examination

History of Present Illness T.T. is a 40-year-old African-American male who presents for a physical examination after urging by his wife. He has been healthy and generally feels well. His only complaint is mild mid-afternoon headaches. He does admit to several episodes of high blood pressure in the past.

Past Medical History Unremarkable

Surgical History Appendectomy

Family History Mother, A&W; father, HTN; five brothers, A&W

Developmental Stage Generativity versus Stagnation

Role-Relationship Married for 20 years. Has two sons, ages 8 and 9, and one daughter, age 12. Works as a salesman and his wife is a nurse

Sleep/Rest Sleeps 6 to 8 hours per night and awakens rested. Uses OTC sleeping pills when he has heavy job demands (about once per week)

Nutrition/Metabolic He is modestly overweight and admits that his diet and business lunch choices could be improved.

Activity/Exercise No regular exercise; plays neighborhood basketball occasionally

Coping/Stress When he gets frustrated, he eats more. T.T. describes moderate job stress. He often reviews problems and opportunities with his wife. He attends church occasionally

Health Management He recently quit smoking after a 1 pack per day history for more than 20 years. Alcohol, 2 or 3 drinks per day with business lunches or at night to unwind. Caffeine, 6 cups of coffee with cream and sugar per day. Exercise, occasionally plays basketball with the children at night

Self-Perception and Values/Beliefs Is feeling stressed with job demands recently. Would like to return to college for a mid-career shift. His family is his major support.

Medications None

Allergies NKMA

Pertinent Physical Findings

Vital Signs Height 6 feet; weight 235 pounds; BMI 32; temperature 98.2° F; pulse 72; respiration 18; blood pressure 190/110 on right arm, 185/108 on left arm, both readings while sitting; blood pressure at end of examination, 170/100 on right arm

HEENT Normocephalic; features are symmetrical. Eyes: PERRLA with intact EOM; funduscopic examination shows "silver wiring" in both eye grounds. Ears: Normal position, no discharge. Nose: Patent nares, no discharge. Oropharynx: Moist membranes, no visible lesions; teeth are in good repair. Neck: Supple and without masses; no bruits and no JVD evident; thyroid is nonpalpable

Skin Numerous macules are present on anterior face, arms, and hands

Heart Tones are clear, rate is regular. No murmurs are appreciated; however, S_2 is increased

Lungs Respirations are symmetrical and clear throughout; no crackles or wheezing

Abdomen Rounded with well-healed scar present in the RLQ of the abdomen, consistent with history of appendectomy. Nontender, with active bowel sounds in all quadrants; no bruits are heard; no masses or organomegaly are apparent.

Extremities No edema, no tenderness; pulses are readily palpable. ROM is normal; crepitus is apparent in the left knee with range of motion.

Neurological   Cranial nerves II-XII grossly intact; no focal deficits noted

Diagnostics

Diagnostic Tests   A CBC drawn the previous day was normal, with WBC 7.2, hemoglobin 14.0 gm/dl, and platelets 151,000/μl. A complete metabolic profile revealed normal sodium, potassium, chloride, BUN, and creatinine; fasting glucose, however, was elevated at 135. Urine analysis was normal.

History Data   Questions specific to the working diagnosis of hypertension include the following:

- Do you have a history of elevated blood pressure, high cholesterol, diabetes, stroke, or heart disease of any kind?
- Does anyone in your family have high blood pressure, high cholesterol, diabetes, stroke, or heart disease?
- Do you have problems with your kidneys?
- Have you had problems with poor circulation?
- What medications are you taking at present? Do you use any herbal therapies, street drugs, or other products to stay healthy?
- Have you had a recent weight gain or weight loss?

- Do you smoke or have you ever smoked? If so, how long did you smoke and how much did you smoke?
- What is a typical meal for you? Describe what you have eaten over the last 24 hours?
- Do you have headaches? Tell me about them.
- Describe common stresses in your life. Do you feel unusually stressed?

A more detailed history of T.T.'s headaches and other symptoms suggestive of hypertension must be gathered. Other common causes of secondary hypertension should be considered (Table 7-1).

Physical Examination Data   The focused examination suggested for hypertension by the JNC VI (1997) includes: (1) two or more repeat measures of blood pressure (both arms) using recommended techniques and recorded standing and supine; (2) baseline measure of height and weight; (3) funduscopic examination (using established classifications for retinal change); and (4) physical examination including particular attention to carotid bruits, thyromegaly, abnormal heart or lung sounds, abnormal masses, pulsations, or bruits in the abdomen; and examination of the extremities for edema, diminished pulsation, and neurosensory change. Attention to sites of end organ involvement of the heart, brain, kidneys, eyes, and peripheral arteries is also an essential part of the physical examination.

Table 7-1
Common Causes of Secondary Hypertension

Disease	Medications	Other
Renal disease	Antidepressants	Alcohol
Primary aldosteronism	Appetite suppressants	Amphetamines
Renovascular disease	Bromocriptine	Anabolic steroids
Cushing's disease	Cyclosporine	Caffeine
Coarctation of the aorta	Estrogen	Cocaine
Pheochromocytoma	Erythropoietin	Lead
	MAO inhibitors	
	Nasal decongestants	
	NSAIDs	
	Oral contraceptives	
	Steroids	
	Sympathomimetics	

From Joint National Committee: The sixth report of the Joint National Committee on prevention, detection, evaluation, and treatment of high blood pressure, *Arch Intern Med* 157(21):2413-2446, 1997.

Differential Diagnosis   There is no differential diagnosis for hypertension. However, it is important to determine whether the hypertension is primary or secondary. About 95% of all hypertension is primary, or essential, meaning that no particular cause can be determined (Tierney, McPhee, and Papadakis, 1999). Secondary causes of hypertension should be ruled out with an appropriate history and physical examination.

Probable Causes of the Presenting Symptoms
Abnormalities in the nervous system or in the hormonal mechanism (renin-angiotensin-aldosterone system) that regulates blood pressure are common causes of primary hypertension. Excessive dietary salt, insulin resistance, and hyperinsulinemia have also been implicated as possible causes. Rarely, genetic factors that involve the renin-angiotensin-aldosterone system, sympathetic nervous system, or kallikrein-kinin system are causative. A defect in naturetic peptide has also been implicated.

Diagnostic Tests   Suggested laboratory testing includes: CBC to assess for possible anemia or RBC abnormalities; urinalysis and renal function tests to detect blood, protein, and casts; electrolyte assessment to detect abnormal values; fasting blood sugar; lipid profile; and uric acid. A baseline ECG is also suggested. Depending on the suspected cause of the symptoms, other diagnostic tests may include CXR, renal ultrasound, echocar-

diogram, and abdominal imaging. However, routine evaluation for suspected primary hypertension does not require extensive testing unless secondary causes are suspected.

Diagnostic Impression   When no other secondary cause for elevated blood pressure is apparent, essential hypertension can be estalished as a working diagnosis. Because glucose levels are abnormal, the contribution of diabetes mellitus must be evaluated and considered in this case. The history of prior hypertension and the presence of retinal change on examination suggest more longstanding disease. Lifestyle choices are likely also contributory in T.T.'s case.

Therapeutic Plan of Care   After confirming physical and laboratory findings, T.T. needs an education and treatment plan that includes: (1) recognition of hypertension as a disease; and (2) specific lifestyle modifications and strategies that are appropriate given his risk profile (Table 7-2). His success with smoking cessation should be applauded and used as motivation to address other needed lifestyle changes. Mrs. T. should be included in any teaching since she seems to be a factor in T.T.'s choice to seek care. Moreover, she likely prepares meals in the home. Because the evidence of "silver wiring" indicates change in retinal arterial diameter, T.T. will be started on medication as well as targeted lifestyle changes. T.T.'s initial high fasting

---

Table 7-2
Risk Stratification and Treatment

Blood Pressure stages (mm Hg)	Risk Group A (No Risk Factors, No TOD/CCD)*	Risk Group B (At Least One Risk Factor, Not Including Diabetes: No TOD/CCD)	Risk Group C (TOD/CCD and/or Diabetes with or without Other Risk Factors)
High-normal (130-139/85-89)	Lifestyle modification	Lifestyle modification	Drug therapy†
Stage 1 (130-139/85-89)	Lifestyle modification (up to 12 mo)	Lifestyle modification‡ (up to 6 mo)	Drug therapy
Stages 2 and 3 (≥160/≥100)	Drug therapy	Drug therapy	Drug therapy

From Joint National Committee: The sixth report of the Joint National Committee on prevention, detection, evaluation, and treatment of high blood pressure, *Arch Intern Med* 157(21):2413-2446, 1997.
Note: Lifestyle modification should be adjunctive therapy for all patients receiving pharmacologic therapy.
*TOD/CCD indicates target organ disease/clinical cardiovascular disease.
†For those with heart failure, renal insufficiency, or diabetes.
‡For patients with multiple risk factors, clinicians should consider drugs as initial therapy plus lifestyle modifications.

glucose levels and persistent modest elevations require further evaluation for diabetes, with diet and exercise favored as an initial therapy. An ophthalmology referral will be made for baseline.

Patient Education and/or Community Resources The JNC VI algorithm for the treatment of hypertension provides an excellent reference for initial therapy and modification (Figure 7-1). While African-Americans are purported to have a better response to calcium channel blockers and diuretics, the choice of antihypertensive agent is better dictated by comorbid disease. The mechanisms of action within a given class of antihypertensives are often similar. Table 7-3 lists oral antihypertensive agents by category. Likewise, side effects are also common among classes of agents. ACE inhibitors preserve renal function in diabetics, improve CHF, and probably decrease LVH. ACE inhibitors may cause cough, which can be an annoying side effect. Beta-blockers slow the pulse rate and work on the renin-angiotensin system, as well as lowering blood pressure by other unexplained mechanisms. They are beneficial in CAD, angina, migraine, and in persons who tend to be tachycardic. Beta-blockers may cause a slight increase in certain lipid factions, as do diuretics. Diuretics may also affect potassium negatively unless combined with a potassium-sparing agent. Calcium channel blockers dilate blood vessels, control cardiac dysrhythmias, and have orthostatic hypotension as a significant side effect. The newest class of antihypertensives, angiotensin receptor blockers, appears to have all of the benefits of ACE inhibitors with fewer side effects. However, more data is still needed regarding the use of these agents. The alpha-receptor blockers are still another consideration. Table 7-4 identifies considerations for individualizing antihypertensive therapy.

For this patient, a logical first choice agent would be an ACE inhibitor. T.T. will be started on Vasotec, 5 mg daily.

Follow-Up Plan T.T. will be followed with blood pressure measurements taken at least weekly by the office nurse. He will be seen for a follow-up in 1 month, with potassium, FBS, BUN, and creatinine repeated at that time. Target lifestyle changes will include: weight reduction; reduced alcohol and sodium intake; planned physical exercise; diabetic education; and dietary education for healthy living, including adequate potassium and calcium intake. Table 7-5 identifies the dietary approaches to stop hypertension (DASH) diet. Eventually, home blood pressure monitoring will be considered.

The JNC VI provides classification of blood pressure for adults over 18. Table 7-6, has recommendations for follow-up based on initial blood pressure measurement for adults.

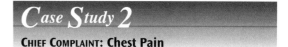

Case Study 2

CHIEF COMPLAINT: Chest Pain

History of Present Illness P.V. is a 60-year-old Caucasion pharmaceutical sales representative who has called the office with complaints of retrosternal chest pain, which he rates as mild in nature. Heavy meals and exertion, such as carrying his display cases up stairs, exacerbate his pain. He denies radiation of his pain, palpitations, sweating, or nausea. He admits to more frequent pain over the last few weeks and increasing "heartburn." He rates his pain as 3 on a numerical scale of 1-10, with 10 representing the most severe pain. Upon questioning he describes the pain as short-lived, lasting less than 5 minutes at a time. He reports that rest or ceasing activity promptly relieves his pain, and therefore he was not overly concerned until the frequency of his pain increased. He has had regular physicals with normal blood pressure readings and normal physical findings. Periodic ECGs have also been unremarkable. He has been told to increase his regular exercise and watch his diet because of elevated cholesterol, modest obesity, and inactivity. He recalls that his "good cholesterol" is a little low and his triglycerides are in question.

Past Medical History Broken R arm age 9

Past Surgical History No surgical procedures

Family History Father deceased at 69 years of CAD; mother is 72, A&W; one uncle with CAD and DM; no cancer, CVA, or HTN in family

Developmental Stage Generativity versus Stagnation

Role-Relationship Married for 27 years; employed for 15 years with present company

Text continued on page 131.

Algorithm for the Treatment of Hypertension

Begin or continue lifestyle modifications

↓

Not at goal blood pressure (<140/90 mm Hg)
Lower goals for patients with diabetes or renal disease

↓

Initial Drug Choices[a]

Uncomplicated Hypertension[b]
Diuretics
β-Blockers

Specific Indications for the Following Drugs
ACE inhibitors
Angiotensin II receptor blockers
α-Blockers
α- and β-Blockers
β-Blockers
Calcium antagonists
Diuretics

Compelling Indications[b]
Diabetes mellitus (type 1) with proteinuria
 • ACE inhibitors
Heart failure
 • ACE inhibitors
 • Diuretics
Isolated systolic hypertension (older persons)
 • Diuretics preferred
 • Long-acting dihydropyridine calcium
   antagonists
Myocardial infarction
 • β-Blockers (non-ISA)
 • ACE inhibitors (with systolic dysfunction)

• Start with a low dose of a long-acting, once-daily drug and titrate dose
• Low-dose combinations may be appropriate

↓

Not at goal blood pressure

↓ No response or troublesome side effects

Substitute another drug from a different class

↓ Inadequate response but well tolerated

Add a second agent from a different class
(diuretic if not already used)

↓

Not at goal blood pressure

↓

Continue adding agents from other classes;
consider referral to a hypertension specialist

[a]Unless contraindicated. *ACE* indicates angiotensin-converting enzyme; *ISA*, intrinsic sympathomimetic activity.
[b]Based on randomized controlled trials.

Figure 7-1 Algorithm for the Treatment of Hypertension. (From Joint National Committee: The sixth report of the Joint National Committee on prevention, detection, evaluation, and treatment of high blood pressure, *Arch Intern Med* 157(21):2413-2446, 1997.)

Table 7-3
Oral Antihypertensive Drugs

Drug	Trade Name	Usual Dose Range, Total mg/day* (Frequency per Day)	Selected Side Effects and Comments*
Diuretics (Partial List)			Short-term: increases cholesterol and glucose levels; biochemical abnormalities: decreases potassium, sodium, and magnesium levels; increases uric acid and calcium levels; rare: blood dyscrasias, photosensitivity, pancreatitis, hyponatremia
Chlorthalidone (G)	Hygroton	12.5-50 (I)	
Hydrochlorothiazide (G)	HydroDIURIL, Microzide, Esidrix	12.5-50 (I)	
Indapamide	Lozol	1.25-5 (I)	(Less or no hypercholesterolemia)
Metolazone	Mykrox, Zaroxolyn	0.5-1.0 (I)	
Loop diuretics			
Bumetanide (G)	Bumex	0.5-4 (2-3)	(Short duration of action, no hypercalcemia)
Ethacrynic acid	Edecrin	25-100 (2-3)	(Only nonsulfonamide diuretic, ototoxicity)
Furosemide (G)	Lasix	40-240 (2-3)	(Short duration of action, no hypercalcemia)
Torsemide	Demadex	5-100 (1-2)	
Potassium-sparing Agents			Hyperkalemia
Amiloride hydrochloride (G)	Midamor	5-10 (I)	
Spironolactone (G)	Aldactone	25-100 (I)	(Gynecomastia)
Triamterene (G)	Dyrenium	25-100 (I)	
Adrenergic Inhibitors			
Peripheral agents			
Guanadrel	Hylorel	10-75 (2)	(Postural hypertension, diarrhea)
Guanethidine monosulfate	Ismelin	10-150 (1)	(Postural hypertension, diarrhea)
Reserpine (G) §	Serpasil	0.05-0.25 (I)	(Nasal congestion, sedation, depression, activation of peptic ulcer)
Central alpha-agonists			Sedation, dry mouth, bradycardia, withdrawal hypertension
Clonidine hydrochloride (G)	Catapres	0.2-1.2 (2-3)	(More withdrawal)

From Joint National Committee: The sixth report of the Joint National Committee on prevention, detection, evaluation, and treatment of high blood pressure *Arch Intern Med* 157(21):2413-2446, 1997.
Note: (G) indicates generic form is available.
*These dosages may vary from those listed in the Physicians' Desk Reference (51st edition), which may be consulted for additional information. The listing of side effects is not all-inclusive, and side effects are for the class of drugs except where noted for individual drugs (in parentheses); clinicians are urged to refer to the package insert for a more detailed listing.
§ Also acts centrally.

Table 7-3
Oral Antihypertensive Drugs—cont'd

Drug	Trade Name	Usual Dose Range, Total mg/day* (Frequency per Day)	Selected Side Effects and Comments*
Adrenergic Inhibitors—cont'd			
Guanabenz acetate (G)	Wytensin	8-32 (2)	
Guanfacine hydrochloride (G)	Tenex	1-3 (1)	(Less withdrawal)
Methyldopa	Aldomet	500-3000 (2)	(Hepatic and "autoimmune" disorders)
Alpha-blockers			Postural hypotension
Doxazosin mesylate	Cardura	1-16 (1)	
Prazosin hydrochloride (G)	Minipress	2-30 (2-3)	
Terazosin hydrochloride	Hytrin	1-20 (1)	
Beta-blockers			Bronchospasm, bradycardia, heart failure, may mask insulin-induced hypoglycemia; less serious: impaired peripheral circulation, insomnia, fatigue, decreased exercise tolerance, hypertriglyceridemia (except agents with intrinsic sympathomimetic activity)
Acebutolol‡†	Sectral	200-800 (1)	
Atenolol (G) ‡	Tenormin	25-100 (1-2)	
Betaxolol‡	Kerlone	5-20 (1)	
Bisoprolol‡	Zebeta	2.5-10 (1)	
Carteolol hydrochloride†	Cartrol	2.5-10 (1)	
Metoprolol tartrate‡	Lopressor	50-300 (2)	
Metoprolol succinate‡	Tropol-XL	50-300 (1)	
Nadolol (G)	Corgard	40-320 (1)	
Penbutolol sulfate†	Levatol	10-20 (1)	
Pindolol (G) †	Visken	10-60 (2)	
Propranolol hydrochloride (G)	Inderal	40-480 (2)	
	Inderal LA	40-480 (1)	
Timolol maleate (G)	Blocadren	20-60 (2)	
Combined alpha- and beta-blockers			Postural hypotension, bronchospasm
Carvedilol	Coreg	12.5-50 (2)	
Labetalol hydrochloride (G)	Normodyne, Trandate	200-1200 (2)	
Direct Vasodilators			Headaches, fluid retention, tachycardia
Hydralazine hydrochloride (G)	Apresoline	50-300 (2)	(Lupus Syndrome)
Minoxidil (G)	Loniten	5-100 (1)	(Hirsutism)

† Has intrinsic sympathomimetic activity.
‡ Cardioselective.

Continued

Table 7-3
Oral Antihypertensive Drugs—cont'd

Drug	Trade Name	Usual Dose Range, Total mg/day* (Frequency per Day)	Selected Side Effects and Comments*
Calcium Antagonists			Conduction defects, worsening of systolic dysfunction, gingival hyperplasia (Nausea, headache)
Nondihydropyridines			
Diltiazem hydrochloride	Cardizem SR	120-360 (2)	
	Cardizem CD, Dilacor XR, Tiazac	120-360 (1)	
Verapamil hydrochloride	Isoptin SR, Calan SR, Verelan, Covera HS	90-480 (2) 120-480 (1)	(Constipation)
Dihydropyridines			
Amlodipine besylate	Norvasc	2.5-10 (1)	
Felodipine	Plendil	2.5-20 (1)	
Isradipine	DynaCirc, DynaCirc CR	5-20 (2) 5-20 (1)	
Nicardipine	Cardene SR	60-90 (2)	
Nifedipine	Procardia XL, Adalat CC	30-120 (1)	
Nisoldipine	Sular	20-60 (1)	
ACE Inhibitors			Common: cough; rare: angioedema, hyperkalemia, rash, loss of taste, leukopenia
Benazepril hydrochloride	Lotensin	5-40 (1-2)	
Captopril (G)	Capoten	25-150 (2-3)	
Enalapril maleate	Vasotec	5-40 (1-2)	
Fosinopril sodium	Monopril	10-40 (1-2)	
Lisinopril	Prinivil, Zestril	5-40 (1)	
Moexipril	Univasc	7.5-15 (1-2)	
Quinapril hydrochloride	Accupril	5-80 (1-2)	
Ramipril	Altace	1.25-20 (1-2)	
Trandolapril	Mavik	1-4 (1)	
Angiotensin II Receptor Blockers			Angioedema (very rare), hyperkalemia
Losartan potassium	Cozaar	25-100 (1-2)	
Valsartan	Diovan	80-320 (1)	
Irbesartan	Avapro	150-300 (1)	

From Joint National Committee: The sixth report of the Joint National Committee on prevention, detection, evaluation, and treatment of high blood pressure, *Arch Intern Med* 157(21):2413-2446, 1997.
Note: (G) indicates generic form is available.

Table 7-4
Considerations for Individualizing Antihypertensive Drug Therapy[a]

Indication	Drug Therapy
Compelling Indications Unless Contraindicated	
Diabetes mellitus (type 1) with proteinuria	ACE I
Heart failure	ACE I, diuretics
Isolated systolic hypertension (older patient)	Diuretics (preferred), CA (long-acting DHP)
Myocardial infarction	Beta-blockers (non-ISA), ACE I (with systolic dysfunction)
May Have Favorable Effects on Comorbid Conditions*	
Angina	Beta-blockers, CA
Atrial tachycardia and fibrillation	Beta-blockers, CA (non-DHP)
Cyclosporine-induced hypertension (caution with the dose of cyclosporine)	CA
Diabetes mellitus (type 1 and 2) with proteinuria	ACE I (preferred), CA
Diabetes mellitus (type 2)	Low-dose diuretics
Dyslipidemia	Alpha blockers
Essential tremor	Beta-blockers (non CS)
Heart failure	Carvedilol, losartan potassium
Hyperthyroidism	Beta-blockers
Migraine	Beta-blockers (non CS), CA (non-DHP)
Myocardial infarction	Diltiazem hydrochloride, verapamil hydrochloride
Osteoporosis	Thiazides
Preoperative hypertension	Beta-blockers
Prostatism (BPH)	Alpha-blockers
Renal insufficiency (caution in renovascular hypertension and creatinine $\geq$ 265.2 μmol/L [3 mg/dL])	ACE I
May Have Unfavorable Effects on Comorbid Conditions*†	
Bronchospastic disease	Beta-blockers§
Depression	Beta-blockers, central alpha-agonists, reserpine§
Diabetes mellitus (types 1 and 2)	Beta-blockers high-dose diuretics
Dyslipidemia	Beta-blockers (non-ISA), diuretics (high-dose)
Gout	Diuretics
2-degree or 3-degree heart block	Beta-blockers,§ CA (non-DHP) §
Heart failure	Beta-blockers (except carvedilol), CA (except amlodipine besylate, felodipine)
Liver disease	Labetalol hydrochloride, methyldopa§
Peripheral vascular disease	Beta-blockers
Pregnancy	ACE I, angiotensin II receptor blockers§
Renal insufficiency	Potassium-sparing agents
Renovascular disease	ACE I, angiotensin II receptor blockers

From Joint National Committee: The sixth report of the Joint National Committee on prevention, detection, evaluation, and treatment of high blood pressure, *Arch Intern Med* 157(21):2413-2446, 1997.
*Conditions and drugs are listed in alphabetical order.
†These drugs may be used with special monitoring unless contraindicated.
ACE I, angiotensin-converting enzyme inhibitors; *BPH,* benign prostatic hyperplasia; *CA,* calcium antagonists; *DHP,* dihydropteridine; *ISA,* intrinsic sympathomimetic activity; *MI,* myocardial infraction; *non-CS,* noncardioselective.

Table 7-5
The Dietary Approaches to Stop Hypertension (DASH) Diet

Food Group	Daily Servings	Serving Sizes	Examples and Notes Food Group to the DASH Diet Pattern	Significance of Each
Grains and Grain Products	7-8	1 slice bread ½ C dry cereal ½ C cooked rice, pasta, or cereal	Whole wheat bread, English muffin, pita bread, bagel, cereals, grits, oatmeal	Major sources of energy and fiber
Vegtables	4-5	1C raw leafy vegetable ½ C cooked vegetable 6 oz vegetable juice	Tomatoes, potatoes, carrots, peas, squash, broccoli, turnip greens, collards, kale, spinach, artichokes, beans, sweet potatoes	Rich sources of potassium, magnesium, and fiber
Fruits	4-5	6 oz fruit juice I medium fruit ¼ C dried fruit ½ C fresh, frozen, or canned fruit	Apricots, bananas, dates, grapes, oranges, orange juice, grapefruit, grapefruit juice, mangoes, melons, peaches, pineapples, prunes, raisins, strawberries, tangerines	Important sources of potassium, magnesium, and fiber
Low-fat or Nonfat Dairy Foods	2-3	8 oz milk 1 C yogurt 1.5 oz cheese	Skim or 1% milk, skim or low-fat buttermilk, nonfat or low-fat yogurt, part-skim mozzarella cheese, nonfat cheese	Major source of calcium and protein
Meats, Poultry, and Fish	2 or less	3 oz cooked meats, poultry, or fish	Select only lean; trim away visible fats; broil, roast, or boil, instead of frying; remove skin from poultry	Rich source of protein and magnesium
Nuts, Seeds, and Legumes	4-5 per week	1.5 oz or ⅓ C nuts ½ oz or 2 Tbsp seeds ½ C cooked legumes	Almonds, filberts, mixed nuts, peanuts, walnuts, sunflower seeds, kidney beans, lentils	Rich source of energy, magnesium, potassium, protein, and fiber

From Joint National Committee: The sixth report of the Joint National Committee on prevention, detection, evaluation, and treatment of high blood pressure, *Arch Intern Med* 157(21):2413-2446, 1997.

Table 7-6

Recommendations for Follow-up Based on Initial Blood Pressure Measurements for Adults

Initial Blood Pressure (mm Hg)*		Follow-up Recommendations†
Systolic	**Diastolic**	
<130	<85	Recheck in 2 years
130-139	85-89	Recheck in 1 year‡
140-159	90-99	Confirm within 2 months‡
160-179	100-109	Evaluate or refer to source of care within 1 month
≥180	≥110	Evaluate or refer to source of care immediately or within 1 week depending on clinical situation

From Joint National Committee: The sixth report of the Joint National Committee on prevention, detection, evaluation, and treatment of high blood pressure, *Arch Intern Med* 157(21):2413-2446, 1997.
*If systolic and diastolic categories are different, follow recommendations for shorter time follow-up (e.g., 160/86 mm Hg should be evaluated or referred to source of care within 1 month).
†Modify the scheduling of follow-up according to reliable information about past blood pressure measurements, other cardiovascular risk factors, or target organ disease.
‡Provide advice about lifestyle modifications.

Text continued from page 124.

Sleep/Rest Sleeps 6½ hours per night and awakens rested. P.V. uses Ambien 5 mg at HS prn for sleep. He usually uses it about twice a month.

Nutrition/Metabolic Eats a large breakfast with eggs and bacon; has a good-sized lunch with meat, potatoes, and a vegetable; and his wife makes a wonderful dinner in the evening. P.V. snacks frequently on candy and sweets.

Activity/Exercise No regular exercise, but works to maintain a small garden with tomatoes and peppers

Coping/Stress Feels occasional stress from work. Has a positive relationship with his wife and talks with her frequently. Uses Xanax prn if the stress gets too bad (usually takes 1 pill two or three times per month). Has not attended church for over 20 years, but feels with his chest pain that he might start attending Sunday services again

Health Management Quit smoking 2 years ago, has 30-pack year prior history; alcohol intake includes 2 to 3 oz bourbon per day; caffeine includes 6 to 10 cups of coffee per day

Self-Perception and Values/Beliefs Feels positive about himself and prides himself in his strong work and family ethic

Medications Multivitamin, vitamin E, ASA 325 mg/day, and occasional Xanax for nerves. Ambien 5 mg at HS prn sleep.

Allergies NKMA

Pertinent Physical Findings

Vital Signs BP 140/90; heart rate 80; respirations 20; weight 207 pounds; height 5 feet 11 inches; BMI 29

General Appearance Well developed, no acute distress, modestly overweight in "apple" distribution

HEENT Unremarkable; no nicking, or signs of increased blood pressure

Lungs Clear to auscultation; no abnormal sounds are heard

Heart Regular, tones are distinct; II-III/VI systolic murmur loudest at the LSB radiating to the neck

Abdomen Obese, no guarding, tenderness or rebound; no hepatomegaly or splenomegaly

Extremities Good peripheral pulses, no edema, no clubbing or cyanosis

Neurological Cranial nerves II-XII are intact; normal examination. No focal weakness is apparent

Diagnostics

Diagnostic Tests ECG is normal; CBC was also within normal limits; a lipid panel showed cholesterol at 245, HDL at 35 and triglycerides at 250

History Data   Questions specific to the chief complaint of chest pain include the following:

- Describe your pain for me. Have you ever had pain like this before?
- Can you rate your pain for me on a scale of 1-10, with 10 representing the worst pain you have ever experienced?
- What were you doing when the pain presented? What makes the pain better? What makes it worse?
- What do you think is causing your pain?
- Do you, or anyone in your family, have a history of chest pain, heart disease, high cholesterol or lipids, diabetes, or stroke?

A careful history will help focus subsequent diagnostics and physical examination to rule out the more serious causes of chest pain efficiently.

Physical Examination Data   The chief complaint of chest pain requires a complete physical examination with attention to all body systems. The patient appearing in acute distress requires emergent transfer.

Differential Diagnosis   Chest pain can present as a chief complaint in a number of disorders. Cardiac causes of chest pain can include angina, pericarditis, myocardial infarction, dissecting aortic aneurysm, and others. The more common causes of noncardiac chest pain include gastrointestinal disorders (such as reflux or ulcer), pneumonia with pleuritis, musculoskeletal pain, spontaneous pneumothorax, pulmonary hypertension, and anxiety. Pulmonary embolism in a traveling salesman, or anyone who sits for extended periods, is a further consideration. Table 7-7 lists the common causes of cardiac chest pain.

Table 7-7 Common Causes of Cardiac Chest Pain Differential Diagnostic Cues			
Diagnosis	**Signs and Symptoms**	**Lab Data**	**Treatment**
Angina	Retrosternal chest pain or burning, "tightness"; may radiate to neck, jaw, left arm and last 10 minutes; worse with exercise, cold, heavy meals, stress; split S2; better with rest	Laboratory studies may be completely normal ECG may be normal	Relieved with rest; responds to sublingual nitroglycerin
Myocardial infarction	Substernal pain "vice-like"; heavy, pressure, constriction; lasts 10 minutes; may be accompanied with SOB, diaphoresis, nausea, and vomiting	ST segment elecation on ECG or depression evolving Q waves, symmetrical inversion of T waves CK-MB elevation; Troponin T, or Troponin I elevation	Requires urgent care for possible thrombolytic therapy, ASA, nitrates, O_2; observation for dysrhythmias, monitoring
Pericarditis	Substernal pain or pain at apex of heart; may radiate; sharp, stabbing pain, "knife-like" Deep breathing, supine position increases pain Friction rub and pulsus paradoxus may be present	ECG may show ST and T changes; CXR may show cardiac enlargement; echocardiogram may show effusion	Restrictive pericarditis with tamponade must be ruled out; referral to emergent care or cardiologist

Table 7-8 lists the common noncardiac causes of chest pain.

Probable Causes of the Presenting Symptoms

P.V.'s symptoms and history are consistent with cardiac-related chest pain. The most likely cause is angina due to an imbalance between oxygen demand and supply.

Diagnostic Tests Expanded laboratory testing would include a CBC, electrolyte panel, lipid panel with total cholesterol, HDL, and triglycerides. Urinalysis is also important. A treadmill will be ordered if the initial ECG is normal; if abnormal, but not diagnostic, a nuclear stress test (e.g., thallium or Cardiolite) or stress echocardiogram should be ordered. If cardiac studies are normal, and no other overt findings are apparent, a gastrointestinal source should be considered. An ultrasound of the gall bladder, liver, and pancreas would be appropriate. Endoscopy may also be helpful as further work-up.

Diagnostic Impression P.V.'s presentation, risk factors, and evaluation suggest angina. The character, duration, and circumstances under which his pain appears support a diagnosis of angina because his pain is consistently associated with activity and promptly relieved by rest. The stable character and location of the pain, and the lack of atypical descriptors such as "crushing" or "knife-like," also support angina. The diagnosis would also be more likely if nitroglycerine, given sublingually, relieved or prevented the distress. The relative absence of other abnormal findings supports an initial diagnosis of angina.

Therapeutic Plan of Care Initial treatment will depend upon degree of suspicion on the ECG. Most CAD is associated with normal laboratory studies, and a stress test is a logical next step. The patient should be cautioned about stressful activity and recurring episodes of pain. P.V. should be given clear direction for accessing medical help during

---

Table 7-8
Noncardiac Causes of Chest Pain Differential Diagnostic Cues

Diagnosis	Signs and Symptoms	Lab Data	Treatment
GI Disorders	Substernal, epigastric; burning, aching, colic-like, nausea or vomiting; worse when lying flat or with meals	ECG is normal; cardiac enzymes are normal;	Responds to antacids, H_2-blockers, or proton pump therapy
Pneumonia With Pleuritis	Pain is more localized, pleuritic in character; area of consolidation on physical examination; SOB, cough, fever, pleural rub	ECG is normal; cardiac enzymes are normal CXR shows infiltrates, area of consolidation	Resolves with treatment of pneumonia
Pulmonary Embolism	Substernal pain; angina-like pain; sudden onset minutes to hours; dyspnea, hypotension, hemoptysis	ECG is normal; cardiac studies are normal; V/Q scan positive for altered perfusion; spiral CT diagnostic for PE, or angiogram	Emergent care referral; systemic anticoagulation; O_2
Musculoskeletal	Variable, aching; movement exacerbates; history of injury or exertion; tender to pressure	Cardiac work-up is normal	Responds to NSAIDs, rest

further diagnostics. Nitroglycerin tablets may be given for use with recurring pain. Long-standing nitrates in an oral or transdermal form could also be considered if his pain is responsive to nitrates. A proton pump or histamine H_2 blocker may also be appropriate while awaiting test results. The basics of healthy eating were discussed and P.V. was placed on an American Heart Association diet. Excess caffeine and alcohol were discouraged. With a positive nuclear test, a prompt referral to a cardiologist for cardiac catheterization is imperative. In this patient, the stress test was positive and a coronary angiogram showed 60% to 70% lesions in three vessels. The cardiologist further noted aortic stenosis, which was consistent with the cardiac murmur heard on initial assessment.

Patient Education and/or Community Resources Written resources from the American Heart Association describing "heart smart" low-cholesterol diet, weight control, and exercise were given to P.V. He was also given the contact number of a local walking club, which he later joined.

Follow-Up Plan P.V. will continue care under the direction of the cardiologist as well as his primary care provider. He was directed for small group education on low-cholesterol diet, exercise, and healthy lifestyle. Target weight loss was established. P.V. was started on a lipid-lowering agent and a beta-blocker. ASA 81 mg/day, vitamin E 400 units/day, and a multivitamin were also ordered. A 3-month follow-up was arranged. A repeat electrolyte panel, lipid panel, and CBC will be obtained at that time. If advance directives have not been addressed, an appropriately-timed discussion of preferences should be arranged.

Case Study 3

CHIEF COMPLAINT: Shortness of Breath

History of Present Illness G.B. is a 66-year-old Caucasian female who complains of dyspnea on exertion, increasing over the last 2 weeks. She admits to significant SOB when attempting to climb stairs. She further describes the need to sleep with two pillows lately, and blames this on her hiatal hernia. She recently notes a feeling of bloating and some mild ankle edema. She has had only an occasional cough, mostly at night. She specifically denies chest pain, chills, fever, night sweats, or sputum production.

G.B. has a remote history of myocardial infarction (15 years ago) that was uncomplicated and not followed. She admits that she has "fallen away" from seeing a doctor on a regular basis. She was known to have high blood pressure in the past, but denies current use of any antihypertensives. She has her blood pressure checked regularly at the grocery store, with readings of 140-150/80-90.

Past Medical History Denies illnesses other than above

Past Surgical History Cholecystectomy age 40

Family History Father deceased at age 40 with CAD; mother deceased at age 70 with CVA; sister aged 63 A&W; brother deceased at age 49 with CAD; denies family history of cancer, no knowledge of cholesterol

Developmental Stage Ego Integrity versus Despair

Role-Relationship Lives independently with her husband. She is retired from the telephone company after 30 years as a senior operator. She describes a loving relationship with her husband and their two daughters, who live nearby.

Sleep/Rest Sleeps about 8 hours a night; describes recent difficulty. Occasionally sleeps in chair for comfort

Nutrition/Metabolic Breakfast, juice and toast or cereal; lunch, soup and salad or sandwich; dinner, meat, vegetables, salad, and dessert. Snacks two or three times a week in the evening, usually chips or cheese and an apple

Activity/Exercise Enjoys walking with a friend in the mall; had to stop walking in the last month due to her SOB

Coping/Stress G.B. describes her husband as her best support. She further indicates a good relationship with her two daughters

Health Management Smoking history, 30 pack-years, quit 10 years ago; denies use of alcohol

Self-Perception and Values/Beliefs Describes herself as independent and hard working; attends church regularly; says she is not uncomfortable expressing her thoughts and feelings

Medications Multivitamin, echinacea, occasional ASA or Advil

Allergies Strawberries

Pertinent Physical Findings

Vital Signs Height 5 feet 5 inches; weight 168 pounds; BMI 28; temperature 98.2° F; heart rate 88; respirations 18; blood pressure 178/98 sitting

General appearance Elderly Caucasian female, appearing older than stated age; mildly dyspneic at rest; skin is sallow and pale

HEENT Normocephalic, features are symmetrical; PERRLA with EOMI, sclera are non-icteric; arteriole/vein (AV) ratio 1:3 with increased light reflex and minor nicking; no hemorrhage or exudates; nares intact, no polyps, no lesions; oral, membranes moist; dentition in good repair; carotids +2 and equal, right with 2/4 bruit, louder as bruit is followed up the neck; slight increase in neck veins measuring 6 cm at 45 degrees; no hepatojugular reflex or unusual pulses or "v" waves; thyroid not enlarged; no adenopathy

Heart PMI is outside the MCL with questionable left ventricular heave; tones are regular S_1 is normal and S_2 is increased; there is a questionable S_3 and S_4. There is a 3/6 mitral regurgitant murmur heard best from the LSB to the apex. No diastolic murmurs are apparent. A soft aortic basal II/VI SEM is heard but without radiation to the neck

Lungs Bibasilar crackles; clear to palpation and percussion; no bronchophony, egophony, or whispered pectoriloquy

Abdomen Soft; nontender; no organomegaly; no palpable masses, guarding, or tenderness. Bowel tones are normal; rectal is unremarkable with brown stool

Neurological Intact; cranial nerves II-XII intact; DTR, gait, Babinski, and mental status are normal; no focal areas of weakness are noted

Extremities Peripheral pulses, equal; 1+ edema is present in both lower extremities to the mid-tibia

Diagnostics

Diagnostic Tests Initial evaluation should include ECG and CXR completed the day of evaluation; oxygen saturation should be checked in the office, and blood should be drawn for a CBC, electrolytes, BUN, and creatinine. A urinalysis should also be obtained. An echocardiogram should be done or scheduled at the first available opportunity. Further diagnostics should include a carotid Doppler, a complete metabolic profile, lipid profile, TSH, and stools for guaiac.

History Data Questions specific to the chief complaint of shortness of breath require a complete review of systems and include the following:

- When did you first notice your shortness of breath?
- Do you feel it is progressing? If so, please explain.
- Do you have a history of problems with your heart, your lungs, or a history of similar symptoms?
- Do you have symptoms such as a rapid heart rate or skipped heartbeats?
- Do you have a history of bleeding, ulcer disease or anemia?
- Have you lost or gained weight?
- Have you ever been told that you have thyroid disease?
- Do you have other medical problems?

Physical Examination Data The focused examination for the chief complaint of shortness of breath includes complete physical examination with attention to cardiovascular examination

Differential Diagnosis Congestive heart failure, chronic lung disease, pulmonary fibrosis, ischemic cardiac disease, cardiomyopathy (Table 7-9)

Probable Causes of the Presenting Symptoms Adequate function of the heart is determined by four factors: (1) heart rate, (2) preload, (3) afterload, and (4) contractility. An abnormality in any factor can cause symptoms of heart failure. G.B.'s signs and symptoms correlate with change in physiologic function of the heart. A common cause is hypertension and associated LVH. Other common causes might be fluid overload, valvular heart disease, and myocardial ischemia (e.g., atherosclerosis or CAD).

Diagnostic Tests The CBC and complete metabolic profile were returned within normal limits. Her oxygen saturation on room air was 91%. The TSH was also normal. Metabolic abnormalities must be ruled out. CXR showed cardiac enlarge-

Table 7-9
Differential Diagnostic Cues for Shortness of Breath

Cause	Nature of Patient	Nature of Symptoms	Associated Symptoms	Precipitating and Aggravating Factors	Ameliorating Factors	Physical Findings	Diagnostic Studies
Acute or Recurrent Dyspnea							
Asthma	Most common cause of recurrent dyspnea in children	Acute dyspnea Episodic May rarely be dyspneic only at night	Cough (indicates asthmatic bronchitis)	Allergens Exercise Noxious fumes Respiratory tract infections Recumbency Exposure to cold or beta blockers		Bilateral wheezing Sibilant, whistling sounds prolonged expiration	Pulmonary function tests: Decreased respiratory flow rates Decreased maximum voluntary ventilation Increased tidal volume Pre- and post-bronchodilator evidence for reversible airway obstruction (>10%)
Pulmonary emboli	Women using birth control pills Patients in postoperative period Long-term recumbent patients Patients with phlebitis Patients in postpartum period	Acute onset of dyspnea	Chest pain Faintness Loss of consciousness	Oral contraceptives Prolonged recumbency		Tachypnea Peripheral cyanosis Low blood pressure Rales Wheezing (usually only on side of emboli) Pleural friction later with pulmonary infarction	Ventilation and perfusion studies Digital subtraction angiography Electrocardiography indicates acute right ventricular strain Pulmonary infarction or effusion on x-ray
Hyperventilation and anxiety	Usually anxious	Acute dyspnea "Sighing" respirations	Lightheadedness Palpitations Paresthesias (especially in perioral region and extremities)	Stress Panic		Signs of anxiety but no signs of dyspnea	Pulmonary function tests are usually normal

Continued

Poor physical conditioning	Obese; Physically inactive	Dyspnea on minimal exertion				Obesity; After exercise pulse slows very gradually	Pulmonary function tests: Decreased total lung capacity; Increased respiratory minute volume; Decreased compliance
Foreign body aspiration	Most common in children; May occur in intoxicated or semiconscious people during eating	Acute dyspnea			Removal of foreign body; Heimlich maneuver	Tachypnea; Inspiratory stridor; Localized wheezing; Suprasternal retraction with respiration; May be unilateral wheezing	Chest radiograph may show atelectasis or the foreign body
Pulmonary edema		Acute onset; Episodic	Dyspnea on exertion; Orthopnea; Paroxysmal nocturnal dyspnea			Gallop rhythm; Rales at bases	Decreased ejection fraction; Chest radiograph shows cardiomegaly with upper lobe redistribution or Kerley's B lines
Pneumothorax	Often a prior history of similar episode; May be familial	Acute onset		Cystic fibrosis; Chronic obstructive pulmonary disease		Decreased or absent breath sounds; Tracheal shift	Chest radiograph shows pneumothorax
Chronic Dyspnea							
Chronic obstructive pulmonary disease	Older adults; Rarely patients under age 30; Most often smokers	Chronic dyspnea; Dyspnea with exertion	Fast rate of recovery to normal respiration after stopping exercise; Leaning forward while seated or supine with head down; History of smoking	Smoking; Exertion; Postural changes have little or no effect	With severe disease patients may obtain some symptomatic relief by leaning forward while sitting	Rapid and shallow respirations	Pulmonary function tests: Spirometry

From Seller RH: *Differential diagnosis of common complaints*, ed 3, Philadelphia, 1996, WB Saunders.

Table 7-9
Differential Diagnostic Cues for Shortness of Breath—cont'd

Chronic Dyspnea—cont'd

Cause	Nature of Patient	Nature of Symptoms	Associated Symptoms	Precipitating and Aggravating Factors	Ameliorating Factors	Physical Findings	Diagnostic Studies
Emphysema		Progressive dyspnea precedes onset of cough Usually no dyspnea at rest				"Pink puffers" Hyperventilated lungs Decreased breath sounds Decreased diaphragmatic movement Increased anteroposterior chest diameter Hyperresonance	Decreased respiratory flow rate Increased tidal volume Decreased maximum voluntary volume Increased residual volume
Chronic bronchitis		Dyspnea not necessarily presenting symptom Cough precedes dyspnea	Persistent, minimally productive cough			"Blue bloaters" Rhonchi	Same as with emphysema Spirometry shows widespread airway narrowing
Congestive heart failure	Older patients	Chronic dyspnea with gradual onset Paroxysmal nocturnal dyspnea Dyspnea remains long after stopping exercise	Edema	Exercise Beta blockers Calcium channel blockers Recumbency Trauma Shock Hemorrhage Anesthesia	Nocturnal dyspnea may be relieved by sitting	Shallow respirations (not necessarily rapid) Edema Hepatomegaly Jugular venous distention Third heart sound Basilar rales	Spirometry Respiratory volume is greater than normal at all exercise levels Pulmonary congestion and cardiomegaly on radiograph

From Seller RH: *Differential diagnosis of common complaints*, ed 3, Philadelphia, 1996, WB Saunders.

ment with evidence of Kerley B lines and cephalization of the vessels, consistent with CHF. ECG showed LVH with a strain pattern, but no acute change that would suggest MI. The echocardiogram confirmed the presence of a dilated LV and LVH with decreased ejected fraction. A mitral regurgitation murmur of moderate degree and thickening of the aortic valve cusps, compatible with aortic sclerosis was seen. A minimal aortic stenosis murmur was also noted. Lipid profile showed total cholesterol of 325; triglycerides of 300; HDL of 40; (LDL is calculated as follows: total cholesterol − HDL − triglycerides/5 = LDL [225 in this case]). Carotid Doppler showed a 60% narrowing on the right. Her stool guaiacs were normal.

Diagnostic Impression G.B.'s clinical and diagnostic presentation (i.e., CXR, echocardiogram, and carotid Doppler) is consistent with a cardiomyopathy contributing to her congestive heart failure. Moreover, she has moderate hypertension and carotid atherosclerosis. Her laboratory profile, with the exception of her lipid profile, is normal. Her lipid profile shows a mixed dyslipidemia.

Therapeutic Plan of Care Therapy for CHF is multimodal and targeted at the likely cause or causes. G.B. can be followed as an outpatient with regularly scheduled in-home nursing assessment. Clear communication between her primary care provider and home nurse will be important to compliance and the treatment outcomes. Initial treatment will include salt restriction (2 to 5 gm/day) and fluid restriction (1500 to 2000 cc/24 hours). She will be placed on ASA, 325 mg daily, and started on a long-acting ACE inhibitor such as lisinopril. She will also be given furosemide 20 mg daily. Her dyslipidemia will be managed with a HMG-CoA inhibitor. Her progress will be followed weekly with a basic electrolyte panel, in-home blood pressures, and daily weights. She will be scheduled for a 2-week office evaluation unless her symptoms require more urgent assessment. Lanoxin will be considered to improve cardiac contractility if her symptoms fail to respond. A beta-blocker such as carvedilol (Coreg) will be considered if other therapy fails. Evaluation of the CHF patient must look at systolic and diastolic function via echocardiogram; consideration of coronary sta-

tus with nuclear or echo scans; and cardiac catheterization, as well as careful long-term follow-up. G.B.'s hypertension must be corrected. Secondary causes of heart failure such as ischemic cardiomyopathy, amyloidosis, thyroid disease, renal or hepatic disease, and anemia must be ruled out.

Patient Education and/or Community Resources G.B. should receive complete instructions and indications for her medications. She will need dietary instruction on a heart healthy diet with specific direction regarding her sodium, cholesterol, fat, and fluid restrictions. Home blood pressure readings will be initially managed by the visiting nurse until acceptable techniques for self-monitoring are learned. Lifestyle changes, including exercise, should be added as her symptoms improve. Community programs for healthy heart living should be considered for both G.B and her family members. Lipid management and follow-up profiles should include muscle and liver enzymes to monitor for side effects of the HMG-CoA inhibitor.

Follow-Up Plan G.B. should be scheduled for a return call as soon as all of her diagnostic tests are back so that a mutual plan can be established. Her hypertension should be monitored in the home and recorded. At intervals, her blood pressure should also be validated in the office. The timeliness of further office visits will depend on her progress. However, she will be scheduled for a visit in 2 weeks and another 1 month after initiation of therapy. At that time, subsequent visits will be established. Electrolyte and renal function will need to be watched.

Case Study 4 Optional Exercise
CHIEF COMPLAINT: Leg Pain

History of present illness K.K. is a 34-year-old Caucasian female who presents to the emergency room complaining of a sore and swollen left leg. She had noticed mild tenderness in her calf for 2 or 3 days prior to seeking care, but paid little attention until she noticed a slight swelling of the foot and ankle. She denies injury to the extremity and prior history of similar symptoms. Her general health has been excellent. She states she returned to

Michigan from Florida 4 days earlier after a 24-hour trip with her husband and 6-year-old daughter. She shared in the driving on the trip.

K.K. has no history of phlebitis and has no open sores. She denies noting any red streaks on her leg. She further denies chest pain; cough; sputum production; hemoptysis; chills, fever, or sweats; or feeling ill in other ways.

Past Medical History   Gravida-3, abortion-2, para 1. Her remaining history is non-contributory.

Past Surgical History   D&C on two occasions following incomplete abortion

Family History   Mother aged 56, A&W with past history of phlebitis; father aged 58, A&W; no siblings. No history of CAD, CVA, or HTN; maternal aunt had deep vein thrombosis (DVT)

Developmental Stage   Intimacy versus Isolation

Role-Relationship   Married for 10 years; has one daughter, 6 years of age, born after two miscarriages. Happy in her relationship with her husband. Her parents live nearby; they have a comfortable relationship and communicate on a regular basis. She is employed as an executive secretary to the superintendent of schools.

Sleep/Rest   Sleep on an average of 8 hours a night; goes to bed after the 11 PM news; awakes without the aid of an alarm around 7 AM

Nutrition/Metabolic   Carefully watches her diet and conscientiously plans nutritious meals. Eats three meals a day. Eats lunch out several times a week. Rarely snacks

Activity/ Exercise   Leads an active lifestyle but does not exercise on a regular basis

Coping/Stress   K.K. admits to significant stress during the loss of two pregnancies; admits she has learned to "count her blessings," and denies difficulty with coping or stress at present. K.K. has several good friends and neighbors that she considers sources of additional support.

Health Management   Smoking history, smoked off-and-on for 10 years, with 8 pack-year history, trying to quit; alcohol, averages one drink per week, mostly wine; caffeine, 3 or 4 cups per day

Self-Perception and Values/Beliefs   Considers her family the focus of her life; comfortable with her success as a wife and mother; does not attend a particular church, but believes in God and considers herself a Christian

Medications   Multivitamins, oral birth control pills

Allergies   NKMA

Pertinent Physical Findings
Vital Signs   Height 5 feet 4 inches; weight 145 pounds; BMI 25; temperature 97.3° F; heart rate 72; respirations 14; blood pressure 134/70

General Appearance   Appears younger than stated age; alert and appropriate

HEENT   Unremarkable; no bruits, no venous distention

Heart   Regular, clear S_1 and S_2; no murmurs; no cardiac enlargement by percussion

Lungs   Clear to auscultation and percussion; no abnormal sounds are heard. No CVA tenderness

Abdomen   No guarding, tenderness, distention, or masses; bowel tones are normoactive

Extremities   Symmetrical pulses; left leg has 1+ edema with mild calf tenderness, no palpable cord, no color change, no temperature change; Homans' sign is positive in left only, right extremity is unremarkable

Diagnostics
Diagnostic Tests   CBC, WBC 6200; hemoglobin 12.7 gm/dL; hematocrit 37.5%; platelet count 247,000; peripheral smear is normal; basic metabolic panel is also normal. Ultrasound Doppler of the left leg is positive for deep vein thrombosis. Because of her family history and miscarriages, a coagulation profile will be drawn. If suspicion is high for an inherited component, antiphospholipid antibodies, lupus anticoagulant, and factor V Leiden may also be requested. Antithrombin III and protein C and S disorders would seem less likely, but may be considered.

Discussion Questions

What type of history data should be collected?

What type of physical data should be collected?

What are the differential diagnoses?

Continued

> *Discussion Questions—cont'd*
>
> *What are the probable causes of the presenting symptoms?*
>
> *What is your diagnostic impression?*
>
> *What is the therapeutic plan of care?*
>
> *What are the patient education and/or community resources?*
>
> *What is your follow-up plan?*

Discussions for optional case study exercises can be found in the accompanying Instructor's Manual.

References

Joint National Committee: The sixth report of the Joint National Committee on prevention, detection, evaluation, and treatment of high blood pressure, *Arch Intern Med* 157(21):2413-2446, 1997.

Seller RH: *Differential diagnosis of common complaints,* ed 3, Philadelphia, 1996, WB Saunders.

Tierney L, McPhee S, Papadakis M: *Current medical diagnosis and treatment,* ed 38, Stamford, Conn, 1999, Appleton & Lange.

Selected Readings

Amsterdam E, Gaziano J, Ockene I: Modifying lipids through lifestyle changes, *Patient Care* Feb. 28 (Suppl):2-10, 1999.

Bennett C, Plum F: *Cecil textbook of medicine,* ed 20, Philadelphia, 1996, WB Saunders.

Duvernoy C, Mosca L: Coronary heart disease in women: why the differences matter, *J Crit Illn* 14(4):209-216, 1999.

Ferri F: *Practical guide to care of the medical patient,* ed 4, St Louis, 1998, Mosby.

Hill M, Merz N, Peters A, Wenger N: Elevated lipid levels in special populations, *Patient Care,* Feb. 28, 1999 (Suppl):22-29, 1999.

Kiley R: *Medical Information on the Internet: a guide for health professionals,* New York, 1998, Churchill Livingstone.

National Cholesterol Education Program: *Second report of the expert panel on detection, evaluation, and treatment of high blood cholesterol in adults (Adult Treatment Panel II), executive summary,* National Institute of Health, Publication No. 93-3096, 1993.

Rakel R: *Saunders manual of medical practice,* Philadelphia, 1996, WB Saunders.

Sackett D, Richardson W, Rosenberg W, Haynes R: *Evidence-based medicine: how to practice and teach EBM,* New York, 1997, Churchill Livingstone.

Seidel H, Ball J, Dains J, Benedict G: *Mosby's guide to physical examination,* St Louis, 1995, Mosby.

Speicher C: *The right test,* ed 3, Philadelphia, 1998, WB Saunders.

Zollo A: Medical secrets, ed 2, Philadelphia, 1997, Hanley & Belfus, Inc.

CHAPTER 8

Gastrointestinal Disorders

Jean Nagelkerk

Case Study 1

CHIEF COMPLAINT: Lower Abdominal Pain with Diarrhea

History of Present Illness M.J. is a 21-year-old Caucasian female who presents with chief complaint of left-sided lower abdominal pain with diarrhea and constipation for 4 months duration. M.J. has 1 to 5 liquid, brown stools per day and is constipated for 1 to 2 days every other week. Often the crampy lower abdominal pain will be relieved by a bowel movement. She is never awakened at night by the pain. Her stools are usually either liquid or semi-formed and brown with an occasional streak of mucus. She is sexually active with three partners in the past 6 months and does not use condoms. M.J. denies blood in her stools, weight loss, laxative use, foreign travel, or change in water source. M.J. reports that food does not aggravate or alleviate these symptoms.

Past Medical History Mild asthma

Past Surgical History Unremarkable

Family History Mother age 51, A&W; father age 62, MI at age 50; brother age 23, A&W

Developmental Stage Intimacy versus Isolation

Role-Relationship M.J. is a college student majoring in computers at the University of Florida in Gainesville. She lives in university housing and has a roommate that she gets along with well. Her parents live in Ohio and call her once a week and e-mail her almost every day. M.J. works about 16 hours per week at the university in the Academic Computing Center. She has dated several different men over the past year.

Sleep/Rest M.J. sleeps about 8 to 9 hours per night and always awakens rested. She does enjoy going out in the evening to parties, social events, or to movies with friends, so her sleep hours vary.

Nutrition/Metabolic Breakfast, either a donut (half of the time) or nothing; lunch, a salad, Mexican food, or a pizza at the university food court; dinner, usually a meat, vegetable, pasta dish, and frozen yogurt at the university center. M.J. likes specialty coffees so usually has 3 or 4 cups per day and also drinks 3 or 4 Diet Cokes. Snacks consist of crackers, sweets, or chips.

Activity/Exercise M.J. consistently works out in the university fitness center 1 hour per day. She usually uses the treadmill, stationary bike, or rowing machine.

Coping/Stress M.J. will call her mother or talk to her roommate if she feels under stress. M.J. enjoys swimming, bicycling, and walking. She does not attend church.

Health Management M.J. does not smoke. She usually has 5 or 6 mixed drinks on the weekend and uses marijuana occasionally. LMP was 2 weeks ago. Her menses last 5 or 6 days and she has a light flow. She is worried about having a sexually transmitted disease because she has been with three partners in the past 6 months without the use of condoms. Her last Pap smear was 9 months ago and was normal. She does not own a firearm and she feels safe in the university housing units. She denies physical or sexual abuse.

Self-Perception and Values/Beliefs M.J. is excited to graduate in 3 months and is looking forward to a career in the computer industry. She has a positive self-image and is looking forward to accomplishing the goals she has set for herself.

Medications Triphasil 1 qd (has used for 3 years); albuterol (Ventolin) 2 puffs qid prn and has been using the medication one or two times a month

Allergies Sulfa: at age 7 had felt as though her throat was closing off and had difficulty swallowing

Pertinent Physical Findings
Vital Signs Height 5 feet 7 inches; weight 135 pounds; BMI 21 (normal BMI = 18.5-24.5); temperature 98.4° F; heart rate 82; respirations 12; blood pressure 120/70

Heart Apical pulse 82, rate regular; no murmurs, S_3, or S_4

Lungs Clear to auscultation

Abdomen Abdomen soft; + bowel sounds, slightly tender over LLQ without guarding or rebound tenderness; no splenomegaly or hepatomegaly

Genital External genitalia with no lesions, discharge or rashes; vaginal mucosa pink and moist; cervix pink, non-parous os, no lesions; no cervical motion tenderness (CMT) or adnexal masses

Diagnostics
Diagnostic Tests Stool for ova and parasites × 3 negative; stools for culture, occult blood × 3, leukocytes, and fecal fat are negative; CBC with ESR, within normal limits; wet mount negative; DNA probe for chlamydia and gonorrhea is negative

History Data Questions specific to the chief complaint of lower abdominal pain with diarrhea and occasional constipation include the following:

- Where is the pain located?
- How long have you had the pain?
- What is the frequency, quality, severity, and duration of the pain?
- What aggravates or alleviates the abdominal pain, constipation, and diarrhea?
- Does defecation relieve the abdominal discomfort? (Tenesmus is the feeling of incomplete emptying and may indicate an inflammatory or infectious cause or carcinoma.)
- Is there a relationship of pain to change in stool consistency and frequency?

- Do you have mucus in your stools?
- Do you have blood in your stools, weight loss (may occur in malabsorption, inflammation, cancer, and hyperthyroidism), or are you awakened at night from pain or diarrhea? (These questions, if answered affirmatively, indicate a potential diagnosis of inflammatory bowel disease [Uphold and Graham, 1998]).
- Do you have bloating, belching, or a sense of fullness?
- What is your usual diet and eating pattern? (Milk may cause lactase deficiency, soft drinks may cause sucrose intolerance.)
- Is there any relationship of stress to your symptoms?
- (If female) When was your last menstrual period? Describe the frequency, amount of flow, and any difficulties you experience during menstruation.
- What medications or other treatments have you used to alleviate symptoms and what was their effectiveness?
- Are you using laxatives? (laxative abuse)
- What medications, herbal products, vitamins, recreational drugs, caffeine, and alcohol are you using? (determine type, amount, and frequency)
- Have you recently traveled outside of the United States? (traveler's diarrhea)
- Have you drunk water from a river or pond?

Physical Examination Data The focused examination for the chief complaint of lower abdominal pain with diarrhea includes: vital signs, heart, lungs, abdomen, and genital (if high risk for sexually transmitted diseases).

Differential Diagnosis Functional bowel syndrome: irritable bowel; inflammatory bowel syndrome: ulcerative colitis and Crohn's disease; lactose intolerance; colonic neoplasia; gynecological problems: pelvic inflammatory disease (PID) and endometriosis; causes of chronic diarrhea, diverticulosis (Table 8-1)

Probable Causes of the Presenting Symptoms Irritable bowel syndrome (IBS) accounts for approximately 50% of the gastrointestinal complaints to primary care providers. Women are twice as

Text continued on page 148.

Table 8-1
Lower Abdominal Pain and Diarrhea Differential Diagnostic Cues

Diagnosis	Signs and Symptoms	Lab Data	Treatment
Functional Bowel Syndrome *Irritable Bowel Syndrome (IBS)* > 3 months duration including intermittent lower abdominal pain and alteration in bowel habits As many as 20% of adults have IBS symptoms Usually begins in adolescence or early adulthood Stress may increase symptoms Symptoms may increase 1-2 hours after eating	Intermittent, crampy lower abdominal pain. Pain often is relieved with defecation. Patient experiences altered bowel habits of >3 bowel movements per day or <3 per week. May have straining, urgency, bloating, abdominal distention, and altered stool consistency	Stools for ova and parasites × 3, CBC with erythrocyte sedimentation rate (ESR) is reflective of inflammation and infection and is nonspecific Fecal leukocytes, stools for culture, stools for occult blood × 3. If severe pain or diarrhea, do flexible sigmoidoscopy If patient is experiencing predominately diarrhea, consider TSH If high risk for a sexually transmitted disease consider a wet mount, DNA probe if + CMT or high risk	Keep food diary with activities to evaluate dietary or psychosocial factors. Trial of lactose-free diet. Avoid flatulogenic foods (see page 148 for listing). Trial of high fiber diet (20-30g/d) (see pages 148-149 for listing) *OR* fiber supplements with psyllium, methylcellulose or polycarbophil. If symptoms persist may use antispasmodic agent given 30-60 minutes before meals (e.g., dicyclomine [Bentyl] 10-20 mg 3-4 × day; *OR* hyoscyamine [Levbid] 0.375 mg/tab 1-2 tab q 4 hours, max 4 tablets qd). Antidiarrheal agents prn (if severe). Consider psychotropic agents (e.g., SSRI) if stress or depression component present. Behavioral modification therapies may assist in decreasing stress.
Inflammatory Bowel Syndrome *Crohn's Disease* Inflammation of any part of the alimentary canal Transmural inflammation, bowel wall & submucosal thickening, linear ulcerations, discontinuous (skip areas), fissures, and fistulas	Insidious onset of intermittent RLQ *OR* periumbilical pain, nonbloody diarrhea, low-grade fever, weight loss, malaise	Lab data is for both ulcerative colitis and Crohn's disease. CBC with ESR, serum albumin (Assesses disease severity and nutritional status. Usually will see anemia, volume depletion and hypoalbuminemia in severe colitis.), stools for ova and parasites (O&P) × 3. Do stools for O&P before barium tests because they interfere with the ability to identify O&P for 1-3 weeks. *C. difficile* toxin, and stools for occult blood × 3, stools for culture, and fecal leukocytes If Crohn's is suspected, an upper gastrointestinal series with a small bowel follow-through (SBFT) is generally ordered. If +, Crohn's disease may show ulcerative areas, fistulas, or strictures. In the small bowel, note segmental narrowing, *string sign* (narrow passage of barium through an inflamed area),	Refer for GI evaluation and management plan for patients with inflammatory bowel syndrome. When the patient is stable or on maintenance medication, co-manage patient care. Well-balanced diet. Trial lactose-free diet if has flatulence or diarrhea. If colonic involvement, give fiber supplement. If obstructive symptoms, place on low-roughage diet. Exacerbations use steroid preparation. 5-aminosalicylic acid agents (e.g., sulfasalazine 1.5-2 g daily) may decrease exacerbations. If unresponsive, may give immunomodulatory drugs (e.g., azathioprine *OR* mercaptopurine). Check blood counts weekly for 1 month, then monthly and discontinue if side effects. Regular diet, eliminate caffeine and gas-producing foods. Fiber supplements. Antidiarrheal agents may be given unless in acute exacerbation, then could precipitate toxic megacolon For distal colitis, topical agents such as mesalamine as a suppository 500 mg bid for proctitis or as an enema 4g at HS for proctosigmoiditis.
Ulcerative Colitis Inflammation of the mucosa of the colon with the rectum almost always involved Inflammation extending continuously (no skip areas) proximally for a variable extent	Lower abdominal cramps with urgency, bloody diarrhea, mucus, anemia, may have mild fever, hypoalbuminemia, and orthostatic hypotension		

and skip areas (normal mucosa interspersed with areas of inflamed mucosa).

In ulcerative colitis, a sigmoidoscopy without cleansing preparation is used to assess the bowel mucosa in the distal colon and rectum.

Ulcerative colitis shows friable mucosa, purulent exudate, ulcers, bleeding and granular tissue.

Barium enema and colonoscopy are not used in acute colitis because they may potentiate toxic megacolon.

With a colonoscopy, mucosal biopsies of the colon or terminal ileum can be taken to determine the extent of the disease and is diagnostic. in 10% of cases it is difficult to differentiate between Crohn's and ulcerative colitis.

In Crohn's, the biopsy would show strictures, segmental involvement of the colon, and ulcers.

In ulcerative colitis, the biopsy would show inflammation without skip areas in the rectum and colon.

Mild to moderate colitis, use oral sulfasalazine **OR** mesalamine.

Severe colitis may require hospitalization for parenteral therapy. Proctocolectomy is required if severe disease and poor control.

Colonic Neoplasia
Risk Factors are age 50 history of adenomatous polyps, history of inflammatory bowel syndrome, family history of colorectal cancer or polyposis syndrome

May be asymptomatic. May have alteration in bowel habits (diarrhea and constipation). Stools 1 for occult blood. May experience fatigue from anemia from chronic gastrointestinal blood loss

Stools for occult blood × 3

Routine screening .50 years of age is sigmoidoscopy q 5 years or colonoscopy if family history of colorectal disease or previous polyps

CBC, liver enzymes.

If suspect colon cancer, do colonoscopy; if cecum is not visualized, follow with barium enema

If 1 colon cancer, draw CEA, CXR, may order abdominal CT (cancer staging). If 1 rectal cancer, get pelvic MRI and endorectal ultrasonography (shows depth of cancer in rectal wall and pararectal lymph nodes)

Referral to oncologist
Surgical resection common
Depending on the stage of the tumor, adjuvant chemotherapy and radiotherapy may be ordered

Continued

Table 8-1
Lower Abdominal Pain and Diarrhea Differential Diagnostic Cues—cont'd

Diagnosis	Signs and Symptoms	Lab Data	Treatment
Gynecological Problems PID	Lower abdominal pain, chills, fever, menstrual irregularities, purulent cervical discharge, cervical and adnexal masses	May use a cervical culture with modified Thayer-Martin media for *N. gonorrhea* **OR** DNA probe for chlamydia and gonorrhea Wet mount CBC with ESR If differentiating gynecological problems, may need pelvic ultrasound HCG test for pregnancy	If mild, can treat outpatient with antibiotic treatment. Examples of treatments include: ofloxacin (Floxin) 300 mg bid × 7 days covers *N. gonorrhea* and *C. trachomatis;* and metronidazole (Flagyl) 500 mg bid × 14 days – covers anaerobes and bacterial vaginitis **OR** ceftriaxone (Rocephin) 250 mg IM × 1 – covers *N. gonorrhea* and doxycycline 100 mg bid × 14 days—covers *C. trachomatis* **OR** cefoxitin (Mefoxin) 2 gm IM—*N. gonorrhea* and some anaerobe coverage **PLUS** Probenecid 1 gram × 1 and doxycycline 100 mg bid × 14 days. If severe, is pregnant, has AIDS, hospitalize for treatment
Endometriosis	Lower abdominal pain with or without back pain, dyspareunia may occur, rectal pain with or without bleeding, infertility, aching pain begins before menses and is worse until flow ceases	Pelvic ultrasound often done Laparoscopy is diagnostic Proctosigmoidoscopy only if bowel involvement (e.g., blood in stool)	Referral to gynecologist for laparoscopy and treatment plan. Medical therapy includes: GnRH analogs (e.g., leuprolide acetate 3.75 mg IM monthly used for 6 months; **OR** danazol 200-400 mg bid used for 6-9 months) to suppress menstruation; **OR** combination oral contraceptive pills 1 qd for 6-12 months to suppress bleeding; **OR** medroxyprogesterone acetate 100 mg IM q2 weeks for 4 doses, then 100 mg q4 weeks for 6-9 months. Surgical interventions for severe cases
Causes of Chronic Diarrhea (Diarrhea lasting 2 weeks or recurrent) Diarrhea is defined as 200 grams produced per day	Usually 5 or more episodes of diarrhea per day, crampy lower abdominal pain	Stools for ova and parasites × 3, fecal leukocytes, stool cultures. Collect 24-hour stool for weight and quantitative fecal fat if diagnosis is elusive or if fat malabsorption is suspected; weight >1000-1500 g suggests secretory process; fecal fat >10 g suggests a malabsorption process	Treatment is aimed at one of the six types of chronic diarrhea: • Osmotic (e.g., lactose deficiency) • Malabsorptive (e.g., intestinal resection) • Secretory (e.g., endocrine tumor) • Inflammatory (e.g., Crohn's disease) • Motility (e.g., IBS) • Chronic infections (e.g., parasitic)

	Signs and Symptoms	Diagnostic Evaluation	Treatment
		CBC, serum electrolytes, albumin. Beta-carotene (levels below 50 ug/dL indicate severe malabsorption) and prothrombin time to assess for malabsorption. Liver function to assess for hepatobiliary disease. Calcium and phosphorus to assess for metabolic condition. TSH and total T_4 to assess for thyroid dysfunction. The above tests will direct your imaging studies (e.g., UGI with SBFT, sigmoidoscopy, colonoscopy)	
Causes of Acute Diarrhea Diarrhea lasting <3 weeks duration Commonly caused by infectious agents, bacterial toxins, or drugs	Noninflammatory diarrhea (viral or toxins affecting the small intestine); presents with large volume watery diarrhea, no bloody stools, N/V, bloating, cramps Inflammatory diarrhea (bacteria, parasites or toxins affecting the large bowel) presents with frequent bloody, small volume stools, fever, abdominal cramps, tenesmus, and fecal urgency	If less than 24-48 hours, no test necessary If diarrhea continues, order stools, O&P × 3 Check for fecal leukocytes; if +, do stool cultures Check for C. *difficile*, especially if has been on antibiotics	Acute diarrhea is usually self-limited and resolves within 5 days. Use oral rehydration therapy (infants: Pedialyte or Rice-lyte for 6 hours then resume formula; children: Gatorade or Pedialyte or Rice-lyte for 6 hours). Stop solids for 12 hours. No dairy products. For children and elderly use the BRAT diet (bananas, rice, applesauce, and toast). Hospitalize if there is severe dehydration, toxicity or severe abdominal pain. Do not give antimotility agents if has fever or bloody stools. For traveler's diarrhea may give ciprofloxacin (Cipro) 500 mg bid **OR** trimethoprim-sulfamethoxazole (Bactrim DS) -160/800 bid × 3-5 days, in some areas, resistance is occurring with Bactrim DS.
Diverticulosis	Intermittent colicky lower left side abdominal pain, flatulence, abdominal distention, altered bowel habits	Barium enema will show diverticula and may show narrowed colon. If stricture or mass noted, schedule colonoscopy to evaluate for malignancy (contraindicated if diverticulitis is suspected). If diverticulitis is suspected, then CT of abdomen (usually have fever, tenderness with diverticulitis)	For diverticulosis, try high-fiber diet (25-35 gms), may need bulk laxative or antispasmodic. Avoid peanuts, popcorn, and seeds If acute exacerbation of diverticulitis is an emergent surgical referral

Note: See CDC guidelines for treatment of sexually transmitted disease for detailed and alternative treatment plans.

Continued from page 143.

likely to seek health care for gastrointestinal complaints and be diagnosed with IBS. IBS is a functional bowel syndrome that consists of a disturbance in intestinal motility and visceral perception. Personal stress often triggers the symptoms of IBS (Castell and Johnston, 1996; Jarrett et al, 1998). Patients who have IBS may also experience anxiety, depression, somatization, or have a personality disorder.

Individuals typically have altered motility and heightened visceral perception. In patients with normal intestinal motility, the colonic contractions and the myoelectric patterns are more consistent and do not have an exaggerated motor response to food. When patients have diarrhea, the flow of fecal material through the ascending and transverse colon is accelerated, whereas individuals with constipation experience delays in fecal material passage (Isselbacher et al, 1994). This is thought to be due to central nervous system control. Individuals with IBS also experience increased sensitivity when the intestines are distended, which may account for part of the abdominal discomfort.

Factors that influence irritable bowel symptoms in some patients include lactose (dairy products), fructose (in common citrus fruit sugar), sorbitol (the substance in sugar-free candy), and malabsorption (Goroll, May, and Mulley, 1995). In addition, caffeine and recreational drugs may be irritants to individuals with IBS. Clinical criteria for IBS consists of continuous or intermittent abdominal discomfort relieved by defecation or associated with alteration in bowel habits for at least 3 months. Additional criteria include altered stool patterns at least 25% of the time with at least two of the following symptoms: alteration in stool consistency; sensation of urgency, straining upon defecation, or a sense of incomplete evacuation; abdominal distention; or mucus expulsion (Goroll, May, and Mulley, 1995).

Diagnostic Tests   CBC with ESR (evaluate for gastrointestinal blood loss, inflammation or infection); ova and parasites (assess for amebiasis such as giardiasis, *Cryptosporidium, Cyclospora*); fecal leukocytes (suggests an inflammatory diarrhea); culture and sensitivity (evaluate for *Campylobacter, Salmonella,* and *Shigella*); and stools for occult blood × 3 (assess for inflammatory bowel syn-

dromes, neoplasms, polyps). If on antibiotics (especially ampicillin, clindamycin, or cephalosporins), do *C. difficile* toxin (Tierney, McPhee, and Papadakis, 1999). The patient may have antibiotic-associated colitis requiring treatment. A flexible sigmoidoscopy is often performed if the patient has severe pain or diarrhea. If there is acute colitis, the mucosa will be friable, edematous, and have erosions. Patients who have acute colitis should not have a colonoscopy during the acute phase because of the risk of colon perforation.

If diarrhea is the main stool type of the patient, consider ordering a thyroid function test. A 24-hour stool collection for weight, electrolytes, and osmolality may be used if diagnosis is elusive or if fat malabsorption is suspected. If the stool weight is >300 grams per day, further evaluation is necessary because this is uncommon in irritable bowel syndrome.

Certain patients are at high risk for a sexually transmitted disease. If the patient is at high risk or has positive cervical motion tenderness (CMT), perform a wet mount and DNA probe.

Diagnostic Impression   M.J. does not present with constitutional signs and symptoms such as fever, weight loss, and malaise. Her symptoms (lower abdominal pain with diarrhea and occasional constipation relieved with defecation, no night symptoms, and lack of bloody stools) characterize irritable bowel syndrome.

Therapeutic Plan of Care   M.J. should begin by keeping a food diary along with a record of her daily activities to evaluate both dietary intake and life events that exacerbate her symptoms. The next step is to have her engage in a 2- or 3-week trial of a lactose-free diet. Avoiding flatulogenic foods (e.g., cabbage, raw onions, coffee, red wine, beer, brown beans, Brussels sprouts, cauliflower, and plums) may help control symptoms.

Should M.J.'s symptoms persist after the lactose trial and the elimination of flatulogenic foods, the next intervention would be to begin a high-fiber diet (20 to 30 g per day) or to institute a fiber supplement with psyllium, methylcellulose, or polycarbophil. Often patients better tolerate the fiber supplement. Foods high in fiber include fruits (e.g., strawberries, apples), vegetables (e.g., green beans), legumes (e.g., garbanzo beans), and whole-grain breads and cereals (e.g., shredded wheat). Caffeine and recreational drugs may exacerbate or cause irritable bowel symptoms, and a trial abstinence from these products may improve the patient's quality of life. If symptoms are persistent and of moderate intensity, a trial of an antispasmodic agent given 30 to 60 minutes before meals (e.g., dicyclomine [Bentyl] 10 to 20 mg three or four times per day) may be useful. Antidiarrheal agents used on an as-needed basis may also be necessary for short bouts of severe diarrhea. In addition, an evaluation of the patient's psychosocial factors may indicate that the use of a psychotropic agent such as a serotonin reuptake inhibitor (SSRI) may be beneficial. Within 1 month of starting a patient on an SSRI you should see a decrease in symptoms if it is working effectively for the patient. Other treatments include relaxation therapies and counseling.

M.J. verbalized concern about having a sexually transmitted disease due to multiple sexual partners. A discussion of safe sexual practices should occur at this visit. HIV testing should be explained and offered.

Patient Education and/or Community Resources
Behavioral modification approaches such as relaxation and counseling may be beneficial for some patients. Discussing lifestyles and how to decrease stress and activities that increase symptoms should be explored. A discussion should be held about the use of alcohol and recreational drugs, with a description of their irritative effects on the patient's symptoms.

Follow-Up Plan   Schedule an appointment in 2 weeks to reassess M.J.'s symptom control. Then schedule appointments every 2 weeks until symptoms are in control. Evaluate in 1 month and reevaluate at 3- or 6-month intervals.

Case Study 2

CHIEF COMPLAINT: Heartburn

History of Present Illness   J.S. is a 42-year-old Vietnamese-American male who presents with chief complaint of severe heartburn that is worse after he eats. These symptoms have been present for 6 months, but the discomfort is getting so bad that he is seeking medical intervention. J.S. reports that the hearburn usually occurs after eating food and lasts for about 1 hour. His diet consists of a variety of foods, although he has eliminated spicy foods because they seem to make the heartburn and indigestion worse. He describes the heartburn as burning substernal pain that radiates to his left arm. J.S. notes that his heartburn is worse with bending, lying down, or reclining in a chair. Activity does not increase or decrease the discomfort. J.S. denies dysphagia, weight loss, and tarry or bloody stools. He has tried over-the-counter antacids with no relief. A neighbor gave him his prescription of Pepcid, which he is using with minimal relief.

Past Medical History   Unremarkable

Past Surgical History   Unremarkable

Family History   Mother age 72, hypothyroidism; father age 75, heart attack at age 45, HTN; brother age 45, heart attack age 44, HTN; brother age 50, coronary artery bypass surgery at age 45; sister age 47, A&W

Developmental Stage   Generativity versus Stagnation

Role-Relationship   Lives in a four-bedroom home in the city with his family, his parents, and his oldest brother and his family. There are 12 individuals who live together with the women staying home to share the household chores. J.S. works in a factory putting small parts together. He has been married for 19 years and has three children.

Sleep/Rest   Falls asleep about 11 PM and awakens at 5 AM to go to work

Nutrition/Metabolic   Breakfast, warm cereal and toast or rice cakes; lunch, rice with vegetables and a piece of fruit; dinner, rice with vegetables and meat, soup, and dessert that usually consists of fruits

Activity/Exercise   Does not engage in regular exercise

Coping/Stress   J.S. is working to save money and buy a home for his family. He talks with his father and brothers when he has problems. J.S. enjoys time with his extended family.

Health Management   Smokes one pack of cigarettes per day × 15 years. Td: Unsure of last tetanus date, but thinks it was when he was in grade school. He has a smoke detector in the house and changes the batteries annually. J.S. drinks two cups of coffee in the morning, two colas in the afternoon, and has two beers in the evening.

Medications   For 6 weeks J.S. has been taking famotidine (Pepcid) 20 mg bid that his neighbor gave him

Allergies   NKMA

Pertinent Physical Findings

Vital Signs   Height, 5 feet 2 inches; weight 136 pounds; BMI 25; temperature 98.2° F; heart rate 66; respirations 12; blood pressure 120/78

Heart   Apical pulse 66, rate regular; no murmurs, S_3 or S_4

Lungs   Clear to auscultation

Abdomen: Abdomen soft; no abdominal bulges noted when head raised; + bowel sounds; slight tenderness over mid-epigastric area; no splenomegaly or hepatomegaly

Diagnostics

Diagnostic Tests   Stools for occult blood are negative × 3; ECG NSR

History Data   Questions specific to the chief complaint of heartburn include the following:

- When did you first experience heartburn?
- How often do you experience heartburn and how long does each episode last?
- Describe the type and location of the discomfort.
- Do you have any radiation of the discomfort? If so, where does the discomfort radiate?
- Is the heartburn aggravated by food?
- Is the heartburn relieved by sitting up, standing, or taking antacids?
- Does activity or exercise aggravate the pain? (This helps differentiate any cardiac symptoms.)
- Are you a smoker? (Smoking decreases the lower esophageal sphincter pressure, increasing symptoms of heartburn.)
- Do you have difficulty swallowing, weight loss, or bloody stools? (These symptoms require further diagnostic evaluation.)
- Do you experience a gaseous feeling or frequent burping?
- Are you often under stress?
- How much caffeine and chocolate do you consume each day?
- Are you taking any nonsteroidal antiinflammatory drugs such as Motrin (NSAIDs)?

Physical Examination Data   The focused examination for the chief complaint of heartburn includes: vital signs, heart, lungs, and abdomen. Vital signs are important indicators of the hemodynamic status of the patient. A systolic blood pressure less than 100 mm Hg (regardless of the heart rate) in a high-risk gastrointestinal patient indicates significant acute blood loss that requires emergent care. A systolic blood pressure more than 100 mm Hg and a heart rate more than 100 beats per minute indicates moderate blood loss (Tierney, McPhee, and Papadakis, 1999). Postural changes of more than 20 mm Hg in systolic blood pressure; or a heart rate increase of more than 20 to 30 beats per minute from supine to standing, in patients at high risk for gastrointestinal bleeding, suggests a 10% to 15% blood loss (Singer, Burstein, and Schiavone, 1996). The supine blood pressure is generally maintained until there is greater than a 20% to 25% blood volume loss. The hematocrit is not a good indicator of acute blood loss because it takes 24 to 72 hours for reequilibration of the intravascular volume.

Differential Diagnosis   Gastroesophageal reflux disease, peptic ulcer disease, gastritis, cardiac chest pain, gallbladder disease (Table 8-2)

Probable Causes of the Presenting Symptoms
Approximately 40% of adults experience heartburn at least one time per month, and about 5% have weekly symptoms. Heartburn is the major complaint of individuals diagnosed with gastroesophageal reflux disease (GERD). Individuals who have esophageal motility disorders, or who have hyposalivation, often have severe GERD. Those who have scleroderma or CREST syndrome (subcutaneous calcinosis, Raynaud's phenomenon, esophageal dysmotility, sclerodactlyly, and telangiectasia) often have complictions from GERD. Smoking and anticholinergic medications decrease salivation and predispose to increased severity of GERD. Foods and medication that decrease LES pressure include chocolate, alcohol, fatty foods, peppermint, onion and garlic oils, calcium channel blockers, xanthines, and beta-adrenergic antagonists. Complications that may occur with GERD

Table 8-2			
Heartburn Differential Diagnostic Cues			
Diagnosis	**Signs and Symptoms**	**Lab Data**	**Treatment**
Gastroesophageal Reflux Disease	Heartburn worse when bending, lying down, or eating large meals; regurgitation; retrosternal or atypical chest discomfort; chronic cough, sore throat; chronic laryngitis	Stools for occult blood × 3 If age <45 and no history of dysphagia, weight or blood loss, may initiate medical management A 4-week trial of medical management is appropriate; if no improvement, then order an upper endoscopy	Avoid lying down 3 hours after meals, meals, elevate the head of the bed on 6-inch blocks. Avoid acidic foods or agents that relax the LES or delay gastric emptying. Avoid bending after eating. Decrease the meal size. Trial of antacids, H_2 antagonists, a promotility drug, or a proton pump inhibitor
Peptic Ulcer Disease Commonly caused by NSAIDs, chronic *H. pylori* infection, or acid hypersecretory states (e.g., Zollinger-Ellison syndrome)	Dyspepsia, dull aching pain may be relieved by food or antacids, awakened by nocturnal pain, may have nausea	*H. pylori* with urease breath test or serum test to assess ulcer pathology Upper endoscopy; if + must follow-up with endoscopy in 12 weeks to document complete healing. If healing is incomplete, suspect malignancy CBC to assess for anemia If severe epigastric pain, order serum amylase to assess pancreatic involvement If suspect Zollinger-Ellison syndrome, order fasting serum gastrin levels	Treatment depends on the cause. If NSAID-induced, discontinue NSAID, use H_2 receptor antagonists, proton pump inhibitors, or sucralfate. For prevention of NSAID-induced ulcers, use misoprostol (Cytotec) 200 micrograms 3-4 × day with meals and at HS. If + *H. pylori* and has a duodenal or gastric ulcer, use an FDA approved treatment option (e.g., omeprazole 40 mg qd + clarithromycin 500 mg tid × 2 weeks; then omeprazole 20 mg qd × 2 weeks **OR** lansoprazole 30 mg + amoxicillin 1 gm bid + clarithromycin 500 mg bid × 14 days (See CDC Guidelines on *H. pylori* in peptic ulcer disease for treatment guidelines (NIH Consensus Conference, 1994). Zoellinger Ellison Syndrome requires referral
Gastritis Examples of causes of gastritis include stress, NSAID-induced, alcoholic, portal hypertension gastropathy, and *H. pylori* gastritis	Epigastric pain, N/V, hematemesis, melena, commonly seen in alchoholics or those who take NSAIDs	Stools for occult blood × 3. With erosive gastritis there is often hematemesis which requires upper endoscopy within 24 hours. *H. pylori* test if persistent epigastric discomfort. SOB × 3.	Refer any patient with bleeding May treat symptomaticaly with either sucralfate (Carafate) 1 g 4 × day **OR** H_2-receptor antagonist (e.g., ranitidine [Zantac] 150 mg bid) **OR** proton pump inhibitors (e.g., omeprazole [Prilosec] 20 mg qd). Eliminate the offending agent if possible (e.g., NSAID, drugs, alcohol, or *H. pylori*)

Continued

Table 8-2
Heartburn Differential Diagnostic Cues—cont'd

Diagnosis	Signs and Symptoms	Lab Data	Treatment
Cardiac Chest Pain	Chest pain that occurs at rest, with exertion or activity, or at night, pain may be substernal and radiate to arms or jaw, dyspnea, diaphoresis, N/V	ECG Cardiac enzyme tests	Transport to hospital for emergency care for acute event
Gallbladder Disease	Severe pain in RUQ or epigastric pain, N/V, fatty foods may precipitate attack, rarely presents with painless jaundice*	Ultrasound of the gallbladder CBC, bilirubin, alkaline phophatase are mildly elevated in acute cholecystitis SGOT, amylase HIDA scan may identify cystic duct obstruction	Surgical intervention

*The combination of RUQ pain, fever, and jaundice is Charcot's triad and is classic for acute cholangitis.

include esophagitis, esophageal strictures, and Barrett's esophagus.

Heartburn is commonly caused by a motility disorder in which reflux sends acid gastric contents into the esophagus, causing varying degrees of mucosal damage (Greene et al, 1996). In many cases, the acid reflux occurs when the lower esophageal sphincter relaxes. The sensation of heartburn may be burning, pain, and warmth or heat in the retrosternal region (Seller, 1996). Atypical heartburn symptoms include chest pain, dysphagia, cough, and respiratory complaints. If regurgitation is prolonged, patients may develop Barrett's esophagitis. In this disorder, the squamous epithelium in the esophagus is replaced by metaplastic columnar epithelium. Approximately 10% of individuals with Barrett's esophagitis will develop adenocarcinoma of the esophagus.

Diagnostic Tests   Patients who present with uncomplicated common symptoms of heartburn can be treated empirically for 4 weeks without further diagnostic work-up. However, J.S. has been having symptoms for 6 months and has a strong family history of cardiac problems. Therefore, he should have an EKG and stress test to rule out cardiac disease. In uncomplicated cases of heartburn there is no need for further diagnostic testing. In patients who present with severe reflux symptoms, an upper endoscopy is the usual procedure for identifying the type and extent of gastroesophageal problems and also offers the advantage of biopsy. The grading of severity of esophageal damage is mild (1) to severe (4). In this case, J.S. should undergo upper endoscopy with biopsy to determine the type and extent of tissue damage. An upper GI is sometimes used to look for strictures, anatomic abnormalities, and gastric webs. The upper GI has limited ability to differentiate between types of lesions; these require an upper endoscopy for identification.

Diagnostic Impression   J.S. presents with heartburn unrelieved by over-the-counter medications and therapeutic doses of an H_2-histamine blocker (Pepcid). He has heartburn after meals. J.S.'s diagnosis is GERD.

Therapeutic Plan of Care For GERD there is a step or phase approach to the treatment of patients.

Step one is lifestyle modifications. The patient is instructed to lose any excess weight (a 10-pound weight loss can decrease heartburn symptoms), avoid lying down after meals, and elevate the head of the bed on 6-inch blocks. Patients should avoid acidic foods such as tomatoes, citrus fruits, spicy foods, and coffee because these increase gastric acids and heartburn symptoms. Patients should avoid substances that delay gastric emptying or relax the LES (such as fatty foods, peppermint, chocolate, alcohol, and smoking). Patients should eat frequent, small meals instead of large portions to decrease the heartburn sensation. They can use antacids (e.g., Maalox TC, Mylanta II, and Gaviscon tablets) to help alleviate heartburn symptoms.

Step two includes the use of H_2-histamine receptor antagonists or promotility agents. Patients who present with frequent typical GERD symptoms should be given a trial of an H_2-histamine receptor antagonist (e.g., ranitidine [Zantac] 150 mg bid or famotidine [Pepcid] 20 mg bid). These medications should be used for 8 to 12 weeks prior to discontinuing. If symptoms reoccur, they may need to be treated continuously or intermittently with medical therapy.

Step three includes the use of proton pump inhibitors such as omeprazole (Prilosec) or lansoprazole (Prevacid). These medications are used for documented erosive esophagitis, reflux complications, atypical reflux symptoms, symptoms unresponsive to other medical therapies, and as first-line treatments by some practitioners because of their efficacy (Tierney, McPhee, and Papadakis, 1999).

J.S. should be instructed on steps one and three treatments. A discussion should be held about smoking cessation and decreasing caffeinated and alcoholic beverages to decrease symptoms of heartburn. J.S. has used both antacids and H_2-histamine receptor antagonists with little relief of symptoms; therefore a trial of omeprazole (Prilosec) 20 mg qd should be instituted.

Patient Education and/or Community Resources A discussion about lifestyle changes should occur at every visit.

Follow-Up Plan Recheck J.S. after 2 weeks. If symptoms are controlled, reevaluate in 6 weeks. After the 6-week recheck, schedule a visit in 3 months.

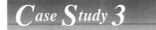

Case Study 3

CHIEF COMPLAINT: Bloody Stools

History of Present Illness C.T. is a 49-year-old African-American male who presents with chief complaint of bloody stools and anal pruritus × 2 weeks. Upon further questioning, he describes the blood occurring after each stool as bright red on the toilet paper with an occasional streak on the stool. He states that he is getting worried because the blood has persisted and he has a family history of colon cancer. C.T. states that the rectal discomfort and itching has increased over the past 2 days. He has been sitting in warm water in his whirlpool tub at home, which helps alleviate the discomfort a little. He states that he typically has a stool every other day and that the stool is brown and formed. About once a month he has constipation, which he relieves by drinking a glass of prune juice. C.T. denies bleeding disorders, liver disease, CHF, abdominal tumors, and anorectal surgery. C.T. does not practice anal-receptive intercourse.

Past Medical History Ankle fracture at age 10; multiple ear infections as a child

Past Surgical History Unremarkable

Family History Father died of colon cancer at age 62; father's oldest brother died of colon cancer at age 65; father's youngest brother had recurring polyps; mother age 79, A&W; sister age 52, breast cancer; sister age 47, A&W; brother age 54, multiple rectal polyps removed

Developmental Stage Generativity versus Stagnation

Role-Relationship Lives with his wife and three children in a three-bedroom home in the suburbs. Enjoys his job as a salesman for a pharmaceutical company.

Sleep/Rest Falls asleep about 11:30 PM and awakens at 7:30 AM rested

Nutrition/Metabolic For breakfast has a donut and coffee while he drives to his first appointment. For lunch he usually has a salad and sandwich with fruit. Dinner is usually with the family and they have chicken or steak, a vegetable, and pasta. Snacks include sweets, chips, and sodas.

Activity/Exercise   Exercises by swimming and using the stationary bicycle every day at a fitness center.

Coping/Stress   C.T. talks to his wife when problems come up, and together they determine the best course of action. He enjoys his job and does not feel pressured at work. He spends many evenings with his children playing and working on homework. C.T. belongs to a golf league that plays once a week. He enjoys swimming, bicycling, and playing basketball with his children.

Health Management   C.T. feels that he takes good care of his health and has a physical at least every other year. He does admit to smoking a cigar three to five times a week, but says he intends to quit. C.T. does not drink alcohol or take recreational drugs.

Medications   C.T. uses Extra Strength Tylenol occasionally for a tension headache.

Allergies   PCN and sulfa, rash

Pertinent Physical Findings
Vital Signs   Height, 6 feet even; weight 191 pounds; BMI 26; temperature 97.6° F; heart rate 76; respirations 12; blood pressure 136/78

Heart   Apical pulse, 76; rate regular, no murmurs, S_3, or S_4

Lungs   Clear to auscultation

Abdomen   Abdomen soft and nontender; + bowel sounds, no masses or organomegaly

Rectal   Four protuberant purple nodules covered with mucosa emerging from the anus, no fissures, skin tags, dermatitis, or fistulas; normal anal tone; prostate smooth with no nodules

Diagnostics
Diagnostic Tests   Digital rectal examination with hemoccult negative stool in the anal vault. Anoscopy shows internal hemorrhoids above the dentate line in the left lateral position.

History Data   Questions specific to the chief complaint of bloody stools include the following:

- How long and how frequently do you have bloody stools?
- Do you experience constipation or diarrhea?
- Do you have pain associated with stools, itching, or burning?
- Do you have a history of bleeding disorders, liver disease, congestive heart failure, or abdominal tumors (Barker, Burton, and Zive, 1999)?
- Have you had anorectal surgery?
- Have you had a previous flexible sigmoidoscopy or colonoscopy?
- (If a female) Are you now or have you ever been pregnant?
- Do you have a family history of hemorrhoids, polyps, or rectal cancer?
- Do you have anal-receptive intercourse?

Physical Examination Data   The focused examination for the chief complaint of bloody stools includes: vital signs, heart, lungs, abdomen, and rectal.

Differential Diagnosis   Hemorrhoids, carcinoma of the anus, rectal prolapse, anal fissures, pruritus ani, anorectal infections, Crohn's disease and ulcerative colitis (Table 8-3)

Probable Causes of the Presenting Symptoms   Hemorrhoids develop from swelling of the submucosal cushions from constant increase in the intraabdominal pressure (Rubin et al, 1996). The hemorrhoid then becomes swollen and is forced through the rectal sphincter. Increased intraabdominal pressure occurs from constipation, pregnancy, heavy lifting, or any form of straining. Hemorrhoids can be categorized in four stages (Tierney, McPhee, and Papadakis, 1999). *Stage I* is confinement in the anal canal. *Stage II* is protrusion during any activity that results in straining; when the activity subsides the prolapse reduces spontaneously. *Stage III* is prolapsed hemorrhoids that require manual reduction. *Stage IV* is chronically prolapsed hemorrhoids. For stage 1 and stage II hemorrhoids, conservative therapeutic management is recommended. In stages III and IV, hemorrhoidectomy is the treatment of choice.

Table 8-3
Bloody Stools Differential Diagnostic Cues

Diagnosis	Signs and Symptoms	Lab Data	Treatment
Hemorrhoids	Bright red blood on toilet tissue, streaked in stool or slight coloration of toilet bowl. May have pruritus, discomfort, or rectal pain.	Digital rectal examination to assess for hemorrhoids, obtain a stool sample for occult blood and to evaluate the rectum. Anoscopy in the office Schedule for a proctosigmoidoscopy to exclude disease in the rectum or sigmoid CBC if fatigued or signs of anemia (rare). If + anemia, need a colonoscopy or BE to exclude disease above the sigmoid colon	High fiber diet Prescribe a psyllium bulk laxative (e.g., Metamucil, Citrucel); for itching and inflammation try Anusol-HC Cream or Wyanoids-HC Ointment 3-4 × day. Suppositories do not work well. Warm sitz baths, cold packs, or witch hazel compresses may provide relief. If hemorrhoid is thrombosed, may lance and remove clot. If hemorrhoids become problematic, may consider surgical intervention.
Carcinoma of the Anus	Bleeding, pain, and/or rectal mass	CT scan and endoluminal ultrasound to determine depth and spread	Refer to an oncologist for treatment, which may include external radiation and chemotherapy. For severe cases may consider abdominoperineal resection
Rectal Prolapse	Mucous discharge, bleeding, rectal incontinence, sphincter damage and prolapsed rectum	None	Refer for surgical correction
Pruritus Ani	Erythema, excoriations, lichenification, eczematous skin	None	Cleanse gently after BMs with nonscented wipes premoistened with lanolin, then gently dry the rectal area. Use cotton balls to absorb mucus. Avoid creams and ointments that may further irritate rectal area
Anorectal Infections *Neisseria Gonorrhoeae*	Burning, itching, tenesmus, mucopurulent discharge	Swabs for Gram stain during anoscopy; cultures from urethra and pharynx in men and cervix in women	Ceftriaxone (Rocephin) 125 mg IM, ciprofloxacin 500 mg PO *OR* ofloxacin 400 mg PO and erythromycin 500 mg qid PO *OR* doxycycline 100 mg bid PO × 7 days

Continued

Table 8-3
Bloody Stools Differential Diagnostic Cues—cont'd

Diagnosis	Signs and Symptoms	Lab Data	Treatment
Anorectal Infections—cont'd			
Syphilis Treponema Pallidum	Primary syphilis chancre, inguinal lymphadenopathy or with secondary syphilis may have condylomata lata	Dark-field microscopy of scrapings from the chance or condyloma. VDRL	Primary and secondary syphilis with rectal involvement: benzathine penicillin G 2.4 million units IM *OR* if PCN allergic give doxycycline 100 mg bid × 2 weeks *OR* tetracycline 500 mg qid × 2 weeks
Chlamydia Trachomatis	Fever, bloody diarrhea, painful perianal ulcerations	Culture of rectal discharge	Tetracycline 250-500 mg PO qid *OR* doxycycline 100 mg bid × 21 days
Herpes Simplex II	Small vesicles in perianal area, constipation, pain, tenesmus	Viral culture or antigen detection assays of vesicular fluid	Active infection may be treated with acyclovir (Zovirax) 400 mg PO 5 × day for 5-10 days
Venereal Warts Condyloma	Itching, bleeding, pain, and warts in or covering rectal area	None	May try topical application of podophyllum resin with small lesions – must protect the unaffected skin with petroleum and dust the treated area with cornstarch or talc. Refer larger lesions. Large lesions may require CO_2 laser surgery or cryotherapy
Anal Fissures	Blood, pain, constipation	None	High fiber diet Fiber supplements Sitz baths Topical anesthetics

Diagnostic Tests Inspect the anal area and rectum and perform a digital rectal examination with hemoccult evaluation. Perform an anoscopy to detect any bleeding internal hemorrhoids. The American Cancer Society recommends screening of asymptomatic individuals with a sigmoidoscopy every 3 to 5 years beginning at age 50. A colonoscopy is recommended for patients who have any of the following: a first-degree relative with colon cancer; a diagnosis of inflammatory bowel disease; adenomatous polyps; or a history of colon, rectal, breast, ovarian, or endometrial cancer. Because he has a strong family history of colon cancer, C.T. should be scheduled for a colonoscopy.

Diagnostic Impression C.T. presents with bright red blood on the toilet paper after a BM and slight rectal discomfort with itching for 2 days duration. These symptoms are characteristic of hemorrhoids.

Therapeutic Plan of Care To help alleviate his rectal discomfort, C.T. should try Anusol HC, applying a thin film two to four times per day. Encourage the use of warm sitz baths for 20 minutes qid prn. C.T. should schedule a colonoscopy. Give him a copy of a high-fiber diet and encourage him to use Metamucil three times a day PO, using 1 rounded teaspoon in 8 oz of water. If he is unable to tolerate the Metamucil, suggest the use of Fiber-Con, an OTC fiber product in tablet form, taken every day with at least 2 liters of fluid.

Patient Education and/or Community Resources The American Cancer Society recommends that all individuals aged 50 and older have stool tested for occult blood. Providing a written handout on a high fiber diet will help C.T. remember the types of foods he needs to eat. He should report any constant or moderate-to-large amounts of bleeding, or increased or intense pain. He can also obtain information by accessing the National Cancer Institute's website at http://www.nci.nih.gov/

Follow-Up Plan C.T. should have a follow-up visit after his colonoscopy to review the test results and discuss the effectiveness of the therapeutic plan of care.

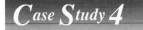

Case Study 4

CHIEF COMPLAINT: Jaundice

History of Present Illness L.M. is a 28-year-old Caucasian male who presents with a chief complaint of jaundice. L.M. states that his girlfriend noticed that his eyes and skin were turning yellow and urged him to seek help. He states he cannot play basketball after work as he usually does because he is so tired. Upon further questioning he states that his stools are clay-colored and that his urine is getting dark. L.M. also describes some RUQ abdominal pain, but attributes it to spicy foods. He also complains that his cigarettes don't taste good anymore. L.M. has multiple sexual partners (six in 6 months) and does not use condoms. He denies receiving blood products, using intravenous drugs or steroids, or having a tattoo.

Past Medical History Acute bronchitis at least twice a year

Past Surgical History Unremarkable

Family History Mother age 62, alcoholic; father age 72, stroke; brother age 34, A&W

Developmental Stage Intimacy versus Isolation

Role-Relationship L.M. enjoys being a mechanical engineer. He is engaged to be married. He lives in an apartment in a large city.

Sleep/Rest Falls asleep at 11 PM and awakens at 7 AM feeling rested.

Nutrition/Metabolic Breakfast, donuts and coffee; lunch, fast food and soda; dinner, frozen dinners. Snacks on chips, sweets, and sodas

Activity/Exercise Tries to run every day for at least 1 mile and play basketball

Coping/Stress He finds his job stressful as it demands frequent temporary assignments out of the state and has many tight deadlines. L.M. has many friends. He enjoys swimming, running, and reading.

Health Management Drinks one or two beers every night to help relax and unwind. Smokes 1½ packs of cigarettes a day for the past 10 years. Unsure of the date of his last tetanus shot. Owns a handgun for protection, but only uses it when he goes to the target range for practice. L.M. is not fearful nor does he feel unsafe: he purchased the handgun in case of the event that an intruder would enter his apartment.

Medications L.M. takes Tylenol Extra Strength, two tablets every 4 to 6 hours almost daily for headaches.

Allergies NKMA

Pertinent Physical Findings
Vital Signs Height 6 feet 2 inches; weight 241 pounds; BMI 31; temperature 99.2° F; heart rate 66; respirations 16; blood pressure 126/82

Skin Fair complexion, skin smooth, moist, cool, good turgor; no edema, lesions, exudates; slight yellow hue; no cyanosis; no abnormal moles, bruising, vascular spiders, or palmar erythema

Heart Apical pulse 66, regular rate and rhythm; no murmur, S_3 or S_4

Lung Lungs clear to auscultation

Abdomen Slightly convex, active bowel sounds, no abdominal bruits, soft, tender over RUQ, liver edge is tender with a 12 cm span, no ascites or splenomegaly, no inguinal lymphadenopathy, no CVA tenderness

Diagnostics

Diagnostic Tests   SGPT/ALT, 157 U/L (0-45); SGOT/AST, 94 U/L (0-45); LDH, 1200 U/L; total bilirubin, 10.1 mg/dl; direct bilirubin, 8.2 mg/dl; alkaline phosphatase, 120 U/L (25-130); protein, 7.6G/dl (6-8.5); albumin 4.0G/dl (3.5-5.3); HBsAg, positive; HBsAb, negative; HBcAb, positive; IgM anti-HAV, negative; Anti-HCV, negative; prothrombin time, 15 seconds; urinalysis—color brown, appearance clear; pH 6.0; bilirubin, large, Protein: 1+; CBC: WBC 4.5 k/ul; RBC 4.79 ml/ul; Hgb 15.7 g/dl; Hct 44.9%; MCV 93.7 fl; MCH 32.5 pg; MCHC 34.6%

History Data   Questions specific to the chief complaint of jaundice include the following:

- How long have you had the jaundice?
- Do you have any other symptoms such as fatigue, loss of appetite, nausea or vomiting, diarrhea, or fever?
- Has your urine turned darker or do you have lighter stools?
- Has any of your friends, co-workers, or sexual partners have similar symptoms?
- What medications (prescription and OTC), herbs, vitamins, and anabolic steroids (body builders) have you taken in the past 2 months?
- Have you ever received any blood products?
- Have you ever used intravenous drugs or received a tattoo?
- Have you been to a foreign country recently?
- Do you eat wild mushrooms?
- Do you have exposure to daycare?
- Are you currently sexually active and do you use condoms? If so, how many partners have you had within the past 6 months? (The incubation period of hepatitis B is 6 weeks to 6 months.)

Physical Examination Data   The focused examination for the chief complaint of jaundice includes: vital signs, skin, heart and lung, and abdomen.

Differential Diagnosis   Viral hepatitis (A, B, C, D, E, G); cholangitis; alcoholic hepatitis; cholestatic jaundice secondary to drugs; autoimmune hepatitis; carcinoma of the pancreas (Table 8-4)

Probable Causes of the Presenting Symptoms   Jaundice occurs from either unconjugated or conjugated bilirubin in the serum. Unconjugated bilirubin results from an overproduction of bilirubin, impaired conjugation of bilirubin, or impaired hepatic uptake of bilirubin. Conjugated bilirubin results when there is extrahepatic biliary obstruction or impaired excretion of bilirubin from the liver. Causes of unconjugated hyperbilirubinemia include hemolytic anemias, drug reactions, and Crigler-Najjar syndrome. Causes of conjugated hyperbilirubinemia include hepatitis, biliary cirrhosis, cholangitis, and industrial toxins.

Diagnostic Tests   Patients who present with a chief complaint of jaundice should have the following diagnostic tests: liver enzymes, serological testing for viral antigens and antibodies (hepatitis panel), CBC, total and direct bilirubin, prothrombin time, and urinalysis. Depending on the presenting symptoms, a liver biopsy may be performed if the prothrombin time is adequate. L.M. should be offered HIV testing because he has had unprotected intercourse with multiple partners.

Diagnostic Impression   L.M. presents with jaundice, fatigue, scleral icterus, clay-colored stools, and dark urine. He is having RUQ discomfort and is avoiding cigarettes. These symptoms, coupled with his laboratory tests, indicate that he has hepatitis B virus (HBV).

Therapeutic Plan of Care   L.M.'s symptoms should be managed and he should be monitored closely. He should avoid vigorous physical activity, eat nutritious meals, stop drinking alcohol, discontinue his Tylenol Extra Strength, and use condoms with intercourse. L.M. should not share personal hygiene items and he should use good handwashing technique. He should encourage his girlfriend to see a health care provider and she should receive hepatitis B immunoglobulin (HBIG) if she is unvaccinated and initiate the HB vaccine.

	Table 8-4		
	Jaundice Differential Diagnostic Cues		

Diagnosis	Signs and Symptoms	Lab Data	Treatment
Viral Hepatitis	For all of the viral hepatitis categories: Fever, dark urine, light stools, fatigue, scleral icterus, hepatomegaly, RUQ tenderness, jaundice (Alexander, 1998).	For all of the viral hepatitis categories: Liver enzymes, serological testing for viral antigens and antibodies (hepatitis panel), CBC, total and direct bilirubin, prothrombin time, urinalysis	Symptom management for all viral hepatitis categories includes: No vigorous physical activities until symptoms are gone; adequate fluids; low-fat, high-carbohydrate diet if low appetite; antiemetics sparingly for vomiting; do not take any hepatotoxic drugs (e.g., narcotics, alcohol); good handwashing and sanitation; safe sex; discourage alcohol use for 6 months; do not share personal hygiene items
Hepatitis A (HAV) Abrupt onset Incubation 15-50 days Transmission oral and sexual No chronic carrier state Infectious 2 weeks before symptoms and 1 week after		IgM anti-HAV = acute infection; IgG anti-HAV = past infection or vaccination	Symptom management: Give 0.02 ml/kg of immune globulin after exposure (within 2 weeks) to all household and sexual contacts Report all daycare outbreaks to the local health department Should not be around daycare until 1 week after onset of illness and jaundice is gone Good handwashing
Hepatitis B (HBV) Insidious onset Incubation 28-160 days Transmission sexual, percutaneous, perinatal, oral Chronic carrier state possible Infectious 4-6 weeks before symptoms to weeks to months (unpredictable)		HBsAg (hepatitis B surface antigen) establishes infection, if persists after the acute illness indicates chronic carrier state Anti-HBs (antibodies to HbsAg) signals recovery and shows up after successful vaccination Anti-HBc (antibody to hepatitis B core antigen) appears after HBsAg and persists indefinitely; Hbe-Ag (hepatitis Be antigen) indicates infectivity	Refer for management. If exposed person and unvaccinated, give HBIG × 1 and initiate HB vaccine Symptom management: Cannot donate blood or blood products; safe sex Prevention of HBV: Prenatal screening for HbsAg. Immunoprophylaxis for those at high risk and universal precautions Refer for management. Treatment for chronic hepatitis B: May use interferon (Intron-A); epivar-HBV (contains lamivudine l00 mg) awaiting FDA approval; must have HIV testing before starting on Epivar-HBV. (If HIV+, could lead to resistant strains of HIV [Prescriber's Letter, 1998]).

Continued

Table 8-4
Jaundice Differential Diagnostic Cues—cont'd

Diagnosis	Signs and Symptoms	Lab Data	Treatment
Viral Hepatitis—cont'd			
Hepatitis C (HCV) Insidious onset Incubation 15-160 days Transmission sexual and percutaneous Chronic carrier state possible Infectivity is same as HBV		Anti-HCV (antibody to hepatitis C virus) present in acute and chronic state	Refer for management. Same treatment as for HBV May try interferon alfa-2b (Intron A) **OR** interferon and ribavirin (Rebetron)
Hepatitis D (HDV) Co-occurs with HBV Insidious onset Incubation 28-140 days Transmission sexual and percutaneous Chronic carrier state possible Infectivity is same as HBV		Anti HDV (antibody to hepatitis D virus) in acute disease	Refer for management. Same treatment as for HBV
Hepatitis E (HEV) Found in developing countries Abrupt onset Mean incubation is 40 days Transmission oral No chronic carrier state Infectivity similar to HAV		No serologic test for HEV	Symptom management Prevention through good sanitation and hygiene
Hepatitis G (HGV) Found in developing countries Insidious onset Incubation questionable Transmission percutaneous Lasts at least 10 years Is a flavivirus			Symptom management

	Table 8-4		
	Jaundice Differential Diagnostic Cues—cont'd		

Diagnosis	Signs and Symptoms	Lab Data	Treatment
Cholangitis	Jaundice, sudden onset of RUQ or epigastric pain, N/V, fever	Ultrasonography Liver function tests, total and direct bilirubin, prothrombin time, alkaline phosphatase, serum amylase	Refer for surgical evaluation or hospitalization for medical treatment
Alcoholic Hepatitis	N/V, jaundice, ascites, anorexia, hepatomegaly, abdominal pain, fever, splenomegaly, encephalopathy	CBC, liver function tests, total and direct bilirubin, prothrombin time, alkaline phosphatase, and serum amylase; ultrasound to rule out biliary obstruction Liver biopsy if prothrombin time is adequate	Stop drinking indefinitely; adequate nutritional intake (high CHO and caloric intake) and vitamins (folic acid and thiamine); may consider methylprednisolone 32 mg/d for I month
Cholestatic Jaundice Secondary to Drugs	Jaundice, RUQ or epigastric pain, N/V, fatigue	CBC, liver function tests, total and direct bilirubin, prothrombin time, alkaline phosphatase, and serum amylase; ultrasound to rule out biliary obstruction Liver biopsy if prothrombin time is adequate	Discontinue the offending drug(s); adequate nutrition; follow with liver function tests
Autoimmune Hepatitis	Jaundice, fever, amenorrhea, fatigue, anorexia, weight loss, hepatomegaly, splenomegaly, spider angiomas, palmer erythema, and extrahepatic symptoms (e.g., arthritis, rash)	CBC, liver function tests, total and direct bilirubin, prothrombin time, alkaline phosphatase, and serum amylase In select patients check alpha1-antitrypsin deficiency	Referral or consultation Corticosteroids, may be combined with azathioprine; usual length of time is 1 year but may require longer and even indefinite treatment
Carcinoma of the Pancreas	Jaundice, LUQ or epigastric pain which may radiate to back, diarrhea, weight loss	Abdominal ultrasound, CT, ERCP; if + will follow with percutaneous needle aspiration for cytological examination Total and indirect bilirubin, alkaline phosphatase, prothrombin time, liver function tests, CBC	Refer for possible surgical intervention Radiation and chemotherapy have limited results, but may be used for palliative treatment

Patient Education and/or Community Resources   A discussion about the causes of HBV, the disease trajectory, and the prognosis should occur. The patient should be cautioned to not consume alcohol for 6 months after symptoms are alleviated and laboratory tests are clear of HBV.

Follow-Up Plan   Reevaluate L.M. in 2 weeks

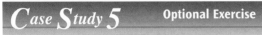

Case Study 5   **Optional Exercise**

CHIEF COMPLAINT: Abdominal Pain

History of Present Illness   S.P., a 17-year-old Caucasian male, presents with chief complaint of abrupt onset of generalized abdominal pain and episodes of vomiting this morning. He began feeling queasy during gym with constant dull periumbilical abdominal discomfort so he went home at 10:30 AM to rest. He ate a snack in hopes of feeling better, but the abdominal discomfort became worse. It is now 3:30 PM and he states he has constant, sharp, stabbing, right-sided abdominal pain that is worse with movement. He has vomited three times, had loose stools twice, and feels like he has a fever. He denies burning or frequency of urination, H/As, abdominal surgery or trauma, inflammatory bowel disease, or recurrent pneumonia. S.P. is sexually active with his girlfriend and they use condoms for birth control.

Past Medical History   Broken right arm at age 7

Past Surgical History   Unremarkable

Family History   Mother age 43, A&W; father age 41, asthma; sister age 15, A&W

Developmental Stage   Intimacy versus Isolation

Role-Relationship   Lives in the suburbs with his mother, father, and sister. S.P. has a girlfriend that he has dated for 1 year. He is actively involved in community activities and plays tennis for the varsity team. S.P. is a senior in high school and works part time at a local movie theatre.

Sleep/Rest   S.P. usually sleeps 7 hours per night during the school week and 8 hours on weekends.

Nutrition/Metabolic   S.P. eats a large breakfast consisting of cereal, fruit, eggs, milk, and orange juice. Lunch includes a sandwich, fruit, chips, cookie, and soda. Dinner is usually with his family and includes a meat, potato dish, and vegetable. He snacks on chips and sweets.

Activity/Exercise   S.P. plays golf in the summer with his friends or father and plays tennis on the varsity team. He enjoys swimming, basketball, and skiing with his friends.

Coping/Stress   S.P. has a positive relationship with his parents and discusses major issues with them. He is planning on attending college and majoring in business. He attends church regularly and is involved in the teen study group once a month.

Health Management   Does not smoke, drink alcoholic beverages, or take recreational drugs. Is up to date on tetanus booster (7/2/98). Does not own a firearm and is not fearful for his personal safety

Medications   Ibuprofen 400 mg every 4 to 6 hours prn for occasional headache or muscle pain

Allergies   NKMA

Pertinent Physical Findings

Vital Signs   Height 5 feet 9 inches; weight 189 pounds; BMI 28; temperature 99.2° F; heart rate 90; respirations 16; blood pressure 124/82

Heart   Apical pulse 90, regular rate and rhythm; no murmurs, S_3 or S_4

Lung   Clear to auscultation

Abdomen   Hypoactive bowel sounds, involuntary guarding when palpation attempted; pain elicited in the RLQ (McBurney's point is midway between the symphysis pubis and the iliac crest); +rebound tenderness, +psoas sign, +obturator sign; no organomegaly

Genital   No inguinal hernias, penis uncircumcised, no discharge, testes descended without masses or tenderness

Rectal   No lesions, masses, or hemorrhoids, normal anal tone, obvious abdominal discomfort with rectal examination; hemoccult negative for occult blood in stool

Diagnostic Tests

Diagnostic Tests   WBC 17,000/uL with shift to the left (neutrophilia); abdominal ultrasound + for visualization of the appendix

Discussion Questions

What type of history data should be collected?

What type of physical data should be collected?

What are the differential diagnoses?

What are the probable causes of the presenting symptoms?

What is your diagnostic impression?

What is the therapeutic plan of care?

What are the patient education and/or community resources?

What is your follow-up plan?

Discussions for optional case study exercises can be found in the accompanying Instructor's Manual.

References

Alexander IM: Viral hepatitis: primary care diagnosis and management, *Nurse Pract* 23(10):13-14, 17-20, 25-26, 1998.

Barker LR, Burton JR. Zive PO: *Principles of ambulatory medicine,* ed 5, Baltimore, 1999, Williams and Wilkins.

Castell DO, Johnston BT: Gastroesophageal reflux disease: Current strategies for patient management, *Arch Fam Med* 5(4):221-227, 1996.

Goroll AH, May LA, Mulley AG: *Primary care medicine: office evaluation and management of the adult patient,* ed 3, Philadelphia, 1995, Lippincott-Raven.

Greene H, Fincher RM, Johnson WP et al: *Clinical medicine,* ed 2, St Louis, 1996, Mosby.

Isselbacher K, Braunwald E, Wilson J et al: *Harrison's principles of internal medicine,* New York, 1994, McGraw Hill.

Jarrett M, Heitkemper M, Cain KC et al: The relationship between psychological distress and gastrointestinal symptoms in women with irritable bowel syndrome, *Nurs Res* 47(3):154-161, 1998.

National Institutes for Health: NIH Consensus Conference: Helicobacter pylori in peptic ulcer disease, *JAMA* 272(1):65-99, 1994.

Prescriber's Letter: *Infectious Diseases,* 5(11):63, 1998

.Rubin H, Voss C, Derksen DJ et al: *Medicine: a primary care approach,* Philadelphia, 1996, WB Saunders.

Seller R: *Differential diagnosis of common complaints,* Philadelphia, 1996, WB Saunders.

Singer AJ, Burstein JL, Schiavone FM: *Emergency medicine pearls,* Philadelphia, 1996, F.A. Davis Company.

Tierney L, McPhee SJ, Papadakis MA: *Current medical diagnosis and treatment,* Stamford, Conn., 1999, Appleton & Lange.

Uphold C, Graham M: *Clinical guidelines in family practice,* Gainesville, Fla., 1998, Barmarrae Books.

Selected Readings

American Academy of Pediatrics: *Red book: report of the committee on infectious diseases,* ed 24, Elk Grove Village, Ill, 1997, Author.

Bensoussan A, Talley NJ, Hing M et al: Treatment of irritable bowel syndrome with Chinese herbal medicine, *JAMA* 280(18):1585-1589, 1998.

Carrico CW, Fenton LZ, Taylor GA et al: Impact of sonography on the diagnosis and treatment of acute lower abdominal pain in children and young adults, *Am J Roentgenol* 172(2):513-516, 1999.

Case AM, Reid RL: Effects of the menstrual cycle on medical disorders, *Arch Intern Med* 158:1405-1412, 1998.

Chaudhry V, Hyser MJ, Gracias VH et al: Colonoscopy: the initial test for acute lower gastrointestinal bleeding, *Am Surg* 64(8):723-728, 1998.

Corrarino KE: Perinatal hepatitis B: update and recommendations, *MCN Am J Matern Child Nurs* 23(5):246-252, 1998.

Malone AJ: Unenhanced CT in the evaluation of the acute abdomen: the community hospital experience, *Semin Ultrasound CT MR* 20(2):68-76, 1999.

CHAPTER 9

Blood Dyscrasias

Ruth Ann Brintnall

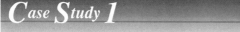

Case Study 1

CHIEF COMPLAINT: Fatigue

History of Present Illness   M.B. is a 37-year-old Caucasian female who presents as a patient new to the office for an employment physical. She has no specific complaints other than a lack of energy. M.B. has recently transferred to the area as a senior customer services representative at a local bank. She describes feelings of unusual fatigue at day's end, in spite of fairly constant work responsibilities. Because of shortness of breath and palpitations, M.B. has recently cut back her distance running. She denies other changes in her health, but with questioning, admits to heavy periods that have persisted since the birth of her last baby. Her menses last 7 to 9 days and are heavy days 1 through 5 with 10 pad changes per day.

Past Medical History   Gestational diabetes with second child

Past Surgical History   Appendectomy 1989; tubal ligation 1995

Family History   Mother and one sister, hypothyroidism; father, HTN; two brothers, ages 32 and 34, A&W

Developmental Stage   Intimacy versus Isolation

Role-Relationship   Single mother with two daughters, ages 6 and 2. She is estranged from her husband. Presently, not sexually active

Sleep/Rest   Sleeps 6 hours per night. M.B. usually falls to sleep at 11:30 PM and awakens at 5:30 AM

Nutrition/Metabolic   Breakfast, coffee; lunch, salad; dinner, meat, potatoes, and vegetables. Rarely snacks or has dessert

Activity/Exercise   M.B. enjoys running. Until recently, she was running 3 to 5 miles per day.

Coping/Stress   M.B.'s parents support her by assisting with childcare and being available for her to talk to and share information. M.B.'s best friend, Candice, also is a strong support.

Health Management   Smoking history quit 2 years ago (5 pack-year history); and drinks alcohol socially (<1 drink per month); does not engage in recreational drug use. Td: 1/27/98

Self-Perception and Values/Beliefs   Enjoys her children, but would like to find a suitable partner in the future. M.B. likes her co-workers and finds her job rewarding.

Medications   None

Allergies   NKMA

Pertinent Physical Findings

Vital Signs   Height 5 feet 6 inches; weight 130 pounds; temperature 98.2° F; heart rate 88; respirations 15; blood pressure 126/64 lying, 122/60 sitting, and 124/66 standing

General Appearance   Healthy appearing female; skin is smooth, dry with pale tone

HEENT   Normocephalic, symmetrical features; PERRLA with intact EOM, conjunctival membranes are pale; oral membranes, moist; nose, ears unremarkable; neck is supple and without adenopathy; thyroid is not enlarged

Heart   Apical rate 88/min, regular with soft systolic murmur, II/VI, loudest at the left sternal border 2nd and 3rd ICS, no radiation

Lungs   Clear to auscultation in all fields; expansion is symmetrical; no abnormal sounds are heard; breasts are without masses, tenderness, or nipple discharge

Abdomen   Soft, non-distended and non-tender to palpation; no hepatosplenomegaly; active bowel sounds all quadrants

Extremities   No edema; nail beds are pale; no clubbing, no spooning

Pelvic   Vaginal mucosa is moist, intact and without unusual discharge; uterus is within normal size, no adnexal masses or tenderness

Diagnostics

Diagnostic Tests   CBC, WBC 5.200; hemoglobin 8.2 g/dL; hematocrit 24.6%; platelet count 403,000 μl; peripheral smear shows microcytic (low corpuscular volume), hypochromic (low hemoglobin concentration) RBCs; no spherocytes are seen; Ferritin <30 ug/L; TIBC (total iron binding capacity) increased; stool guaiac (for possible source of anemia) negative three times.

History Data   Questions specific to the chief complaint of lack of energy include the following:

- When did you first notice lack of energy?
- Do you feel it is progressing?
- How has your lack of energy affected your daily activities?
- Do you have a prior history of similar symptoms?
- Do you have a history of blood loss, peptic ulcer disease, vomiting of blood (hematemesis), or black stools?
- Do you have a history of abnormally long or heavy periods or blood in your stools (guaiac positive)?
- Do you have a history of repeated blood donations or unusual fatigability?
- Do you have symptoms such as racing heart rate, dyspnea, or breathlessness on exertion?
- Do you have an eating disorder or crave unusual food (pica)?
- Do you have a history of alcoholism, inflammatory disorders, or chronic infection?
- Do you have a family history of anemia?
- What do you typically eat in a 24-hour period?

Physical Examination Data   The focused examination for the chief complaint of lack of energy includes: Vital signs, general appearance, HEENT, heart, lung, abdomen, extremities, and pelvic.

Differential Diagnosis   Iron deficiency anemia and the less common causes of microcytic anemia include: the anemia of chronic disease; the thalassemias; and, rarely, sideroblastic anemia (Table 9-1)

Probable Causes of the Presenting Symptoms

Initial assessment of MCV is especially helpful to differentiate the anemias. Table 9-2 classifies anemias by MCV and lists common causes of microcytic, normocytic and macrocytic anemia. An adult patient is considered anemic if the HCT <41%; HGB <13.5g/dl in males or HCT <37%; HGB <12 g/dl in females (Tierney, McPhee, and Papadakis, 1999). Anemias are classified based on their pathophysiological cause (i.e., destruction, loss of RBCs, or decreased production of RBCs) or on their cell size. Iron deficiency anemia (IDA) reveals small (microcytic), pale (hypochromic) RBCs with a decrease in iron stores.

In America, the most common cause of microcytic anemia by far is iron deficiency anemia. In fact, iron deficiency anemia is the most common form of anemia worldwide. Many patients are asymptomatic at the time of diagnosis, and their anemia is discovered as an incidental finding. Blood loss in adults is a frequent cause of iron deficiency and occurs when the loss of iron exceeds dietary intake. IDAs are slow in onset and stimulate compensatory mechanisms, so symptoms develop gradually or are minimal until significant anemia (HCT <30) develops. IDA in early childhood or adolescence usually is related to dietary factors or growth spurts.

In M.B., suspicion for the common sources of blood loss (such as gastrointestinal loss from ulcer, or tumor) does not seem high. Her normal physical examination and the absence of significant other history point to her menstrual loss as the most likely cause of her iron-deficient state. Moreover, her laboratory results and history corroborate the picture of iron deficiency anemia. Her low ferritin level and elevated TIBC reflect depleted iron stores. Cell indices show a low mean corpuscular volume (MCV), which occurs as red blood cell formation continues with deficient iron supplies. Eventually, anisocytosis and poikilocytosis (variations in size and shape of the red blood cells) occur because the building blocks for healthy cell forma-

Table 9-1
Common Anemias Differential Diagnostic Cues

Diagnoses	Signs and Symptoms	Lab Data	Treatment
Iron Deficiency Anemia	Fatigue, weakness, HA, dizziness; perhaps SOB on exertion, orthostatic hypotension, pale skin tones; history of blood loss; may have no symptoms	Microcytic, hypochromic anemia; decreased serum ferritin, increased TIBC, decreased serum iron	Oral iron replacement, diet teaching on iron rich foods, and education on the side effects of iron Treat cause of deficiency
Anemia of Chronic Disease	Weakness, fatigue, HA, orthostatic hypotension, SOB with exertion, underlying chronic inflammation or malignancy. Check for GI blood loss	Hypochromic or normochromic anemia; increased serum ferritin, decreased TIBC, decreased serum iron	Control chronic disease as able; ACD will usually not respond to administration of iron; erythropoietin may be of value but therapy is costly. May require no treatment unless severe; transfuse if severely anemic
Thalassemia, Alpha and Beta	May have heterozygous or homozygous form, thus thalassemia minor or major. May be alpha or beta Weakness, HA, chronic fatigue splenomegaly; minor have mild symptoms; major have more pronounced symptoms	Normochromic anemia; basophilic stippling, target cells, nucleated RBCs on peripheral smear May have increased stainable iron in bone marrow and increased hyperplasia Low MCV, iron studies are normal	Should be diagnosis of exclusion with Asian, African, Mediterranean origin Genetic counseling Distinguish from iron deficiency anemia and other hemoglobinopathies Severe forms may require regular transfusions, folate Splenectomy for hypersplenism; iron chelators under investigation for hemosiderosis
Sideroblastic Anemia	May have no specific symptoms other than those of anemia	MCV may be normal, increased or low Diagnosis is made by bone marrow revealing increased iron stores and ringed sideroblasts; serum iron is usually high, high transferrin	May not respond to therapy; occasionally, pyridoxine may be given; transfusion may be required for severe anemia; erythropoietin not usually helpful

Table 9-2
Classification of Anemias by MCV

Normocytic (Normal MCV)	Microcytic (Decreased MCV)	Macrocytic (Increased MCV)
Numerous causes, including • Normal variant (diagnosis of exclusion) • Acute hemorrhage • Anemia of chronic illness • Dilutional anemia • Liver disease (e.g., hepatitis, cirrhosis) • Uremias • Hemoglobinopathies (e.g., sickle cell, hemoglobin C disease) • HIV-related anemia	• Iron deficiency • Thalassemia, alpha or beta • Anemia of chronic disease • Sideroblastic anemia, acquired or congenital	Megaloblastic • Vitamin B_{12} deficiency • Folate deficiency Nonmegaloblastic • Myxedema • Chemotherapy • Myelodysplastic disease • Aplastic anemia • Alcoholism Hemolytic anemias

tion are not available. M.B.'s platelet count is within the normal range, but elevations can occasionally be seen in severe iron deficient states.

Diagnostic Tests   For this patient, the probability of an uncomplicated anemia is likely and existing laboratory data favors this conclusion. Further diagnostic tests at this point are not compelling until conventional treatments are tried. If M.B. failed to improve on iron replacement therapy, other tests might include serum iron, iron saturation, oral iron absorption test, hemoglobin electrophoresis, and peripheral smear for sideroblasts.

Diagnostic Impression   The initial diagnostic tests for anemia include CBC with differential, ferritin, TIBC, and stools for guaiac. M.B.'s presentation and history are typical of iron deficiency anemia secondary to excessive menstrual blood loss. Her peripheral blood smear reveals microcytic, hypochromic cells and supports the diagnosis of iron deficiency anemia. A practical approach to this common condition, seen in as many as 20% of adult women, is to begin therapy without further extensive testing. Table 9-3 shows laboratory findings for select iron deficiency anemias.

Therapeutic Plan of Care   The therapy for iron deficiency anemia requires restoration of the body's iron stores. Oral iron supplements in the form of ferrous sulfate are inexpensive and usually well tolerated. Ferrous sulfate 325 mg given three times a day provides an abundant source of iron to restore body needs. Continued therapy for 6 months is recommended to correct anemia and renew depleted iron stores (Rakel, 1996; Tierney, McPhee, and Papadakis, 1999). If necessary, supplemental iron doses are started slowly and gradually increased. The addition of vitamin C may aid absorption. Reticulocytosis should be seen within a week, indicating new erythrocytosis. After 3 to 4 weeks, an increase in hemoglobin should be seen. Very rarely, intolerance or refractoriness to oral iron is seen. Parenteral iron should be considered with care and should be reserved for use after alternate forms of oral iron (such as ferrous gluconate and ferrous fumarate) are tried. Iron dextran IV may be preferred to Imferon.

Further attention to M.B.'s heavy menses will be required, and a complete work-up should be planned to determine the cause. She should receive complete dietary instruction for an iron-rich diet. Likely side effects of iron therapy (such as constipation, diarrhea, and black stools) should be reviewed. Written medication and dietary handouts will help to reinforce teaching and promote compliance at home. M.B. should be cautioned to keep her iron tablets (and all medications) out of the

Table 9-3
Key Anemia Tests and Findings

	Serum Iron	TIBC	Serum Ferritin	Peripheral Smear	Hemoglobin Electrophoresis	Bone Marrow	Other
Iron deficiency anemia	Decreased	Increased	Decreased	Hypochromin	Normal	Erythroid hyperplasia No stainable iron	Increased free erythrocyte protoporphyrin (FEP) History of blood loss Diagnosis of exclusion
α Thalassemia	Increased	Normal or increased	Normal or increased	Basophilic stippling, target cells, nucleated RBCs, normochromia	Normal	Erythroid hyperplasia Increased stainable iron	Asian type more severe African type less severe
β Thalassemia	As above	As above	As above	As above	Increased Hemoglobin A Minor: 3%-7% Major: 7%-90%	As above	Mediterranean ethnic groups Minor mild symptoms and hemolysis Major: more severe iron overload
Sideroblastic anemias	Increased	Normal or decreased	Increased	Dimorphism: microcytic and normocytic RBCs, basophilic stippling	Normal	Erythroid hyperplasia Increased stainable iron Increased number of ringed sideroblasts, vacuolated RBCs	FEP increased
Anemia of chronic diseases	Decreased	Decreased	Increased	Hypochromia or normochromia	Normal	Increased stainable iron	Underlying chronic inflammation, malignancy

From: Rakel R: *Saunders manual of medical practice*, Philadelphia, 1996, WB Saunders.

reach of her children due to the toxicity of these preparations.

Patient Education and/or Community Resources M.B. is a new patient in the office and should be informed regarding office routines, suggested physical examinations, preventive screening, immunizations, and healthy living. She should be encouraged to honestly report new or changing symptoms and be assured of attention to her concerns. Her understanding of iron-rich foods should be reviewed at her return appointment. M.B. should be instructed to take her iron supplement with juices containing vitamin C to promote absorption, and avoid taking it with other medications that might alter absorption (for example, antacids or antibiotics). The rationale for follow-up of heavy menses should be explained. If heavy bleeding persists, an ultrasound of the pelvis will be scheduled for evidence of thickening of the endometrium or the presence of fibroids. Birth control pills or progesterone may be considered to regulate periods.

Follow-Up Plan M.B. should be scheduled for a CBC and reticulocyte count in 10 days to 2 weeks. A follow-up office appointment in 4 weeks is suggested to follow progress. If her laboratory studies show a response, and she is tolerating her iron supplements, she can be seen in 1 month. A phone follow-up is encouraged soon after iron therapy is started to ensure compliance.

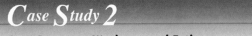

Case Study 2

Chief Complaint: Weakness and Fatigue

History of Present Illness R.T. is a 62-year-old Caucasian female with a 20-year history of rheumatoid arthritis. She presents with progressive weakness and fatigue over the last month. An office assessment reveals no significant change in her physical examination in spite of the fact that her last scheduled visit was more than 5 years ago. R.T. reports that she has not required medical intervention since joining a local alternative therapy group. She confesses that over the last few weeks she has had to resume regular dosing of ibuprofen due to increasing pain and stiffness. She adds that her fa-

tigue has caused her to cancel evening volunteer activities. Her laboratory profile shows an anemia, with hemoglobin of 8.9 g/dl. Her peripheral smear reveals normocytic cells, with a borderline normal MCV at 80 fl. She denies recent dietary change or weight loss, change in bowel habits, history of vomiting blood or blood in stool, or easy bruising.

Past Medical History Benign essential hypertension, rheumatoid arthritis, hemorrhoids; gravida 3, para 3

Past Surgical History Hysterectomy and bilateral oophorectomy 1979; T&A age 5

Family History Mother, HTN; father, HTN; brother age 55, A&W; brother age 61, HTN; sister age 65, hypothyroidism; daughter age 24, A&W; son age 26, A&W; daughter age 28, hypothyroidism

Developmental Stage Ego Integrity versus Despair

Role-Relationship A retired secretary, R.T. lives alone. Completed high school. Widowed. Travels with female friends and often goes to plays and church meetings. Baby-sits the grandchildren on weekends when her son and daughter-in-law have plans.

Sleep/Rest Falls asleep at 10 PM and awakens at 6 AM

Nutrition/Metabolic Breakfast, tea and toast; lunch, sandwich, fruit, and dessert; dinner, meat, vegetable and potato (may be frozen dinners or may make dinner herself)

Activity/Exercise Uses a stationary bicycle each day for 15 minutes. For the past month she has not been consistently using the bicycle because of fatigue.

Coping/Stress Attends a Baptist church every week and is active in the women's club. Socializes with the ladies and has several friends from church that go out to eat and invite each other over. Her son calls her weekly to make sure everything is okay.

Health Management Smoking and alcohol, none

Self-Perception and Values/Beliefs Feels a sense of accomplishment and enjoys her friends and activities. Is very concerned about her ability to manage her activities of daily living with the extreme fatigue.

Medications Ibuprofen 400-800 mg, three times daily; natural progesterone yam-based cream daily; had been prescribed Vasotec 5 mg qd, but ran out of pills and stopped taking them; also has taken a special pill for her rheumatoid arthritis, but quit it because she felt better; and a multivitamin, l tablet daily

Allergies Sulfa causes rash

Pertinent Physical Findings

Vital Signs Height 5 feet 3 inches; weight 121 pounds; temperature 97.7° F; heart rate 72, regular; respiratory rate 16; blood pressure 135/76 sitting, right arm

General Appearance Appears stated age; appears pale and fatigued, but not in acute distress; reliable historian

Skin Seborrheic keratoses are evident on anterior and posterior chest; skin tones are pale

HEENT Unremarkable other than mild pallor in conjunctival membranes; no icterus is seen; oropharynx is clear; neck is supple without thyromegaly or obvious adenopathy; no jugular vein distention (JVD) is present.

Lungs Clear with symmetrical expansion and good exchange of air; no adventitious sounds are apparent

Heart Regular, with distinct S_1 and S_2; a II/VI murmur, loudest at the LSB, is present; no radiation is appreciated

Abdomen rounded, but soft and non-distended; no organomegaly; bowel sounds are readily audible

Extremities Interosseus wasting with a swan neck deformity of both hands is apparent. Grasp is impaired bilaterally with grip strength at 3/5. Gross sensation and spontaneous movement are symmetrical. Crepitus is apparent in both knees, greater on the right. Range of motion is reduced; motion provokes discomfort and reports of stiffness. No cyanosis, clubbing, or edema is present. Rectal: tone is normal, with negative guaiac

Neurological Unremarkable; reflexes are symmetrical. No focal deficits are apparent

Diagnostics

Diagnostic Tests Diagnostic tests revealed low serum iron, low TIBC with normal serum ferritin and reticulocyte count. Second and third guaiacs were negative

History Data Questions specific to the chief complaint of weakness and fatigue include the following:

- When did you first notice your weakness and fatigue? How have your symptoms changed your lifestyle?
- Have you noticed a rapid heart rate or shortness or breath? Are your symptoms worse with exertion?
- Do you have a history of other significant medical illness, low blood counts, or times when you noted excessive bleeding?
- What medications and therapies are you taking? What about past medications?
- Does anyone in your family have symptoms similar to yours?
- What is a typical diet for you?
- Do you think that you have been exposed to anything that might be harmful, such as chemicals or toxic materials?

The patient should be asked specifically about treatment, past and present, with medications known to be myelosuppressive, such as methotrexate.

Physical Examination Data The focused examination for the chief complaint of fatigue and weakness is dictated by careful attention to history, onset and associated symptoms. Fatigue and weakness occur commonly and may represent an array of illnesses. Therefore, persistent fatigue requires a complete physical examination with attention to all body systems.

Differential Diagnosis Anemia of chronic disease, iron deficiency anemia, occult blood loss, and multifactorial anemia (See Table 9-1 for additional details.)

Probable Causes of the Presenting Symptoms R.T. has a clinical picture consistent with the anemia of chronic disease (ACD). A chronic inflammatory disease, such as rheumatoid arthritis, is the likely cause. Other chronic diseases associated with ACD include cancer and inflammatory disorders. ACD should be considered in patients with known chronic illness who present with anemia.

Iron deficiency anemia or folic acid deficiency can present along with ACD and confuse the clinical picture. Suspicion for multiple causes should be considered when the anemia is pronounced. Occult malignancy, chronic infection, and inadequate nutrition must be considered when anemia persists. Patients with ACD have adequate iron stores but have impaired iron utilization by the bone marrow. Sequestration of iron within the reticuloendothelial system blocks iron availability and makes inadequate iron available for red cell production in spite of adequate stores.

Diagnostic Tests Initial tests ordered for R.T. include CBC with differential, TIBC, ferritin, reticulocyte counts, and stools for guaiac. Serial CBCs should be followed for progress. A pathologist should evaluate the peripheral smear. If anemia persists, a B_{12} and folate level, and a repeat reticulocyte counts should be requested. LDH and haptoglobin would be helpful to determine if hemolysis is present. A complete metabolic profile and thyroid function tests should also be considered for persistent anemia. Renal and liver function should be assessed.

Diagnostic Impression In light of known chronic illness and lack of other significant laboratory findings, the most likely cause of this mild anemia is ACD. The anemia of chronic disease is characterized by modest declines in hemoglobin to 8 to 10 g/dl. Hemoglobin levels less than 7 g/dl are unusual and require further investigation. An impaired response to erythropoietin is also seen in ACD, although purified recombinant erythropoietin (epoetin alfa) has been shown to be effective in managing some anemias associated with inflammatory chronic disease. Of note, the anemia seen with chronic renal failure results from a different mechanism and is, in general, more pronounced.

Therapeutic Plan of Care The ACD may require no treatment if it is relatively asymptomatic. The anemia associated with inflammatory disease may best respond to treatment of the underlying disease. Iron supplements are not effective for this disorder. Persistent and symptomatic anemia may require red blood cell transfusion. Erythropoietin 10,000 units subcutaneously may be tried three times a week for 6 to 12 weeks and then reevaluated; however, therapy is extremely expensive. Lifestyle modifications to minimize fatigue and promote optimal health should be reviewed.

Patient Education and/or Community Resources R.T. should be scheduled for a complete physical examination soon, and the chronicity of her disease should be discussed. Treatment goals should be mutually determined. She should be strongly encouraged to continue her nonsteroidal antiinflammatory agents (NSAIDs) and, depending on her response, be informed that other agents may be needed to control her symptoms. An H_2 blocker may be added. COX-2 agents should be considered if NSAIDs cause distress and/or to fail to control symptoms. The basics of healthy eating should be reviewed. Conversations regarding alternative therapies should be encouraged and attempts to work within her belief system should be a part of her plan of care.

Follow-Up Plan R.T. will be scheduled for follow-up and complete physical examination within 1 month. An appointment will be arranged sooner if her laboratory work-up proves abnormal. Otherwise, a telephone appointment to review diagnostics and progress at home will be scheduled in 2 weeks. At that time, laboratory findings will be shared and questions that may have surfaced since her intitial evaluation will be answered.

Case Study 3

CHIEF COMPLAINT: Profound Fatigue, Swollen Glands

History of Present Illness J.P. is a 41-year-old Hispanic male who calls the office requesting an urgent office visit for profound fatigue and swollen glands. He says that his fatigue has progressed to the point that he is unable to keep up his work schedule at a local discount store and requests a written work release to keep from losing his job. In spite of attempts to get extra rest, J.P. reports that he awakes tired and has been unable to fully recover from an upper respiratory infection which began more than 6 weeks ago. He reports recurrent fevers to 101° F and a recent weight loss of 10 pounds, as well as a decline in his usually hearty appetite.

Past Medical History   Unremarkable

Past Surgical History   Surgery on his R knee at age 16

Family History   Mother, DM; father, HTN; sister age 40, DM; sister age 38, A&W; brother age 44, A&W

Developmental Stage   Generativity versus Stagnation

Role-Relationship   Married for 9 years. Has a 7-year-old son. Junior college graduate in business. Works as a bookkeeper for a local discount store.

Sleep/Rest   For the past couple of months J.P. has been sleeping from 9 PM until 8 AM and napping when he has a chance

Nutrition/Metabolic   For the past few months he has not felt like eating much. He picks at his food and may eat a partial bowl of oatmeal in the morning, a sandwich for lunch, and a small dinner consisting of beans, rice, and chicken with fresh vegetables.

Activity/Exercise   Unable to engage in a daily exercise program secondary to progressive and prolonged fatigue.

Coping/Stress   J.P. feels he is under a great deal of stress with his job on the line and his poor health. He doesn't feel well at all and is constantly fatigued and tired. His wife and both of their families have been available to help them. His family attends a local Roman Catholic church weekly.

Health Management   Smoking history: nonsmoker at present, smoked 1 year <5 cigarettes/day as a teen; alcohol: drinks an occasional beer. Does not use recreational drugs

Self-Perception and Values/Beliefs   J.P. has a positive view of the world and enjoys his family. His extended family provides great support and comfort.

Medications   Multivitamin, daily

Allergies   PCN (has difficulty breathing)

Pertinent Physical Findings

Vital Signs   Height 5 feet 11 inches; weight 170 pounds; temperature 100.4° F; heart rate 112; respiratory rate 20; blood pressure 110/58 on right arm while lying recumbent

General Appearance   Ill-appearing, Hispanic male with pale skin tones; appears fatigued with prominent circles under eyes

HEENT   Normocephalic, with symmetrical features; PERRLA with EOMI; pale conjunctival membranes; pale oral mucosa with petechia evident in posterior pharynx; nose, ears are unremarkable; neck with bilateral, bulky adenopathy greater in right anterior cervical chain

Lungs   Diminished in both bases with occasional crackle right base; no wheezes, no rhonchi

Heart   Regular, tones are distinct. II-III/VI murmur, non-radiating, at LSB

Abdomen   Soft, non-distended; spleen tip is palpable LUQ; liver edge is palpable with mild tenderness RUQ; no guarding or rebound; bowel sounds are normoactive

Extremities   several ecchymotic areas are present on forearms, LLE; pale palmar creases; nail beds are pale; no clubbing or spooning of nails

Diagnostics

Diagnostic Tests   Office CBC reveals white blood cell count of 62,000, hemoglobin of 7.2 gm/dl, hematocrit of 22 %, and platelet of 21,000 u/dl; 30% blasts are apparent on the peripheral smear

History Data   Questions specific to the chief complaint of profound weakness and fatigue include the following:

- When did you first notice your symptoms? How have your symptoms changed your daily routines?
- Tell me about your health, in general. Have you had significant medical ilnessess or ever required on-going care by a medical professional?
- Have you had recent infections, fever, weight loss, sweating, swollen glands, breathlessness with exertion, or unexplained bruising?

Physical Examination Data   The comprehensive history and physical examination for vague physical complaints includes a complete blood workup with CBC, peripheral smear, electrolytes, complete metabolic profile, and urinalysis.

Differential Diagnosis   The most probable differential diagnoses are leukemias, myeloproliferative disorders, and aplastic anemia. The leukemias and myeloproliferative disorders can be complex and life threatening; when suspected, they should be evaluated and managed by a skilled hematologist (Table 9-4). Other diagnostic considerations should include marrow failure secondary to nonhematopoietic tumor. When lymphadenopathy or splenomegaly dominate, infectious disease, autoimmune disease, HIV, and other malignancies should be considered.

Probable Causes of the Presenting Symptoms
The clinical presentation and diagnostic testing is suggestive of a leukemia or myeloproliferative disorder. Urgent referral to a hematologist for diagnosis and treatment is indicated.

Diagnostic Tests   Initial diagnostic tests for J.B. should include CBC with differential. Further testing is best left to the discretion of a hematologist. A bone marrow biopsy with core biopsy will assist in the diagnosis. Additional studies on the marrow specimen, such as histochemical, cytochemical, and immunologic staining and phenotyping; flow cytometry; karyotypic analysis; and analysis of cerebrospinal fluid may also be re-

quested. Other diagnostics may include: complete metabolic panel; liver function profile; renal function profile; coagulation studies (prothrombin time, partial thromboplastin time, DIC panel); and blood cultures.

Diagnostic Impression   J.P.'s symptoms are troubling. His symptoms reflect an acute disruption in normal hematopoiesis, likely an acute leukemia. The white blood cell differential examination shows an abnormal ratio of blasts, or immature cells. An abnormal crowding of leukemic cells in the bone marrow has likely caused the low hemoglobin, low platelets, and high (but dysfunctional) white blood cell counts. Urgent referral for diagnosis and treatment is essential. Subsequent evaluation by a hematologist will define the nature of his disease and appropriate treatment. While this patient appears to have an acute leukemia, the leukemias represent an array of disorders that are characterized by an abnormal proliferation and differentiation in one of the cell lines of the marrow. Leukemia can originate from myeloid or lymphoid cell lines; it can present as acute or chronic. Common presentation of symptoms can be found in Figure 9-1.

Depending on the type of leukemia and the degree of leukemic burden, common symptoms in-

Table 9-4
Characteristics of Common Leukemias

Type of Leukemia	Acute Myeloid (AML)	Acute Lymphoid (ALL)	Chronic Myeloid (CML)	Chronic Lymphoid (CLL)
Presentation	Adults 82% Children 10%	Children 85% Adults 15%	Adults >50	Adults 25-45
CBC				
• Leukocytes	Myeloblasts, elevated	Lymphoblasts, elevated	Elevated, mature myeloid cells; may have decreased leukocytes	Elevated lymphocytes
• Hemoglobin	Decreased	Decreased	Decreased	Decreased
• Platelets	Decreased	Decreased	Decreased	Decreased
Other	Auer rods		Philadelphia chromosome	
Treatment	URGENT referral	URGENT referral	Referral; goal WBC <20,000	Referral; treat according to stage

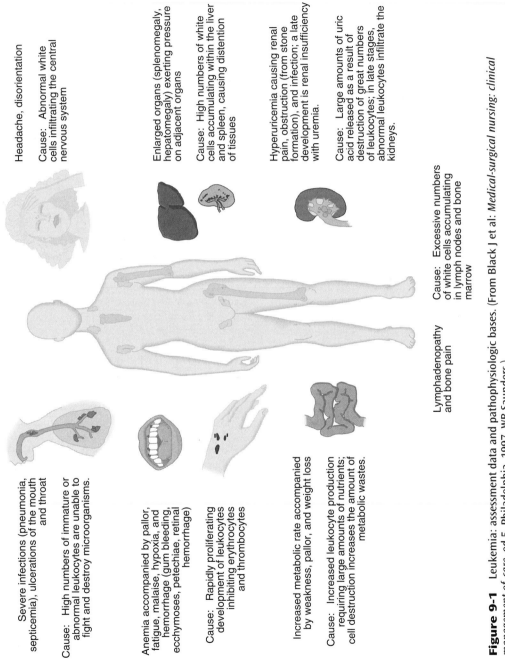

Headache, disorientation

Cause: Abnormal white cells infiltrating the central nervous system

Enlarged organs (splenomegaly, hepatomegaly) exerting pressure on adjacent organs

Cause: High numbers of white cells accumulating within the liver and spleen, causing distention of tissues

Hyperuricemia causing renal pain, obstruction (from stone formation), and infection; a late development is renal insufficiency with uremia.

Cause: Large amounts of uric acid released as a result of destruction of great numbers of leukocytes; in late stages, abnormal leukocytes infiltrate the kidneys.

Lymphadenopathy and bone pain

Cause: Excessive numbers of white cells accumulating in lymph nodes and bone marrow

Severe infections (pneumonia, septicemia), ulcerations of the mouth and throat

Cause: High numbers of immature or abnormal leukocytes are unable to fight and destroy microorganisms.

Anemia accompanied by pallor, fatigue, malaise, hypoxia, and hemorrhage (gum bleeding, ecchymoses, petechiae, retinal hemorrhage)

Cause: Rapidly proliferating development of leukocytes inhibiting erythrocytes and thrombocytes

Increased metabolic rate accompanied by weakness, pallor, and weight loss

Cause: Increased leukocyte production requiring large amounts of nutrients; cell destruction increases the amount of metabolic wastes.

Figure 9-1   Leukemia: assessment data and pathophysiologic bases. (From Black J et al: *Medical-surgical nursing: clinical management of care*, ed 5, Philadelphia, 1997, WB Saunders.)

clude: fatigue, abnormal bleeding, infection, weight loss, adenopathy, weakness, bone pain, headache, nausea and vomiting, and central nervous system changes, such as confusion.

Therapeutic Plan of Care J.P. requires an immediate hematology referral for appropriate diagnosis and management of his care. He and his family need a thorough explanation of the likely reasons for his symptoms and the rationale for urgent care. Ideally, a telephone referral and evaluation can be arranged while J.P. waits in the office. Following referral, careful follow-up with J.P. is essential for continuity of care. If leukemia is confirmed, hospital admission for induction for systemic chemotherapy will be required. While the primary care provider is an essential part of the team, the rigors of systemic induction therapy for leukemia require the expertise and vigil of a hematologist and comprehensive health team.

Patient Education and/or Community Resources The treatment of leukemia requires a coordinated team effort, and it is essential that J.P. feel that he is a part of the team. Knowledge of the disease, required treatment, and stategies to promote adaptation to the diagnosis of leukemia are essential. A coordinated multidisciplinary team effort with ongoing education, dictated by the readiness of J.P. and his family, is ideal. The Leukemia Society of America has excellent written resources and websites. Community support is often linked during hospitalization. Local American Cancer Society support groups are also available during treatment.

Follow-Up The multidisciplinary team should continue to follow J.P. after discharge. Home care referrals should be a part of planned follow-up. Multiple chemotherapy treatments and hospital admissions will be required to achieve remission. For certain leukemias, bone marrow transplant may be the treatment of choice. Contact and continuity from the multidisciplinary team (including primary care provider, hematologist, nurses, dietitian, social worker, clergy, clinical pharmacist, physical therapist, home health care worker, and others) will provide safe and supportive care during treatment.

Case Study 4 Optional Exercise
Chief Complaint: Abdominal Pain and Fever

History of Present Illness J.W. is a 20-year-old African-American male with known sickle cell disease, diagnosed in infancy. He awoke this morning with a fever of 102.5° F with pain in his left side and abdomen. His cough, previously unproductive, has worsened and is now productive of yellow to tan mucus in modest amounts. He notes mild shortness of breath when compared to the previous day. He is concerned that his recent upper respiratory infection is progressing and fears that his infection has triggered a sickle cell crisis. He describes a history of more than 20 hospital admissions for sickle cell crisis, most during his childhood.

Past Medical History Sickle cell disease
Past Surgical History None
Family History His biological sister has sickle cell trait, the genotype of his half sister is unknown; mother and father with sickle cell trait
Developmental Stage Intimacy versus Isolation
Role-Relationship J.W. resides at home with his mother and two younger sisters. Both girls have been home from school with sore throats and fevers. J.W. attends junior college, part time. He works at a local fast food restaurant.
Sleep/Rest Usually feels rested when he awakes, unless he is hospitalized and disturbed by the noise. Sleeps 6 to 8 hours per night, denies naps, use of sleeping medication, or nightmares
Nutrition/Metabolic Eats cereal for breakfast, fast food for lunch and whatever anyone cooks for dinner. Eats lots of snack foods and enjoys ice cream
Coping/Stress J.W. describes his chronic illness as the major stressor in his life. Feels he is now over "being mad" and is in control of his health. Copes by "shooting hoops" or sharing with his best friend. Has recently returned to church and sings in the choir. He is concerned that he had to slow down in school with all the hospitalizations and is behind in his schoolwork.
Health Management He reports only occasional alcohol intake and does not smoke
Self-Perception and Values/Beliefs Describes himself as a "good man." At times he feels betrayed

by his body and frustrated with his illness. Denies depression, sadness, but admits to hopelessness at times when he has a flare of his illness

Medications Folic acid and multivitamin

Allergies None

Pertinent Physical Findings

Vital Signs Height 5 feet 9 inches; weight 156 pounds; temperature 102.3° F; heart rate 104; respirations 24; blood pressure 136/80

General Appearance Appears younger than stated age; seems uncomfortable but not in acute distress

HEENT Normocephalic. Eyes, PEERLA with intact EOM, sclera are clear. Ears, TMs are pearly gray with cerumen evident in canals, bilaterally. Neck is supple, with several nodes >1 cm present in the left anterior, cervical chain. Nose, both nares are patent, no discharge is apparent. Oropharynx, membranes are clear and moist; the posterior pharynx shows mild erythema, no exudates

Cardiothoracic Respiratory excursion is normal; however, crackles are apparent in the left posterior field extending to mid-thorax; a deep inspiration provokes discomfort on left. Increased fremitus is appreciated in the left base. Heart is regular and tachycardic at 102, but tones are distinct. A systolic murmur grade III/VI is present and loudest at the base; no radiation is evident

Abdomen Appears slightly distended with diffuse tenderness; some guarding with palpation, no rebound. Bowel sounds are present in all quadrants. No masses are present; spleen is palpable

Extremities Gross sensation and motor strength are symmetrical; joint tenderness is present at the right elbow and left knee upon palpation; further ROM deferred due to discomfort. Chronic joint changes are apparent.

Neurological Fully alert and appropriate; cranial nerves II-XII are intact; DTR are WNL; no areas of focal weakness are noted.

Diagnostics

Diagnostic Tests CBC reveals hemoglobin of 7.0 g/dl with hematocrit of 21; WBC is 14,000; platelets are WNL. Office CXR shows moderate cardiomegaly and infiltrates in the left lung base. Urinalysis shows no WBCs, nitrates, or leukocyte esterase; specific gravity is low at 1.004. Oxygen saturation on room air is 90%.

Discussion Questions

What type of history data should be collected?

What type of physical data should be collected?

What are the differential diagnoses?

What are the probable causes of the presenting symptoms?

What is your diagnostic impression?

What is the therapeutic plan of care?

What are the patient education and/or community resources?

What is your follow-up plan?

Discussions for optional case study exercises can be found in the accompanying Instructor's Manual.

References

Rakel R: *Saunders manual of medical practice,* Philadelphia, 1996, WB Saunders.

Tierney L, McPhee S, Papadakis M: *Current medical diagnosis and treatment,* ed 38, Stamford, Conn., 1999, Appleton & Lange.

Selected Readings

Dailey J: *Dailey's notes on blood,* ed 3, Arlington, Mass., 1996, Medical Consulting Group.

Ferri F: *Practical guide to care of the medical patient,* ed 4, St Louis, 1998, Mosby.

Mascara M, Czar P, Hebda T: *Internet resource guide for nurses and health care professionals,* Menlo Park, CA, 1999, Addison Wesley.

U.S. Department of Health and Human Services: *Clinical practice guideline # 6: sickle cell disease: screening, diagnosis, management, and counseling in newborns and infants* (AHCPR Publication No. 93-0562), Rockville, Md., 1993, Author.

Speicher C: *The right test,* ed 3, Philadelphia, 1998, WB Saunders

Wood M, Bunn P: *Hematology/oncology secrets,* St Louis, 1994, Mosby.

CHAPTER 10

Urogenital Disorders

Jean Nagelkerk

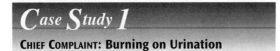

Case Study 1

CHIEF COMPLAINT: Burning on Urination

History of Present Illness T.N. is a 27-year-old Caucasian female who presents with chief complaint of burning on urination. She has had frequent urination with urgency for 2 days duration. T.N. does not experience burning on her labia with urination. She has a mild ache in the right side of her back and feels miserable. She has not taken her temperature but says she feels warm at times. She denies N/V, chills, diarrhea, constipation, and increased vaginal discharge. T.N. is in a monogamous relationship with her husband. She has just returned from her honeymoon. She consistently uses a diaphragm for contraception. Her menses are regular every 28 days and last 5 days. LMP: 1/1/99 (1 week ago). T.N. has a negative STD history.

Past Medical History Reports one UTI 2 years ago and used an antibiotic with resolution

Past Surgical History LEEP procedure 7 years ago for abnormal PAP smear (Papanicolaou test)

Family History Mother, age 60, HTN, hysterectomy age 41 for heavy bleeding; father, age 65, DM; brother, age 30, A&W; sister, age 32, DM

Developmental Stage Intimacy versus Isolation

Role-Relationship T.N. has just returned from her honeymoon and lives with her new husband who is an auto mechanic. They reside in a one-story, two-bedroom home with her 3-year-old daughter. T.N.'s husband enjoys her daughter and takes time to play with her each day. Her daughter's biological father does not visit or play an active role in her care.

Sleep/Rest Falls to sleep at 11 PM and awakens rested at 6 AM. Occasionally will take an OTC sleeping pill in order to get to sleep if she is stressed at her job (about once per month).

Nutrition/Metabolic Breakfast, a diet breakfast bar; lunch, fast food at a local shop; dinner, tries to prepare a well-balanced meal for the family with fruits, vegetables, meat, and pasta. N.T. admits to snacking heavily on "junk foods" and enjoys sweets, chips, and candy.

Activity/Exercise Leisure activities include reading and playing with her daughter. Denies routine exercise

Coping/Stress Feels she has an adequate support system. Discusses problems with her mother and/or husband. Does not attend church. Does not feel that work is too stressful.

Health Management Last Td was when she was in grade school. Last Pap smear was 5 years ago. Alcohol, has one or two mixed drinks at parties or restaurants (about once a week). Denies recreational drug use

Self-Perception and Values/Beliefs Feels satisfied with her life. Enjoys her daughter and is pleased to be married to her new husband

Medications None

Allergies Quinolones produce a rash

Pertinent Physical Findings

Vital Signs Height 5 feet 9 inches; weight 182 pounds; BMI 27; temperature 99.8° F without antipyretic; heart rate 76; respirations 16; blood pressure 130/82

Heart Apical pulse 76, rate regular, no murmurs, S_3, or S_4

Lungs Clear to auscultation

Abdomen Abdomen soft and nontender; + bowel sounds; no splenomegaly or hepatomegaly; slight superpubic tenderness; mild + CVA tenderness with percussion

Genital External genitalia with no lesions, discharge or rashes; no CMT or adnexal masses; vaginal mucosa pink and moist; cervix pink, parous os, no lesions; scant amount of clear discharge in vaginal vault

Diagnostics

Diagnostic Tests Urine dip + for leukocytes and nitrites; microscopically there is >5 leukocytes per high power field (40×); wet mount negative; urine C&S and Pap smear collected

History Data Questions specific to the chief complaint of burning on urination include the following:

- When did you begin to feel burning on urination?
- Do you have nausea and vomiting, abdominal pain, back pain, fever, chills, or diarrhea?
- Do you have vaginal or urethral discharge?
- Do you have blood in your urine, constipation, or diarrhea?
- Do you feel burning with urination or burning when urine passes over the labia (may indicate herpes simplex infection)?
- Do you have a history of diabetes, kidney stones, sexually transmitted diseases, immunosuppression, or (if a male) prostatic hyperplasia?
- What type of contraception do you use? Do you use it 100% of the time?
- When was your last normal menstrual period?
- Any history of UTIs or kidney infections?
- What treatments did you receive for your UTI and were they effective?

Physical Examination Data The focused examination for the chief complaint of burning on urination includes: vital signs, heart, lung, abdomen, and genitalia (pelvic examination for a female and a prostate examination for a male)

Differential Diagnosis Urinary tract infection, acute pyelonephritis, vulvovaginitis, pelvic in-

flammatory disease, prostatitis (in males), bladder cancer, acute cervicitis, urethritis (gonococcal and nongonococcal, in males) (Table 10-1)

Probable Causes of the Presenting Symptoms
The symptoms of frequent urination and urgency are caused by uropathogens that have ascended from the rectum to the vagina with colonization in the introitus and distal urethra (Kelley, 1997). Urinary tract infections are either acute or chronic. Acute infections usually are associated with a single microorganism, with coliform bacteria responsible for most of the infections. Chronic infections generally have two or more bacteria responsible for the infection. A urinary tract infection (UTI) can be categorized as either lower or upper. Lower UTIs involve the mucosa, such as in the case of a simple cystitis. Upper UTIs involve the soft tissue, such as in the case of pyelonephritis or prostatitis. Infections of the lower urinary tract are characterized by no or low grade fever, urgency, and burning. Infections of the upper urinary tract are characterized by fever of >101° F, chills, flank pain, and dysuria.

Diagnostic Tests Urine dip (to screen for infection), urine C&S (to isolate causative organism), wet mount (to rule out vulvovaginal *Candida, Trichomonas vaginalis,* or bacterial vaginitis), Pap smear (has not had one in 5 years and has a history of LEEP procedure and abnormal Pap), and cervical cultures or swabs for gonorrhea and chlamydia. Diabetic screening is important given T.N.'s strong family history (both her father and sister have diabetes).

Diagnostic Impression T.N.'s complaints of frequent urination with urgency and mild CVA tenderness with percussion are probably caused by a lower UTI. Due to the mild CVA tenderness, a longer course of antibiotic therapy would be recommended.

Therapeutic Plan of Care A 10-day course of trimethoprim-sulfamethoxazole (Bactrim) DS bid is an appropriate treatment. T.N. should increase fluids to a minimum of 2 liters per day and protect herself from the sun while on the medication. T.N. should also receive a Td at this visit to update her immunizations. She should be scheduled for a re-

Table 10-1
Burning Upon Urination Differential Diagnostic Cues

Diagnoses	Signs and Symptoms	Lab Data	Treatment
Urinary Tract Infection Risk Factors • History of recent UTI • Pregnancy • Failure to void after intercourse • Use of diaphragms • Increased sexual activity (women) • Immunosuppression • Lack of circumcision in men • Homosexuality (men) Criteria for symptomatic UTI is 10^2 pathogens per ml; traditionally, 10^5 pathogens per ml has been used	Dysuria, urinary urgency, frequency, suprapubic discomfort, may have hematuria	Urine dip + for leukocytes and nitrites. Microscopic examination of urine sediment >5 leukocytes by high power. Urine C&S if a recurrent infection, child, or male. Imaging only if recurrent infections, child, male, pyelonephritis, or suspect anatomical abnormality Most common organisms are gram-negative bacilli, with *E. coli* the most common. Others include *Klebsiella pneumoniae* and *Proteus mirabilis* In young, sexually active females, the second most common cause of UTI is *Staphylococcus saprophyticus*. In elderly and those who have had instrumentation, *Enterococcus faecalis* (gram +) is probable	Uncomplicated UTI: May initiate single dose or 3-day therapy. Trimethoprim-sulfamethoxazole (Bactrim DS) 160/800 mg bid × 3 days **OR** trimethoprim (Trimpex) 100 mg bid **OR** nitrofurantoin (Macrodantin) 100 mg qid **OR** ciprofloxacin (Cipro) 250-500 mg bid × 3 days. Recurrent UTIs, give medicine for 7-10 days. If >3 UTIs in 1 year, use prophylaxis: either single dose med after intercourse **OR** prophylactic antibiotic qd or three times a week (e.g., trimethoprim-sulfamethoxazole 40/200 mg ½ tablet regular strength at HS). Warm sitz baths prn. Increase fluids to 8-10 glasses qd, drink cranberry juice. May use a urinary analgesic if needed (e.g., phenazopyridine [Pyridium] 200 mg tid prn with meals) and if on antibiotic 2 days only (may stain underwear and soft contact lenses)
Acute Pyelonephritis	Chills, fever (>101° F), N/V, diarrhea, flank pain, urinary urgency, frequency, dysuria, tachycardia, +CVA tenderness	Urine dip + for leukocytes and nitrites. Microscopic examination of urine sediment >5 leukocytes by high power. Urine C&S. May order abdominal radiograph to check for obstruction, anatomical abnormalities of urinary tract, or calculi. Renal ultrasound to evaluate kidneys. In children a voiding cystourethrogram is commonly done after first UTI to evaluate for structural abnormalities: done after treatment	May hospitalize children and men, especially if vomiting or if they have a toxic appearance, because they tend to have a higher likelihood of structural abnormality. Hospitalize women for severe infections for IV antibiotic and further diagnostic test (e.g., CBC, blood cultures if indicated). Consult with physician for outpatient treatment and give trimethoprim-sulfamethoxazole (Septra) DS tablet bid × 14 days **OR** ciprofloxacin (Cipro) 250-500 mg bid × 14 days. Recheck in 24 hours; if no improvement, hospitalize and do imaging studies. Take follow-up cultures at 2 weeks and 3 months
Vulvovaginitis The most common causes of urinary symptoms are*: • Trichomonas vaginalis	Malodorous, frothy yellow-green discharge; pruritus, vaginal erythema, and possibly red macular lesions on cervix	Wet mount with saline: pH >4.5 and motile organisms with flagella; endocervical cultures	Metronidazole (Flagyl) 2-g single dose **OR** 500 mg bid × 7 days. No alcohol while on medicine. Treat partners

Note: For a detailed discussion of sexually transmitted disease treatment plans, see Centers for Disease Control and Prevention: Guidelines for treatment of sexually transmitted disease, *MMWR Morb Mortal Wkly Rep* 47 (No. RR-1), 1998.
*Dysuria may be due to urethritis or inflammation of external tissues (splash phenomenon).

Continued

Table 10-1
Burning Upon Urination Differential Diagnostic Cues—cont'd

Diagnoses	Signs and Symptoms	Lab Data	Treatment
Vulvovaginitis—cont'd			
• Candida vaginitis	Dyspareunia, burning vaginal discharge, vulvar pruritus	Wet mount with 10% KOH; filaments and spores present	Topical (e.g., clotrimazole [Gyne-Lotrimin] 100 mg vaginal suppository × 7 days) **OR** fluconazole (Diflucan) 150 mg PO × 1 dose
• Bacterial vaginosis	Increased amounts of grayish, frothy vaginal discharge; often the vaginal discharge is malodorous (fishy); pH is 5.0-5.5	Wet mount with 10% KOH; whiff test + for fishy odor; clue cells present	Metronidazole 500 mg bid × 7 days **OR** metronidazole gel (0.75%, 5 grams) bid × 5 days **OR** metronidazole 2 grams PO × 1; **OR** clindamycin 300 mg PO bid × 7 days
Pelvic Inflammatory Disease	Mild to severe lower abdominal pain, dysuria, menstrual irregularities, purulent cervical discharge, chills, fever, cervical and adnexal tenderness Diagnostic criteria: lower abdominal pain, adnexal pain, or CMT Additional criteria: Temp >100.9° F; abnormal vaginal or cervical discharge, elevated sed rate, elevated C-reactive protein; +GC or *C. trachomatis*	Endocervical culture, but treat empirically	Determine need for hospitalization and IV antibiotics. Outpatient treatment: ofloxacin (Floxin) 400 mg bid and metronidazole (Flagyl) 500 mg bid × 14 days **OR** cefoxitin (Mefoxin) 2g IM and probenecid 1 g PO **OR** ceftriaxone (Rocephin) 250 mg IM plus doxycycline 100 mg bid × 14 days. Treat partners
Prostatitis			
Acute	Irritative voiding symptoms, fever, suprapubic pain, very tender on rectal examination, + urine culture. Prostate is often tender, boggy, and may be swollen†	CBC, urine dip, urine culture. Acute prostatitis is usually caused by gram-negative rods (e.g., *E. coli* and *Pseudomonas* species)	For severe cases, hospitalization may be required. Outpatient treatment: data indicate that using a fluoroquinolone such as norfloxacin, ciprofloxacin, ofloxacin cover uropathogenic bacteria and *Chlamydia* and *Mycoplasma* species. Some practitioners prefer trimethoprim-sulfamethoxazole (Bactrim) DS bid × 4-6 weeks. If urinary retention, do not catheterize: needs a percutaneous suprapubic tube
Chronic‡	Irritative voiding symptoms, dull, poorly defined suprapubic	Segmented culture of urine and expressed prostatic secretions (EPS). Bacteria in	Trimethoprim-sulfamethoxazole (Bactrim) DS bid × 6-12 weeks. Bactrim is the drug of choice because

Note: For a detailed discussion of sexually transmitted disease treatment plans, see Centers for Disease Control and Prevention: Guidelines for treatment of sexually transmitted disease, *MMWR Morb Mortal Wkly Rep* 47 (No. RR-1), 1998.
†Do not vigorously massage prostate; this may result in bacteremia.
‡Gram-negative rods common, but also may be a gram-positive organism.

Table 10-1			
Burning Upon Urination Differential Diagnostic Cues—cont'd			
Diagnoses	**Signs and Symptoms**	**Lab Data**	**Treatment**
Chronic‡—cont'd	discomfort, + expressed prostatic secretions.	first and midstream specimen suggests cystitis; 10 × bacteria in EPS and voiding post-prostatic bacterial prostatitis; EPS and VPPM with WBC, but no bacteria suggests nonbacterial prostatitis. Other tests as indicated (e.g., BUN/creatinine [renal function], pelvic radiographs, or transrectal ultrasound [prostatic calculi])	it diffuses into the prostate. Other medications include cephalexin, a quinolone, or erythromycin
Bladder Cancer Risk factors include smoking and occupational exposures to industrial dyes or solvents (e.g., painters)	Gross or microscopic hematuria is the major symptom. May have urinary frequency and urgency	Urine dip; urinalysis; urine for cytology; cystoscopic examination. Imaging may be used in select cases (e.g., intravenous urography, ultrasound, CT or MRI – all show filling defects). Staging may entail a CXR, abdominal and pelvic CT, or radionuclide bone scan	Transurethral resection is typically the treatment of choice. Intravesical chemotherapy, radiotherapy and chemotherapy are additional treatment options.
Acute Cervicitis§ *Chlamydia trachomatis*	Asymptomatic or watery urethral or cervical discharge, slight discomfort, dysuria	Direct immunofluorescence assay, enzyme linked immunoassay **OR** DNA probe of cervical sample	Tetracycline or erythromycin 500 mg qid or doxycycline l00 mg bid × 7 days **OR** azithromycin 1 g dose × 1.
Gonorrhea	Purulent, profuse urethral/cervical discharge, dysuria, fever, rash	Cultures of affected orifices. Offer HIV testing and syphilis testing.	Treat empirically: ceftriaxone (Rocephin) 125 mg IM, cefixime (Suprax) 400 mg **OR** ciprofloxacin (Cipro) 500 mg. Spectinomycin 1 g IM × 1 if allergic to PCN
Urethritis‖ Gonococcal (caused by *Neisseria gonorrhea*)	Purulent urethral discharge, dysuria	Culture	Ceftriaxone (Rocephin) 250 mg IM × 1 **OR** ofloxacin (Floxin) 400 mg × 1 **OR** ciprofloxacin (Cipro) 500 mg × 1.
Nongonococcal (most common cause is *Chlamydia trachomatis*)¶	Urethral discharge is watery, some dysuria	Direct immunofluorescence assay, enzyme-linked immunoassay **OR** DNA probe.	Doxycycline 100 mg bid × 10 days **OR** ofloxacin (Floxin) 300 mg bid × 10 days **OR** azithromycin (Zithromax) 1 gram × 1 dose

‡Gram-negative rods common, but also may be a gram-positive organism.
§When managing acute cervicitis treat for both gonorrhea and *Chlamydia trachomatis*.
‖Urethral discharge in male patients.
¶Ureaplasma urealyticum second common. Trichomonas vaginalis and herpes simplex virus are less common causes.

turn visit to evaluate the condition of her diaphragm.

Patient Education and/or Community Resources Patient education for T.N. should include a review of the physiological relationship of UTIs to sexual activity. After urinating, she should wipe front to back to avoid introducing pathogens from the rectal area into the urethra. She should be instructed to remove her diaphragm 6 to 8 hours after sexual intercourse. Discuss with her the importance of voiding after intercourse to decrease the risk for a subsequent UTI. Should T.N. have repeated UTIs with a diaphragm, she may need to consider another method of birth control. Encourage T.N. to increase her fluid intake to 8 to 10 glasses of water per day and to drink cranberry juice. Instruct the patient to avoid a full bladder and to completely empty during voiding.

Follow-Up Plan T.N. should have a return visit to recheck her urine and evaluate the proper fitting and condition of her diaphragm. She should be encouraged to schedule an annual physical examination given her history of an abnormal Pap smear.

For those who present with uncomplicated UTI, follow-up is indicated for return symptoms or if the patient does not improve. At this time you would follow-up with urinalysis and, if indicated, urine culture.

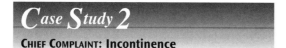

Case Study 2

CHIEF COMPLAINT: Incontinence

History of Present Illness S.R. is a 65-year-old Caucasian female who presents with chief complaint of incontinence. She describes her incontinence as losing small amounts of urine each time she coughs, sneezes, or laughs. S.R. states that she feels so uncomfortable about losing urine that she often wears a mini pad to protect her clothing. S.R. can wait approximately 5 to 10 minutes after she experiences the urge to void. Once she initiates her urine stream she cannot stop until she has voided completely. She admits to frequency when she drinks large amounts of fluids. Denies dysuria, hes-

itancy, hematuria, or dribbling. S.R. has constipation about one time per week. She uses prunes with some success. She is sexually active with her husband and experiences some dryness. She uses tap water occasionally as a lubricant during sexual intercourse. LMP: Age 51. Gravida: 5; Para: 5; All vaginal births; episiotomies performed during the first three deliveries. No other trauma to the perineal area.

Past Medical History HTN

Past Surgical History Cholecystectomy at age 25

Family History Mother deceased at age 83 from natural causes; father deceased age 72 after a stroke, HTN; brother age 65, HTN and hyperlipidemia; sister age 62, A&W; sister age 68, HTN, breast cancer

Developmental Stage Ego Integrity versus Despair

Role-Relationship A retired accountant, S.R. lives with husband in a small condominium. She travels with her husband and has dinner at least two times per week at a local restaurant. She is a member of a synagogue. She has one son, age 40, who is married and has two children ages 8 and 10. S.R. talks with her son or daughter-in law once per week. They live 25 miles away and visit every other month.

Sleep/Rest S.R. sleeps 8 hours per night and awakens rested.

Nutrition/Metabolic Breakfast includes tea and toast; lunch, a sandwich and piece of fruit; dinner, some pasta, meat, and vegetables. Snacks on sweets, crackers, or fruit

Activity/Exercise Hobbies include knitting, sewing, and volunteering for community service at a local health department. Has no planned exercise, but walks ½ mile per day as she completes her normal activities

Coping/Stress Talks with her husband if she has a major decision or feels stressed. States she does not have a stressful lifestyle. Enjoys traveling

Health Management Smokes 1 pack of cigarettes per day; alcohol, one glass of white wine at HS. Does not have a living will or advanced directive. Is not physically or emotionally abused. Has a smoke detector and CO_2 monitor in her condominium. Last Pap smear and mammogram 3 years ago. Td: 3/12/96.

Self-Perception and Values/Beliefs Is content, but would like to do more for the community.

Medications Hydrochlorothiazide 25 mg one qd; multivitamin with iron one qd

Allergies PCN

Pertinent Physical Findings

Vital Signs Height 5 feet 6 inches; weight 155 pounds; BMI 25; temperature 97.2° F; heart rate 80; respirations 18; blood pressure 138/72

General Appearance Alert and oriented to time, place and person; well-nourished and well-groomed; speech clear; coordinated movements; stable gait; in no apparent distress

Breasts Symmetrical, no tenderness, enlargement, dimpling, or masses, no nipple discharge or axillary lymphadenopathy

Heart Heart rate 80 with regular rate and rhythm, no murmurs, no S_3 or S_4; PMI 5th ICS-LMCL

Lungs Clear to auscultation and equal bilaterally, no adventitious breath sounds, resonant throughout lung fields

Abdomen: Slightly protuberant, active bowel sounds, no abdominal bruits, soft, no masses or organomegaly, nontender, no inguinal lymphadenopathy, no CVA tenderness

Genital External genitalia with no lesions, swelling or discharge; perineal muscles weak; no urethral discharge; vaginal mucosa pale pink with loss of folds and slightly dry; cervix pink with no lesions; no adnexal masses or CMT; small cystocele noted

Rectal No masses or lesions, small external hemorrhoids noted, hemoccult negative stool in anal vault, normal anal tone

Extremities: Pink, warm, without edema, no varicosities; bil negative Homan's sign; dorsalis pedis and radial pulses 2+ bil equal; joints without evidence of ligamentous laxity, effusions, erythema or swelling

Neurological: CN II-XII grossly intact, DTR 2+ bil symmetrical, muscular strength intact bil, no atrophy or tremors, Romberg negative, sensation intact to light touch and pinprick, able to heel-to-toe-walk

Diagnostics

Diagnostic Tests Urinalysis negative; BUN/creatinine normal; post-voiding residual (PVR) 45 ml (<45 is normal bladder emptying; >200 is indicative of retention)

History Data Questions specific to the chief complaint of incontinence include the following:

- How often do you experience incontinence?
- Do you ever wear a pad to catch urine leakage?
- Do you ever have difficulty getting to the bathroom to urinate?
- Once you have the urge to urinate, how long can you hold it?
- Are you frequently constipated?
- How much fluid do you drink? Do you drink many caffeinated beverages? Do you take diuretics?
- Do you have pain on urination, hesitancy, awaken to urinate, frequency, blood in your urine, or dribbling?
- How many pregnancies, miscarriages, and abortions have you had?
- Were your deliveries vaginal or cesarean section?
- If a vaginal birth, did you have an episiotomy?
- Have you started any new medications? (Methyldopa, prazosin, phenothiazines, diazepam and diuretics aggravate stress incontinence, whereas alpha-adrenergic agents, androgens, calcium channel blockers, anticholinergics, and sympathomimetic agents cause urinary retention [Seller, 1996].)

Physical Examination Data The minimum examination for chief complaint of incontinence includes mental status, neurological, musculoskeletal, abdominal, pelvic, and rectal. A complete history and physical examination is preferred.

Differential Diagnosis Stress incontinence, urge incontinence, overflow incontinence, functional incontinence (Table 10-2)

Probable Causes of the Presenting Symptoms Stress incontinence occurs with activities that increase intraabdominal pressure such as coughing, bending, sneezing, and laughing. Urethral sphincter insufficiency occurs when pelvic floor laxity causes the proximal urethra and bladder neck to herniate through the pelvic floor with increased pressure, thereby creating unequal pressure to the

Table 10-2
Incontinence Differential Diagnostic Cues

Diagnoses	Signs and Symptoms	Lab Data	Treatment
Stress Incontinence Causes include weakness of the pelvic floor and trauma or surgery causing urethral sphincter weakness Multiparity and vaginal deliveries of large babies are also risk factors for weak pelvic floors.	Leakage of small amounts of urine with coughing, laughing, or sneezing	Urine dip to screen in office; urinalysis and C&S if irritative symptoms; BUN/creatinine if suspect retention Post-voiding residual either by catheterization or ultrasound	Kegel exercises. Routine voiding schedule. If constipation, chronic cough, or obesity, must address pelvic floor issues. If atrophic vaginitis, treat with hormone therapy. May try alpha-agonist (e.g., pseudoephedrine 30-60 mg tid *OR* phenylpropanolamine 75 mg bid. Can try imipramine (Tofranil) 10-25 mg qd-tid. Periurethral injection of collagen may be helpful. Surgery for bladder neck suspension
Urge Incontinence*	Usually large amount of urine leakage from the inability to wait to void	Urine dip to screen for leukocytes, blood, glucose, and protein. Urinalysis and C&S if +. BUN and creatinine. If hematuria, order urine cytology. Do post-voiding residual (PVR); if + may consider additional tests like cystometry, urodynamics, uroflowometry, or video-urodynamics	Bladder training Scheduled toileting or prompted voiding. May trial bladder relaxant drug therapy like propantheline (Pro-Banthine) 7.5-30 mg 3-5 × day; oxybutynin (Ditropan) 2.5-5 mg tid; imipramine (Tofranil) 10-25 mg qd-tid; doxepin (Sinequan) 10-25 mg qd-tid. Periodically check PVR because of the side effect of urinary retention with meds. May trial detrol (tolterodine tartrate) 2 mg bid, may reduce to 1 mg bid
Overflow Incontinence Resulting from detrusor instability of bladder outlet or urethral obstruction Causes are drugs, constipation, SCI, BPH, cancer, MS, cystocele or uterine prolapse Other causes include post-surgical and post-radiation treatment for BPH or prostate cancer	Usually small amounts of urine leakage	Urine dip to screen for leukocytes, blood, glucose, and protein. Urinalysis and C&S if +. BUN and creatinine. If hematuria, order urine cytology. Do post-voiding residual (PVR); if + may consider additional tests like cystometry, urodynamics, uroflowometry, or video-urodynamics. PSA if suspect prostatic problems	Any obstruction requires surgical removal. Catheterization either intermittent or indwelling
Functional Incontinence†	Urination or leakage of urine	Physical examination is key. Order diagnostic tests as appropriate	Try voiding schedules or prompted voiding. Use bedside commode or make other environmental alterations. Use protective pads. May require catheter

* There is bladder or detrusor hyperactivity. Causes include lower urinary tract conditions like cancer, cystitis, stones, or obstruction. Other causes include central nervous system disorders like stroke, dementia, multiple sclerosis, Parkinson's, and spinal cord injury.
†Resulting from dementia or immobility.

urethra and incontinence (Greene et al, 1996). Stress incontinence can be aggravated by atrophic vaginitis.

Urinary incontinence is a major problem for the elderly. Approximately 40% of the elderly experience some degree of urinary incontinence. Urinary incontinence is embarrassing for many individuals, and may even lead to isolation and loneliness. Problems created by incontinence include skin breakdown, urinary tract infections, falls, and depression. When assessing urinary incontinence it is important to remember to evaluate the patient for reversible causes. Kelley (1997) describes an acronym that identifies several reversible causes of incontinence: DRIP (*d*elirium, *r*estricted mobility, *r*etention, *i*nfection, *i*nflammation, *i*mpaction, *p*olyuria, and *p*harmaceuticals).

Diagnostic Tests   Urine dip (to screen for nitrates, leukocytes, blood, glucose, and protein); urinalysis and C&S (if + for microorganisms); BUN and creatinine; if hematuria, order urine cytology; do post-voiding residual (PVR), if + may consider additional tests like cystometry, urodynamics, uroflowmetry or video-urodynamics

Diagnostic Impression   S.R.'s chief complaint of incontinence with coughing, sneezing, and laughing is indicative of stress incontinence. The atrophic vaginitis, constipation, and diuretic use aggravate the incontinence.

Therapeutic Plan of Care   S.R. is menopausal and is not on any hormone replacement therapy (HRT). Starting her on Premarin 0.625 mg and Provera 2.5 mg qd is a good choice to manage the atrophic vaginitis. S.R. may also choose to use a lubricant such as Astroglide or KY Jelly during sexual intercourse. In addition, S.R. should be taught to do Kegel exercises a minimum of 10 $\times$ qid, holding the contraction for 10 seconds and then relaxing. S.R. is constipated and should increase the fiber in her diet, increase fluid intake to 2 liters per day, and increase the number and quantity of fruits and vegetables in her diet. She may need to add a bulk agent such as Metamucil or FiberCon qd to alleviate the constipation. Consider switching her blood pressure medication from a diuretic to an ACE inhibitor such as fosinopril sodium (Mono-

pril) initially 10 mg qd (20 to 40 mg qd is the usual maintenance dose). Stop the diuretic 2 to 3 days before beginning the ACE inhibitor.

Patient Education and/or Community Resources   Patient education needs include information on incontinence, HRT, Kegel exercises, and possibly bladder training, as well as other treatments for incontinence. Provide S.R. with *Understanding incontinence: a patient guide,* published by the U.S. Department of Health and Human Services (AHCPR Pub. No. 96-0684; to order, phone (800) 358-9295).

Follow-Up Plan   S.R. should return to your office in 4 to 6 weeks to evaluate the effects of HRT, constipation management, and Kegel exercises. If she continues to experience problems with incontinence, a trial of an alpha-adrenergic agonist may be instituted, along with bladder training and planned toileting. In addition, discuss annual flu vaccination and pneumococcal vaccination (she is age 65 and has a smoking history). S.R. should schedule a mammogram because it has been 3 years since her last one and her sister has breast cancer. Information regarding a living will and advanced directive should be given to S.R. because she has not completed one.

Case Study 3
CHIEF COMPLAINT: Urinary Hesitance and Decreased Urine Stream

History of Present Illness   R.S. is a 72-year-old Caucasian male who presents with chief complaint of urinary hesitance and decreased stream. He states that for the past year he has been having a hard time starting to urinate, that he cannot void completely, and that he must void more often than in the past. His urine stream is weak, and he gets up at least twice a night. R.S. has not noticed blood in his urine. He said he has tried drinking more fluids (2 liters per day, limiting his intake to 8 to 12 ounces in the evening), but that it does not help. R.S. is administered the American Urological Association Index and his score is 14. (A score of 14 indicates moderate obstructive symptoms.) He feels fine otherwise and has no other complaints.

Past Medical History R.S. states that he has some arthritis, but that it doesn't bother him unless it is rainy. Otherwise, he has a negative medical history.

Past Surgical History T&A at age 13

Family History Father deceased at age 62, automobile accident; mother deceased age 72, natural causes; sister age 78, A&W; brother age 70, Parkinson's disease

Developmental Stage Ego Integrity versus Despair

Role-Relationship R.S. lives in a ranch home with his wife who is 60 years old. His wife works at the local high school as an office secretary. R.S. attends a nondenominational church regularly. He has one daughter, age 30, who has Down syndrome and lives at home. She works 8 hours per week in a work program. R.S. is a retired furniture maker.

Sleep/Rest Falls asleep at 11 PM and awakens at 7:30 AM rested. Does not use sleep aids

Nutrition/Metabolic Breakfast, oatmeal, eggs, or peanut butter on toast; lunch, a sandwich, soup, or salad; dinner, a full, well-balanced meal. Rarely snacks. Enjoys his evening dessert

Activity/Exercise R.S. is very active and walks 1 to 2 miles per day. He enjoys visiting neighbors on his walks. His hobbies include cooking, woodwork, and volunteering at the church.

Coping/Stress R.S. does not feel he has a great deal of stress. He does worry about his daughter's care when he and his wife should pass away. R.S. has a close relationship with his wife and talks with her about problems or concerns.

Health Management Smoking, R.S. quit smoking 10 years ago and never felt better. Alcohol, drinks a beer each night. Caffeine, 1 cup of coffee for breakfast. Td: 8/18/89. Has a living will

Self-Perception and Values/Beliefs Feels he has had a very good life. Enjoys spending time with his wife and daughter

Medications Ibuprofen (Motrin) 200 mg prn for arthritis pain (usually takes 2 pills twice a week)

Allergies NKMA

Pertinent Physical Findings

Vital Signs Height 6 feet 2 inches; weight 210 pounds; BMI 27; temperature 98.2° F; heart rate 82; respirations 16; blood pressure 160/95 (standing), 154/92 (sitting)

General Appearance Alert and oriented to time, place, person, and situation; well-nourished and well-groomed; in no apparent distress

Heart Apical pulse 80 with regular rate and rhythm; no murmurs, S_3 or S_4; PMI at 5th ICS-LMCL

Lungs Clear to auscultation

Abdomen Soft, nontender abdomen with active bowel sounds in all quadrants. No masses or organomegaly, no inguinal lymphadenopathy, no CVA tenderness

Genital Penis circumcised, no discharge, testes descended without masses or tenderness

Rectal No masses, lesions or hemorrhoids, hemoccult negative stool in anal vault, normal anal tone; prostate smooth with no nodules, firm, nontender, mildly enlarged with median sulcus obliterated. (When the distal margins of the prostate gland cannot be felt, there is usually enlargement of three or more times normal size [Goroll, May, and Mulley, 1995].)

Neurological CN II-XII grossly intact, DTR +2 bil symmetrical, muscular strength intact bil, no atrophy or tremors, Romberg negative, sensation intact to light touch and pinprick, able to heel-to-toe walk

Diagnostics

Diagnostic Tests Urinalysis within normal limits; BUN, 10 mg/dl; creatinine, 0.9 mg/dl; PSA, 2.8 ug/L

History Data Questions specific to the chief complaint of urinary hesitancy and decreased force of urine stream include the following (Administer the American Urological Association Symptom Index [Table 10-3]):

- Have you had urological surgery?
- Do you have diabetes mellitus or multiple sclerosis? (These may cause neurogenic bladder.)
- Are you on cold or sinus medications or anticholinergic drugs? (These may aggravate the symptoms of benign prostatic hyperplasia [BPH].)
- Are you having any pain, bloody urine, anorexia, or weight loss? (These symptoms may be caused by bladder cancer.)

Table 10-3
American Urological Association Symptom Index for Benign Prostatic Hyperplasia

Questions to Be Answered	Not at All	Less Than One Time in Five	Less Than Half the Time	About Half the Time	More Than Half the Time	Almost Always
1. Over the past month, how often have you had a sensation of not emptying your bladder completely after you finish urinating?	0	1	2	3	4	5
2. Over the past month, how often have you had to urinate again less than 2 hours after you finished urinating?	0	1	2	3	4	5
3. Over the past month, how often have you found you stopped and started again several times when you urinated?	0	1	2	3	4	5
4. Over the past month, how often have you found it difficult to postpone urination?	0	1	2	3	4	5
5. Over the past month, how often have you had a weak urinary stream?	0	1	2	3	4	5
6. Over the past month, how often have you had to push or strain to begin urination?	0	1	2	3	4	5
7. Over the past month, how many times did you most typically get up to urinate from the time you went to bed at night until the time you got up in the morning?	0	1	2	3	4	5

Sum of seven circled numbers equals the symptom score. A score of 0-7 indicates mild symptoms that should be periodically reevaluated. A score of 8-19 indicates moderate symptoms in which treatment options should be offered. A score of 20-35 indicates severe symptoms in which treatment options should be offered.

From Barry JM et al: The American Urological Association Symptom Index for benign prostatic hyperplasia, *J Urol* 148(5):1549-1557, 1992.

Physical Examination Data   The minimum examination for chief complaint of urinary hesitancy and decreased force of urine stream includes: vital signs, heart, lungs, abdomen, genital and rectal, and neurological (focused)

Differential Diagnosis   Ureteral stricture or obstruction, neurogenic bladder, benign prostatic hyperplasia, prostate or bladder cancer, urinary tract infection, prostatitis (if pain with palpation of prostate gland) (Table 10-4)

Table 10-4
Urinary Hesitancy and Decreased Stream Differential Diagnostic Cues

Diagnoses	Signs and Symptoms	Lab Data	Treatment
Ureteral Stricture or Obstruction	Decreased urinary output at a single voiding with alternating polyuria hesitancy, weak urinary stream, palpable bladder	Kidney-ureter-bladder film (KUB); ultrasound is the procedure of choice if screening for obstruction	Refer to urologist. May require prostatectomy, urethral dilation, or an endoscopic urethrotomy
Neurogenic Bladder*	Frequency, urgency, incontinence	Urinalysis, BUN/creatinine, BS. Urodynamic evaluation to evaluate bladder and urethral function (e.g., cystometry, flow rate and flow electromyography studies, electromyography, video studies, and spinal evoked potentials)	Refer to urologist for evaluation. Therapies may include medications or surgical intervention. Catheterization may be required
Benign Prostatic Hyperplasia	Weak urinary stream, hesitancy, intermittent stream	Urinalysis, PSA, BUN/creatinine Additional tests may be ordered based on other symptoms (e.g., IVP if suspect stones, plain film of abdomen for suspected urinary tract calculi) Post-void residual urine for assessing moderate-severe symptoms Uroflowmetry is useful in assessing severe BPH	Mild symptoms suggest limiting fluids after dinner, avoid medications that increase symptoms, and avoid alcohol or caffeine. Moderate-to-severe symptoms, may opt for treatment with medications such as an alpha blocker (e.g., terazosin [Hytrin] 2-10 mg qd, give at HS, SE postural hypotension adjust slowly starting at 1 mg titrate slowly over 30 days; doxazosin mesylate [Cardura], 1 mg qd at HS,

Note: See Case 1 on pages 177-182 for information on bladder cancer, urinary tract infection, and prostatitis.
*Requires a focused neuro-urologic examination of perianal pinprick sensation, bulbocavernosus reflex, and relaxation and contraction of the anal sphincter. This provides data on S2, S3, and S4.

Probable Causes of the Presenting Symptoms
Benign prostatic hyperplasia is hyperplasia of tissue in the periurethral and transitional zones. BPH has a multifactorial etiology that includes the role of aging and sex hormones. Growth of the prostate gland is quite static until the male reaches puberty, at which time it grows rapidly and becomes adult size (about the size of a walnut) at 20 ± 6 g (Kelley, 1997). In later years the prostate may again increase in size, which can create hyperplasia and cause varying degrees of urethral obstruction. Patients with BPH may experience obstructive symptoms (e.g., decreased urine stream, hesitancy, and intermittent stream) or irritative symptoms (e.g., urgency, frequency, and nocturia) (Tierney, McPhee, and Papadakis, 1999).

Diagnostic Tests   Urinalysis (screening for infection, hematuria, proteinuria, PSA (to screen for prostate cancer), and BUN/creatinine (to assess kidney function)

Table 10-4
Urinary Hesitancy and Decreased Stream Differential Diagnostic Cues—cont'd

Diagnoses	Signs and Symptoms	Lab Data	Treatment
Benign Prostatic Hyperplasia —cont'd			double dose q 2 weeks if necessary to maximum 8 mg qd; *OR* tamsulosin HCl [Flomax] 0.4 mg with a meal, may increase to 0.8 mg qd in 2-4 weeks if no improvement; *OR* finasteride [Proscar], 5 mg qd). Other options include balloon dilation, transurethral resection of prostate, transurethral incision of the prostate, or prostatic stints. Saw palmetto 160 mg bid may reduce urinary symptoms associated with BPH (controversial)
Cancer: Prostate	Usually asymptomatic, may have varying degree of urinary retention, digital rectal exam may be positive for nodule or induration	PSA, urinalysis, BUN/creatinine Transrectal ultrasound with guided If suspect metastasis, may order radionuclide bone scan	Referral to urologist. Treatment may include radiation or radical prostatectomy for local disease. Regionally advanced disease may consider a combination of radiation, surgery, and hormonal therapy. For metastatic disease may consider androgen blockade by using orchiotomy or an antiandrogen with an LHRH agonist

Diagnostic Impression R.S. has classic obstructive symptoms (BPH) of decreased urine stream, increased urine frequency, and nocturia. His symptoms are classified as moderate on the American Urological Association Symptom Index.

Therapeutic Plan of Care R.S. has moderate symptoms of BPH. Treatment for R.S.'s moderate symptoms include limiting large amounts of fluids after dinner, avoiding medications that increase his obstructive symptoms, and limiting caffeine and alcohol (diuretic effect). In addition, because of R.S.'s elevated blood pressure (BP), ordering Hytrin 1 mg at HS and gradually increasing dose to maintenance of 5 to 10 mg per day will help bring his BP down and alleviate some of his obstructive symptoms. Inform the patient that postural hypotension is a potential side effect of Hytrin, so that he will need to rise slowly from a standing or sitting position. Taking the medication at HS may also minimize this side effect.

Patient Education and/or Community Resources   Patient education consists of describing BPH to R.S. and providing him a copy of *Treating Your Enlarged Prostate,* a patient teaching guide available from the Agency for Health Care Policy and Research. To order by phone, call (800) 358-9295.

Follow-Up Plan   R.S. should return in 2 to 4 weeks to have his BP and obstructive symptoms reevaluated. R.S. has verbalized concerns about the care of his daughter upon his death. Assist R.S. with exploring potential options for her care in the community.

Case Study 4

CHIEF COMPLAINT: Scrotal Pain

History of Present Illness   T.J. is an 18-year-old African-American male who presents with chief complaint of a 4-day history of gradual onset of one-sided scrotum pain. T.J. states it is painful and tender, and worse when walking or lifting. He denies any trauma. Upon further questioning he states that he has some discomfort with urination and a small amount of thick yellow discharge at the end of his penis. He is not experiencing any nausea or vomiting and he is not running a fever. T.J. is sexually active and has had three partners in 4 months. T.J. is unaware of any of his partners having any problems. He does not use condoms and is unsure of what birth control the women used. He is a high school student active in football and basketball.

Past Medical History   Unremarkable

Past Surgical History   None

Family History   Mother, age 39, and father, age 40, A&W; sister, age 12, ADHD

Developmental Stage   Identity versus Role Confusion

Role-Relationship   T.J. "doesn't want to be tied down," so he dates several girls. Has many friends and hangs around with them often. He enjoys movies, playing pool, and hanging out with his friends. T.J. plans on attending college when finished with his senior year.

Sleep/Rest   On school nights falls asleep at 11 PM and awakens at 6:30 AM; on weekends he stays out with his friends until after midnight and sleeps until 11 AM or noon

Nutrition/Metabolic   Breakfast, French toast, cold cereal, or eggs with orange juice and milk; lunch, whatever is on the school's hot lunch program; dinner, eats with his family. Snacks on chips, pizza, sweets, and candy

Activity/Exercise   Is very active with training for football and basketball. Spends approximately 1 to 3 hours per day conditioning and practicing

Coping/Stress   Talks with friends about any problems. Feels he has a good relationship with his parents

Health Management   Nonsmoker. Alcohol, drinks beer and mixed drinks on the weekend. Recreational drugs, has tried street drugs (e.g., smoking marijuana, snorting cocaine, and using IV drugs), but doesn't anymore because he had a bad experience and felt like he was going to die. Td: 7/14/98.

Self-Perception and Values/Beliefs   Enjoys life, has many friends, and is actively involved in sports. Attends church because his parents insist

Medications   Has experimented with using steroids, but stopped when he learned that they could have bad side effects

Allergies   NKMA

Pertinent Physical Findings

Vital Signs   Height 5 feet 9 inches; weight 176 pounds; BMI 26; temperature 98.8° F without antipyretic; heart rate 66; respirations 12; blood pressure 132/82

Heart   Apical pulse 66 with regular rate and rhythm, no murmurs, clicks, S_3 or S_4

Lungs   Clear to auscultation

Abdomen   Flat, soft, nontender, active bowel sounds; no masses or organomegaly; no inguinal lymphadenopathy, no CVA tenderness

Genital   Penis uncircumcised, slight yellow discharge at meatus, erythematous urethra; testes descended with no masses or nodules, left testicle tender upon palpation with epididymis slightly enlarged and tender; scrotal skin is slightly erythematous; elevation of the left testis relieves the pain (+Prehn's sign)

Rectal   No masses, lesions or hemorrhoids; normal anal tone; prostate smooth, nontender, no nodules or enlargement

Diagnostics

Diagnostic Tests Urinalysis shows pyuria; urine C&S sent; collect chlamydial test; gonococcal culture of urethral discharge prior to obtaining urine specimen; and Gram stain of urethral discharge

History Data Questions specific to the chief complaint of scrotal pain include the following:

- Did the pain develop gradually or suddenly?
- Is the pain unilateral or bilateral?
- Do you have any nausea or vomiting?
- Do you have any urethral discharge, or are you running a fever?
- Have you experienced any trauma or injury?
- Are you sexually active? If so, how many sexual partners do you have?
- Do you have any new sexual partners?
- Has any of your sexual partners had any pelvic discomfort or urinary symptoms?

Physical Examination Data The focused examination for the chief complaint of scrotal pain includes: vital signs, heart, lungs, abdomen, genital, and rectum.

Differential Diagnosis Testicular torsion, epididymitis, testicular tumor, orchitis, hydrocele, testicular trauma, varicocele (Table 10-5)

Probable Causes of the Presenting Symptoms Epididymitis is caused by an organism that spreads in a retrograde fashion along the vas deferens (Hurst, 1996). The organism may be spread from a urinary tract infection, the posterior urethra, or seminal vesicles (Uphold and Graham, 1998). Epididymitis is an inflammatory process that can occur at any time during the lifespan, but is more common in adulthood. When children get epididymitis, it is most commonly associated with a urinary tract infection caused from a structural lesion in the urinary tract or from a urological surgery requiring catheterization. In males 20 to 40 years of age, epididymitis is usually caused by a sexually transmitted disease, with the most common causative organisms being *Neisseria gonorrhoeae* and *Chlamydia trachomatis*. In older males, epididymitis is usually associated with urinary tract infections, instrumentation, or surgery with a gram-negative enteric organism.

Diagnostic Tests Urinalysis, urine C&S, Gram stain of urethral discharge, chlamydia test, gonococcal culture of urethral discharge

Diagnostic Impression T.J. presents with gradual onset of unilateral scrotal pain, dysuria, + Prehn's sign, and urethral discharge. T.J. has also had three partners in 4 months. The likely cause of the symptoms is acute epididymitis.

Therapeutic Plan of Care T.J. should be treated empirically for gonorrhea and chlamydia. He should receive azithromycin (Zithromax) 1 gram PO and cefixime (Suprax) 400 mg PO. A discussion about sexually transmitted diseases should occur at this meeting, and he should notify his partners so that they can seek treatment.

Patient Education and/or Community Resources A discussion on birth control methods and types and clinical course of sexually transmitted diseases should occur with T.J. Safer sexual practices should be reviewed. He should be offered HIV testing. Health teaching on alcohol consumption and driving should be discussed.

Follow-Up Plan T.J. should return if his symptoms do not resolve. He should also return for annual visits and prn.

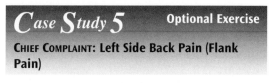

Case Study 5 **Optional Exercise**

CHIEF COMPLAINT: Left Side Back Pain (Flank Pain)

History of Present Illness J.K. is a 32-year-old Caucasian male who presents with chief complaint of sudden onset of severe localized left-sided back pain approximately 8 hours ago. He states that the pain is gripping and almost constant. He is not experiencing dysuria, urethral discharge, or bloody urine. He doesn't recall any injury to his back and does not have a history of kidney stones. J.K. denies any stressful exercise or activities. He has no nausea or vomiting. J.K. states that he feels he is

Table 10-5
Scrotal Pain Differential Diagnostic Cues

Diagnoses	Signs and Symptoms	Lab Data	Treatment
Testicular Torsion	Abrupt onset of unilateral testicular pain. It is often reported after a minor injury, but can occur anytime. N/V in 50% of patients. No fever, urethral discharge, or dysuria	Surgical exploration. If uncertain, may order technetium nuclear scan scand (shows decreased perfusion) or Doppler ultrasound (shows absent testicular artery pulsation) Scrotal ultrasound is used to evaluate a scrotal mass and trauma.	This is a urological emergency and requires immediate action. (Within 6 hours of the torsion, damage to the testes takes place.) Consult with the physician for proper intervention. Immediate surgery is required to correct the torsion.
Epididymitis	Gradual onset of unilateral testicular pain and tenderness, dysuria, and urethral discharge; fever may occur; pain may increase with standing or walking	Urinalysis; urine C&S, Gram stain of urethral discharge, *Chlamydia* test, gonococcal culture of urethral discharge. In men >40 years, collect expressed prostatic secretions. If unable to differentiate between testicular torsion, consult with physician and consider ordering Doppler ultrasound, scrotal ultrasound, or radionuclide scrotal imaging.	Men <40 years old, treat with broad-spectrum agent (e.g., trimethoprim-sulfamethoxazole [Bactrim] 40 mg/kg/d bid × 10-14 days. After treatment, reculture urine and conduct diagnostic tests to assess for structural lesion For STD, treat empirically (e.g., doxycycline l00 mg bid × 10 days **OR** azithromycin [Zithromax] 1 gram PO × 1 and ceftriaxone [Rocephin] 250 mg IM × 1) In men >40 without STD symptoms, treat with trimethoprim-sulfamethoxazole (Septra) DS bid × 10 days or quinolone (e.g., levofloxacin [Levaquin] **OR** ciprofloxacin [Cipro] 500 mg bid × 10 days). If associated with bacterial prostatitis, continue treatment at least 4 weeks. Symptomatic treatment: bed rest, scrotal support, scrotal elevation, sitz bath, and pain medication (e.g., NSAIDs)
Testicular Tumor*	Either painless presentation of a nodule on the testicle or heaviness in the scrotum. May also present with acute testicular pain (10%) from intratesticular hemorrhage or a secondary hydrocele (5%-10%)	Scrotal ultrasound. Human chorionic gonadotropin, alpha-fetal protein, and LDH	Urological referral for evaluation and potential surgical intervention. Depending on the tumor stage and type, may have a radical orchiectomy and/or retroperitoneal irradiation (Stage I or IIa) or primary chemotherapy (Stage III). In select cases may use surveillance, but must meet criteria

*A risk factor is a history of cryptorchism.

Table 10-5
Scrotal Pain Differential Diagnostic Cues—cont'd

Diagnoses	Signs and Symptoms	Lab Data	Treatment
Orchitis†	In mumps orchitis, the scrotum is swollen and tender. Fever up to 104° F is common. No dysuria. Occurs about 3 days after parotitis Symptoms of bacterial orchitis are the same as mumps, but with dysuria. May also have flank pain and malaise, N/V In tuberculosis orchitis, there is scrotal mass, pain, and/or discharging sinus. May also have malaise, loss of weight, high fever	Urinalysis. If suspect mumps, get acute and convalescent serum viral titers. If suspect Tb, get Tb test	Bed rest. Local heat. Support. Meds for pain and fever. Mumps, follow at office, will need to hospitalize if scrotal abscess Bacterial orchitis, give appropriate antimicrobials and supportive care; evaluate need for hospitalization Tuberculosis, long-term treatment and follow-up, tuberculin medications
Hydrocele	Scrotal swelling that is nontender. May feel a dull ache. Transillumination shows a fluid-filled mass with light passing through the mass	Scrotal ultrasound	May do nothing if symptoms absent. If it bothers the patient, causes a pain, or has dermatitis, may do surgical repair
Testicular Trauma	Sudden onset of scrotal pain and swelling, may have ecchymosis	Scrotal ultrasound	Scrotal support and elevation
Varicocele	Scrotal swelling. May feel heaviness or dull pain that is worse with heavy lifting. Pain may radiate to inguinal area	Examine patient standing and lying – veins are not felt when lying, but are palpable when standing. If veins stay palpable when lying, suspect obstruction No diagnostic tests usually needed. May order IVP for abrupt onset of varicocele may have venous obstruction or renal carcinoma If infertility is a problem, need a complete infertility workup.	Consult about new onset varicoceles: testing is indicated. If classical variocele, can assess annually. If a problem for the patient, may need surgical intervention

†Can be caused by mumps, bacterial (from urethral instrumentation, prostatic surgery, or UTIs), or tuberculosis.

running a fever. J.K. has not had the desire to drink or eat during the past few hours.

Past Medical History Genital herpes diagnosed at age 27

Past Surgical History T&A age 9; myringotomy age 7

Family History Mother age 57, asthma; father age 60, HTN; sister age 30, asthma

Developmental Stage Intimacy versus Isolation

Role-Relationship J.K. is married to Melissa and lives in a two-story home in the suburbs. J.K. has one daughter, age 9 years old, who lives with his ex-wife and visits once a week and every other weekend. He and Melissa have two daughters, ages 2 and 4. Melissa has a 7-year-old son from her first marriage who lives with them. J.K. is a mechanical engineer for a local company. J.K. enjoys his daughters and blended family and tries to spend as much time with them as possible. He acknowledges that there is some jealousy among the girls when they all get together.

Sleep/Rest Falls to sleep at 10:30 PM and arises at 5:30 AM feeling rested. Does not use sleep aids

Nutrition/Metabolic J.K. is a vegetarian, and tries to eat healthy foods as much as possible. Breakfast, a donut and cup of coffee; lunch, his wife makes him a salad, yogurt, and fruit; dinner, pasta dishes, potato dishes, or casseroles with vegetables, bread, and fruit. Snacks on fruit, raw vegetables, and sweets

Activity/Exercise Feels he is too busy with work and children to exercise

Coping/Stress When he is stressed he takes a walk or goes out with his male friends for a beer. He discusses major problems with his wife or else solves them alone. He doesn't feel he has time for church, but his wife and daughters attend regularly. His hobbies include skiing in the winter and golfing or swimming in the summer.

Health Management Smoker, smokes 1 pack of cigarettes per day for 14 years; alcohol and recreational drugs, none. States he experimented with cocaine for about 6 months, but quit a year ago

Self-Perception and Values/Beliefs J.K. is pleased to have purchased a nice home in the suburbs and he enjoys time with his daughters. He does state that he feels bad that his first marriage didn't work, and at times finds it difficult to blend the families together. However, he is optimistic that things will work out very well over time.

Medications None
Allergies NKMA

Pertinent Physical Findings

Vital Signs Height 6 feet 1 inch; weight 219 pounds; BMI 29; temperature 100.2° F without antipyretics; heart rate 88; respirations 18; blood pressure 142/90

Heart Heart rate 88, regular rate and rhythm, no murmurs, no S_3 or S_4

Lung Clear to auscultation

Abdomen Active bowel sounds, soft, negative rebound, pain to deep palpation over the left side of the abdomen, no masses, no splenomegaly or hepatomegaly, no inguinal lymphadenopathy; + left side CVA tenderness

Back No paraspinal tenderness, full ROM of back; reflex + 2 in lower extremities, gait stable; able to maintain flexion and extension of lower extremities against resistance

Diagnostics

Diagnostic Tests Urine dip, large amount of blood, negative for leukocytes; a plain radiograph of the kidneys, ureters, and bladder (KUB) shows calcifications in the left kidney; IVP shows a 5-mm stone in the left kidney with blunted calyces, indicating hydronephrosis.

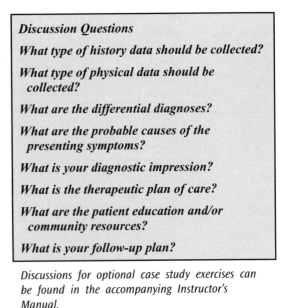

Discussion Questions

What type of history data should be collected?

What type of physical data should be collected?

What are the differential diagnoses?

What are the probable causes of the presenting symptoms?

What is your diagnostic impression?

What is the therapeutic plan of care?

What are the patient education and/or community resources?

What is your follow-up plan?

Discussions for optional case study exercises can be found in the accompanying Instructor's Manual.

References

Barry JM et al: The American Urological Association Symptom index for benign prostatic hyperplasia, *J Urol* 148(5):1549-1557, 1992.

Centers for Disease Control and Prevention: Guidelines for treatment of sexually transmitted disease, *MMWR Morb Mortal Wkly Rep* 47 (No. RR-1), 1998.

Goroll AH, May LA, Mulley AG: *Primary care medicine: office evaluation and management of the adult patient,* ed 3, Philadelphia, 1995, Lippincott-Raven.

Greene H, Fincher RM, Johnson W et al: *Clinical medicine,* St Louis, 1996, Mosby.

Hurst JW: *Medicine for the practicing physician,* Stamford, Conn., 1996, Appleton & Lange.

Kelley W: *Textbook of internal medicine,* ed 3, Philadelphia, 1997, Lippincott-Raven.

Seller R: *Differential diagnosis of common complaints,* Philadelphia, 1996, WB Saunders.

Tierney L, McPhee SJ, Papadakis MA: *Current medical diagnosis and treatment,* Stamford, Conn., 1999, Appleton and Lange.

Uphold C, Graham M: *Clinical guidelines in family practice,* Gainesville, Fla., 1998, Barmarrae Books.

U.S. Department of Health and Human Services: *Understanding incontinence: a patient guide* (AHCPR Pub. No. 96-0684), Rockville, Md., 1996, Author.

Selected Readings

American Academy of Pediatrics: Practice parameter: the diagnosis, treatment, and evaluation of the initial urinary tract infection in febrile infants and young children, *Pediatrics* 103(4 Pt 1):843-852, 1999

Falagas ME, Gorbach SL: Practice guidelines: urinary tract infections, *Infectious Disease Clinical Practice* 4:241-257, 1995.

Gilbert DN, Moellering RC, Sande MA: *The Sanford guide to antimicrobial therapy,* ed 29, Dallas, 1999, Antimicrobial Therapy Inc.

Lipsky BA: Prostatitis and urinary tract infection in men: what's new; what's true? *Am J Med* 106(3):327-334, 1999.

CHAPTER 11

Women's Health

Jean Nagelkerk

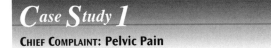

Case Study 1

CHIEF COMPLAINT: Pelvic Pain

History of Present Illness   L.T., a 25-year-old African-American female, presents with chief complaint of pain with intercourse. She states that the pain started 2 weeks ago and has not gone away. She also reports dysuria and sharp pain off and on in her perineum for the past 2 days, which is "driving her crazy." L.T. has also noticed some small bumps in one spot in her perineal area. She has tried position changes with sexual intercourse with no relief. She has douched, been eating yogurt, and drinking cranberry juice to relieve the discomfort. She has not had any N/V, abdominal discomfort, or abnormal bleeding. She has noticed an odorous yellow discharge after sexual intercourse. She is in a monogamous relationship (2 years) with her husband. L.T. is suspicious that her husband may be involved with an old girlfriend.

Past Medical History   Unremarkable

Family History   Mother age 60, breast cancer; father age 72, HTN; sister age 33, A&W; brother age 33, A&W

Developmental Stage   Intimacy versus Isolation

Role-Relationship   L.T. confides in a coworker when she has problems. L.T. and her husband rent a one-bedroom apartment. L.T. enjoys her time with her husband, but is concerned that he is working long hours and seems to be distancing himself from her.

Sleep/Rest   Sleeps 6 to 8 hours per night and awakens rested. Uses OTC sleeping pills when has heavy job demands (about once per month)

Nutrition/Metabolic   She is overweight and admits that her diet and snacking could be improved. Often snacks on chips, chocolates, and sweets

Activity/Exercise   No regular exercise; walks around her neighborhood occasionally

Coping/Stress   Works as a CPA in a local accounting firm. Tax season often produces job stress with long hours and a heavy workload. Reviews problems with her friends and husband. Attends church occasionally

Health Management   L.T. does not smoke or consume alcoholic beverages. She admits to drinking 8 cups of coffee per day with cream and sugar. Td: last immunization was in grade school. L.T. consistently uses seatbelts and has a smoke detector in her home.

Self-Perception and Values/Beliefs   Describes herself as overweight. Is interested in losing weight. Is very concerned that her husband may be having an affair, but does not want to confront him about this possibility

Medications   She uses Lo-Ovral 1 qd for birth control.

Allergies   NKMA

Pertinent Physical Findings

Vital Signs   Height 5 feet 4½ inches; weight 180 pounds; BMI 31; temperature 98.8° F; heart rate 82; respirations 16; blood pressure 138/88

General Appearance   African-American female, alert and oriented × 4 well-developed, well-nourished and groomed, in no apparent distress

Heart   Apical pulse 82, rate regular, Grade II systolic murmur best heard at LMCL 5th ICS

Lungs   Clear to auscultation

Abdomen   Abdomen soft, +BS, slightly tender over lower abdomen. No organomegaly. No rebound tenderness

Genitalia   No femoral or inguinal lymph-adenopathy. External genitalia with clusters of vesicular lesions on the labia majora bilaterally. Vaginal mucosa is pink and moist. Cervix pink, non-parous with copious yellow, thick discharge, friable; +CMT, mild discomfort with bimanual, uterus not enlarged, no adnexal masses

Diagnostics
Diagnostic Tests   Wet mount, many WBCs; urine, negative; viral culture for herpes simplex, chlamydia, and gonorrhea + (test results were available 2 days after patient encounter). HIV and syphilis testing declined by patient. (Because the patient is positive for gonorrhea, chlamydia, and herpes simplex virus, she should be counseled to reconsider her decision to decline HIV and syphilis testing, especially since she reports she is monogamous but unsure of her husband's fidelity.)

History Data   Questions specific to the chief complaint of pelvic pain include the following:

- Are you having any vaginal discharge, abnormal bleeding, pelvic pain, or urination problems?
- Are you experiencing fever or chills?
- Are you having pain with intercourse? If so, is the pain with initial penetration or pain with deep thrusting penetration?
- What is the date of your LMP?
- Do you use any barrier method of protection?
- Have you or your sexual partner ever been treated for a STD?
- Are you using any contraception? If so, what kind?
- What was the date of your last sexual encounter, and how many sexual partners do you have? How many sexual partners does your partner have?
- Are you having vaginal, oral, and/or anal intercourse?
- Do you use sexual aids or instruments?
- Do you engage intravenous drug use, share needles, or exchange sex for drugs?
- Do you use hot tubs frequently?
- Have you had sex against your will?
- Do you have painful menses or heavy flow?

- Have you been hit, kicked, slapped, or punched?

Physical Examination Data   The focused examination for chief complaint of pain with intercourse includes vital signs, heart, lung, abdomen, and genital (femoral and inguinal lymphadnopathy).

Differential Diagnoses   Acute cervicitis (*Chlamydia trachomatis* and gonorrhea); genital ulcer disease (*Herpes simplex,* primary syphilis, chancroid, *Lymphogranuloma venereum*), condyloma acuminata, pelvic inflammatory disease, acute vaginitis (*Trichomonas,* candida, bacterial vaginosis), foreign body (Table 11-1)

Probable Causes of the Presenting Symptoms L.T. has two diagnoses causing her discomfort. She has a polymicrobial infection of the upper genital tract from *N. gonorrhea* and *C. trachomatis.* These sexually transmitted organisms create an inflammatory condition and can cause scarring and damage in the upper genital tract leading to infertility and chronic pelvic pain (Uphold and Graham, 1998). L.T. also has contracted genital herpes. Herpes simplex virus type 1 generally creates oral lesions, but can be found in the genital area. Herpes simplex virus type 2 creates genital lesions. Due to changes in sexual behavior, approximately 40% of cases of newly acquired genital herpes are caused by HSV-1 (Tierney, McPhee, and Papadakis, 1999).

Diagnostic Tests   Wet mount; viral culture; DNA probe of cervical samples; urine, HIV, and syphilis testing. Echocardiogram for Grade II systolic murmur evaluation to rule out mitral valve prolapse

Diagnostic Impression   L.T. complains of dyspareunia, +CMT, and malodorous yellow discharge, all of which support a diagnosis of acute cervicitis. L.T. also complains of sharp pain in the perineum and dysuria, which commonly occur with genital herpes.

Therapeutic Plan of Care   Gonorrhea and chlamydia commonly co-occur, so L.T. should be treated for both. L.T. could be given an injection of ceftriaxone (Rocephin) 125 mg and take

Text continued on page 202.

Table 11-1
Pelvic Pain Differential Diagnostic Cues

Diagnosis	Signs and Symptoms	Lab Data	Treatment*
Acute Cervicitis *Chlamydia trachomatis* Co-infection with gonorrhea common so treat for both Leading cause of infertility in United States	May be asymptomatic or watery urethral or cervical discharge, slight discomfort unless has progressed to PID then painful	Use direct immunofluorescence assay, enzyme linked immunoassay, or DNA probing of cervical samples	Tetracycline **OR** erythromycin base 500 mg qid or doxycycline 100 mg bid × 7 days **OR** azithromycin 1 g dose × 1. For those who are pregnant, erythromycin is the drug of choice. Treat sexual partners
Gonorrhea Gram-negative intracellular diplococci may occur in pharynx cervix, urethra, or rectum Co-infection with chlamydia common, so treat for both	Purulent, profuse urethral/cervical discharge, dysuria, fever, rash	Cultures of affected orifices Offer HIV testing and syphilis testing	Treat empirically Ceftriaxone (Rocephin) 125 mg IM; cefixime 400 mg × 1, ciprofloxacin (Cipro) 500 mg × 1 plus azithromycin 1 g (treatment for chlamydia) × 1 **OR** doxycycline 100 mg bid × 7 days. Spectinomycin 2 g IM × 1 if allergic to PCN. Treat sexual partners
Genital Ulcer Disease *Herpes simplex* Typically HSV I = oral and HSV II = genital infection; however this is not definitive Incubation = 2-12 days	Burning, hyperesthesia, pain, dysuria, itching, low-grade fever, small grouped vesicles on an erythematous base, lymphadenopathy and tenderness. Primary episode viral shedding is about 12 days and healing of lesions takes 21 days. Recurrent episode viral shedding is about 7 days and lesions heal in about 5 days.	ELISA Testing. Viral Culture = most definitive; negative culture does not mean no herpes because lesions may be dried or drying.	Primary outbreak: acyclovir (Zovirax) 200 mg po 5 × day or 400 mg tid; valacyclovir (Valtrex) 1000 mg bid **OR** famciclovir (Famvir) 250 mg tid × 7-10 days (severity based) Recurrences: acyclovir (Zovirax) 200 mg 5 × day or 400 mg tid × 5 days; valacyclovir (Valtrex) 500 mg bid × 5 days; **OR** famciclovir (Famvir) 125 mg bid × 5 days Prophylaxis if 6 or more occurrences in a year: acyclovir (Zovirax) 400 mg bid; valacyclovir (Valtrex) 500 mg qd; famciclovir (Famvir) 250 mg bid. After 1-year trial, take off medication to see if herpes recurrence. If herpes recurrence, can use over several years if needed.
Chancroid	Painful ulcers, tender inguinal adenopathy, larger ulcer often with exudate	Culture for *Haemophilus ducreyi,* culture or antigen test for HSV, darkfield examination or direct immunofluorescence	Azithromycin (Zithromax) 1 gm × 1 **OR** ceftriaxone (Rocephin) 250 mg IM × 1 **OR** ciprofloxacin (Cipro) 500 mg bid × 3 days **OR** erythromycin base 500 mg qid × 7 days. Follow up in 3-7 days.

*When treating pregnant patients, it is necessary to check the pregnancy category of all drugs being used in treatment.

Table 11-1
Pelvic Pain Differential Diagnostic Cues—cont'd

Diagnosis	Signs and Symptoms	Lab Data	Treatment
Chancroid—cont'd		test for *Treponema pallidum*	Patients should experience decreased symptoms in 3 days and ulcer will be healing in 7 days. Treat partners if had sexual contact during the 10 days prior to onset of symptoms.
Granuloma inguinale (donovanosis) Organism is an intracellular Gram-negative bacterium (*Calymmatobacterium granulomatis*) Relapse may happen 6-18 months after therapy Rare in United States	Painless, progressive, highly vascular ulcer, no regional lymphadenopathy, bleeds easily	Visualization of dark-staining Donovan bodies on tissue preparation or biopsy. Test for other STDs	Trimethoprim-sulfamethoxazole (Bactrim DS) bid × 3 weeks or longer until ulcer is healed **OR** doxycycline 100 mg bid × 3 weeks or until healed **OR** ciprofloxacin (Cipro) 750 mg bid × 3 weeks or until healed **OR** erythromycin base 500 mg qid × 3 weeks or until healed. Follow up until ulcers healed. Treat partners if sexual contact within 60 days of patients symptoms.
Lymphogranuloma venereum Uncommon in the United States Cause is serovars L1, L2, and L3 of *C. trachomatis*	Heterosexual men: unilateral tender inguinal or femoral lymphadenopathy. Women or homosexual men: proctocolitis or inflammation of the perirectal or perianal lymphatic tissues. May have strictures or fistulas	Serology and by exclusion of other causes of genital ulcers and lymphadenopathy	Doxycycline 100 mg bid × 21 days **OR** erythromycin base 500 mg qid × 21 days. Treat partners if sexually active 30 days prior to patient's symptoms. May need to drain buboes
Primary syphilis Secondary (rash, mucocutaneous lesions) Tertiary (cardiac, neurological, ophthalmic, auditory, gummatous lesion)	Ulcer or chancre	Darkfield examination and direct fluorescent antibody tests of lesion exudates or tissue is confirmatory. Presumptive testing includes nontreponemal (VDRL and RPR) – usually correlates with disease activity and treponemal (FTA-ABS and MHA-TP)	Treatment for primary syphilis: benzathine penicillin G 2.4 million units IM × 1. Test for HIV. Partners within 90 days of diagnosis should be treated; if >90 days and testing is unavailable, treat. Long-term sexual partners should be evaluated and treated appropriately. Follow-up is at 6 and 12 months (sooner if follow-up may be problematic). If PCN allergies may give doxycycline 100 mg bid × 2 weeks **OR** tetracycline 500 mg qid × 2 weeks.

Continued

Table 11-1
Pelvic Pain Differential Diagnostic Cues—cont'd

Diagnosis	Signs and Symptoms	Lab Data	Treatment*
Genital Warts *Human papillomavirus virus* 20 types of HPV are associated with the genital tract Types 6 and 11 commonly cause visible genital warts Types 16, 18, 31, 33, and 35 are associated with cervical dysplasia Removal of warts does not eliminate virus Intra-anal warts are most often seen in those who practice receptive anal intercourse	Visible genital warts, usually nonpainful unless irritated	None unless: • Diagnosis is in question • Warts do not respond to treatment • Patient is immunocompromised • Warts are pigmented or indurated or ulcerated (then biopsy)	Patient-applied modalities: podofilox 0.5% solution or gel – apply to wart bid × 3 days then no treatment 4 days (safety in pregnancy is not established). May repeat 4 cycles. Wart area should be <10 cm^2 with no more med than 0.5 ml qd **OR** imiquimod 5% cream – apply at HS 3 × week for up to 16 weeks, wash with mild soap and water 6-10 hours after applied (safety in pregnancy has not been established). Provider treatments: cryotherapy **OR** podophyllin resin 10%-25% in compound of tincture of benzoin – apply small amount to wart and air dry wart area >10 cm^2 or <0.5 ml of med, wash off well 1-4 hours after treatment. Repeat weekly if needed. **OR** TCA (many providers prefer over podophyllin) or BCA 80%-90% — paint area around wart with K-Y jelly or Vaseline then apply small amount of medication to wart and dry. Use powder with talc or sodium bicarbonate to remove unreacted acid. Repeat weekly if needed **OR** surgical excision or laser ablation
Pelvic Inflammatory Disease *Polymicrobial infection of the upper genital tract* Typically associated with *N. gonorrhea* and *C. trachomatis* and endogenous organisms Risk Factors = IUD, smoking, douching, multiple sex partners Increases the risk of infertility, ectopic pregnancies	May be mild or severe. Lower abdominal pain, menstrual irregularities, purulent cervical discharge, chills, fever, cervical and adnexal tenderness Minimum diagnostic criteria: lower abdominal pain, adnexal pain, or CMT Additional criteria: Oral temperature >101° F, abnormal vaginal or cervical discharge,	Endocervical culture, but treat empirically	Determine need for hospitalization for IV antibiotics: • Those who have acute PID • Where other diagnoses must be ruled out (appy or ectopic or tubo-ovarian abscess) • If unable to follow or failed outpatient therapy • Severely ill (N/V, high fever) • Pregnancy • Young age (12-15 years old) • Immunodeficient Outpatient treatment: ofloxacin (Floxin) 400 mg bid + metronidazole (Flagyl) 500 mg bid × 14 days **OR** cefoxitin (Mefoxin)

*When treating pregnant patients, it is necessary to check the pregnancy category of all drugs being used in treatment.

Table 11-1
Pelvic Pain Differential Diagnostic Cues—cont'd

Diagnosis	Signs and Symptoms	Lab Data	Treatment
Pelvic Inflammatory Disease—cont'd	elevated erythrocyte sedimentation rate, elevated C-reactive protein, laboratory results + for *N. gonorrhoeae* or *C. trachomatis*		2 g IM + probenecid 1 g PO bid × 1 + doxycycline 100 mg bid × 14 days **OR** ceftriaxone (Rocephin) 250 mg IM + doxycycline 100 mg bid × 14 days Treat sexual partners
Acute Vaginitis			
Trichomonas Vaginalis	Malodorous, frothy, yellow-green discharge; pruritus; vaginal erythema, and possibly red macular lesions on the cervix "strawberry cervix"; may have strong odor after intercourse	Wet mount with saline: pH >4.5 and motile organisms with flagella Endocervical cultures	Metronidazole (Flagyl) 2 g single dose **OR** 500 mg bid × 7 days (may be more effective). No alcohol while on medicine due to the Antabuse effect. Metronidazole can cause GI upset and produces a metallic taste in the mouth. Patients should be told of the side effects so they are not surprised and discontinue the medication. Treat sexual partners
Vulvovaginal candidiasis Risk factors • DM • AIDS • Pregnancy • Antimicrobial treatment	Dyspareunia, burning, thick and chunky vaginal discharge, vulvar pruritus	Wet mount. 10% KOH improves visualization of yeast by disrupting cellular material (CDC, 1998)	Topical treatments such as clotrimazole (Gyne-Lotrimin) 100 mg vaginal tablet × 7 days **OR** miconazole 200 mg vaginal suppository × 3 days **OR** fluconazole (Diflucan) 150 mg PO × 1 dose. Terconazole 0.4% cream 5 g intravaginally × 7 days **OR** terconazole 0.8% cream 5 g intravaginally × 3 days effective against *Candida glabrata* and *Candida tropicalis*)
Bacterial vaginosis Polymicrobial disease not considered sexually transmitted	Grayish-white malodorous vaginal discharge, pH 4.5, + whiff test	Wet mount with 10% potassium hydroxide check whiff test and saline to check for clue cells + Amine (whiff test)	Metronidazole (Flagyl) 500 mg bid × 7 days **OR** clindamycin vaginal cream 2%, 5 g intravaginally qd × 7 days; **OR** metronidazole gel (0.75%, 5 g) bid × 5 days. Alternatives = metronidazole 2 g PO × 1 **OR** clindamycin 300 mg PO bid × 7 days.
Foreign Body in Posterior Cul de Sac Commonly a retained tampon	Pain in lower abdomen, cramps, malodorous vaginal discharge, dyspareunia	None	Remove foreign body

Text continued from page 197.

azithromycin 1 g × 1 dose. Her sexual partner should also be treated. In addition, L.T. also has a primary outbreak of herpes simplex. She should be started on acyclovir (Zovirax) 200 mg PO 5 × day × 10 days. An adult tetanus injection should be administered.

Patient Education and/or Community Resources   Reportable conditions include gonorrhea, syphilis, chancroid, lymphogranuloma venereum, and chlamydia. In most states, reports are sent to the local health department. For L.T., patient education on sexually transmitted diseases is important. Specifically, patient education about the herpes simplex virus, its treatment and infectious nature during the viral shedding periods, is necessary. The risk of shedding the virus during the asymptomatic period is unclear and should be discussed with the patient. The use of condoms does not work well to protect against herpes simplex because they only cover the penile shaft and not the pubic area where lesions usually occur. L.T. should discontinue douching to protect the normal healthy vaginal environment. In future visits, discuss healthy lifestyle because L.T.'s BMI is 31 and she drinks 8 cups of coffee with sugar and cream daily. Follow-up with health promotion at each scheduled visit.

Back up contraception may be used during antibiotic treatment when the patient is on oral contraceptives. L.T. should not have intercourse until after she and her partner have completed treatment. HIV testing is recommended for any patient who has acquired a sexually transmitted disease.

Follow-Up Plan   Schedule a return visit for a complete physical examination and health promotion. Treatment failure is rare. Have the patient return if symptoms do not resolve or reoccur.

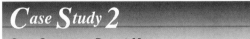

Case Study 2

CHIEF COMPLAINT: Breast Mass

History of Present Illness   N.R. is a 53-year-old Hispanic female who presents with chief complaint of breast mass. She states that she noticed a lump in her breast about 6 months ago, but waited to see if it would go away. N.R. relates that the mass is nontender, hard, and fixed. She has not had a menstrual period since she was 50 years old and is currently taking Prempro (0.625 mg/2.5 mg) 1 tablet qd. Her hot flashes are controlled and she has no vaginal dryness.

Past Medical History   HTN; migraine H/As controlled by Motrin 800 mg q8 hours prn

Past Surgical History   Unremarkable

Family History   Father age 78, HTN; mother age 77, breast cancer; sister age 52, type 2 diabetes; sister age 55, HTN

Developmental Stage   Generativity versus Stagnation

Role/Relationship   Occupation: Nurse. N.R. lives with her 55-year-old husband who is an accountant. She has a daughter age 20 and son age 25, both attending college and in good health. N.R. and her husband live in a two-story home and often travel.

Sleep/Rest   N.R. sleeps 8 hours per night and feels rested.

Nutrition/Metabolic   Eats three well balanced meals per day. Is concerned about her weight and eats healthy foods. Snacks include fresh fruits and vegetables, whole grains, and fruit drinks. She often juices at home

Activity/Exercise   N.R. and her husband either walk or swim 30 to 45 minutes per day. They enjoy being outdoors and exercising together.

Coping/Stress   N.R. uses meditation as a coping strategy. She shares most concerns with her husband or a close friend.

Health Management   Smoked 1 pack a day for 25 years, quit 5 years ago. Mammogram, negative 14 months ago. Pap, 12 months ago was within normal limits. Td: 1/21/99

Medications   Prempro (0.625 mg/2.5 mg) 1 tablet qd. Univasc 7.5 mg qd; Motrin 800 mg q8 hours prn for migraine headaches

Allergies   PCN: rash

Pertinent Physical Findings

Vital Signs   Height 5 feet 6 inches; weight 155 pounds; BMI 25; temperature 98.2° F; heart rate 76; respirations 12; blood pressure 124/78

Breasts: Symmetrical, no tenderness, enlargement, or nipple discharge. R breast, 1 cm hard, fixed mass in upper outer quadrant at 11 o'clock 4 cm from nipple with slight dimpling. L breast, no masses. Lymph nodes, no palpable supraclavicular, infraclavicular or axillary lymphadenopathy

Heart Apical pulse 76, rate regular, no murmurs, S_3 or S_4

Lungs Clear to auscultation

Diagnostics

Diagnostic Tests Mammogram shows clustered polymorphic microcalcification in the upper outer quadrant of the R breast.

History Data Questions specific to the chief complaint of breast mass include the following:

- Do you do breast self-examination (BSE)? If so, how often?
- Have you had any trauma to the breasts?
- How long have you had the breast lump?
- Does the lump stay the same or get bigger and then smaller?
- Does the breast mass change in size before and after menses? (Asked if the patient has menses)
- Do you have any nipple discharge? (If so, is it spontaneous or expressed? What is the type of discharge?)
- Have you had previous breast masses, surgery, or needle aspirations?
- Are you on digoxin, phenytoin, or oral contraceptives?
- When was your last mammogram (for comparison purposes)?

The risk factors for breast cancer should be assessed. The risk factors are: Early menarche (before age 12) and late natural menopause (after age 50); nulliparous; full-term pregnancy after age 35; family history of breast cancer in a first-degree relative especially if premenopausal or bilateral breast disease (Rubin, Voss, Derksen et al, 1996; Tierney, McPhee, and Papadakis, 1999; Uphold and Graham, 1998). Other factors that increase the risk of breast cancer include DES exposure in utero or a personal history of ovarian or endometrial malignancy.

It is important to elicit the patient's concerns and feelings regarding the breast mass. Often, this is a very frightening experience for a woman.

Physical Examination Data The focused examination for chief complaint of breast mass includes: vital signs, breast, and lymph nodes. (Examine for solitary or multiple lesions; location, consistency, and extent of mass; movable or fixed on chest wall; displacement or retraction of nipple; retraction or dimpling of skin overlying mass; palpable lymph nodes – axillary, supra/infra clavicular.) R.T. has a history of mild hypertension so an examination of the heart and lung is included.

Differential Diagnoses: Fibrocystic breast disease, fibroadenoma of the breast, nipple discharge, cancer of the breast, mastitis, Paget's carcinoma (Table 11-2)

Probable Causes of the Presenting Symptoms Cancer of the breast is a proliferation of malignant cells from the breast epithelium (Hurst, 1996). Five percent of breast cancer is hereditary. In women with a personal history of breast cancer, the chances of developing a second primary breast cancer increases 1% per year.

Diagnostic Tests The American Cancer Society recommends a baseline mammogram between the ages of 35 and 40; an annual or biennial mammogram starting at age 40; and after age 50, an annual mammogram (Report of the U.S. Preventive Services Task Force, 1989). N.R.'s diagnostic mammogram showed clustered polymorphic microcalcification in the upper outer quadrant of the right breast (something that is often indicative of malignancy). She should be scheduled for a breast biopsy. Seller (1996) notes that mammograms miss 10% to 15% of lesions; therefore, biopsy of suspicious masses should be performed.

Diagnostic Impression N.R. presents with a nontender, hard, fixed mass. She is postmenopausal and on estrogen therapy. These are classical signs of a breast carcinoma.

Therapeutic Plan of Care N.R. should be referred for a surgical biopsy of the breast mass regardless of results of the mammogram. Treatment will depend on the analysis of the breast biopsy.

> **Table 11-2**
> Breast Mass Differential Diagnostic Cues

Diagnosis	Signs and Symptoms	Lab Data	Treatment
Fibrocystic Breast Disease	Multiple bilateral cyclic fibroglandular breast changes with cyclic pain. Pain and size increase during premenstrual phase of cycle. Common in 30-50 age group	None unless differentiating a carcinoma, then mammography or sonography (useful in determining a cystic versus solid mass in young women). If still unclear, may do fine needle aspiration (FNA) to confirm cystic nature and remove fluid, which may alleviate pain. If fibroadenoma is diagnosed by FNA, refer for surgical excision.	Avoid trauma to breasts. Wear a well fitting brassiere (may also need at night). Take vitamin E 400-800 IU qd. Avoiding caffeine and chocolate may be helpful. Decreased caffeine intake can affect fibrocystic development (Russel, 1989). HRT may be tried **OR** danazol 100-200 mg bid PO, but there are many side effects (e.g., acne, hirsutism, edema).
Fibroadenoma of the Breast	Discrete round, rubbery movable, nontender mass. Common in 20-30 age group	Must differentiate between cyst and carcinoma. If under 30, do ultrasonography. May need fine needle aspiration (FNA) or excisional biopsy	Differentiating cyst from cancer. If cancer, will need surgical intervention with follow-up by medical and radiation oncologist
Nipple Discharge *Galactorrhea* Caused by factors outside the breast Causes include OCP, psychotropics (e.g., imipramine), antihypertensives (e.g., reserpine), methyldopa, pituitary adenomas, brain tumors, thyroid disorders, sexual stimulation, pregnancy	Usually bilateral spontaneous milky discharge that is not related to lactation	Serum prolactin level, TSH, test for occult blood of nipple discharge. If hyperprolactinemia, get CT of pituitary fossa to check for pituitary micro- or macroadenoma. Refer to neurosurgeon if either is found. Mammogram if over 30; ultrasonography if under 30	If medication induced, discontinue the offending agent. If hypothyroidism, treat. If hyperprolactinemia, may be treated with bromocriptine or surgical intervention.

| Table 11-2 | | | |
| Breast Mass Differential Diagnostic Cues—cont'd | | | |
Diagnosis	Signs and Symptoms	Lab Data	Treatment
Nipple discharge from ductal system disorders	Intraductal Papilloma = small, nonpalpable benign tumor in the mammary duct, spontaneous serous or serosanguineous nipple discharge	Occult blood test of nipple discharge, cytology of nipple discharge, mammogram	Refer for surgical intervention
	Duct ectasia = straw-colored, green, or brown discharge, non-cyclic breast pain	Mammogram, occult blood test of nipple discharge	Surgical intervention — wedge excision
Cancer of the Breast Mean age of breast cancer is 60 Alcohol intake, having a first-degree relative with breast cancer, and a high-fat diet may increase the risk of breast cancer. Risk factors include female gender, older age, menarche before age 11 or after age 14, onset of menopause after 55 (Uphold and Graham, 1998)	Single, nontender, fixed, firm mass. Later skin or nipple retraction, dimpling, pain, axillary lymphadenopathy	Mammogram. If a mass, must refer for biopsy	Refer for surgical evaluation and treatment and possible consultation with medical and radiation oncologist
Paget's Carcinoma	Pink or red eczematous areas with hyperkeratosis, itching of the nipple, superficial erosions	Mammogram. Biopsy of the eroded area	Refer for surgical evaluation
Mastitis	Warm, red, tender, swollen area, often on outer quadrant of breast. May have low-grade fever and malaise	None. May perform C&S but seldom done	Dicloxacillin sodium 250-500 mg q 6 hours × 10 days **OR** cephalexin (Keflex) 250-500 mg qid × 10 days. Tylenol 325-650 mg PO q 4 hours (max 4 g) prn. Ice or warm packs prn. Continue breast-feeding, begin on the unaffected breast and proceed to affected one (Younkin and Davis, 1998)

Patient Education and/or Community Resources Provide support for the patient and her family. Should the patient be diagnosed with breast cancer, provide the names of resources such as the American Cancer Society, Betty Ford Breast and Cancer Screening Center, and the local breast cancer organizations. If the patient has fibrocystic breast disease, provide a handout on caffeine content in beverages and foods. Provide breast self-examination and mammography literature. If the patient is on hormone replacement therapy and menses have ceased, encourage her to do breast self-examination on the first day of every month. This provides a monthly cue for the patient to remember to do breast self-examination. For patients who smoke, discuss smoking cessation and treatment options to assist them in quitting. Provide them with literature on smoking cessation and identify support groups in their area. Identify individuals who are supportive and can assist the patient in smoking cessation.

Follow-Up Plan Routine follow-up for annual and prn visits. Review the pathology and the consultant reports to make sure patient is being evaluated and her options are discussed. (Some healthcare providers keep a file system to remind them to follow up on specific patient management plans.) The surgeon often has the patient return to review the results of the pathology report, and if there is a malignancy, they will make recommendations for scheduled follow-up care.

Case Study 3
CHIEF COMPLAINT: Prolonged, Heavy Menses

History of Present Illness D.S. a 42-year-old Caucasian female, presents with chief complaint of irregular, prolonged, heavy menses for 9 months duration. She reports that her menses are no longer regular, but may last from 8 to 14 days and have a 30-day cycle. D.S. feels tired all of the time. Her LMP was 11/29/98, lasting 12 days. The first 4 days were heavy and she changed a super tampon every 2 hours. On days 5 to 8 she had a light flow, changing a maxi pad every 4 hours. On the final 4 days, there was spotting, so she used a mini pad. Birth control: her husband has had a vasectomy. They have a monogamous marriage.

Past Medical History Iron deficiency anemia as a teenager and with her pregnancies.

Past Surgical History T&A at age 5 years

Family History Adoptive father and mother, A&W; no siblings. Further medical history unavailable

Developmental Stage Generativity versus Stagnation

Role/Relationship D.S. is a registered nurse who is currently a homemaker. Her husband is a pediatrician. She has three children ages 4, 6, and 9. Her parents visit often and care for the children so that she can shop and spend quality time with her husband.

Sleep/Rest Sleeps 8 hours per night except when her husband is on call; then, the telephone often awakens her. She awakens rested.

Nutrition/Metabolic D.S. is a gourmet cook and prides herself on her healthy, attractive, and varied meals.

Activity/Exercise Exercises 30 to 45 minutes daily at a health spa. Has a scheduled visit with a personal trainer once per week

Coping/Stress Feels she has a very happy life, enjoys her children and husband. Shares concerns with her mother and her husband

Health Management Drinks 1 to 3 glasses of wine at HS every day. Nonsmoker. Td: 5 years ago; Pap smear 2 years ago was normal. Mammogram, baseline at age 40

Medications Vitality for women vitamins, 1 qd

Allergies NKMA

Pertinent Physical Findings

Vital Signs Height 5 feet 7 inches; weight 135 pounds; BMI 21; temperature 98.2° F; heart rate 76; respirations: 12; blood pressure 120/80

General Appearance Caucasian female, alert and oriented $\times 4$, well-developed and nourished, in no apparent distress

Heart Apical pulse 76, rate regular, no murmurs, no S_3 or S_4

Lungs Clear to auscultation

Abdomen Abdomen soft, nontender, +BS, no organomegaly

Genitalia External genitalia with no lesions, swelling or discharge. No urethral discharge. Vaginal walls without lesions and pink. Cervix is pink with no lesions, scant amount of old blood at the os, uterus anteflexed. No adnexal masses or CMT

Rectal Posterior wall of uterus smooth, no masses. No hemorrhoids, lesions or fissures, no masses or tenderness. Stool for guaiac tests negative

Diagnostics
Diagnostic Tests Pap smear is within normal limits. HCG, negative; pelvic ultrasound, normal. CBC: Hgb, 12.0; Hct, 36; RBC, 4.1 million/ul; differential within normal limits; WBC, 7.2; platelets, 155,000; TSH, 1.2 mg/dl; FSH, 22. Endometrial biopsy is normal

History Data Questions specific to the chief complaint of irregular, prolonged, heavy menses include the following:

- What is the date of your last menstrual period? What is the length of your menses and how heavy is your menses?
- Do you have any clots during menses?
- How many pads or tampons do you use per day?
- Do you have any cramping or abdominal pain?
- Are you sexually active and/or pregnant?
- What do you use for birth control?
- Do you have any pain or bleeding with or after intercourse?
- How many sexual partners do you have?
- How many sexual partners does your partner have?
- Have you ever had a STD?
- Elicit obstetrical history (times pregnant, live births, stillbirths, miscarriages, abortions, and ectopic pregnancies; also vaginal or cesarean section deliveries and complications).
- What is your sleep pattern?
- What is your stress level?
- Do you have fever, chills, N/V, diarrhea, or vaginal discharge?

Physical Examination Data The focused examination for the chief complaint of menstrual irregularity includes: vital signs (check orthostatic BPs if concerned about increased blood loss); neck (examine thyroid); skin (examine for evidence of bleeding disorders [e.g., petechiae or ecchymosis]); heart and lung, abdomen, genitalia, and rectal (speculum examination: observe cervix for polyps, erosions, lesions because these may contribute to vaginal bleeding)

Differential Diagnoses Pregnancy (abortion, ectopic pregnancy), benign neoplasm (fibroid, polyp, endometriosis), cancer (endometrial or cervical), sexually transmitted disease, foreign body, thyroid dysfunction, blood dyscrasia, dysfunctional uterine bleeding (Table 11-3)

Probable Causes of the Presenting Symptoms Normal menses last approximately 4 days with a range of 2 to 7 days. The normal blood loss during menstruation is 40 ml. Blood loss greater than 80 ml per menses is abnormal and may cause anemia.

Dysfunctional uterine bleeding (DUB), the probable cause, is a term used when all other diagnoses are excluded. DUB is caused by an overgrowth of endometrium that results from estrogen stimulation with lack of adequate progesterone (Tierney, McPhee, and Papadakis, 1999). Anovulatory bleeding commonly occurs from estrogen withdrawal or estrogen breakthrough bleeding. Heavy bleeding is often associated with high levels of estrogen. High levels of estrogen are seen in polycystic ovarian syndrome, obesity, immature hypothalamic-pituitary axis (in adolescence), and in late anovulation (in perimenopause) (Speroff, Glass and Kase, 1994).

Terms describing menstrual disturbances are important to know when documenting the patient's symptoms. Table 11-4 lists the common terms used in charting. D.S. is having menometrorrhagia — excessive, frequent, irregular bleeding.

Diagnostic Tests Pregnancy test, CBC, TSH, Pap smear, endometrial biopsy, FSH, LH, pelvic ultrasound (endovaginal probe is best method to check endometrial thickness and uterine structures), STD cultures as appropriate

Diagnostic Impression D.S. has menometrorrhagia, which may be attributed to dysfunctional uterine bleeding. However, all differential diagnoses must be ruled out before diagnosing her con-

Table 11-3
Menstrual Irregularities Differential Diagnostic Cues

Diagnosis	Signs and Symptoms	Lab Data	Treatment
Pregnancy	Amenorrhea, nausea, fatigue, breast tenderness and enlargement	Pregnancy test (quantitative) Pelvic examination Transvaginal ultrasound	Prenatal blood work, prenatal vitamins, and schedule prenatal visits. Offer HIV testing
Spontaneous abortion >50% of women with vaginal bleeding will have a spontaneous abortion in the first trimester	Vaginal bleeding (scant pinkish-brown to large amount of red), cramping or abdominal pain, pelvic pressure, nausea	Pelvic ultrasound. Depending on amount of bleeding, may order CBC. May order serial quantitative serum B-human chorionic gonadotropin (decreasing or low levels indicate a problem)	If first trimester and bleeding heavily, needs emergent attention. If spotting, prescribe bed rest and no coitus, tampons, or douching until resolved. If less than 8 weeks, may pass spontaneously. May need to reassess with ultrasound to check for residual tissue. If >8 weeks, D&C. Rho Gam if indicated
Ectopic pregnancy	Amenorrhea or spotting, pain in lower quadrant, adnexal mass	Quantitative serum pregnancy test (HCG), CBC, and emergency pelvic or transvaginal ultrasound	Refer for emergent surgical intervention **OR** medical intervention (methotrexate)
Benign Neoplasm *Leiomyoma of the uterus (fibroid)*	Irregular enlargement of the uterus, heavy or irregular menses, pelvic pressure	CBC, pelvic ultrasound	If the patient has severe anemia, may use Depo-Provera (medroxyprogesterone acetate) 150 mg IM q 28 days **OR** danazol 400-800 mg/d May consider myomectomy or hysterectomy if problematic. In pregnancy, fibroids tend to enlarge and may cause complications.
Polyp	Abnormal vaginal bleeding and discharge	Endometrial sampling and microscopic evaluation of the polyp to rule out endometrial disease	Removal of polyp with uterine packing or ring forceps Endometrial sampling
Endometriosis	Lower abdominal pain with or without back pain, dyspareunia, rectal pain with or without bleeding, aching pain begins before menses and is worse until flow ceases	Pelvic ultrasound Laparoscopy is diagnostic Proctosigmoidoscopy if bowel involvement	Refer to OB/GYN for laparoscopy treatment plan. Medical therapy includes: GnRH analog **OR** danazol **OR** combination OCPs **OR** medroxyprogesterone acetate. Surgical intervention for severe cases

See Case Study 1 (p. 196) for information on sexually transmitted diseases and foreign body.

Diagnosis	Signs and Symptoms	Lab Data	Treatment
Cervical Cancer Preventative measures include: • Regular Pap smears • Limit number of sexual partners • Use condoms • Stop smoking Cervical infection with the human papillomavirus (HPV) has a strong correlation with cervical dysplasias and cancers.	Often asymptomatic, but may have spotting or bleeding after intercourse	Pap smear from non-menstruating female from the squamocolumnar junction. Colposcopy with biopsy and endometrial sampling. (See Table 11-5 for management of abnormal Pap smears)	Treatment depends on the results of the biopsy. Treatment modalities include: LEEP, cryosurgery, CO_2 laser, loop resection, conization of cervix. Follow-up is often every 3 months with Pap smears $\times$ 2 years, then q 6 months $\times$ 1 year.
Endometrial Cancer Important to rule out with abnormal vaginal bleeding in peri- and post-menopausal women	Abnormal vaginal bleeding. Late stage may have pelvic discomfort	Endocervical and endometrial sampling May do ultrasound to determine the thickness of the endometrium	Refer for surgical intervention, which usually consists of hysterectomy and bilateral salpingo-oophorectomy
Hypothyroidism	Menorrhagia, fatigue, weakness, cold intolerance, hair thinning, dry skin, constipation, muscle cramps	Screening TSH	Levothyroxine qd. Based on TSH levels
Blood Dyscrasia	Abnormal prolonged, heavy, irregular menses, bruising, petechiae	CBC, platelet count, partial thromboplastin time, prothrombin time, and bleeding time	Refer to hematologist
Dysfunctional Uterine Bleeding >70% to 80% of DUB is associated with anovulation. It is more likely to occur when the HPO axis declines in function in females between 40 and 50 years old	Heavy, prolonged, irregular menstrual bleeding, fatigue. Occurs secondary to anovulatory cycles associated with pre- and perimenopause.	CBC, Pap smear, TSH, FSH Pelvic ultrasound if indicated. Cervical biopsy if indicated. Get endometrial biopsy	Medroxyprogesterone acetate 10 mg $\times$ 10-14 days starting on day 15 of the cycle. Repeat $\times$ 3 cycles. **OR** combination OC given 4 pills day 1 then 2 pills days 2-5 then 1 pill daily through day 20 then withdrawal bleeding. Then usual dose 1 qd $\times$ 3 cycles

Table 11-4
Terminology for Describing Menstrual Disturbances

Term	Menstrual Disturbance
Amenorrhea	Absence of menses
Menometrorrhagia	Excessive, frequent, irregular bleeding
Oligomenorrhea	Infrequent menses occurring at periods of greater than 35 days
Menorrhagia	Excessive flow and duration of menses at regular intervals
Ovulatory bleeding	Spotting at midcycle
Intermenstrual bleeding	Bleeding at any time within the normal menstrual cycle
Metrorrhagia	Irregular bleeding
Hypomenorrhea	Light menstrual flow in the normal cycle
Polymenorrhea	Menses occurring at 21 days or less

dition as DUB. D.S.'s diagnostic tests were all negative, therefore she is being treated for DUB.

Therapeutic Plan of Care D.S. could be started on a combination oral contraceptives 1 tablet qd (low dose monophasic so same amount of hormone is given daily instead of fluctuating levels as in the bi- or triphasic preparations). For the patient who is actively bleeding, start with 4 tablets day 1, then 2 tablets days 2-5, then 1 tablet to day 20, then withdrawal bleed. Then start on 1 qd × 3-6 cycles or longer if patient desires oral contraception. Or Provera 10 mg days 16-25 every month may be used or 3 to 6 cycles. Some women prefer to take Provera 10 mg 1 tablet qd days 1-10 of the month because the first day of the new month is a memory trigger to help the patient remember to take the medication. The patient should also understand that using Provera is not contraceptive and that she must use a form of contraception (e.g., condoms, diaphragm). Neither the Provera nor a history of probable anovulatory cycles will provide adequate protection against unwanted pregnancies.

Patient Education and/or Community Resources Patient education should cover the cause and course of the dysfunctional uterine bleeding.

Follow-Up Plan Schedule a follow up examination in 2 weeks to discuss test results and medication response. If bleeding has decreased and is light, schedule follow-up visit in 1 to 3 months. If bleeding persists, schedule sooner. In addition, D.S. should have routine annual breast and pelvic examinations including a Pap smear. D.S. should also have a mammogram because she is over 40 years of age.

Management of Abnormal Pap Smears: The cytological reports from laboratories vary in their reporting of descriptive findings. The system most widely used is the Bethesda System. The cytological report will include a classification, a description of any abnormal cells, and indicate if the human papillomavirus (HPV) is present. The report will indicate if the specimen is adequate and if it is normal. If the sample is abnormal, a recommendation for further diagnostics will be included.

- Atypical squamous cells of undetermined significance (ASCUS) are cells that are atypical.
- ASCUS indicates a need to further investigate why the cells are atypical. The term low-grade squamous intraepithelial lesion (LSIL) indicates mild dysplasia or HPV
- High-grade squamous intraepithelial lesions (HSIL) indicates moderate to severe dysplasia or carcinoma in situ (CIS).
- Table 11-5 describes the management of abnormal Pap smears.

Case Study 4   **Optional Exercise**

CHIEF COMPLAINT: Nausea

History of Present Illness S.N., an 18-year-old Caucasian female, presents with chief complaint of nausea for 1 week duration. After further questioning she reports that her breasts are tender, she feels like she may have the flu, she is tired, and cannot remember the exact date of her LMP. Her

Table 11-5
Management of Abnormal Pap Smears

Category	Description	Treatment
Inadequate sample	Sample was not prepared correctly or there were too few cells to be evaluated	Repeat Pap smear in 6-8 weeks; earlier testing increases the chances for a false-positive result because of poor reparation from previous test. If postmenopausal and inadequate sample, consider topical vaginal estrogen cream for 4-6 weeks and repeat the Pap smear 1-2 weeks after completion.
Normal Sample	Adequate cells were present to determine normalcy; Class I	Repeat Pap smear annually
Infection caused by trichomonad, fungal organism, *Gardnerella*, actinomyces, HSV, chlamydia	Benign cellular changes; Class II	Treat infections identified through symptoms or with Pap smear results Repeat Pap smear in 3 to 6 months; if normal repeat annually. If HSV suspected, do herpes culture for confirmation. Repeat Pap annually. If patient is older than 35 years with IUD and actively colonized actinomyces without symptoms remove IUD and recheck Pap smear in 3 months. If symptomatic with PID, refer for IUD removal and possible IV antibiotics.
Reactive/reparative changes caused by mechanical or chemical irritation, infectious process of chlamydia and gonorrhea, viral infections, posttraumatic repair or invasive carcinomas	Benign metaplasia from inflammatory process and the repair of the tissues by the body's natural defenses; Class II	If gonorrhea or chlamydia, treat and repeat Pap smear in 1 year. With inflammatory changes of unidentified origin, repeat Pap smear in 6 to 12 weeks. If continued inflammatory changes, refer for colposcopy. If postmenopausal and has atrophic vaginitis and Pap smear shows ASCUS or LSIL, treat with topical estrogen vaginal cream for 4-6 weeks and repeat Pap smear. If asymptotic, no further treatment and do routine Pap smears. If IUD, changes are usually benign, routine follow-up is recommended.
Squamous intraepithelial lesions (SIL) caused by cellular changes from HPV, mild to moderate dysplasia, or CIS	Atypical cellular or nucleus changes These changes could be from benign irritation, malignant changes, or HPV infection; Class III May be reported as ASCUS, LSIL, or HSIL	Refer for colposcopy and biopsy with possible surgical intervention. Repeat intervention. Repeat Pap smear q 3 months.
Severe, high-grade or squamous cell carcinoma	Severe dysplasia showing malignancy and CIS; Classes IV and V	Refer to gynecologist
Gland cell abnormalities caused by bacteria, HPV, or adenocarcinoma; common in postmenopausal or anovulatory premenopausal women	Benign endometrial cells or atypical glandular cells may be a sign of exfoliation of cells if endometrial hyperplasia or carcinoma is advancing	Refer to gynecologist

Reprinted with permission from Fenstermacher K, Hudson BT: *Practice guidelines for family nurse practitioners,* Philadelphia, 1997, WB Saunders.

last menstrual period was about 2 months ago. She lives with her parents who are concerned about her illness and encouraged her to see a health care provider. She is sexually active with her 18-year-old boyfriend who is a high school senior and is using withdrawal for contraception. S.N. has no chills, fevers, or any recent illnesses. She has never had a Pap smear. Sexual History: First partner for both S.N. and her boyfriend.

Past Medical History   Unremarkable

Past Surgical History   Unremarkable

Family History   Mother age 42, hypothyroidism; father age 46, A&W; brother age 16, A&W

Developmental Stage   Identity versus Role Confusion

Sleep/Rest   Usually sleeps 8 hours per night, but the last month has been sleeping 9 to 10 hours to feel rested.

Nutrition/Metabolic   Breakfast includes a donut and glass of milk; lunch is usually a hot lunch she takes to school. For dinner she eats with her parents. Meals usually includes pasta, vegetables, meat, and a dessert. Snacks include candy, fruit, crackers, and chips. S.N. drinks 2 to 5 cola products per day.

Activity/Exercise   S.N. practices for cheerleading 1 hour twice a week and usually cheers at one or two games per week. She enjoys swimming, walking, and biking. Is engaged in one sport per season

Coping/Stress   S.N. is a high school senior who is consistently on the honor roll and is a cheerleader for the varsity team. She feels very close to her parents and boyfriend. Talks to her close friends and boyfriend about concerns. Religion: Jehovah's Witness.

Health Management   Td: 1 year ago. Usually does not see a health-care provider unless she is really sick. Has had her sports physical examinations at the local high school. Does not perform routine breast self-examination and is unsure how to do this

Self-Perception and Values/Beliefs   S.N. has a positive self-image and enjoys life. She is very happy with her academic achievement and is excited about attending college to pursue a baccalaureate degree in education. Her goal is to teach 4th grade students in a local school.

Medications   None
Allergies   None

Pertinent Physical Findings

Vital Signs   Height 5 feet 5 inches; weight 135 pounds; BMI 23; temperature: 97.6° F; heart rate 76; respirations 12; blood pressure 110/70

Neck   Supple without JVD or thyromegaly, no cervical lymphadenopathy, trachea is midline.

Heart   RRR at 76, without murmurs, no S_3 or S_4, PMI 5th ICS-LMCL

Lungs   Clear to auscultation and equal bilaterally, no adventitious breath sounds, resonant throughout lung fields

Breast   Symmetrical, mild tenderness and fullness, no dimpling, or masses, no nipple discharge, no axillary lymphadenopathy

Abdomen   Slightly rounded, active bowel sounds, no abdominal bruits, soft, no masses or organomegaly, nontender, no inguinal lymphadenopathy, no CVA tenderness

Genitalia   External genitalia with no lesions, discharge, or rashes; vaginal mucosa pink and moist, no CMT or adnexal masses, cervix soft with bluish color, fundus palpated below symphysis pubis

Diagnostics

Diagnostic Tests   + Urine pregnancy test

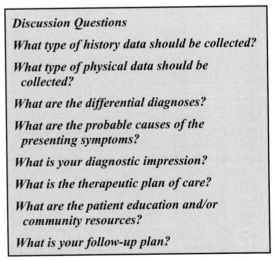

Discussion Questions

What type of history data should be collected?

What type of physical data should be collected?

What are the differential diagnoses?

What are the probable causes of the presenting symptoms?

What is your diagnostic impression?

What is the therapeutic plan of care?

What are the patient education and/or community resources?

What is your follow-up plan?

Discussions for optional case study exercises can be found in the accompanying Instructor's Manual.

References

Centers for Disease Control and Prevention: *1998 Guidelines for treatment of sexually transmitted diseases* 47(RR-1), Atlanta, 1998, United States Department of Health and Human Services.

Fenstermacher K, Hudson BT: *Practice guidelines for family nurse practitioners,* Philadelphia, l997, WB Saunders.

Hurst JW: *Medicine for the practicing physician,* Stamford, Conn., 1996, Appleton & Lange.

U.S. Preventative Services Task Force: *Guide to clinical preventative services,* Baltimore, 1998, Williams and Wilkinson.

Rubin H, Voss C, Derksen DJ et al: *Medicine: a primary care approach,* Philadelphia, 1996, WB Saunders.

Russel LC: Caffeine restrictions as initial treatment for breast pain, *Nurs Pract* 14(2):36-37, 40, 1989.

Seller RH: *Differential diagnosis of common complaints,* Philadelphia, 1996, WB Saunders.

Speroff L, Glass R., Kase N: *Clinical gynecologic endocrinology and fertility,* Baltimore, 1994, Williams and Wilkinson.

Tierney L, McPhee SJ, Papadakis MA: *Current medical diagnosis and treatment,* Stamford, Conn., 1999, Appleton & Lange.

Uphold C, Graham, M: *Clinical guidelines in family practice,* Gainesville, Fla., 1998, Barmarrae Books.

Younkin EQ, Davis MS: *Women's health: a primary care clinical guide,* Norwalk, Conn., 1998, Appleton & Lange.

Selected Readings

Bravender T, Emans SJ: Menstrual disorders. Dysfunctional uterine bleeding, *Pediatr Clin North Am* 46(3):545-553, 1999.

Dealy MF: Dysfunctional uterine bleeding in adolescents, *Nurse Pract* 23(5):12-13, 16, 18-20, 1998.

Ford K, Marcus E, Lum B: Breast cancer screening, diagnosis, and treatment, *Dis Mon* 45(9):335-405 1999.

Sedlacek TV: Advances in the diagnosis and treatment of human papillomavirus infections *Clin Obstet Gynecol* 42(2):206-220, 1999.

Volpe CM, Raffetto JD, Collure DW, Hoover EL, Doerr RJ: Unilateral male breast masses: cancer risk and their evaluation and management, *Am Surg* 65(3):250-253, 1999.

CHAPTER 12

Dermatological Disorders

Katherine Barbee

Case Study 1

CHIEF COMPLAINT: Acne

History of Present Illness M.R. is a 15½-year-old Caucasian male, accompanied by his mother, who presents with a chief complaint of "problems with acne." He reports that he first noticed a few "pimples" when he was 14½ years old. At the time he didn't need to use any special cleansers or creams and washed only with Dove soap. However, over the past 6 months he has been having more pimples, mostly on his face with a few scattered on his anterior chest, shoulders, and upper back, some have been large and lasting 5 to 7 days. The larger pimples can be tender and painful, are usually filled with "pus" and he often "pops" them. He has been using OTC salicylic acid products such as Clearasil but reports that they don't seem to be helping. His mother also reports that he has wanted to stay home from school on several occasions and has declined social invitations because he is embarrassed when his skin is "really bad."

Past Medical History Exercise induced asthma, allergic rhinitis, ADHD

Past Surgical History Bilateral myringotomy with tympanostomy tubes inserted × 3 at ages 12 mos, 2½ yrs and 4½ yrs

Family History Mother and father A&W with no history of severe acne; two brothers and two sisters, all older, with no history of severe acne (all other family members experienced mild acne vulgaris in teens and early 20s, none with any residual scarring)

Developmental Stage Identity vs. Role Confusion

Role-Relationship Lives with his parents and one older brother (other siblings in college or living on their own). Attends local public high school as a 10th grader, does fair in school and enjoys playing on the JV football team

Sleep/Rest Sleeps 6 to 8 hours a night but at times has difficulty falling asleep or awakens after only 4 to 5 hours sleep and is unable to return to sleep

Nutrition/Metabolic Generally eats two or three meals a day and snacks often. Usually has cold cereal and juice for breakfast; lunches often in the school cafeteria on french fries and pizza or hamburger; dinner, eats meal that his mother prepares (usually a meat, vegetable or salad, and a starch). Snacks on chips, microwave sandwiches, occasional fruit, ice cream, and soda. Consumes milk with his breakfast cereal and at lunch

Activity/Exercise Rides his bike to school and in the neighborhood, works out with the football team and in the weight training room at school. In his leisure time he prefers to watch TV or play video games or hang-out with his friends. He vacations at the beach for 2 to 3 weeks each summer.

Coping/Stress Has recently become less open with his family and tends to withdraw to his room or sulk when he is frustrated. Has been in several fights with his friends when he feels they are teasing him about his skin or about being chubby. His teachers report that he occasionally comes to class "with a chip on his shoulder" and sits in the back of the room slumped at his desk with his head down. His mother reports that he recently talks less with his friends on the phone and spends more time alone in his room.

Health Management Denies tobacco, alcohol or recreational drug use. Immunizations are up to date on MMR, polio, tetanus, and hepatitis B. He had chickenpox at 7 months. He rarely uses sunscreen because he "tans easily."

Self-Perception and Values/Beliefs M.R. reports feeling ugly and fat because of his skin and weight problems. He states that "it's no wonder I don't have a girlfriend."

Medications Albuterol MDI prn, OTC antihistamines prn, Adderall 20 mg BID

Allergies Allergic to sulfa antibiotics, penicillin drugs, and Ceclor

Pertinent Physical Findings

Vital Signs Height 5 feet 10 inches; weight 210 pounds; BMI 30; temperature 98.4° F; blood pressure 112/72; pulse 68; RR 14

General Appearance Alert, oriented × 3, mood withdrawn with head down, answering questions initially with one or two words, appears angry when describing feelings about skin appearance; moderately obese, casually dressed, 15½-year-old Caucasian male

Skin Coloring is fair with medium brown hair and hazel eyes. The patient has some fine facial hair on his upper lip but has not started shaving. Multiple closed and open comedones appear on the cheeks, forehead, and chin with inflamed papules and papulopustules also scattered on cheeks, forehead, and chin. Anterior chest, bilateral shoulders, and upper back appear with scattered inflamed papules and open comedones. Three discrete pustules are apparent on the upper back, as well as one on left shoulder. There is also violaceous scarring on bilateral cheeks. No cysts, nodules, or sinus tracts are apparent. No sinus tracts or local induration palpated. Neck: No enlarged or tender lymph nodes. No thyromegaly, nodules, or tenderness

Diagnostics
Diagnostic Tests None

History Data Demographic information is important when evaluating any dermatological complaint. Age, race, and gender may help initially in limiting your differential diagnoses. Acne vulgaris is most common among teens and young adults in their 20s, although it may persist into later adulthood, more commonly extending into adulthood in females than in males. Rosacea and perioral dermatitis are more common in adults up to mid-50s age group. Acne vulgaris and nodulocystic acne development is associated with circulating androgens. They therefore have a higher incidence and are often more severe in males, whereas rosacea and perioral dermatitis have a higher incidence in females. Acne vulgaris is more common in Caucasian people and less common among people of African and Asian descent. Work and recreational habits impact dermatological conditions. Working in hot, greasy surroundings such as commercial kitchens or machine shops may increase the likelihood of acne vulgaris, as does wearing occlusive cosmetics or hats. Sun exposure and sun protection are important data to collect since many dermatologic preparations can cause photosensitivity.

Questions specific to the chief complaint of acne include the following:

- What do the lesions look like?
- Where are the lesions?
- Describe the types of pimples you are having. Are they mostly whiteheads, blackheads, or are they pus-filled pimples/zits?
- How long have you been experiencing acne?
- Have the pimples changed in character or number since they began?
- What treatments have you tried (determine whether scarring is secondary to "popping the pimples" and what OTC products have been used with consistency)?
- What is your normal skin care (including soap used and any harsh rubbing or scrubbing)?

For female patients, obtain a menstrual history. Acne vulgaris may be associated with hormonal imbalances such as polycystic ovaries.

Physical Examination Data The focused examination for the chief complaint of acne includes: vital signs, general appearance, and a skin and lymph node assessment. If the patient is female, assess for any virilization features such as facial hair, excess upper body weight, and deepened voice. Also assess the thyroid gland for any enlargement, nodules, or tenderness.

Differential Diagnoses Conditions that may present with lesions on the face and upper chest and back include acne vulgaris (mild, moderate), nodulocystic or severe acne vulgaris, rosacea, perioral dermatitis, infectious folliculitis, furunculosis/abscess formation, and tinea barbae (Table 12-1).

Probable Causes of the Presenting Symptoms
Acne vulgaris is the most common dermatological presenting complaint in primary care (Meredith PV et al, 2000) (Figure 12-1). It occurs most often in adolescence (age 10 to 17 years in females, 14 to 19 years in males) and more often in males than in females. It also tends to occur in a more severe form in males.

Acne vulgaris is a disorder of the pilosebaceous unit and results from excess sebum production, abnormal keratinization (comedogenesis), proliferation of *P. acnes,* and an inflammatory response (Figure 12-2). Excess sebum production is associated with increased circulating androgens, a condition associated with puberty and with some pathological states such as polycystic ovary disease. The pilosebaceous units that are most often affected by acne vulgaris are those of

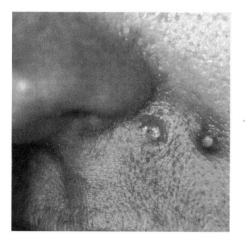

Figure 12-1 Acne vulgaris – the face, upper chest, and back are most commonly affected. Pilosebaceous units become obstructed, forming characteristic comedones, closed comedones, or pustules. (From Meredith PV et al: *Adult primary care,* Philadelphia, 2000, WB Saunders.)

the face, upper back, anterior chest, and shoulders. When evaluating your patient for acne vulgaris it is important to expose the upper body, protecting a patient's privacy with an open back gown. Natural light is optimal for evaluating the skin, but when not available it is helpful to have ceiling lighting so as not to cast any shadows on the skin. Tangential lighting is important when evaluating for raised lesions such as would be found in nodulocystic acne.

Not only does acne vulgaris adversely affect an adolescent's skin, it may have a profound impact on a teen's self-image. Several studies have looked at the impact of acne on an adolescent's attitude and outlook on life (Pearl et al, 1998; Gupta MA, Gupta AK, 1998; Anderson and Rajagopalan, 1998). All suggest that acne has a negative effect on a teen's self-perception and outlook on life, and impact negatively on the ability to participate in or receive pleasure from social activities. Successful treatment of acne is also correlated with improved ability to enjoy social activities and improved self-perception. When evaluating a patient with acne it is important to screen for a negative self-image and depression and to address the psychosocial needs of your patient.

Diagnostic Tests Cultures are usually not warranted in the evaluation of acne vulgaris. This is a diagnosis that is generally made based on the clinical presentation of comedogenic lesions. Whereas other conditions (such as rosacea, perioral dermatitis, or folliculitis) may present with an "acneform" cluster of lesions on the face and upper torso, only acne vulgaris presents with comedones. Rosacea was referred to even in the recent past as "acne rosacea" or "adult form acne," but these terms are no longer considered acceptable because it produces no true comedogenic lesions. Cultures may be helpful in cases where more than one type of lesion is present, or when a patient's acne suddenly worsens after being treated with systemic antibiotics. In this case there is likely to be a secondary infection as a result of prolonged antibiotic use, and culture and sensitivity may narrow antibiotic options. However, even in this situation, cultures are usually not done because treatment with either TMP-SMX or ampicillin after stopping the previous antibiotic is often successful.

Table 12-1
Acne Differential Diagnostic Cues

Diagnosis	Signs/Symptoms	Lab Data	Treatment
Acne Vulgaris Mild Moderate Nodulocystic	Basic lesions: open and closed comedones, papules, and pustules Mild acne-open comedones (blackheads), closed comedones (whiteheads), papules, pustules Moderate acne includes all of the aforementioned lesions as well as inflamed papules Nodulocystic acne includes basic lesions of acne vulgaris with nodulocystic lesions and sinus tract formation under the skin	None unless there is extensive suppuration, in which case a CBC would be warranted to rule out sepsis	Gentle washing bid with mild soap (Dove, Basis, Neutrogena) Keratolytic topical agents — 2.5%, 5%, or 10% Benzoyl Peroxide gel qd to bid. May cause inflammation or drying, therefore start with lowest dose and increase as tolerated Topical antibiotics for inflamed papules or papulopustules exert antiinflammatory and antibiotic effect against *P. acnes*. 1% or 2% erythromycin or clindamycin 1% gel, solution, lotion (Cleocin T) For severe or persistent cases add comedolytic agent: topical tretinoin (Retin-A) 0.025% to 0.1% cream or 0.025% to 0.01% gel (potential side effects include photosensitivity, dry skin and mucous membranes, headache, cheilitis, nausea, vomiting, arthralgias and myalgias, rash, and fatigue) or adapalene 0.1% gel (Differin) qd to bid (potential side-effects include photosensitivity, rash, dryness and pruritus, and stinging). Start with lowest dose then increase gradually PO antibiotics for antiinflammation, antibiotic activity against *P. acnes*. Tetracycline or erythromycin drugs 50 to 250 mg qd to tid. Potential side effects range from mild symptoms of dyspepsia, diarrhea, allergic urticaria, photosensitivity to more severe symptoms of lupus-like syndromes, and pseudotumor cerebri (both associated with tetracycline drugs) Isotretinoin (Accutane), a systemic retinoid, indicated in severe nodulocystic acne. Refer to dermatologist. Potential side effects: teratogenicity, excessive drying of skin and mucous membranes, nausea/vomiting, abdominal pain, lab abnormalities, thinning of hair, conjunctivitis, petechiae, nail brittleness, cheilitis

Continued

Table 12-1
Acne Differential Diagnostic Cues—cont'd

Diagnosis	Signs/Symptoms	Lab Data	Treatment
Rosacea	Papules and tiny pustules with episodic flushing and telangiectases, mainly on the cheeks and nose. No comedones. Late symptoms include hyperplasia and lymphedema with possible rhinophyma. Possible conjunctivitis and blepharitis	None	Avoid flushing triggers such as hot liquids, alcohol, spicy foods, emotional stress, exposure to sun/wind, medications such as niacin 0.75% topical metronidazole, erythromycin, or clindamycin bid PO tetracycline or erythromycin 250 mg qd to tid with topical in severe or persistent cases
Perioral Dermatitis	Papules and papulopustules on erythematous base, mainly in the perioral region (sparing the vermilion border) may include glabella, forehead, periorbital regions	None	0.75% topical metronidazole bid PO tetracycline derivatives 100-500 mg qd to bid indicated for persistent lesions
Infectious Folliculitis Infection of the hair follicle with bacterial, viral or fungal agents Commonly caused by *S. aureus* but may be caused by tinea or herpes simplex virus	Papules and pustules confined to the perifollicular region May be surrounded by an erythematous halo Distinguishing characteristic of folliculitis from acne is the absence of comedones in folliculitis	Gram stain of exudate (Gram negative in cases of folliculitis secondary to prolonged antibiotic use) KOH prep to assess for tinea cultures (including a viral for herpes)	Bacterial folliculitis: • Mupirocin (Bactroban) ointment bid-tid × 7-14 days • PO dicloxacillin, cephalexin or erythromycin 250-500 mg qid • Ciprofloxacin 500 mg bid for *pseudomonas* • Secondary to prolonged treatment of acne vulgaris – d/c antibiotic, start ampicillin 250 mg qid or SMX-TMP qid, continue with benzoyl peroxide and isotretinoin

Diagnostic Impression   M.R. is an adolescent male with multiple facial and upper torso lesions including open and closed comedones, inflamed papules, and papulopustules. There are no nodulocystic lesions or sinus tracts apparent. He has tried first level acne treatment without success, leading to the diagnosis of moderate acne vulgaris.

Therapeutic Plan of Care   M.R. and his mother should be educated about acne vulgaris and myths such as effect of diet on acne should be dispelled. Educating both M.R. and his mother may address his feelings of low self-esteem if he and his family are able to appreciate the common nature of the disorder, its association to puberty, and the po-

Table 12-1
Acne Differential Diagnostic Cues—cont'd

Diagnosis	Signs/Symptoms	Lab Data	Treatment
Infectious Folliculitis —cont'd Pseudofolliculitis barbae affects mostly African-American males and results from penetration of the skin by sharp shaved hairs. It is often complicated by *S. aureus*. Can complicate acne vulgaris in patient treated with antibiotics for extended period.			
Furunculosis/ Abscess Formation/ Carbuncles Deep-seated local infection Most often secondary to *S. aureus*	Inflammation and induration Central necrotic plug Tenderness and pain Lymphadenopathy	Cultures are usually not indicated. Most lesions are colonized with *S. aureus*	Hot, moist compresses × 10 min qid PO cephalexin, dicloxacillin, or erythromycin 250-500 mg qid 7-14 days Septic patients: IV ceftriaxone 1 gm qd × 5-7 days
Tinea Barbae Dermatophytic trichomycosis with invasion of the hair follicle	Pustules with surrounding erythema Scaling, annular patches with or without alopecia Lymphadenopathy	Usually none KOH prep identify buds and hyphae Woods light may cause lesions to fluoresce green Fungal cultures identify fungus	Spectazole cream bid × 2-4 weeks PO itraconazole 100 mg bid **OR** terbinafine 200 mg qd **OR** fluconazole 100 mg bid × 10-14 days

tentially successful treatments available. Education is also important in eliciting M.R.'s participation in the course of treatment. Prescribe medications either alone or in combination. Initially prescribe a keratolytic agent such as benzoyl peroxide in 2.5%, 5%, or 10% gel or lotion qd to bid. Because these preparations may be drying and/or irritating to the skin, it is best to start with the lowest potency preparation (2.5% lotion) qd. After 7 to 10 days, irritative symptoms should have regressed and the dose may then be increased to bid. In conjunction with benzoyl peroxide, a topical antibiotic may be helpful in decreasing inflammation and exerting an antibacterial effect on *P. acnes*. Prescribe either

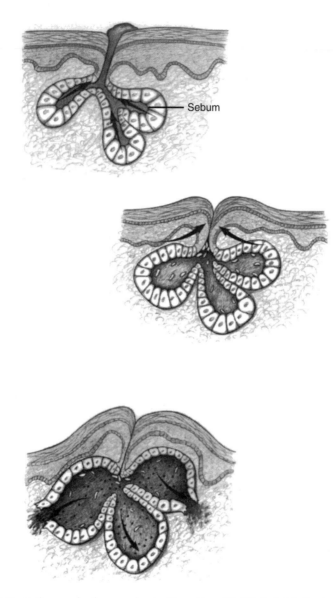

Figure 12-2   Pathogenesis of acne vulgaris. (From Meredith PV et al: *Adult primary care,* Philadelphia, 2000, WB Saunders.)

topical erythromycin 1% or 2% gel (Ery-stat) or clindamycin gel (Cleocin T). For increased ease of treatment and improved compliance, a combination benzoyl peroxide antibiotic gel (Benzamycin topical) is available. At subsequent visits a decision should be made whether to add third and/or fourth lines of treatment. If improvement is not appreci- ated after 4 to 6 weeks, add a topical comedolytic agent such as tretinoin (Retin-A) or adapalene (Differin) qd to bid. These preparations are also drying and potentially irritating and should also be started at the lowest dosage and qd. Increase dosage strength and frequency as tolerated. Creams are generally less irritating than gels, and each preparation comes in a range of dosage strengths from 0.01% to 0.1%. Another approach for persistent or more involved cases would be to add an oral antibiotic to the daily regimen. This may be done in place of the topical antibiotic or prior to trying the topical comedolytic agent. When there is acne involvement of the back, shoulders and chest, oral antibiotic treatment is often considered as a first line approach since it is more difficult to adequately treat these areas with topical agents alone. The oral antibiotics generally considered are tetracycline derivatives (e.g., minocycline 50 to 250 mg qd to tid, tetracycline 150 to 250 mg qd to tid, doxycycline 100 to 200 mg qd to bid, or erythromycin 250 to 500 mg qd to qid). Oral antibiotics are usually tolerated well enough to start at the higher dose and more frequent dosing schedule until symptoms are improving; then they can be tapered down to a maintenance dose. Allergies and potential side effects need to be considered prior to prescribing any drugs. Side effects may range from mild symptoms of dyspepsia and or diarrhea to potential photosensitivity (tetracycline derivatives) or more severe pseudotumor cerebri (tetracycline derivatives) or lupus-like syndrome (tetracycline derivatives). Both of these more severe reactions usually will disappear when the drugs are stopped, but there exists the potential for negative sequelae associated with both syndromes.

Patient Education and/or Community Resources As mentioned earlier, patient education is very important in dispelling any myths about acne and in encouraging cooperation and compliance. Understanding the common nature of acne and its association with puberty may help improve the patient's self-esteem while dealing with this unpleasant condition. Teaching the patient about proper skin care may help to prevent later scarring that may occur from "popping pimples" or roughly abrading lesions with harsh scrubbing. It is also important to stress the need for sun protection because many of the acne treatments have a potential to cause photosensitivity and/or severe sunburns. Presenting education programs in local schools or providing information in the schools or in your office is a helpful way to educate teens about acne and its treatment. It may also be helpful in providing an opening for patients to feel comfortable discussing their acne and their feelings about it. The

American Academy of Dermatology (AAD) maintains a website entitled ACNENET that is both educational and supportive, providing an avenue for patients to communicate with representatives of the AAD and receive feedback.

Follow-Up Plan Revisits for reevaluation should not be scheduled any closer than every 4 to 6 weeks. Improvement is usually not appreciated during the first 2 to 3 weeks of any of the above treatment options. More frequent reevaluation may therefore frustrate the patient with expectations of unrealized improvement. Adding or changing medications prior to a 4- to 6-week trial may eliminate effective treatment options too early in the course. On the other hand, having the patient revisit every 4 to 6 weeks allows the practitioner to evaluate the treatment effectiveness and assess the patient's emotional response to treatment. As mentioned earlier, low self-esteem and depression can complicate acne vulgaris, and practitioners need to be aware of this potential and provide appropriate intervention as indicated.

Acne vulgaris treatment is commonly prolonged, lasting several months to several years. Treatment usually needs to span the years of adolescence and may need to be extended into early adulthood. Once an acceptable level of control has been reached, it is appropriate to decrease some of the medications. Since the comedolytic agents are particularly drying and may be irritating, weaning the patient off of these preparations would be the first step. If the patient continues to do well after stopping the tretinoin or adapalene, then the next step would be weaning off of either the topical keratolytic and/or antibiotic. Some patients require a low maintenance dose of the oral antibiotics for several years to prevent recurrence of acne.

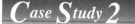

Case Study 2

CHIEF COMPLAINT: Brown Patches on Face

History of Present Illness F.A. is a 63-year-old Caucasian male who presents with a chief complaint of pink and tan patches on his face. He has worked as a construction site supervisor for the past 20 years. Prior to that he worked as a laborer for the same company. He has had these patches for about 3 years, but recently noticed a new and larger patch on his left forehead. His wife is worried because it appears to have a roughened surface. F.A. denies any sensation of pain, pruritus, or dysesthesia, but reports some tenderness when the patch is palpated or rubbed. He denies any exudate, but reports that he awakened one morning with dried blood on his pillow that he assumed came from scratching the area in his sleep. He has tried no treatments and admits that his usual practice of skin care consists of washing his face with mild soap and warm water during his morning and evening shower. He offers that he is not particularly worried about these "spots" on his face since he assumes that they are "just age spots. I wouldn't be here if my wife wasn't nagging me about it."

Past Medical History   Hypertension and gouty arthritis

Past Surgical History   T&A at age 8

Family History   Both parents died in their late 70s of cardiac related disorders. One sister is A&W. No known family history of any skin cancers, but only his mother shared his fair skin and reddish-blond hair and she avoided the sun her entire life. His father and sister have olive skin, dark hair and eyes, and tan easily. He does not come from a family of "sun worshippers."

Developmental Stage   Integrity vs. Despair

Role-Relationship   Lives with his wife of 43 years in a three-bedroom house in the suburbs. He bought a lot on the river 5 years ago where he and family and friends often go to get away and do some fishing. His one son, aged 40, is also a construction worker for the same company. He has one daughter, aged 37, who is married and works in a bank in another city. F.A. has five grandchildren. His son has two daughters and F.A. sees them several times a week since his son lives in the same development and they often socialize or share meals. He sees his daughter's two sons and one daughter about once a month when their family comes for the weekend. He reports feelings of great happiness and pride in his family and satisfaction with his ability to "get through the lean times when the children were little." He and his wife often "take the grandkids for a weekend to let the younger ones have some fun."

Sleep/Rest   Sleeps 6 to 7 hours a night, going to bed after the 10 o'clock news and awakening to the alarm at 5:30 AM. He denies any difficulty sleeping and reports feeling rested.

Nutrition/Metabolic   Eats three meals a day. His wife usually does the cooking, preparing eggs and bacon for breakfast and packing him two cold cut sandwiches, chips, cookies, and coffee for lunch. She also prepares dinner, usually a meal of meat, potatoes, and bread. He loves desserts and says his wife bakes cakes and pies two or three times a week. He rarely eats snacks other than eating salted nuts when he drinks his two beers after work.

Activity/Exercise   Leisure activities involve playing 18 or 36 holes of golf on the weekends, fishing with his family, and working in the yard.

Coping/Stress   Denies any stress in his life over the past 15 to 20 years. Early in his marriage he argued a lot with his wife over money issues, but feels things are better now. He no longer attends the Baptist church to which his family belongs. "I let my wife do all the praying now. I really don't miss the church."

Health Management   Drinks two or three beers daily and a six-pack on the weekends. Smokes 1 to 1½ packs of cigarettes a day and has done so for 50 years. Immunizations: Td 9/95

Self-Perception and Values/Beliefs   Is pleased with his life and proud that he has managed to attain some financial security in spite of having to struggle earlier in life. He feels committed to his wife and children and is happy that he can help his children now with childcare.

Medications   Sustained-release verapamil 180 mg qd, indomethacin 25 mg tid for acute gout, occasional acetaminophen for headache

Allergies   NKMA

Pertinent Physical Findings

Vital Signs   Height 5 feet 9 inches; weight 162 pounds; BMI 23; temperature 98.2° F; pulse 68; RR 12; blood pressure 128/78

General Appearance   Alert and oriented × 3, pleasant and relaxed, casually dressed 63-year-old Caucasian male with thinning strawberry blond hair and blue eyes, in NAD

Skin   Fair coloring, skin phototype (SPT) II (Table 12-2)

Table 12-2
Skin Phototypes Based on Sun Sensitivity

Skin Type	Sunburn and Tanning History
I	Always burns easily; rarely tans
II	Always burns easily: tans minimally
III	Burns moderately; tans gradually and uniformly to a light brown color
IV	Burns minimally, always tans well to moderate brown color
V	Rarely burns; tans profusely to dark brown color
VI	Rarely burns; deeply pigmented black color

From Meredith PV et al: *Adult primary care*, Philadelphia, 2000, WB Saunders.

Face Multiple, discrete, adherent, scaly, reddish-tan, oval and round lesions ranging from 8 to 12 mm with roughened surfaces scattered on the forehead, temples, nose, and neck. No surrounding inflammation or induration is apparent. A 1.2-cm lesion on the left forehead superior to and not contiguous with the left eyebrow appears darker tan with a significantly roughened surface. This lesion alone is tender to palpation. No exudate or bleeding is apparent.

Scalp No suspicious pigmented lesions are apparent.

Upper extremities Few scattered similar reddish-tan oval lesions discretely scattered on dorsum of both wrists. Distinct tan lines apparent above both elbows and multiple tan 1 to 2 mm freckles cover both arms.

Torso and lower extremities Multiple light tan 1-2 mm freckles on torso, clustered more heavily on back and on both legs and dorsum of both feet. Tan lines exist at mid-thigh level bilaterally and freckles are increased in number below the tan lines. No suspicious appearing larger, raised, or scaly lesions appear on any body surfaces other than his face and upper extremities.

Diagnostics

Diagnostic Tests Biopsy of large lesion on forehead and three to five other lesions will be helpful in confirming the diagnosis.

History Data Questions specific to the chief complaint of an abnormal lesion on the face include the following:

- What is the appearance of the concerning lesion and what is different or worrisome about this lesion to you and/or your family?
- Describe the typical state of your skin and what has changed to cause you concern.
- How long have you been aware of the unusual skin lesions? Have any of them recently changed in character?
- Do any of the lesions tend to fade or disappear?
- Is there any numbness, tingling, burning, itching, or pain associated with the lesions? Is there any exudate or bleeding from the lesions?
- Have you experienced any unexplainable weight loss or decreased energy?
- Have you tried any treatments for your skin?
- Do you practice any sun exposure precautions? What is your typical level of sun exposure?
- Is there any family history of skin cancers or precancerous skin lesions?

Look for "red flags" when eliciting a history. Red flags for skin lesions include prolonged unprotected sun exposure, especially for patients with SPT I and II; new or changing lesions; large (greater than 6 mm), multicolored/variegated, raised, or irregularly shaped lesions; and a personal history or family history of cutaneous carcinomas.

Physical Examination Data The focused examination for the chief complaint of an unusual skin lesion includes vital signs, general appearance, and a thorough examination of the skin. A more complete physical examination is not necessary unless indicated by history or general appearance of the patient, including vital signs.

Differential Diagnosis The most common conditions that can present as pigmented facial lesions include actinic keratosis/solar keratosis, seborrheic keratosis, and cutaneous carcinomas (including BCC, SCC, and MM) (Table 12-3).

Table 12-3
Pigmented Facial Lesion Differential Diagnostic Cues

Diagnosis	Signs and Symptoms	Lab Data	Treatment
Actinic/Solar Keratosis Middle aged to elderly Males >females SPT I, II, and III. Rare in SPT IV and extremely rare in dark-skinned and East Indian races Frequent and/or prolonged unprotected sun exposure is a strong risk factor Precursor to squamous cell carcinoma	Single or multiple discrete lesions Dry, roughened and scaly surface Adherent patches Only on sun-exposed skin Remain for months to years, may disappear May be tender May bleed if surface disturbed	Biopsy is necessary to rule squamous cell carcinoma. This can be done by the primary care provider or dermatologist	Prevention is of utmost importance and should be encouraged even after diagnosis to avoid future lesions Topical 5% 5-fluorouracil cream several days to weeks Cryotherapy (liquid nitrogen) alone or followed by 3 day course of 5% 5-fluorouracil Excision of large or nodular lesions
Seborrheic Keratosis Benign epithelial tumor Very common Hereditary – probably autosomal dominant Usually occurs from third decade and throughout lifetime	Skin colored to tan, scattered or discrete macules initially Progress to brown, black or gray round/oval papules or patches "stuck on," possibly greasy, warty surface with plugged follicles called "horn cysts" Isolated or generalized on face, trunk, arms	Biopsy of warty appearing lesions, either by the primary care provider or dermatologist, is necessary to rule out Bowen's disease or squamous cell carcinoma	Electrocautery after evaluation has ruled out atypical cells Cryosurgery with or without subsequent curettage. This may, however, increase the likelihood of recurrences.
Carcinomas *Basal cell* Most common skin cancer Slow growing, rarely metastasizes More frequent in 4th decade and up	Always involves a hair follicle Papule or nodule with pearly appearance Rolled border with prognostic umbilicated center ("rodent bite ulcer")	Biopsy. In the case of suspected malignant melanoma there are specific criteria for biopsy because depth of invasion of the tumor is the best prognostic indicator of the disease (Breslow's	Treatment for all types of cutaneous carcinomas includes: • Excision • Cryosurgery • Electrodesiccation

Probable Causes of the Presenting Symptoms

More than 5 million Americans have actinic keratoses lesions (American Academy of Dermatology, 1999). Many of these cases may progress to squamous cell carcinomas because the affected individuals do not seek evaluation and treatment of their lesions in the early stages. Forty percent of squamous cell carcinomas begin as actinic keratoses (AAD, 1999). Most such lesions occur in fair-skinned people who have prolonged unprotected sun exposure. F.A. possesses such characteristics, and the lesions on his face and upper extremities are consistent with actinic keratosis (Figure 12-3).

Diagnostic Tests Actinic keratosis can be diagnosed based on clinical appearance of a lesion,

Table 12-3
Pigmented Facial Lesion Differential Diagnostic Cues—cont'd

Diagnosis	Signs and Symptoms	Lab Data	Treatment
Carcinomas—cont'd			

Men >women
SPT I, II, and III
Prior radiation a risk
  factor
	Color pink, red, brown,
	  blue, black
	Discrete, round, or oval
	  lesions
		depth). It is used to
		predict risk of metastasis,
		 risk of recurrence, and
		overall survival
		probability. Survival rates
		correlate with the depth in
		millimeters of melanoma
		invasion from epidermis
		to deepest part of tumor.
		Lymph node biopsy
		should also be done in
		cases of malignant
		melanoma.
			• Radiation therapy may
			  be an alternative if
			  excision or microsurgery
			  is not possible, depending
			  on the site of the lesion
			  or when the lesion
			  involves periocular region
			• Chemotherapy may be
			  indicated for patients with
			  high-risk melanomas

Squamous cell
Involves skin or
  mucous membranes
Risk factors: sun
  exposure, certain
  chemicals, HPV,
  ionizing radiation
SPT I and II
In dark skinned persons
  with exposures other
  than sun
More common after age
  50
Male > female
Bowen's disease: type of
  SCC resembling
  psoriasis plaque
	Slow growing
	Indurated papules,
	  plaques or nodules
	Thick adherent keratotic
	  scaling, crusting or
	  ulceration
	Round, oval or
	  umbilicated
	Common on sun exposed
	  areas		

Malignant Melanoma
Most often lethal,
  accounting for 75% of
  all skin cancer deaths
Occurs in middle
  adulthood (30-60)
SPT I and II, rare in
  darker skinned
Positive family history
Unprotected sun
  exposure a risk
	Melanoma – 5 cardinal
	  signs (ABCDE):
	• Asymmetry
	• Border is irregular
	  often scalloped
	• Color is mottled brown,
	  black, blue, gray/pink
	• Diameter is >6 mm
	• Elevation		

but it is almost impossible to distinguish actinic keratosis from squamous cell carcinoma solely on appearance. For this reason, any suspicious lesions should have a biopsy, with treatment based on biopsy results.

Diagnostic Impression   F.A. meets the demographic features associated with sun damaged skin lesions. He has SPT II skin and has had prolonged unprotected sun exposure. The skin lesions that are concerning him are consistent with actinic keratosis in that they are reddish-tan, oval, slightly raised lesions on the face and arms with a roughened, scaly surface that is prone to bleed when abraded. The lesion on his forehead is also mildly tender.

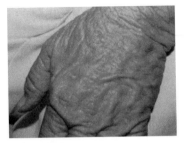

Figure 12-3 Actinic keratoses – resulting from chronic sun exposure, these can lead to squamous cell carcinoma. (From Meredith PV et al: *Adult primary care,* Philadelphia, 2000, WB Saunders.)

Therapeutic Plan of Care Because of the difficulty in making a definitive diagnosis of actinic keratosis versus squamous cell carcinoma solely on clinical appearance, a biopsy is indicated. If no atypical cells suggestive of squamous cell carcinoma are found, the treatment plan could include excision of worrisome lesions, cryosurgery, electrodesiccation, and/or topical application of 5-fluorouracil.

Patient Education and/or Community Resources The risk of unprotected sun exposure can not be overemphasized and needs to be continually addressed. Patients need to understand the importance of avoiding prolonged sun exposure, particularly during the peak hours of UV ray presence from 10 AM to 3 PM. Wearing protective clothing such as hats, long-sleeved shirts, and long pants should be encouraged. When sun exposure is anticipated, it is important to wear a sunscreen with a minimum of 15 SPF. All sunscreens should be reapplied every 2 hours, even those that claim to be waterproof. All health-care providers should provide information on safe skin care in their offices as a matter of policy, and also refer patients to literature available in the form of pamphlets or on websites that address healthy skin. The American Academy of Dermatologists and the American Academy of Family Practice maintain websites with updated information on skin protection and cancer risks. Providing education to local schools, churches, and community organizations is another outreach activity for health-care providers committed to preventive health care.

Follow-Up Plan Once all lesions have healed after treatment, the patient regularly follows up every 6 to 12 months.

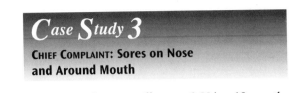

Case Study 3

CHIEF COMPLAINT: Sores on Nose and Around Mouth

History of Present Illness O.V. is a 19-month-old Hispanic male who is brought in by his mother with a chief complaint of sores on his nose and around his mouth for 2 weeks. The mother reports that she first noticed a few "red bumps" on the end of his nose 2 weeks ago. Since that time a rash developed on his nose and upper lip. The area has continued to enlarge and now includes his entire mouth and lower nose. The area started oozing a golden exudate and began to crust over. O.V. does not seem to be bothered by it unless his mother tries to wash it. His mother has tried no treatments other than washing it with soapy water. She denies any recent URIs, fever, lethargy, or difficulty sleeping or eating. No one else at home has similar symptoms.

Past Medical History OM × 2 during his first year; otherwise unremarkable

Past Surgical History None

Family History Parents A&W, no siblings

Developmental Stage Autonomy vs. Shame and Doubt

Role-Relationship O.V. lives with parents in a two-bedroom apartment. Both parents work and he goes to a baby-sitter during the day. The sitter has two children of her own and also baby-sits for five other children, ranging in age from infancy to 5 years.

Sleep/Rest Sleeps in a crib 8 to 9 hours a night and takes one 2-hour nap every day at the sitter's. Mother reports that he has always been a good sleeper as long as he has his pacifier or a bottle of juice in his crib with him.

Nutrition/Metabolic Eats three meals and two or three snacks a day. Generally eats breakfast and lunch at the sitter's, cold cereal and milk for breakfast and soup or sandwich for lunch; cookies, peanut butter crackers, or fruit for morning and afternoon snack. At home the family usually eats together, often having rice and beans. O.V. still drinks two 8-ounce bottles of whole milk a day and two or three 8-ounce bottles of juice drink a day.

Activity/Exercise   Active and generally happy baby, according to his mother. "He runs around all the time."

Coping/Stress   He is generally a happy and easy-going baby, according to his mother. He plays well with the other children at the sitter's. He rarely cries but will want to be held if he is shy or hurt.

Health Management   Immunizations are UTD including Hib, DTaP, polio, MMR, and varicella

Medications   None

Allergies   NKMA

Pertinent Physical Findings

Vital Signs   Height 30 inches; weight 22 pounds; temperature 98.3° F (otic probe); pulse 88; RR 20; blood pressure 80/46

General Appearance   Well-nourished, active, 19-month-old Hispanic male in NAD. Playing and readily smiling and "talking" with mother and practitioner.

HEENT   Normocephalic, hair full, soft, clean and curly. Ears: canals clear, TMs pearly gray, + cone of light bilaterally. Eyes: sclera clear, conjunctiva pink, no exudate. Nose: crusted lesions partially occluding bilateral nares; nasal mucosa mildly inflamed adjacent to crusted lesions, otherwise pink and moist, no exudate. Oropharynx: pink, no lesions or exudate

Neck   Supple, mild lymphadenopathy in the anterior cervical chain

Lungs   CTA A&P bilateral

Cardiac   Regular rate and rhythm, S_1 and S_2 normal, no S_3 or murmur

Abdomen   Soft, no hepatosplenomegaly, masses or tenderness

Skin   Plaques of shiny crusting on top of coalesced vesicles on erythematous base with honey-colored exudate on face from tip of nose, including nares, upper lip, and surrounding mouth. No other lesions are apparent on full body inspection.

Diagnostics

Diagnostic Tests   None

History Data   Questions specific to a chief complaint of a skin rash on a toddler's face should be directed to the parent or adult caretaker who brings the child in. These include the following:

- When did the rash start?
- Where did you first notice the rash, and has it progressed to other areas of the body?
- Does the rash appear the same now as it did in the beginning or has it changed?
- Does the child appear to have any pain or itching?
- Does the child appear to be uncomfortable (for example, crying or moaning) as a result of the rash?
- Are there any systemic symptoms such as fever, lethargy, or a decreased desire or ability to eat or sleep?
- Does the child have any other apparent illnesses such as a cold, cough, runny nose, excess tearing or oozing from his eyes, or painful ears?

Be on the alert for red flags when eliciting a history from the mother. Red flags for toddler skin rashes include fever >101.4° F assessed orally, axillary, or by otic probe; localized inflammation or edema; difficulty breathing or swallowing secondary to occlusion due to edema or enlarged lymph nodes; dehydration secondary to decreased oral intake and/or fever; or unusual lethargy. The Yale Observation Scale or "Look Test" is an excellent tool for evaluating the seriousness of illness in a child (McCarthy PL et al, 1985). This scale utilizes six criteria of behavior and appearance that are rated as normal, moderate illness, or severe illness. The practitioner can then formulate diagnostic and intervention strategies in accordance with the child's immediate health status.

Physical Examination Data   The focused examination for the chief complaint of a facial skin lesion in an infant or small child is more inclusive than if a similar presentation occurred in an older child or adult. This should include a general assessment of vital signs and appearance, a complete HEENT examination to look for other foci of illness, an assessment of lymph nodes, a cardiac and pulmonary assessment, and an abdominal examination. The skin examination includes the area identified by the patient and/or parent as well as a general assessment of the skin to look for any other sites of involvement or any other clues to diagnosis.

Differential Diagnoses Conditions that may present with localized crusted lesions on the face of a toddler include impetigo; *Herpes simplex;* and secondary impetiginization of preexisting dermatoses such as tinea cruris, atopic or contact dermatitis, and psoriasis (Table 12-4).

Probable Causes of the Presenting Symptoms Dermatological complaints account for 20% to 30% of all pediatric office visits (Hurwitz, 1993). Impetigo (Figure 12-4) is one of the most common skin infections in children (Fox, 1997) and is contagious. It is a superficial infection of the skin at a site of a break in the skin integrity. This break may be a prior skin lesion such as an insect bite or varicella lesion, or it may be as a result of trauma to the skin such as a laceration or excoriation. Maceration of the skin from prolonged pacifier sucking may make the skin more prone to impetigo. Impetigo occurs more often in summer months, in children under 6 years of age, and in lower socioeconomic groups.

Diagnostic Tests Skin lesions rarely require diagnostic tests on initial presentation. Diagnosis is generally based on the history and clinical presentation. Treatment is usually initiated based on such a diagnosis, with follow-up for reevaluation encouraged in 5 to 7 days unless symptoms are worsening. If no improvement is seen at the initial follow-up visit, diagnostic tests are indicated to rule out any other possible etiologies. Direct microscopic examination of exudate and/or skin scrapings is an office procedure that can give immediate information to guide further treatment. If symptoms persist in spite of the treatment based on microscope examination, then cultures of the lesion are useful in identifying or eliminating possible etiologies. However, cultures and sensitivities take days to weeks to produce results and so are not often done.

Diagnostic Impression O.V. presents with skin lesions on his face that have progressed over the past 2 weeks to their current state of crusted coalesced vesicles with a honey-colored exudate on an erythematous base. These lesions are present around the nose and mouth. This presentation is most consistent with common impetigo, either resulting from *S. aureus* or group A streptococcus.

Therapeutic Plan of Care O.V. should be prescribed Burow's solution compresses tid to loosen

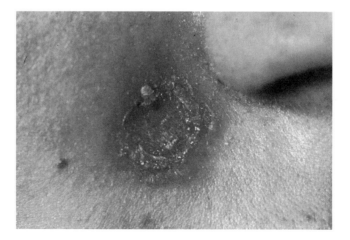

Figure 12-4 Impetigo – bacterial superinfection of a facial lesion produced the purulent, golden-yellow crust. *S. aureus* or group A beta-hemolytic streptococcus is the usual causative pathogen. (From Meredith PV et al: *Adult primary care,* Philadelphia, 2000, WB Saunders.)

Table 12-4
Differential Diagnostic Cues for Facial Lesions in a Toddler

Diagnosis	Signs and Symptoms	Lab Data	Treatment
Impetigo *Common impetigo* Superficial bacterial infection with *S. aureus,* group A beta-hemolytic strep, or mixed May be primary or secondary Requires break in normal skin Common in young children Contact sports such as wrestling may predispose athletes May lead to cellulitis or lymphangitis Possible sequela include glomerulonephritis (streptococcus)	Discrete or confluent vesicles Yellow or honey-colored crusting Erythematous base Self-inoculation leads to satellite lesions Regional lymphadenopathy Pruritus Fever	Gram-stain = intracellular cocci in chains or clusters w/in neutrophils Cultures for *S. aureus* or group A beta-hemolytic streptococcus +/− leukocytosis Anti-DNAse + in prior group A streptococcus	Burow's solution compresses to clean and remove crusts Topical mupirocin 2% ointment tid for 5 to 14 days Systemic antibiotics with activity against *S. aureus* and group A beta-hemolytic streptococcus such as dicloxacillin 12.5 to 50 mg/kg/day, erythromycin 40 mg/kg/day, cephalexin 40 mg/kg/day or cefaclor 20 mg/kg/day, all for 10 days
Bullous impetigo Caused by staphylococci Produces exotoxins Causes staph scalded-skin syndrome	Vesicles and bullae containing clear yellow exudate on normal appearing skin		
Ecthyma Extends into the dermis Develops in lesions that have been neglected	Ulceration with thick adherent crust Painful and/or tender induration		
Herpes Simplex Viral skin infection Usually occurs on mucous membranes but may occur on intact skin as in herpes gladiatorum, which is common among wrestlers Recurrent	Grouped vesicles on erythematous base Vesicles ulcerate and become crusted Prodromal tingling Regional lymphadenopathy Fever and malaise	Tzanck smear with microscopic examination demonstrates giant, multinucleated cells Cultures of exudate or crusting	Burow's solution compresses tid to alleviate discomfort Acyclovir 5-10 mg/kg qid for 5-10 days
Impetiginization of Preexisting Dermatoses Primary lesions could be: • Atopic dermatitis • Contact dermatitis • Dermatophytosis • Psoriasis • Chickenpox	Symptoms similar to common impetigo Need to treat underlying condition if present and would benefit from treatment	Microscopic evaluation: Gram stain for bacteria KOH preparation for tinea Tzanck smear for virus Cultures for *S. aureus,* Group A strep, fungus, and/or virus	Treat bacterial infection same as impetigo Treat underlying dermatoses as indicated

the crusts, and be started on either topical mupirocin 2% ointment tid or an oral antibiotic such as dicloxacillin 12.5 mg/kg/day in four divided doses for 10 days or cephalexin 40 mg/kg/day in four divided doses for 10 days.

Patient Education and/or Community Resources   Impetigo is a contagious superficial skin infection that takes advantage of a break in the integrity of the skin. Family education is essential to alert the parents to the need for adequately treating the infection and decreasing the likelihood of spreading the infection or infecting others. The following instructions should be given in written form and also explained in detail to the parents/caregivers:

- Complete the 10-day course of antibiotic even if the rash has cleared or the rash has disappeared.
- Good handwashing is essential for the infant and all caregivers to prevent the spread of the infection to other parts of the body and to other individuals.
- Trim fingernails of the child to prevent scratching and transporting bacteria elsewhere.
- Check household members and those with whom the child has close contact, particularly the baby-sitter, the baby-sitter's family, and other children in the baby-sitter's care.
- The child should not go to the baby-sitter's until lesions have cleared or until the child has been on antibiotics for 48 hours.
- Launder clothing and linens in hot water and avoid sharing sleeping arrangements until lesions have cleared.
- Clean and/or replace all pacifiers, bottles, toothbrushes, and toys.

Follow-Up Plan   Reevaluate in 5 days unless symptoms worsen in the interim. Advise the mother to observe for any worsening of the lesions or any signs of fever, malaise, lethargy, decreased appetite, or unwillingness to eat or drink. Also instruct the mother to call immediately if dark-colored urine, decreased urinary output, or edema occur because these may be signs of glomerulonephritis secondary to group A streptococcal in-

fection. If she notices any symptoms suggestive of a worsening condition she should schedule an emergency reevaluation sooner than scheduled. If no improvement is seen on the scheduled reevaluation visit, then diagnostic tests are indicated including cultures and sensitivity. If O.V. was originally prescribed topical mupirocin, then starting him on oral antibiotics is indicated. If he was started on oral antibiotics and has shown no improvement but is no worse, then awaiting the results of the culture and sensitivity is appropriate.

Case Study 4   **Optional Exercise**

CHIEF COMPLAINT: Pruritic Rash on Neck and Anterior Chest

History of Present Illness   K.W. is a 22-year-old African-American female who presents with the chief complaint of rashes on her neck and anterior chest. The rashes are sometimes worse than at other times, often pruritic, and appear as a clustering of tiny red bumps. The rashes sometimes get so bad that they ooze a clear substance. When the bumps get better and no longer itch, the area still looks different than her normal skin. It stays darker and rougher than her normal skin and feels slightly "swollen." She first remembers getting these rashes when she was in middle school. In the past she has tried cocoa butter, benadryl topical cream, and cold water. She says the creams "didn't really help but they stopped the itching a little." The cold water also stops the itching for a while.

Past Medical History   Unremarkable

Past Surgical History   None

Family History   Both parents are in their 40s and A&W; two sisters and one brother also A&W

Developmental Stage   Intimacy vs. Isolation

Role-Relationship   K.W. lives with her boyfriend and 2-year-old daughter in a rented apartment. She works as a secretary for the local government, a job that she says is "OK, it pays fine." She hopes to return to school to study computers in hopes of moving ahead in her job.

Sleep/Rest   Sleeps 7 to 8 hours a night, falling asleep about 10 PM and rising at 6 AM to her alarm clock. K.W. denies any problems falling asleep and reports feeling rested on most days.

Nutrition/Metabolic Eats two or three meals a day with snacks. Typically buys a hot "breakfast sandwich" at fast food restaurant on her way to work; eats pizza or a hamburger, also from fast food restaurant, for lunch; and snacks in the evening unless her boyfriend cooks. Her daughter eats all her meals at the daycare center. K.W. doesn't really like to cook so has never learned.

Activity/Exercise Leisure activities include shopping at the mall, going to local clubs on the weekends, and watching TV.

Coping/Stress K.W. reports that she turns to one of her sisters and her best girlfriends when she is having troubles. She rarely attends her family church any longer, but does visit her parents on a regular basis.

Health Management Smokes cigarettes, 1 pack per day; drinks two or three drinks when she goes out on weekends; and uses marijuana every couple of weeks with her boyfriend. She is currently sexually active with her boyfriend only, believes he has no other partners, and gets Depo-Provera every 3 months for contraception. She and her partner do not use condoms. She sees her gynecologist once a year for her examination and Pap smear and is up to date on all immunizations including MMR, OPV, hep B, varicella, and Td. She has never had an HIV test.

Self-Perception and Values/Beliefs K.W. feels OK about her life, believing that she does OK by her daughter and her boyfriend.

Medications Depo-Provera q 3 months, acetaminophen occasionally for a headache

Allergies NKMA

Pertinent Physical Findings

Vital Signs Height 5 feet 5 inches; weight 135 pounds; BMI 22; temperature 98.3° F; pulse 72; RR. 14; blood pressure 110/72

General Appearance Well developed 22-year-old African-American female in NAD; alert and oriented × 3, pleasant and relaxed, dressed casually, and cooperating fully in history taking

Skin Medium to dark brown in pigment; 1.5 cm hyperpigmented, lichenified, oval patches on lateral aspects of neck just below ear lobes. Anterior chest appears with 2 distinct hyperpigmented circular patches 2 cm in diameter at the midclavicular lines just above the breasts with superficial clusters of erythematous micropapules and microvesicles. Slight oozing is apparent on both chest patches. No excoriation, pustules, or nodules present. Positive dermatographia demonstrated.

Lymph Nodes No regional lymphadenopathy discovered

Diagnostics
Diagnostic Tests None

Discussion Questions

What type of history data should be collected?

What type of physical data should be collected?

What are the differential diagnoses?

What are the probable causes of the presenting symptoms?

What is your diagnostic impression?

What is the therapeutic plan of care?

What are the patient education and/or community resources?

What is your follow-up plan?

Discussions for optional case study exercises can be found in the accompanying Instructor's Manual.

References

American Academy of Dermatology: Patients urged to seek treatment for actinic keratosis, Press Release, April 28, 1999, AAD website.

Anderson R, Rajagopalan R: Responsiveness of the Dermatology-specific Quality of Life (DSQL) instrument to treat for acne vulgaris in a placebo-controlled clinical trial, *Qual Life Res* 7(8):723-734, 1998.

Fox JA: *Primary health care of children,* St Louis, 1997, Mosby.

Gupta MA, Gupta AK: Depression and suicidal ideation in dermatology patients with acne, alopecia areata, atopic dermatitis and psoriasis, *Br J Dermatol* 139(5):846-850, 1998.

Hurwitz S: *Clinical pediatric dermatology,* Philadelphia, 1993, WB Saunders.

McCarthy PL et al: Predictive values of abnormal physical examination findings in ill appearing febrile children, *Pediatrics* 76(2):167-171, 1985.

Meredith PV et al: *Adult primary care,* Philadelphia, 2000, WB Saunders.

Pearl A, Arroll B, Leollo J et al: The impact of acne: a study of 195 adolescents' attitudes, perception and knowledge, *N Z Med J* 111(1070):269-271, 1998.

Suggested Readings

Burns CE et al: *Pediatric primary care: a handbook for nurse practitioners,* Philadelphia, 1996, WB Saunders.

Charlesworth EN: Allergic skin disease: atopic dermatitis as a prototype, *Prim Care* 25(4):775-790, 1998.

De Groot AC: Fatal attractiveness: the shady side of cosmetics, *Clin Dermatol* 16(1):167-179, 1998.

Feldman SR et al: Destructive procedures are the standard care for treatment of actinic keratoses, *J Am Acad Dermatol* 40(1):43-47, 1999.

Fitzpatrick TB et al: *The color atlas and synopsis of clinical dermatology,* New York, 1997, McGraw-Hill.

Ferrera PC et al: Dermatologic problems encountered in the emergency department, *Am J Emerg Med* 14(6):588-601, 1996.

Gordon ML et al: Care of the skin at midlife: diagnosis of pigmented lesions, Geriatrics 52(8):56-58, 67-68, 1997.

Hay WW, Hayward AR, Levin MJ, Sondheimer JM: *Current pediatric diagnosis and treatment,* Stamford, Conn., 1999, Appleton & Lange.

Manzani BM et al: Contact sensitization in children, *Pediatr Dermatol* 15(1):12-17, 1998.

Mirrelbronn MA et al: Frequency of pre-existing actinic keratosis in cutaneous squamous cell carcinoma, *Int J Dermatol* 37(9):677-681, 1998.

Schwartz RA: Premalignant keratinocytic neoplasms, *J Am Acad Dermatol* 35(2 Pt 1):223-242, 1996.

Singleton JK: Pediatric dermatoses: three common skin disruptions in infancy, *Nurse Pract* 22(6):32-33,37, 43-44, 1997.

Sober AJ et al: Precursors to skin cancer, *Cancer* 75(2 suppl):645-650, 1995.

Tierney LM, McPhee SJ, Papadakis MA: *Current medical diagnosis and treatment,* Stamford CT, 1998, Appleton & Lange.

Weisshaar E et al: Effect of topical capsaicin on the cutaneous reactions and itching to histamine atopic eczema compared to healthy skin, *Arch Dermatol Res* 290(6):306-311, 1998.

Whited JD et al: Primary care clinicians' performance for detecting actinic keratosis and skin cancer, *Arch Intern Med* 157(9):985-990, 1997.

CHAPTER 13

Neurological Disorders

Jean Nagelkerk

Case Study 1

CHIEF COMPLAINT: Headache

History of Present Illness P.G. is a 25-year-old Caucasian female who presents with chief complaint of right-sided (unilateral) throbbing headache with photophobia and nausea and vomiting for 6 months duration. She has at least 2 headaches a month that begin in the afternoon, last 8 to 12 hours, and do not resolve until she sleeps. Lying in a dark, quiet room is most restful. P.G. is unable to work with the headaches. Her last H/A was yesterday morning at 4 AM and she feels she cannot get relief from them. P.G. is becoming worried about her H/As because she has been awakened five times over a 2-week period in the early morning with throbbing right-sided headaches accompanied by vomiting. She has tried Tylenol, aspirin, Motrin, and Excedrin Migraine with minimal pain relief. P.G. rates her H/A as number 8 on a 0-10 scale with 0 being no pain and 10 being the most severe pain. The headaches have increased over the past 2 weeks. She denies head trauma or medication changes. Her LMP was 5/12/99. She has a 28-day cycle with a light, 5-day flow. Until the H/As began awakening her 2 weeks ago, she felt she was getting adequate sleep and was rested upon awakening. She has been under increased pressure at work because her co-worker, another legal secretary, is on maternity leave. An additional stressor is that her husband is on a long-term assignment (3 months) in Hong Kong, leaving her the sole caregiver for their child.

Past Medical History Fracture of right arm in 1977

Past Surgical History Unremarkable

Family History Maternal grandmother, mother, and brother have a history of migraine headaches; father, + colon cancer; sister, A&W; maternal grandfather and paternal grandmother, HTN; paternal grandfather, Parkinson disease

Developmental Stage Intimacy versus Isolation

Role-Relationship P.G. is a legal secretary for a small law firm. She is married × 3 years to a sales representative who often travels 1 or 2 days per week. They have a 2-year-old daughter. The family lives in a large city in an apartment complex. P.G. has very few friends and no family in the area because they moved to Chicago from Florida 1 year ago. The family is able to visit relatives once a year.

Sleep/Rest Typically sleeps 8 hours per day (10 PM to 6 AM), but has been awakened for the past 2 weeks at approximately 4 AM with severe H/As and vomiting

Activity/Exercise P.G. has the major responsibility for their daughter's care. She attends a health club three or four times per week for a 1-hour exercise workout, but has been unable to exercise for the past 2 weeks due to H/A

Coping/Stress Feels a little more stress than usual with her husband in Hong Kong and an increased workload at her place of employment. Does have a busy schedule, but tries to exercise routinely

Health Management Smokes 1 pack of cigarettes per day × 7 years; alcohol, will order a glass of wine once or twice a week when out for dinner with her husband

Medications P.G. takes acetaminophen (Tylenol), aspirin (Bayer), ibuprofen (Motrin), and Excedrin Migraine every 4 to 6 hours prn when she experiences H/As. She purchases whichever product is on sale at the grocery store to relieve her H/As. She has been on oral birth control for 1

year (levonorgestrel 0.10 mg, ethinyl estradiol 20 mcg – Alesse).

Allergies   None

Pertinent Physical Findings

Vital Signs   Height 5 feet 5 inches; weight 150 pounds; BMI 25; temperature 98.6° F; heart rate 88; respirations l6; blood pressure 110/74

General Appearance   Alert and oriented to time, place, person, and situation; well groomed, speech clear, expression appropriate, coordinated movements, rubbing the R side of head

HEENT   Head, normocephalic, without evidence of trauma, lesions, or tenderness; face, symmetrical; Snellen eye exam, R 20/20; L 20/20; L pupil is 5 mm and R pupil is 3 mm; PRRLA; EOMs intact; fundoscopic: optic discs sharp, well defined, cream color, no exudates or hemorrhages. Ears: TMs gray, landmarks intact with distinct cone of light; Rinne, AC greater than BC au, Weber without lateralization; TMJ, no crepitus or dysfunction; nose, patent bilaterally, septum midline, pink mucosa, no discharge, polyps or sinus tenderness; throat, oral mucosa pink, moist, no lesions, tonsils 2+, uvula midline; teeth, present, straight, with few fillings

Neck   Supple without JVD, carotid bruits, thyromegaly, no cervical lymphadenopathy, trachea is midline

Heart   Apical pulse 88, regular rate and rhythm, no S_3 or S_4, PMI 5th ICS-MCL; radial, pedal, and femoral pulses 2+ and equal bilaterally

Lungs   Clear to auscultation

Neurological   CN II-XII grossly intact, DTR 2+ bil symmetrical, muscular strength intact bil, no atrophy or tremors; Romberg negative, sensation intact to light touch and pinprick; able to heel-to-toe walk; negative Kernig's sign

Diagnostics

Diagnostic Tests   CT of head with contrast: negative

History Data   Questions specific to the chief complaint of headache include the following:

- Where are your headaches located (for example, band around your head, bilateral, unilateral)?
- What type of headache is it (for example, dull, throbbing, pulsating)?

- How severe is this headache on a scale of 0 to 10, with 0 being no pain and 10 being the most severe pain?
- What time of day do these headaches usually occur?
- Is sleep affected?
- How often do the headaches occur?
- How long do the headaches last?
- What aggravates of precipitates an attack?
- Do certain foods such as chocolate, caffeine, alcohol, hot dogs, or Chinese foods; or stress, exercise, or menses cause the headaches or make them worse?
- What medications are you taking, both prescribed, OTC, and herbal (birth control pills can aggravate headaches)?
- How much caffeine or alcohol are you drinking?
- Are your headaches associated with a flash of light, noise, or altered sensation?
- Do you have any visual disturbances?
- Do you have nausea or vomiting, tearing, light sensitivity, noise sensitivity, or blind spot in the visual field?
- Do you have loss of function of an extremity or any other physical sign with your headaches?
- Have you had trauma to your head?
- Have you recently had an upper respiratory infection?
- Do you have allergic rhinitis?
- When was your last dental visit or eye examination?
- Have you been treated for a psychiatric disorder?

Physical Examination Data   The focused examination for the chief complaint of headache includes vital signs, general appearance, HEENT, neck, heart, lungs, and neurological

Differential Diagnoses   Tension headache, migraine headache, cluster headache, brain tumor, meningitis, TMJ, subarachnoid hemorrhage, cervical radiculopathy* (Table 13-1)

---

*Other possible differential diagnoses include sinusitis, abscess from poor dental health, sleep disturbance, and subdural hematoma from trauma.

Table 13-1
Headache Differential Diagnostic Cues

Diagnoses	Signs and Symptoms	Lab Data	Treatment
Tension Headache Related to stress A common cause is muscle contraction	Vicelike or tight, bandlike pressure around the head, bilateral, non-throbbing (dull pressure), intense around the back of the neck or head, generalized. Symptoms worse as the day progresses and absent when removed from the situation. During weekends there usually is relief from the H/As	None unless suspect infection, aneurysm, brain lesion, temporal arteritis, trauma, TMJ, cervical radiculopathy, stroke, or other abnormality; then order diagnostic tests	Try relaxation, massage, biofeedback, exercise, and stress management. May use acetaminophen, aspirin, or NSAIDs. Caution with the use of too much medication which may cause rebound H/A. With chronic H/As, evaluate for anxiety and/or depression, may trial a serotonin reuptake inhibitor or amitriptyline (Elavil)
Migraine Headache May have family history of migraines Triggers include stress, foods, alcohol, menstruation, OCPs, sleep disturbance, or missing meals Migraines are either with aura (classic migraine =old term) or without aura (nonclassic aura = old term) May use prophylaxis if >2 attacks per month (e.g., beta blockers, calcium channel blocking agents, tricyclic antidepressants)	Unilateral, throbbing H/A, nausea, vomiting, photophobia, phonophobia, and blurring of vision	Same as tension H/A	Mild H/A = Take at onset aspirin *OR* Excedrin Migraine 2 tabs q6 hours max 8 tabs qd *OR* NSAIDs (e.g., naproxen sodium [Anaprox] 275 mg 2 tabs then 1 tab q6-8 hrs *OR* oxaprozin [Daypro] 600 mg-1.2 gm qd) Moderate-severe H/A = sumatriptan (Imitrex) SQ give 6 mg at onset then repeat if needed in 1 hour max 2 doses in 24 hrs; PO 25-100 mg at onset then 2nd dose 2 hrs after 1st then q 2 hrs max with PO is 300 mg/day (if injection was also used, then max PO is 200 mg/day); if intranasal, give 5-20 mg then repeat q 2 hrs, max 40 mg/day and 4 H/A in 30 days. Other meds (see Table 13-2) include zolmitriptan (Zomig), dihydroergotamine mesylate (DHE 45, Migranal), Midrin, and analgesics and sedatives (used infrequently).
Cluster Headache If prophylaxis is needed may use verapamil (Calan), lithium, methysergide, propranolol, prednisone	Severe unilateral periorbital H/A, may have ipsilateral nasal congestion, Horner's syndrome, redness of eye, lacrimation, rhinorrhea; H/As last 15 minutes-2 hours	Same as tension H/A	Many of the same medications and dosages used for migraine H/As are used for acute attacks of cluster H/As. SQ sumatriptan (Imitrex) 6 mg *OR* dihydroergotamine (DHE) 1-2 mg IM *OR* ergotamine tartrate (Cafergot) 1 suppository rectally

Continued

	Table 13-1		
	Headache Differential Diagnostic Cues—cont'd		

Diagnoses	Signs and Symptoms	Lab Data	Treatment
Cluster Headache —cont'd			**OR** 100% oxygen at 7L/min for 15 minutes **OR** butorphanol tartrate (Stadol NS) 1 mg spray in one nostril
Brain Tumor	H/A, nausea, vomiting, seizures, fatigue, personality changes	CT with contrast **OR** MRI of head	Refer to neurosurgeon for evaluation and potential surgical intervention. Irradiation and chemotherapy may also be implemented.
Meningitis	H/A, stiff neck, fever, +Kernig and Brudzinski signs, CNS changes	CT if suspect space-occupying lesion (papilledema, coma, seizures); otherwise CBC with diff, LP with examination of cell count, glucose, protein, smear, blood cultures, CXR	Hospitalization for IV antibiotics and supportive care (e.g., steroids, mannitol, mechanical ventilation if necessary)
TMJ	H/A, ear pain, facial tenderness, mandibular joint click, facial asymmetry	None	Soft diet, no gum chewing, use of bite guard, avoid grinding teeth, NSAIDs prn, refer to dentist or oral surgeon
Subarachnoid Hemorrhage	Excruciating H/A, "worse H/A ever experienced," sudden onset, N/V, loss of/or altered consciousness	CT of head; it is quickly performed and sensitive in identifying hemorrhages	Hospitalization, surgical evaluation, bed rest with no activity or straining
Cervical Radiculopathy	H/A, neck pain, numbness and tingling in hands and fingers, unilateral altered sensation in upper extremity	Cervical x-rays, MRI	May try conservative therapy such as NSAIDs, limiting activities, and short-term trial of neck immobilization. If unsuccessful, refer. May need surgical evaluation

Probable Causes of the Presenting Symptoms

There are several different theories about what causes *primary headaches*. Primary headaches result from traction or inflammation of pain sensitive structures, increased muscle contraction, and alteration in neuronal function in the brain. Examples of primary headaches include cluster, migraine, tension, and postraumatic headaches.

For a long time the vascular hypothesis was thought to account for the cause of migraines. Vascular dilation created increased pressure on pain receptors in the large veins, venous sinuses, and ex-

Table 13-2
Medications Commonly Used for Migraine Management

Medication	Dosage	Contraindications	Side Effects
Zolmitriptan (Zomig) Selective serotonin 5-HT 1D Receptor Agonist	Initially 2.5 mg or lower, may repeat after 2 hours, max 10 mg qd. The safety of treating more than 3 H/As in 1 month has not been determined.	History of MI, ischemic heart disease, Prinzmetal's angina or uncontrolled hypertension. Do not use with vasoconstrictive drugs, within 24 hours of ergotamine derivatives, or within 2 weeks of monoamine oxidase inhibitors. May cause serotonin syndrome with SSRI medications. Pregnancy category C	Flushing, throat discomfort, discomfort, neck and chest tightness, and tingling, nausea, and somnolence
Ergotamine Tartrate (Ergot Alkaloid) Different Routes of Administration: Oral = Wigraine Sublingual = Ergostat Suppository = Cafergot	Wigraine (ergotamine tartrate 1 mg + caffeine 100 mg); oral = 2 at onset; then 1 every ½ hour prn max 6 per attack and 10 per week. Ergostat (ergotamine tartrate); sublingual 2 mg; may repeat q 30 minutes. Max 6 mg per attack and 10 mg per week. Cafergot (ergotamine tartrate 2 mg + caffeine 100 mg); rectal suppository 1 suppository per rectum. May repeat in 1 hour. Max 2 per day and 5 per week	Should be 5 days between different routes of administration. Coronary or peripheral vascular disease, hypertension, impaired hepatic or renal function. Pregnancy category X. Do not use within 24 hours of sumatriptan, zolmitriptan, other 5-HT 1 agonists, or other ergot type drugs. Avoid within 2 weeks of MAOIs	Tachycardia, bradycardia, vasoconstrictive complications, numbness, pain, weakness of extremities, nausea and/or vomiting, diarrhea, dizziness
Dihydroergotamine Mesylate (DHE 45, Migranal) = Ergot	DHE 45 (dihydroergotamine mesylate) 1 mg/ml injectable. 1 ml IM or IV at onset; then 1 ml after 1 hour prn. Max 2 ml IV or 3 ml IM per episode. Max total doses 6 ml per week Migranal (dihydroergotamine mesylate 4 mg/ml) 0.5 mg/spray; nasal spray contains caffeine. One spray each nostril at onset, may repeat in 15 minutes prn. Max 6 sprays in 24 hours. Max 8 sprays per week	Contraindicated in ischemic heart disease, coronary artery vasospasm, myocardial ischemia, peripheral artery disease uncontrolled hypertension, basilar or hemiplegic migraine. Pregnancy category X. Precaution in elderly. Do not give within 24 hours of sumatriptan, zolmitriptan, other 5-HT1 agonists, or ergot type drugs. Not within 2 weeks or MAOIs	Supervise first dose. Congestion, burning sensation, dryness, paresthesia, dizziness, somnolence, myocardial and peripheral vascular ischemia or vasoconstriction, rhinitis, diarrhea

Note: Children's Motrin or Children's Tylenol are often very effective for treatment of migraine headaches in children. Prophylaxis may also be used with children and may include propranolol hydrochloride (Inderal) or cyproheptadine (Periactin).

Continued

Table 13-2
Medications Commonly Used for Migraine Management—cont'd

Medication	Dosage	Contraindications	Side Effects
Sumatriptan (Imitrex) Selective serotonin 5-HT 1D receptor agonist Different Routes of Administration: oral, subcutaneous, or nasal spray	Imitrex SQ give 6 mg at onset, then repeat if needed in 1 hour. Max 2 doses in 24 hours. ***OR*** PO give 25-100 mg. 50 mg dose very effective at onset, then second dose 2 hours after first. Then q 2 hours. Max PO is 300 mg/ day (if injection was also used, then max PO is 200 mg/day) ***OR*** Intranasal 5-20 mg at onset of H/A. Then repeat q 2 hours. Max 40 mg/day. Safety has not been established for treating more than 4 H/As in a 30-day period.	History of ischemic cardiac disease, cerebral vascular disease, or peripheral vascular disease. Uncontrolled hypertension or hemiplegic migraine. During or within a 2 week period after stopping MAOIs. Use with SSRIs may cause weakness, hyperreflexia, and coordination problems. Do not give within 24 hours of ergot drugs (methysergide, dihydroergotamine). The first dose of injectable Imitrex should be supervised and some authorities recommend monitoring with an ECG.* Pregnancy category C	Flushing, chest discomfort, fatigue, increased blood pressure, drowsiness, throat discomfort, sweating, anxiety, H/A, acute MI, dysrhythmias, coronary vasospasm, cerebrovascular disorders
Rizatriptan Benzoate (Maxalt) 5-HT 1B/1D Agonist Different routes of administration: Oral = 5 and 10 mg tablets MAXALT-MLT (disintegrating peppermint flavored tablets) 5 mg and 10 mg tablets	Initially 5 or 10 mg. May repeat after 2 hrs. Max 30 mg/day. Safety has not been established for treating more than 4 H/As in a 30-day period.	History of MI, ischemic heart disease, Prinzmetal's angina or uncontrolled hypertension. Do not use if has basilar or hemiplegic migraine. Do not use with vasoconstrictive drugs, within 24 hours of ergotamine derivatives, or within 2 weeks of monoamine oxidase inhibitors. May have interactions with SSRIs	Dizziness, jaw pressure, nausea, H/A, asthenia, paresthesias

Note: Children's Motrin or Children's Tylenol are often very effective for treatment of migraine headaches in children. Prophylaxis may also be used with children and may include propranolol hydrochloride (Inderal) or cyproheptadine (Periactin).
*May consider monitoring with ECG if possibility of unrecognized coronary disease, especially in postmenopausal women, men who are 40 years or older, individuals who are hypertension, smokers, and those with a strong family history of cardiac problems.

tracranial arteries resulting in pain (Kelley, 1997). The neurogenic hypothesis describes a set of neuronal events that triggers changes in the neurotransmitters, resulting in changes in the vessels and blood flow (Goroll, May, and Mulley, 1995). Serotonin receptors play a key role in the neurogenic hypothesis.

Secondary headaches are caused by an underlying organic cause (Goroll, May, and Mulley, 1995; Uphold and Graham, 1998). It is reported that 2% to 5% of headaches are from secondary causes. Examples of secondary headaches include brain lesions, TMJ syndrome, temporal arteritis, infections, metabolic disorders, acute angle glaucoma, trigeminal neuralgia, and subarachnoid hemorrhage.

Table 13-2
Medications Commonly Used for Migraine Management—cont'd

Medication	Dosage	Contraindications	Side Effects
Rizatriptan Benzoate —cont'd		Propranolol increases rizatriptan action. Pregnancy category C	
Naratriptan HCL (Amerge) 5-HT 1B/1D receptor agonist	PO 1 mg or 2.5 mg with fluids. May repeat once after 4 hours. Max 5 mg/24hrs. Safety has not been established for treating more than 4 H/As in a 30-day period.	History of MI, ischemic heart disease, Prinzmetal's angina or uncontrolled hypertension. Do not use with vasoconstrictive drugs, within 24 hours of ergotamine derivatives or within 2 weeks of monoamine oxidase inhibitors. May develop serotonin syndrome with SSRI use. Monitor cardiac function with long term use. Supervise first dose. Some authorities recommend monitoring ECG in patients who have a chance of having unrecognized coronary disease.* Pregnancy category C	Dizziness, throat pressure, neck tightness, drowsiness, fatigue, paresthesias
Midrin (Isometheptene mucate 65 mg + dichloralphenazone 100 mg + acetaminophen 325 mg) = sympathomimetic + sedative + analgesic	For tension H/A give 1-2 tabs every 4 hours. Max 8 daily. For migraine H/A give 2 tablets, then q 1-hour prn. Max 5 per 12 hours.	Contraindications include glaucoma, severe renal, cardiac, hypertensive or hepatic disease. Do not give if on MAOIs or within 2 weeks of MAOIs.	Drowsiness, dizziness, rash, sympathomimetic effects

*May consider monitoring with ECG if possibility of unrecognized coronary disease, especially in postmenopausal women, men who are 40 years or older, individuals who are hypertension, smokers, and those with a strong family history of cardiac problems.

When evaluating for secondary causes of headaches, identify the probable mechanism of the headache and use assessment and diagnostic data to determine the cause and treatment plan. For example, when an elderly patient presents and complains of a headache, review the patient's history for chronic condition such as diabetes, hypertension, and hyperlipidemia that may be associated with a higher risk of stroke. Should the patient present with symptoms of fever or nuchal rigidity, evaluate for meningitis. Evaluate the presenting problem of headache with visual disturbance for possible narrow angle glaucoma. When the patient reports pain with neck movement, an evaluation for cervical problems should be conducted. Patients who present with "the worst headache ever" should be evaluated for a subarachnoid hemorrhage. Often, individuals with brain tumors report pain that is worse in the morning and aggravated by straining.

Diagnostic Tests   The intensity and severity of P.G.'s symptoms require collaborative management of the patient's care with a physician. For P.G., a CT with contrast should be ordered because of the anisocoria, H/A and vomiting, and increasing frequency and intensity of the headaches. According to Wiest and Roth (1996), patients who have neurological defects, severe H/As, or first-time seizures commonly have a CT with contrast to rule out an intracranial space-occupying lesion. A CT with a positive intracranial mass will show a low-attenuation lesion with edema surrounding the mass (Wiest and Roth, 1996). Anisocoria is normal in 5% of the general population. However, if this has not been documented previously, consider a CNS lesion (Jarvis, 1996). Typically, no tests are ordered unless symptoms point to a cause other than migraines. If infection is suspected, consider a CBC with differential. If the WBC count is elevated, consider an LP and blood cultures. If an aneurysm is suspected, order a CT of the head without contrast. If a brain lesion is suspected, order a CT with contrast or MRI of the head. If temporal arteritis is suspected, order a sed rate and refer for a temporal artery biopsy. If there was trauma to the head, order a CT of the head. For TMJ syndrome, no tests are usually necessary. Occasionally, an x-ray of the temporomandibular joint is ordered. For patients who present with symptoms of cervical radiculopathy, order cervical x-rays and, if needed, a MRI. If stroke is suspected, order a CT of the head without contrast.

Diagnostic Impression   It is important to consult with a physician, given P.G.'s presentation, to rule out a CNS lesion. The CT was negative. P.G. reported a unilateral, throbbing H/A with photophobia, nausea, and vomiting. Resting in a dark room is most helpful. She has a strong family history of migraines. Therefore, the most likely cause of her symptoms is migraine cephalgia. However, because this patient presents with undocumented anisocoria, awakening with vomiting, and increased intensity of H/As, a referral to a neurologist for evaluation is in-

dicated. A neurological referral is indicated when the patient does not experience relief from the therapeutic plan of care, when the patient's symptoms intensify or additional symptoms occur, and when neurological deficits occur.

Patients who present with "the worst headache ever," focal neurological deficits, vomiting without nausea, or intense and unrelenting headache, may have complicating factors or underlying pathology and consultation or referral to a specialist is recommended. Diagnostic tests may need to be conducted immediately to rule out a subarachnoid hemorrhage, and appropriate interventions need to be promptly implemented.

Therapeutic Plan of Care   After a more serious intracranial pathology is ruled out, the neurologist and nurse practitioner can collaborate on a plan of care. P.G. is experiencing migraine H/As >2 × month. P.G. should discontinue her OCPs and determine an acceptable alternative birth control method. She should be started on prophylactic medication such as propranolol HCl (Inderal LA) 80 mg qd. A prescription for sumatriptan (Imitrex) nasal spray 20 mg at onset of H/A. Repeat in 2 hours if needed with a maximum of 40 mg/day and 4 H/As in 30 days may be trialed.

Patient Education and/or Community Resources   It is important to discuss the cause, trigger factors, and treatment options for patients who experience H/As. Having the patient begin a headache diary is helpful to evaluate any triggers that exacerbate or initiate a headache. It is also useful in evaluating the type and frequency of H/A, the alleviating and aggravating factors, and the treatment effectiveness. Reviewing the headache diary at follow-up visits will assist in identifying effective methods for treatment.

The nurse should discuss with P.G. the potential triggers for migraine headaches, such as foods high in tryptophan (including red wine, chocolate, and ripe cheeses). Foods high in nitrates (such as hot dogs) and foods with monosodium glutamate (such as Chinese dishes) may also trigger migraines. Alcohol and beverages with caffeine may also potentiate headaches. With female patients, it is important to evaluate birth control practices because oral contraceptives may potentiate headaches and should be discontinued. Progesterone-only pills may be tried. Other triggers may include stress or menstruation. Triggers are patient-specific, and a careful headache diary may help eliminate these individual triggers.

Medications play a central role in the treatment of migraine headaches, but overuse may actually create rebound headaches and make the problem worse. Careful discussion of a multi-faceted treatment approach to the patient's management of their headaches is important. Discussing the role of medications, side effects, and frequency of use is important for controlling headaches. Encouraging the patient to develop a treatment plan that fits into his or her lifestyle is useful. The treatment plan may include regularly scheduled exercise, establishing regular meal times, using biofeedback to help control the headaches, and using relaxation therapy to decrease stress.

Other treatment options include topical ice to the forehead or back of the neck; reclining in a dark, quiet environment; avoiding triggers that stimulate or potentiate headaches; and instituting stress reduction techniques to limit, if possible, stressful situations. Should anxiety or depression be a presenting feature, evaluating this component and then exploring the use of medications and counseling may help eliminate factors that potentiate the headaches.

There are several Internet sources that provide information on migraine headaches. The American Council for Headache Education has a website (http://www.achenet.org/) to provide education for people experiencing headaches. Glaxo-Wellcome, Inc. offers a patient education website (http://www.migrainehelp.com/) that discusses headache triggers and symptoms, and provides a diagnostic screening. The Migraine Foundation website (http://www.niagrara.com/migraine/) serves approximately 3 million Canadian citizens suffering from migraine headaches by providing patient education and awareness.

Follow-Up Plan   P.G. should schedule a return visit in 2 weeks for reevaluation of the H/As with the prescribed treatment plan. P.G. should be alerted to the warning signs and symptoms of serious H/As, and be instructed when to call the office should problems arise. If there is no relief from the

H/A, the patient should return sooner. Then the patient should follow up in 4-6 weeks and prn after this visit if the H/As are controlled.

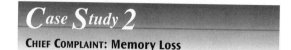

CHIEF COMPLAINT: Memory Loss

History of Present Illness   S.N. is an 87-year-old Caucasian male who presents with his daughter for chief complaint of memory loss. S.N.'s primary care provider retired 6 months ago and he is reluctant to see a new clinician. His daughter wants him to have a complete physical examination because he has been gradually losing memory over the past 2 years and she is worried about him driving. She states that he can no longer remember what happened yesterday, but can remember events that happened years ago. S.N. still drives a car, but he says he only drives during the daylight and not in heavy traffic. He feels he can drive safely and can remember the way to familiar places like the grocery store and favorite restaurants. He has asked that his daughter pay his bills and make all of his appointments. S.N. feels that he is fine and forgets "little things" on occasion, but nothing of importance. His daughter is worried because he became lost on the way home from the grocery store a week ago. S.N. does not feel it is a problem because he rarely drives. S.N. has no history of psychiatric or neurological problems or head trauma. He denies any recent or past falls. S.N.'s daughter is concerned that he may fall during the winter when it is icy and slippery outside. There is no family history of Alzheimer's or dementia.

Past Medical History   Broken wrist, hypertension of 10 years duration

Past Surgical History   Appendectomy at age 26 and T&A at age 12

Family History   Mother, died of colon cancer at 82; father, died of natural causes at 92; brother, 92, HTN; sister, 85, migraine H/As; sister, 82, Parkinson's; daughter and son, A&W

Developmental Stage   Ego Integrity versus Despair

Role-Relationship   S.N. lives with his 85-year-old wife in a two-story house that they have owned for 65 years. S.N.'s wife does not drive. She is able to clean their clothes and wash dishes. He has a daughter who lives ½ mile away and a son who lives 2 miles away. He attends church regularly on Sunday. He is social, but rarely goes anywhere other than family gatherings about four or five times a year. At these gatherings he talks about events that occurred years ago and focuses on himself. In the past, S.N. was a good conversationalist and was very interested in what others were doing. He was an accountant for a small construction company. S.N. and his wife have visitors, mainly relatives, about six times a year.

Sleep/Rest   S.N. falls to sleep after the 11 PM news. For the past 3 months he has been awakening at night for no apparent reason and is unable to return to sleep. His wife gives him a diphenhydramine HCl (Benadryl) pill to help him sleep. He sleeps until 7 AM and naps throughout the day.

Nutrition/Metabolic   S.N. will not cook food anymore; he will occasionally microwave prepared foods or eat things in the refrigerator. S.N. and his wife receive Meals on Wheels 6 days a week. Their daughter and son alternate having them over for dinner on Sundays. Their daughter buys them groceries each week. S.N. and his wife have 1 cup of coffee for breakfast.

Activity/Exercise   S.N. walks to the mailbox each day to get his mail. When the weather is nice, he walks a mile per day. In the past few months, S.N. has not paid much attention to how often his clothes are changed, and is bathing less frequently.

Coping/Stress   S.N. and his wife are appreciative of all the help their children give them. Neither husband nor wife cleans the house because it's too much for them. Their daughter and her husband clean for them.

Health Management   Nonsmoker; alcohol, has at least one drink per night. Daughter reports that he is drinking at least 1 or 2 strong mixed drinks per night.

Medications   Diphenhydramine HCl (Benadryl) at night and terazosin (Hytrin) 2 mg qd

Allergies   NKMA

Pertinent Physical Findings
Vital Signs   Height 5 feet 10 inches; weight 195; BMI 28; temperature 98.2° F; heart rate 76;

respirations 18; blood pressure 110/70 lying, 120/78 standing

General Appearance   Alert and oriented to time, place, person, and situation. Well nourished. Clothes clean. Speech clear, movements are coordinated. In no apparent distress. Appropriate behavior. Mini mental status 17/30. Becker Depression Scale is within normal limits.

Integument   Skin, moist, warm, thin, decreased turgor, no edema, lesions, or exudate. Nails, nail beds pink and smooth, capillary refill less than 3 seconds, no clubbing, nails short and slightly brittle

HEENT   Head, normocephalic, without evidence of trauma, lesions, or tenderness. Face, symmetrical, expression appropriate. Eyes, PERRLA, optic discs sharp, well defined, cream color, no exudates or hemorrhages, vessel nicking and copper wire arteries noted. EOMs intact. Visual acuity, 20/30 OU with glasses. Bilateral arcus senilis. Ears, pinnae have no lesions or scaling, TMs pearly gray, landmarks intact with distinct cone of light. Rinne, AC greater than BC au. Weber without lateralization

Neck   Supple without JVD, carotid bruits, or thyromegaly, no cervical lymphadenopathy, trachea is midline

Chest   Clear to auscultation and equal bilaterally, no adventitious breath sounds, resonant throughout lung fields

Cardiovascular   Apical pulse 72, regular rate and rhythm, no S_3 or S_4, PMI 5th ICS-LMCL, radial, pedal, and femoral pulses 2+ and equal bilaterally

Breast   No masses or axillary lymphadenopathy

Abdomen   Round, active bowel sounds, no abdominal bruits, soft, no masses or organomegaly, nontender, no inguinal lymphadenopathy, no CVA tenderness

Genitalia   Penis uncircumcised, no discharge, testes descended without masses or tenderness

Rectal   No masses or lesions; few external hemorrhoids; hemoccult negative stool in anal vault; normal anal tone; prostate smooth with no nodules, slightly enlarged

Extremities   Pink, warm, without edema, few varicosities bilateral lower extremities, bil negative Homans sign, dorsalis pedis and radial pulses 2+ bil =, joints without evidence of ligamentous laxity, effusions, erythema, or swelling

Neurological   CN II-XII grossly intact, DTR 2+ bil symmetrical, muscular strength intact bil, no atrophy or tremors, Romberg neg, sensation intact to light touch and pinprick, able to heel-to-toe walk

Diagnostics

Diagnostic Tests   HCT 44%, HGB 14.6 g/dl, RBC 4.8 million/ul, MCV 83 u^3, MCH 28 pg, MCHC 33%, WBC 5800/ul, sedimentation rate 30 mm/hr, urinalysis negative, TSH 4.6 mU/L, B12 245 pmol/L, syphilis serology negative, BS 89, Na 139 mEq/L, K 4.2, Cl 101 mEq/L, CO2 24, anion gap 6, calcium 4.9 mEq/L, creatinine 1.2 mg/dl, ALT 11 U/L, AST 16 U/L, CT head: diffuse cortical atrophy and widening of the sylvian fissure, HIV negative, ECG NSR

History Data   Questions specific to the chief complaint of memory loss include the following:

- Do you think you have a memory problem, or have others noticed it?
- Do you have trouble remembering current events and appointments, or remembering to pay bills?
- Is your memory loss getting worse or staying the same?
- Did your memory loss begin gradually or suddenly?
- Did you or others notice your memory loss all of the time or only at certain times of the day and/or night?
- When did you first notice a memory loss problem?
- Does anyone in your family have a problem with memory loss?
- Do you have a history of psychiatric problems, neurological conditions, or any head trauma?
- Have you ever been or are you afraid of being hit or hurt by anyone?
- Have you been the victim of a violent attack?
- Are you lonely?
- How often do you leave your home or have people visit you?
- Do you have a history of hypertension, stroke, or coronary heart disease?
- What medications, either prescription, OTC, or herbal, are you taking? (Medications such

as antihistamines, narcotic analgesics, benzodiazepines, anticholinergics, tricyclic antidepressants, anticonvulsants, cimetidine [Tagamet], and Parkinson's medications can cause toxicity in the elderly because these patients are more sensitive to the side effects of medications.)

- Any recreational drug use?
- Do you drink alcoholic beverages?
- Do you drink beverages with caffeine?

Elicit the history data from the patient and a significant other if possible. Other information that should be collected includes a complete history with functional assessment (see Chapter 2 for complete history information). Evaluate the patient's ability to perform activities of daily living and assess falls or risk of falling. In addition, it is important in the elderly population to evaluate depression as well as a test for memory.

Physical Examination Data   The focused examination for the chief complaint of memory loss includes a complete physical examination with particular attention on the vital signs, hearing and vision screen, and neurological examination with mini-mental examination, heart and lung assessment.

Differential Diagnoses   Dementia, depression, delirium, Parkinson's disease (Table 13-3)

Probable Causes of the Presenting Symptoms Alzheimer's disease is the most common form of dementia. It is rare in middle-aged individuals but extremely common in the frail elderly. It is estimated that as many as 47% of persons over the age of 85 may have Alzheimer's (Henderson, Benton, and Paganini-Hill, 1998). There is an autosomal dominant pattern of familial inheritance of Alzheimer's in only 20% of the population. In those with familial inheritance, researchers have found involvement of at least 3 chromosomes (1, 14, and 21). A specific allele in chromosome 19 (apolipoprotein E4) seems to be associated with a higher incidence of Alzheimer's. In Alzheimer's disease there are neurofibrillary tangles and loss of synapses in the cerebral cortex. The neurofibrillary tangles are the result of intraneuronal accumulations of filamentous materials that tend to oc-

Table 13-3
Memory Loss Differential Diagnostic Cues

Diagnosis	Signs and Symptoms	Lab Data	Treatment
Dementia Cortical dementia 30%-50% are caused by Alzheimer's disease (AD) 30% are caused by multiple strokes (multi-infarct dementia often have a history of vascular disease or hypertension) 20%-30% are caused by a mixed etiology including alcoholism and trauma	Progressive memory loss over weeks to months, becoming lost, inability to manage personal finances, using lists to remember tasks and activities	CBC, sedimentation rate, urinalysis, TSH, B_{12}, syphilis serology, BS, electrolytes, calcium, creatinine, liver function (these labs are to eliminate inflammation, infection, vitamin deficiency, endocrine disorders), CT head (prominent cortical atrophy in AD is common but not diagnostic), HIV, ECG if indicated	Discussion of social, living arrangements and legal issues is important. Encouraging the patient to establish a power of attorney, making decisions about operating a motor vehicle, and discussing housing arrangements are important. Explore the option of getting on a waiting list for a good nursing home or dementia care facility. Establish routines and regular meals. Treat depression with low doses of antidepressants (especially the SSRIs). Treat hallucinations and delusions with low doses of neuroleptics. For patients with AD, two cholinesterase inhibitors are available. Donepezil (Aricept) 5 mg/day, may increase to 10 mg/day after 1 month. Side effects include N/V, diarrhea, insomnia, fatigue, anorexia. Tacrine (Cognex) is available starting at 10 mg qid (max 40 mg qid). N/V are common side effects. Monitor liver enzymes at baseline, every other week to week 16 and then every 3 months
Delirium May be taking multiple medications Causes include infections, metabolic disorder, stroke, brain tumor, subdural hematoma	Abrupt memory loss over hours to days, sundowner syndrome (worse at night), disorientation, hallucinations, delusions, changes in levels of consciousness. A thorough ROS is essential	Laboratory tests are aimed at the suspected cause of the underlying disorder. If a UTI is suspected, a urine dip and culture may be ordered. If a cerebral disorder is suspected, a CT or MRI of the head may be ordered. If a metabolic order is suspected, electrolytes, liver enzymes, and BS may be ordered	Treat the underlying cause. Delirium is an urgent condition and should be treated promptly
Depression May co-exist with dementia	Memory loss, depressed mood, difficulty concentrating, sleep disturbance, loss of interest in surroundings, fatigue. More rapid decrease	TSH, CBC, RBS and urine toxicology. ECG if using TCAs. Geriatric Depression Scale or Beck Depression Scale	Psychotherapy and medications are often used. The most common medications prescribed are TCAs, SSRIs, and MAOs (third line treatment with dietary restrictions). TCAs have anticholinergic side effects and may exacerbate prostatism; overdoses are

Table 13-3
Memory Loss Differential Diagnostic Cues—cont'd

Diagnosis	Signs and Symptoms	Lab Data	Treatment
Depression —cont'd	in function than is typical in degenerative dementia. Mini-mental state examination typified by lack of effort rather than total inability to perform. Drawing and spatial concepts preserved		lethal and are contraindicated in patients with suicidal ideation, cardiac conduction problems, and narrow-angle glaucoma. SSRIs are usually first line treatment because they are well tolerated and do not have the anticholinergic SE.
Parkinson Subcortical dementia Motor disturbances are early with only mild cognitive impairment May have co-existing Parkinson's with another problem (e.g., depression, dementia)	Memory loss (late symptom) gait disturbance, attention problems, tremor, rigidity, bradykinesia, postural instability, mild decline in intellectual function, expressionless face, resting tremor. A common early presentation in young patients is tremor. Early presentation in elderly patients is gait dysfunction and akinesia (Goetz and Pepper, 1999).	None unless ruling out other disorders. May screen for other disorders using CBC, chemistry profile, and urinalysis. Imaging study possible to evaluate for lesion or infarction	A neurologist typically develops a treatment plan and the NP co-manages and monitors the patient. Early disease often does not require medication treatment. Physical or speech therapy may be indicated. Some individuals may prescribe selegiline (Eldepryl). Typical dose is 5 mg (not to exceed 10 mg) once a day. Cannot take meperidine with this med. If exceed 10 mg, cannot have tyramine foods. Mild disease often tries a dopamine sparing approach. For older patients or those with advanced disease, may try monotherapy with L-dopa (low-dose). With others may try dopamine agonist monotherapy (e.g., pergolide (Permax), bromocriptine (Parlodel), ropinirole (Requip), pramipexole (Mirapex). May use amantadine (Symmetrel) starting dose 100 mg bid as an alternative; it is effective with bradykinesia and tremor. Anticholinergic drugs are useful in controlling tremors and may be used in monotherapy or added to an agonist or levodopa. Examples include trihexyphenidyl (Artane) starting dose is 1 mg qd, may increase over weeks to 2 mg tid; **OR** benztropine mesylate (Cogentin), starting dose is 0.5 mg at HS may increase to I mg bid. Carbidopa/levodopa (Sinemet or Sinemet CR [controlled release]) is often used in moderate disease. A new medication that may be used is tolcapone (Tasmar), a catechol-O-methyl transferase inhibitor. Dosage is 100-200 mg tid (max dose 600 mg qd).

cur in the memory centers like the hippocampus and temporal lobe. Another characteristic feature of Alzheimer's disease is the identification of intracortical clusters of thickened neurons, called neuritis, surrounded by amyloid fibrils. Impairment of cholinergic transmission is also present. There is atrophy of the brain and enlargement of the ventricles.

Diagnostic Tests Screening tests should be conducted to rule out any reversible causes of memory loss. A CBC, sedimentation rate, urinalysis, TSH, B_{12}, syphilis serology, BS, electrolytes, calcium, creatinine, and liver functions should be ordered.

Diagnostic Impression S.N. is on diphenhydramine HCl (Benadryl) 50 mg at HS. Benadryl is a sedating antihistamine that may cause disorientation in the elderly patient. He is also drinking one or two "heavy" drinks per night. S.N. has progressively, over several years, been losing his ability to manage his own personal care, financial resources, and plan for future needs. He has memory impairment and is unable to carry out all activities of daily living. Therefore, a likely diagnosis to consider is Alzheimer's disease for this patient.

Therapeutic Plan of Care S.N. discontinued the use of Benadryl at nighttime and stopped his alcohol intake with no improvement of memory function. S.N. should be referred to a neurologist for evaluation and development of a treatment plan and the NP can co-manage his care. The neurologist may recommend starting S.N. on donepezil (Aricept) 5 mg qd and increasing to 10 mg/day after 1 month. If donepezil is started, it is important to document mental status with clock drawing and other objective tests that the clinician can use to re-evaluate the patient's symptoms at specific intervals. Side effects such as nausea, vomiting, diarrhea, insomnia, fatigue, and anorexia should be discussed with the patient and his daughter. A discussion about the safety of driving, making appropriate living arrangements, and establishing a power of attorney is important.

Patient Education and/or Community Resources Establishing routines, regular meals, and a consistent, safe environment is important for pa-

tients diagnosed with Alzheimer's. Encourage daily exercise, which often has a positive impact on mood and behavior and may improve sleep. Try to establish routines and creative activities to encourage expression from individuals and also to enhance mood. Provide reading materials and encourage them to keep in touch with historical events. Do not provide too much stimulation because this can cause increased confusion and depressed mood. Arrange family gatherings to include S.N., and provide prompts to assist him with the conversation. Encourage the patient and his family to discuss durable power of attorney for a family member and the patient's wishes regarding invasive, life-prolonging procedures. Family should also discuss plans for care of the patient when his condition deteriorates, including options for placement if his care at home becomes to onerous to maintain with day help. There are many resources for patients and families with Alzheimer's disease. The Alzheimer's Association is a good resource for families (1-800-272-3900). Some patients may opt to try a more natural approach to improve their memory by using a herbal therapy such as ginkgo (Ginkgo Biloba).

Follow-Up Plan Follow-up initially with an appointment in 1 month to see how the effects of the medication and lifestyle adjustments are working. Include the daughter in the discussions, and assist her in discussing her feelings and responsibilities. Subsequent appointments will need to be scheduled every 3 months to provide support, education, and follow-up.

*C*ase *S*tudy *3*

PRESENTING PROBLEM: Unilateral Weakness and Numbness

History of Present Illness R.S. is a 67-year-old Caucasian male who presents with a complaint of a single episode of abrupt onset of right-sided weakness and numbness that lasted for 2 hours yesterday afternoon at work when he was using the computer. He was able to move his right arm and leg during this period, but it was weaker than normal. R.S. was waiting for the clinic doors to open and is very scared. He is worried that he will have another stroke and end up paralyzed. He had a brain attack (stroke) 2 years ago. R.S. denies head trauma, recreational drug use, alcoholism, cancer, or cigarette smoking. He denies experiencing a H/A, dysarthria, dysphagia, or visual disturbances. He has been on anticoagulation therapy since his first brain attack occurred 2 years ago. When questioned about his medications, he states he has not taken his isosorbide mononitrate (Imdur) every day because he no longer can afford to purchase this medication. R.S. stated that he was going to ask for help with getting this medication at his regular visit that is scheduled for next week. He states that he has taken all of the other medications on schedule.

Past Medical History Hypertension for 20 years, hyperlipidemia for 15 years, diabetes mellitus for 11 years, cardiomyopathy diagnosed 2 years ago, and brain attack 2 years ago

Past Surgical History Cholecystectomy in 1965

Family History Father, fatal Stroke at 65; mother, deceased at 72, colon cancer; son, HTN; daughter, A&W

Developmental Stage Ego Integrity versus Despair

Role-Relationship R.S. lives with his wife who is 65 years old.

Sleep/Rest R.S. goes to sleep at 11 PM and awakens at 6 AM. He does not experience insomnia or nightmares. Since he started the Hytrin for his high blood pressure he does not have to get up to urinate at night.

Nutrition/Metabolic States he has 3 meals per day plus 2 snacks. He tries to avoid desserts and candies because of his DM. He usually has oatmeal and toast in the morning; a sandwich and fruit for lunch; and potatoes, meat, and vegetables for dinner.

Activity/Exercise R.S. walks with a cane due to residual weakness from the stroke. He works part time (16 hours per week) at a local auto body shop entering parts orders into the computer. He is able to carry out all activities of daily living. He no longer drives since his stroke.

Coping/Stress R.S. has a 65-year-old wife who drives, cooks, and cleans. Their daughter and

son live within 5 miles of them and visit at least once per week. Religion: Catholic (attends services weekly)

Health Management Nonsmoker. Alcohol, drinks socially. Td: 1/95

Self-Perception and Values/Beliefs R.S. is adapting to the use of a cane and to the weakness in the right side of his body. He is very worried about having another stroke and being left paralyzed.

Medications Isosorbide mononitrate (Imdur) 30 mg qd, lisinopril 20 mg and hydrochlorothiazide (Zestoretic 20/25) 25 mg, warfarin (Coumadin) 5 mg qd, insulin (Novolin) 70/30 - 65 units subcutaneous qAM and 50 units subcutaneous in the PM, and simvastatin (Zocor) 20 mg at HS, and 2 weeks ago began taking vitamin C 1 gram bid

Allergies NKMA

Pertinent Physical Findings

Vital Signs Height 6 feet 2 inches; weight 233 pounds; BMI 30; temperature 98.2° F; heart rate 82; respirations 18; blood pressure 180/98 standing, 172/94 lying

General Appearance Alert and oriented to time, place, person, and situation. Overweight. Clothes clean and neat. Speech clear, movements are coordinated, and gait is stable

Funduscopic PERRLA, EOMs intact, optic discs sharp, well defined, cream color, no exudates or hemorrhages. Vessel nicking and copperwiring noted

Neck Supple without JVD, left carotid bruit audible, no cervical lymphadenopathy, trachea is midline

Heart Apical pulse 82, regular rate and rhythm with grade II systolic murmur best heard at 5th ICS-LMCL with no radiation, no S_3 or S_4, PMI 5th ICS-LMCL, radial, pedal, and femoral pulses 2+ and equal bilaterally

Lungs Clear to auscultation and equal bilaterally, no adventitious breath sounds, resonant throughout lung fields

Neurological Mini-mental status score 27/30, CNII-XII grossly intact, L side: DTR 2+, muscular strength intact, no atrophy or tremors, sensation intact to light touch and pinprick R side: DTR 3+, slight atrophy of extremities, able to close hand, decreased strength and grip, decreased strength in lower extremity, unsteady without the use of a cane, sensation on R side is altered: able to feel pressure and touch, - Babinski

Diagnostics

Diagnostic Tests   CT of head: There are three old lacunar infarctions in the basal ganglia region on the left. Prothrombin time (PT): 18.9, INR 1.8, carotid Doppler: moderate stenosis to the right carotid and moderate to severe stenosis, 55% to 60% of the internal carotid artery on the left side with normal flow in the common carotid and external carotid

History Data   Questions specific to the chief complaint of unilateral weakness and numbness include:

- What part of your body did you experience weakness and numbness?
- Were you able to move the affected extremity?
- Did you fall or lose balance?
- Did you or do you have a headache?
- What was the intensity, length, and frequency of the weakness and numbness?
- How rapidly did the weakness and numbness occur? (Symptoms from brain tumors tend to occur over a longer time, whereas stroke symptoms occur more suddenly.)
- Have you had any other occurrences?
- What were you doing when you felt the numbness and weakness?
- Were there any associated symptoms such as difficulty swallowing (dysphagia), difficulty speaking clearly (dysarthria), headache, or visual disturbances?
- Have you had any trauma to your head (including motor vehicle accidents or falls)?
- Are you on anticoagulation therapy?
- Do you have a past history of cancer?
- Do you use recreational drugs? (IV drug users may develop brain abscesses.)

Review the *risk factors for stroke* with the patient: hypertension, diabetes, cigarette smoking, hyperlipidemia, AIDS, recreational drugs, alcoholism, family history of stroke, advanced age, atrial fibrillation, carotid artery stenosis, LVH on ECG, TIAs, and lack of exercise (Goetz and Papper, 1999).

Physical Examination Data   The focused examination for the chief complaint of unilateral weakness and numbness includes vital signs, general appearance, fundoscopic examination, neck (assess for carotid bruits), heart (include peripheral pulses), lungs, neurological examination

Differential Diagnoses   Transient ischemic attack, brain attack, subdural hematoma, brain tumor, multiple sclerosis, and brain abscess (Table 13-4)

Probable Causes of the Presenting Symptoms   Transient ischemic attacks (TIAs) are abrupt focal neurological deficits that last less than 24 hours and commonly occur over a period of minutes (Isselbacher, Braunwald, Wilson et al 1994). This is the most likely cause of this patient's symptoms. The usual cause of a TIA is either an ischemic (80%) or a hemorrhagic (20%) event. Ischemic events are caused by vascular occlusion. This can be due to an embolism from the heart or atherosclerotic vessel; a thrombosis; or, rarely, due to a substantial decrease in circulation to the brain from hypotension. Hemorrhagic events are caused by either subarachnoid or intraparenchymal hemorrhage. Other causes of TIAs include inflammatory arterial disorders (e.g., giant cell arteritis, systemic lupus erythematosus), heavy recreational use of sympathomimetic drugs (e.g., cocaine, amphetamines), or hematological disorders (e.g., sickle cell, polycythemia, severe anemia) (Rubin, Voss, Derksen et al, 1996; Tierney, McPhee, and Papadakis, 1999).

Approximately 30% of patients who have a transient ischemic attack will subsequently have a brain attack. The patient presentation with brain attack is highly variable, based upon the location of the cerebral injury. Symptoms may include subtle weakness, speech alterations or personality changes, paralysis, and coma.

Diagnostic Tests   Tests include a CBC (for infection, anemia, thrombocytopenia), FBS (for hypo- or hyperglycemia), sedimentation rate (for inflammation such as temporal arteritis), cholesterol (for hyperlipidemia), serologic test for

Table 13-4
Unilateral Weakness and Numbness Differential Diagnostic Cues

Diagnosis	Signs and Symptoms	Lab Data	Treatment
Transient Ischemic Attack (TIA)	Symptoms are dependent upon the nature and location of the cerebrovascular event. Acute onset of a focal neurologic deficit. The neurological deficit will resolve completely within 24 hours. Recovery often occurs within a few minutes. Symptoms may be motor or sensory or both. If ischemia is in the carotid region may experience weakness and/or numbness in the contralateral side. If ischemia in the vertebrobasilar region may have vertigo, ataxia, speech or disturbance, visual disturbance, or sensory alterations on one or both sides.	CBC, FBS, sedimentation rate, cholesterol, serologic test for syphilis, ECG, CXR. Holter monitoring if a cardiac rhythm problem. CT of head to assess for hemorrhage, lesions, or abscess. If carotid bruits assess with carotid duplex ultrasonographic scan	Need immediate evaluation because of potential for brain damage with delayed treatment. Emergency care transportation Management may entail a carotid endarterectomy if patient has blockage of >70% and is a surgical candidate. If atrial fibrillation is present, use anticoagulation if not contraindicated. Often patients are instructed to take aspirin 325 mg qd **OR,** if unable to tolerate, ticlopidine (Ticlid) 250 mg bid (requires monitoring CBC–baseline, then every 2 weeks for the first 3 months of therapy and then for 2 weeks after it is discontinued; also check CBC if suspect any hematological changes); **OR** Plavix may be used.
Brain Attack (Stroke) Third leading cause of death Strokes may be ischemic (80%) or hemorrhagic (20%)	Acute onset of a neurological deficit. The neurological deficits reflect the area of the brain involved. Warning signs of stroke include difficulty thinking and communicating, speech and visual disturbances, weakness of the affected arm and leg.	Stat CT of head	Emergent care. Transport to emergency facility. Effective treatment for acute stroke requires intervention within 3 hours of onset. Prognosis is poorer if consciousness is lost.
Subdural Hematoma Common cause is head trauma which causes a slow bleed	Assess mental status for slowness, confusion, and memory disturbance. H/A, personality change, or drowsiness.	CT of Head. May need cervical spine x-rays if injury with neck pain or deficit. Assess for skull fracture with any head injury. Signs of	Refer for urgent evaluation and care. Surgical evacuation is the usual intervention

Continued

	Table 13-4		
	Unilateral Weakness and Numbness Differential Diagnostic Cues—cont'd		

Diagnosis	Signs and Symptoms	Lab Data	Treatment
Subdural Hematoma—cont'd Symptoms can take up to 6 weeks to develop		basilar skull fracture include raccoon sign (bruising around orbits), battle sign (blood in the external auditory canal), and CSF in the ear or nose (check for glucose content).	
Multiple Sclerosis Highest incidence is with young adults Autoimmune condition Most common in temperate climates May have a genetic component with the HLA-DR2 antigen	Transient weakness, numbness, unsteadiness. Double vision, disequilibrium, or urinary symptoms of hesitancy or urgency.	MRI of head. The foramen magnum region should be evaluated to rule out Arnold-Chiari malformation (inferior poles of the cerebellum and the medulla enter the foramen magnum into the spinal canal).	A neurologist should be consulted for a management plan. 50% will not have significant disability within 10 years. With exacerbations, high dose corticosteroids are given (Prednisone 60-80 mg qd for 1 week with a 2-3 week taper). Methylprednisolone 1 gram IV × 3 days may be given with exacerbations followed by the oral corticosteroids. In patients who have frequent relapses – beta interferon or subcutaneous copolymer 1 may be initiated.
Brain Abscess Common organisms include streptococci, staphylococci, and anaerobes May arise as a sequel of ear or nose disease	Drowsiness, H/A, confusion, focal neurological defect, fatigue, inattention	CT of head	Refer for urgent care. Treatment usually includes intravenous antibiotics and surgical drainage. May treat medically if abscess is <2 cm. If intracranial edema often will give dexamethasone.

syphilis, ECG (for cardiac dysrhythmias), CXR (for abscess or tumor). If a cardiac rhythm disturbance is suspected, order a halter monitor or event monitor. CT scan of the head is important to assess for hemorrhages, lesions, or abscesses. If there is a carotid bruit, order a carotid duplex ultrasonographic scan or spiral CT scan.

Diagnostic Impression This patient presents with a transient episode of right-sided unilateral numbness and weakness. The most probable cause is a transient ischemic attack.

Therapeutic Plan of Care This patient needs immediate evaluation at an emergency care center. A CT of the head should be ordered. The clinician should conduct an in-depth assessment to evaluate for cardiac rhythm disturbances, carotid bruits, and neurological deficits. Lab work should be drawn as discussed under diagnostic tests. A neurologist should evaluate this patient and develop a plan of care.

Due to the fact that R.S. is on warfarin (Coumadin), it is important to monitor his PT as expressed as INR (this is the internationally accepted standard for monitoring warfarin therapy). His PT should be evaluated in 1 week because it takes several days for the warfarin therapy to reach a new steady state (long elimination of half-lives of warfarin). If the level is therapeutic, then the PT should be rechecked in 2 weeks. If stable, recheck every 4 to 6 weeks.

The neurologist will most likely recommend that R.S. be put on high intensity warfarin therapy. High intensity therapy is used for those patients who have a mechanical valve replacement and those who have thromboembolic recurrence even with adequate anticoagulation. The goal for high intensity therapy is the prolongation of prothrombin time to an INR of 2.5 to 3.0. Because R.S.'s INR was 1.8, he needs to increase his Coumadin and discontinue the vitamin C. Low-intensity warfarin therapy is used for those patients who need prevention for or have a thromboembolic disease. The goal for low-intensity warfarin therapy is an INR of 2.0 to 3.0.

R.S. needs to take his isosorbide mononitrate (Imdur) daily as prescribed to get his BP in an acceptable range. The NP can assist R.S. in getting the medications he needs by using community resources, a prescription assistance service from a pharmaceutical company, or aid the patient in applying for the appropriate assistance programs. The NP should again discuss the importance of proper BP maintenance to help R.S. prevent brain and heart attacks.

Patient Education and/or Community Resources Patient education should focus on the cause, treatment, and lifestyle changes that are applicable. Patients who have carotid stenosis and are not on Coumadin, and are not surgical candidates, should receive aspirin, ticlopidine, or Plavix.

A risk factor evaluation should be undertaken for those patients at high risk for stroke. Evaluate and manage hypertension, smoking, excess alcohol intake, obesity, lack of exercise, and consumption of a high-fat diet. For patients with hypertension and diabetes, it is important to provide an effective treatment plan because the likelihood of a stroke is substantial higher for patients with these conditions. Individuals who would like additional information on strokes and TIAs may contact the National Stroke Association at 1-800-787-6537; or use the Internet to access information from the National Stroke Association at http://www.stroke.org.

Follow-Up Plan Follow-up will depend on the cause of the transient ischemic attack. If there is a substantial carotid blockage, surgical intervention will need to be undertaken. If there is cardiac emboli from atrial fibrillation, refer to a cardiologist for evaluation and treatment as indicated.

R.S. should have his warfarin (Coumadin) increased to 6 mg qd. His PT and INR should be redrawn in 1 week and his BP checked. He should discontinue his vitamin C 1 gram qd because it can interfere with the absorption of warfarin. R.S. should be cautioned about taking garlic pills and vitamin K tablets because these may interfere with the warfarin. A transesophageal echocardiogram may be ordered to determine if there is a cardiac source of embolus and the status of his cardiac function. R.S.'s test revealed no cardiac source of embolus, with normal left ventricular size with diminished left ventricular systolic function. There was mild to moderate mitral regurgitation and mild left atrial enlargement. The test indicated mild aortic valve sclerosis with minimal aortic insufficiency from moderate descending aortic plaquing.

R.S. should have return visits every 3 months to monitor his diabetes through physical assessment and laboratory evaluation (FBS, HgbA1c). He should be reminded to have an annual eye examination by an ophthalmologist for proper eye care. A periodic reassessment of diet, exercise, and proper technique for insulin administration and a review of dosages should take place. In addition, an evaluation of his BP and medications should be conducted. He also has hyperlipidemia, so this should be monitored by evaluating a fasting lipid profile and periodically evaluating the liver enzymes (side effect of many of the medications prescribed for hyperlipidemia). For immunizations, he should receive a pneumovax and an annual influenza vaccine.

R.S'.s care is complex and requires close management and collaboration with appropriate health care professionals (e.g., neurologist, dietitian, ophthalmologist, cardiologist) for a therapeutic plan of care. A comprehensive approach to patient management requires regularly scheduled visits to provide quality care and optimize patient outcomes.

*C*ase *S*tudy *4* Optional Exercise

CHIEF COMPLAINT: Seizure

History of Present Illness R.J., a 21-year-old Caucasian male, presents to your office with chief complaint of jerking of his extremities and loss of consciousness. He states that a month ago he was eating at a restaurant with his girlfriend and he fell out of his chair jerking and lost consciousness. His girlfriend wanted to take him to the emergency room, but he didn't feel it was necessary. R.J. is now concerned because the same thing happened yesterday when he was playing cards with his buddies. He describes a heightened sense of smell and increased nervousness prior to the onset of jerking. He was incontinent and fatigued after both episodes. He lay down for a few hours before he felt okay. R.J. stated that bystanders told him that he was unconscious only for a minute or two. The jerking movements were on both sides equally. There is no family history of epilepsy.

Past Medical History Broken leg at age 10; no history of head injuries, brain attack, or meningitis

Family History Mother, migraine H/As; father, A&W; maternal grandmother, HTN

Developmental Stage Intimacy versus Isolation

Role-Relationship R.J. lives in a three-bedroom apartment with two of his male friends. Has been dating his girlfriend, Jan, for 1 year. Works as a truck driver

Sleep/Rest Roommate tells him he snores at night when he is really tired. Falls asleep at midnight and awakens at 6 AM.

Activity/Exercise Plays sports year-round. Swims in the summer, plays basketball, and skis in the winter

Coping/Stress When he gets real stressed, will drink with his buddies to relax. At other times his girlfriend and he will go to the movies or out for dinner. He is very worried about his recent "spells" because he drives a truck for a living.

Health Management Nonsmoker. Drinks socially from 1 to 6 cans of beer when he gets together with his friends, about two times per week. He has passed out only on one occasion when drinking with his buddies. He doesn't really feel his drinking is a problem, nor does he need a drink when he awakens. Occasionally experiments with recreational drugs (i.e., marijuana and cocaine) with his friends

Self-Perception and Values/Beliefs Is very happy with his employment and his lifestyle. Enjoys his girlfriend and wants to settle down in a few years

Medications Multivitamin 1 qd

Allergies NKMA

Pertinent Physical Findings

Vital Signs Height 6 feet 4 inches; weight 221 pounds; BMI 27; temperature 98.2° F; heart rate 66; respirations 14; blood pressure 122/82

General Appearance Alert and oriented × 4, well-groomed, well-nourished. Coordinated movements with stable gait

HEENT Head, normocephalic, without trauma. Face, symmetrical, smiling. PERRLA, EOMs intact; funduscopic, optic discs sharp, well defined, cream color, no exudates or hemorrhages. Ears, TMs gray with distinct cone of light. Nose, clear.

Throat, oral mucosa pink, moist, no lesions; tonsils 2+; Neck, no cervical lymphadenopathy or carotid bruits. Neck supple. Thyroid WNL

Heart Apical pulse 66 regular rate and rhythm, no S_3 or S_4. Radial, pedal, and femoral pulses 2+ and equal bilaterally

Lungs Clear to auscultation

Neurological CN II-XII grossly intact, DTR 2+ bil symmetrical, muscular strength intact bil, no atrophy or tremors, Romberg negative, sensation intact to light touch and pinprick; able to heel-to-toe walk

Diagnostics

Diagnostic Tests EEG, spiked waves showing generalized abnormality; CT of the head, negative; HCT, 46%; HGB, 15.0 g/dl; RBC, 4.9 million/ul; MCV, 90 u3; MCH, 30 pg; MCHC, 34%; WBC, 7200/ul; ALT, 12U/L; AST, 17 U/L; toxicology screen, negative

---

Discussion Questions

What type of history data should be collected?

What type of physical data should be collected?

What are the differential diagnoses?

What are the probable causes of the presenting symptoms?

What is your diagnostic impression?

What is the therapeutic plan of care?

What are the patient education and/or community resources?

What is your follow-up plan?

Discussions for optional case study exercises can be found in the accompanying Instructor's Manual.

References

Goetz C, Pepper E: *Textbook of clinical neurology,* Philadelphia, 1999, WB Saunders.

Goroll AH, May LA, Mulley AG: *Primary care medicine,* ed 3, Philadelphia, 1995, Lippincott-Raven.

Henderson VW, Benton D, Paganini-Hill A: Alzheimer's disease and other dementias in the older woman, *Aging: The Female Patient* 23:19-24, 1998.

Isselbacher, Braunwald, Wilson, Martin, Foci and Kasper: *Harrison's Principles of Internal Medicine,* ed 13, New York, 1994, McGraw-Hill

Jarvis C: *Physical examination and health assessment,* ed 2, Philadelphia, 1996, WB Saunders.

Kelley W: *Textbook of internal medicine,* ed 3, Philadelphia, 1997, Lippincott-Raven.

Rubin H, Voss C, Derksen DJ et al: *Medicine: a primary care approach,* Philadelphia, 1996, WB Saunders.

Tierney L, McPhee SJ, Papadakis MA: *Current medical diagnosis and treatment,* Stamford, Conn., 1999, Appleton & Lange.

Uphold C, Graham M: *Clinical guidelines in family practice,* Gainesville, Fla., 1998, Barmarrae Books.

Wiest P, Roth P: *Fundamentals of emergency medicine,* Philadelphia, 1996, WB Saunders.

Selected Readings

Kelley R: CT versus MRI for stroke, *Patient Care* 33(6):175-182, 1999.

Le Bars PL, Katz MM, Berman N et al: A placebo-controlled, double-blind, randomized trial of an extract of Ginkgo biloba for dementia, *JAMA* 278(16):1327-1332, 1997.

Marin P: Pharmacological management of migraine, *J Am Acad Nurse Pract* 10(9):407-412, 1998.

CHAPTER 14

Musculoskeletal Disorders

Jean Nagelkerk

Case Study 1

CHIEF COMPLAINT: Low Back Pain

History of Present Illness W.M. is a 32-year-old Caucasian male who presents with chief complaint of low back pain of 8 days duration. W.M. reports constant, sharp, lower back pain with movement and extreme pain with bending since he felt a pop in his back while he was lifting and replacing parts in his car. He has dull, nagging pain in his lower back when sitting and lying. He does not experience shooting pain, loss of sensation, or weakness in his extremities. He has full bowel and bladder control. He works as a manager for a building retail store. His job often requires the lifting of boxes ranging from 5 to 50 pounds. He has only experienced one other episode of low back pain a year ago. At that time he saw a chiropractor who adjusted his back. He took over-the-counter ibuprofen and felt fine in a week. W.M. reports that this episode of back pain is worse. He has seen a chiropractor twice for manipulations, and each time his back has felt worse. The pain has lasted for 8 days and he is worried that there is something seriously wrong with his back.

Past Medical History Unremarkable

Past Surgical History T&A at age 13; appendectomy at age 21

Family History Mother, 58, and father, 60, both A&W; brother, age 34, asthma

Developmental Stage Intimacy versus Isolation

Role-Relationship W.M. lives with his wife of 10 years in a two-story house. They have one son, age 2, and two daughters, ages 4 and 8. W.M. enjoys his job as a manager of a building retail store. Both his and his wife's parents visit often and help with childcare.

Sleep/Rest Sleeps 7 hours a night. W.M. usually falls to sleep at 11:30 PM and awakens at 6:30 AM.

Nutrition/Metabolic Eats three meals per day with snacks. Typically eats oatmeal for breakfast, eats a packed lunch with a sandwich, chips, and fruit for lunch, and eats with his family for dinner (meat, potato, and vegetable). Snacks on fruit and sweets.

Activity/Exercise Leisure activities include reading, swimming, and bicycling. Keeps active with fixing the house and caring for the yard.

Coping/Stress When he is frustrated about activities, he will discuss them with his wife or work in the yard. Attends services at a Christian Reformed Church every Sunday. In the winter, he works on woodwork projects for a hobby.

Health Management Drinks a beer on the weekend. Nonsmoker. Immunizations: Td 4/99

Self-Perception and Values/Beliefs Is pleased with his life and how he is able to purchase a home and enjoy his wife and children.

Medications Acetaminophen (Tylenol) prn

Allergies NKMA

Pertinent Physical Findings

Vital Signs Height 5 feet 11 inches; weight 215 pounds; BMI 30; temperature 98.2° F; heart rate 72; respirations 12; blood pressure 122/76

General Appearance Alert and oriented to time, place, person, and situation; speech clear, dressed casually, gait steady.

Heart Apical pulse 72 regular rate and rhythm, no S_3 or S_4, PMI 5th ICS-MCL; radial, pedal, and femoral pulses 2+ and equal bilaterally

Lungs Clear to auscultation

Abdomen Active bowel sounds, no masses, no abdominal bruits, soft, no organomegaly or inguinal lymphadenopathy, no CVA tenderness

Back Thoracic curve convex and lumbar curve concave. Spinous processes are straight and nontender. Paravertebral muscles in the lumbar region (L2-L4) are tender to palpation. Able to perform complete ROM, but has discomfort with flexion at 35 degrees, lateral flexion at 30 degrees, and rotation at 25 degrees. Muscular strength of lower extremities equal and intact bilaterally, no atrophy or tremors

Neurological Ankle and patellar deep tendon reflexes 2+ bilateral, symmetrical. Sensation intact to light touch and pinprick. Bilateral foot dorsiflexion and great toe dorsiflexion strong and symmetrical. Able to walk on toes and heels. SLR is negative

Diagnostics
Diagnostic Tests None

History Data Questions specific to the chief complaint of low back pain include the following:

- Where is the exact location of your back pain?
- Describe the type and intensity of your back pain. Is the pain constant, intermittent, dull, aching, or shooting?
- Was the onset of your back pain sudden? (If the pain is abrupt without injury, include dissecting aortic aneurysm in your differential diagnoses.)
- Do you have any pain shooting down either or both legs (radicular pain), weakness in extremities, loss of sensation, numbness or tingling, or gait disturbance (neurological deficits)?
- Do you have diminished or lack of sensation in your genital and/or rectal area (perineal anesthesia), bladder, or bowel dysfunction?
- Have you lifted anything heavy or experienced a traumatic injury recently (including MVA)?
- What are your limitations in activities?
- What type of physical activity do you do daily?
- Do you have a history of back pain, cancer, recent lumbar puncture, infection, or use of corticosteroids?
- Have you had a fever, burning upon urination, or persistent pain unrelieved by resting or lying flat?

- What makes your back feel better? What makes your back pain worse?

Stiffness in the morning that is relieved by activities may indicate an inflammatory condition or ankylosing spondylitis. Symptoms that are worse with standing and are better with sitting may indicate spinal stenosis. Pain that is worse with sitting may indicate a lumbar disk herniation. Look for "red flags" when eliciting the history. *Red flags* for low back include: age >50 or <20, trauma, weight loss, fever, history of cancer, pain that wakes the client during night or pain with rest, and medication history (steroid use).

Physical Examination Data The focused examination for the chief complaint of low back pain includes vital signs, general appearance, heart, lungs, abdomen, back, and neurological (plus rectal if there is "saddle anesthesia" or cauda equina syndrome).

Differential Diagnosis Conditions that often present without radicular pain include acute muscle strain, ankylosing spondylitis, spondylolisthesis, malingering, and osteomyelitis. Conditions that usually present with radicular pain include herniated nucleus pulposus, spinal stenosis, fracture, and spinal metastasis (Table 14-1).

Probable Causes of the Presenting Symptoms Approximately 80% of Americans will experience low back pain at least once in their lifetimes (Tierney, McPhee, and Papadakis, 1999). Each year, 20% to 30% of the adult population has at least a single episode of low back pain (Richardson and Iglarsh, 1994). Back pain that lasts longer than 6 weeks is chronic in nature. Chronic low back pain is one of the most common causes of disability. In fact, in the working population below age 45, the most common disability from on-the-job activities is low back pain. Often employers will require their employees who complain of work-related back pain to be evaluated by a health-care provider to prevent further disability. The risk factors for low back pain include obesity, smoking, inactivity, sports (e.g., gymnastics, football), and occupational activities that involve heavy lifting, prolonged sitting, or repetitive twisting

Text continued on page 260.

Table 14-1
Low Back Pain Differential Diagnostic Cues

Diagnosis	Signs and Symptoms	Lab Data	Treatment
Muscle Strain Acute	Usually immediate onset of low back pain; may have pain in buttocks or upper part of thighs; may feel as if something gave way or popped in lower back	None	First 24 hours, conservative treatment with ice or cold packs for 20 minutes qid prn Then local warm, moist heat or warm baths and the use of antiinflammatory agents (e.g., naproxen [Naprosyn] 500 mg bid prn with food *OR* ibuprofen [Motrin] 600-800 mg q 6-8 hours prn with food). Muscle relaxants (e.g., cyclobenzaprine [Flexeril] 10 mg qd-tid prn *OR* methocarbamol [Robaxin] 1.5 grams qid prn *OR* metaxolone [Skelaxin] 800 mg three or four times a day prn) have shown limited efficacy for muscle relaxation and should be reserved for patients who fail NSAIDs and then only used sparingly for short periods (1-2 weeks). Muscle relaxants should be avoided in the elderly due to the potential for falls. Back exercises and back care should be discussed and instructions given (see patient education section on pages 262-265). Bed rest should not be routinely prescribed; if it is prescribed, limit to 2 days if possible to prevent muscle deconditioning. Avoid the use of analgesics if possible, otherwise may use for controlling the initial acute pain (severe) for 1-2 days
Ankylosing Spondylitis Associated with HLA-B27 Axial arthritis Young men are generally more often affected than women (3:1)	Gradual onset of morning spinal stiffness partially relieved by activity; persistence of pain for 3 months or more; diminished chest expansion; decreased spinal flexion	Spinal x-rays. May show narrowing of the sacroiliac joint spaces and reactive sclerosis. Later stages will show fusion of the sacroiliac joint spaces. ESR, HLA B27 typing	NSAIDs such as indomethacin (Indocin), piroxicam (Feldene) to control pain and decrease stiffness; physical therapy is useful to preserve joint functioning and spinal movement. Swimming is advocated. In severe or unremitting cases, may refer to a rheumatologist to evaluate the short-term use of antibiotic therapy or immunosuppressant therapy
Herniated Nucleus Pulposus Most common site (95%) is disk herniation at L4-L5 and L5-S1	L5 nerve root irritation results in LBP that radiates to the dorsum of the foot, weakness of	Plain x-rays may be done if conservative treatment failure. MRI is useful for detailed	Unless there are neurological losses (e.g., weakness, cauda equina syndrome), a course of conservative therapy is tried for 6-12 weeks. Conservative treatment includes NSAIDs, regimented exercise program, physical therapy,

Table 14-1
Low Back Pain Differential Diagnostic Cues—cont'd

Diagnosis	Signs and Symptoms	Lab Data	Treatment
Herniated Nucleus Pulposus—cont'd			
Symptoms depend on the level of the injury Sciatica is a hallmark of nerve root irritation Most commonly occurs in young and middle-aged adults Muscular weakness or atrophy may occur	great toe, and numbness in the great toe region. S1 nerve root irritation results in LBP with numbness and paresthesia in the buttock, posterior thigh, calf, and lateral aspect of the ankle and foot. In general, radicular pain is piercing and shooting in nature and worse with sneezing, coughing, or a Valsalva maneuver. DTR may be decreased or absent in the affected nerve root distribution.	anatomical imaging. CT may also be used, but is less sensitive for imaging cauda equina tumors or intradural lesions. Radionuclide bone scanning is often done when suspecting osteomyletitis or metastasis.	and activity modification Surgical referral if there is a neurological deficit. Should avoid the use of narcotics for chronic back pain; strong analgesic agents should be reserved for acute and reversible causes of pain for short periods
Spondylolisthesis Forward subluxation of a vertebrate Common causes in adults are degenerative changes and arthritis In children, sports causing hyperextension such as gymnastics, diving, or weightlifting	Chronic low back pain and discomfort. May have pain radiating into the thighs. May have tenderness over the spondylolisthetic joint. Patient may present with tight hamstrings	Plain x-rays MRI or CT if indicated	Conservative therapy with warm, moist heat, NSAIDs **OR** analgesics, and back and hamstring stretching exercises. May need to schedule regular rest periods and activity modifications. Rarely will use spine immobilization for short periods of time (a corset or brace is used to stabilize the spine while the patient is instructed on how to strengthen the musculature; the orthotic device is removed once a day to work on strengthening the musculature). Refer to surgeon for evaluation of spinal fusion if treatment failure (rarely needed)

Continued

	Table 14-1		
	Low Back Pain Differential Diagnostic Cues—cont'd		

Diagnosis	Signs and Symptoms	Lab Data	Treatment
Spinal Stenosis Degenerative changes resulting in narrowing of the lumbar nerve canals	Often bilateral pain in the buttock, thigh, or leg. Pain is elicited by walking or prolonged standing. Rest or flexion of the spine may improve pain. May be able to walk uphill with less discomfort than downhill	Magnetic resonance scanning and electromyographic studies	Most often conservative. Use of NSAIDs, activity modifications, and light exercises. Surgical intervention will occasionally be required. Epidural glucocorticoid injections may occasionally be used by specialists as adjunct to therapy for patients experiencing spinal stenosis or disk injury (for those with severe lumbar radiculopathy).
Fracture Causes may be acute trauma, stress fractures in young athletes, post-menopausal osteoporosis, metastatic carcinoma	Acute localized pain. May have weakness or inability to move legs. Pain to ambulate or any movement	Lumbosacral spinal films. If suspect cancer, order CBC, erythrocyte sedimentation rate, urinalysis. If cancer suspected, may consider bone scan	Immobilize and refer depending on the cause of the fracture
Malingering Often poor response to conservative therapy Tends to occur in higher rates for those who use alcohol excessively, dislike their jobs, and who describe pain patterns that are inconsistent with dermatomal patterns	May report a myriad of symptoms. Usually includes LBP with radiculopathy symptoms. Usually the description of the pain and neurosensory distribution is not consistent with dermatomal patterns and the SLR is not positive as well as discrepancies on the heel and toe walking assessments	None Wadell's signs* (5) are indicative of nonorganic pathology. Individually they do not indicate a problem, but 3 or > indicate it is unlikely the patient will respond to treatment of the back. The 5 signs are: (1) abnormal sensation – tender over broad area to light touch; (2) nonanatomic neuro exam; (3) distraction – seated versus lying SLR; (4) simulation –	Conservative management of the the LBP. In addition, determine alcohol use, job dislike, or other issues influencing the patient's chief complaint. May need a referral for alcohol detoxification or counselingdepending on the patient's needs.

*It is important to rule out any external causes of low back pain including herpes zoster (may have radicular symptoms), abdominal aortic aneurysm, penetrating ulcer (usually has a history of peptic ulcer disease), endocarditis (history of cardiac murmur), renal disease, pelvic inflammatory disease, and prostatitis.

Table 14-1
Low Back Pain Differential Diagnostic Cues—cont'd

Diagnosis	Signs and Symptoms	Lab Data	Treatment
Malingering—cont'd		pain with whole body rotation and light pressure to top of head; and (5) behavior of grimacing, groaning, or inappropriate affect.	
Spina Metastasis History of cancer Commonly from carcinoma of the prostate, breast, lung, multiple myeloma or lymphoma	Low back pain that is not relieved by rest or lying in the supine position. Pain often occurs around the clock with little relief.	Plain x-rays for suspected metastasis might show bone lysis or sclerosis. MRI useful if suspecting cauda equina tumor and will show early metastasis. Radionuclide bone scanning is useful to detect early metastasis or osteomyelitis.	Refer to oncologist for treatment options. Radiation is commonly employed. In select patients a combination of radiation and surgery may be elected.
Osteomyelitis Adults are most commonly affected Typically has a history of recurrent urinary tract infections Common in diabetics and may occur in intravenous drug abusers, alcoholics, immunosuppressed	Fever, chills, low back pain. Pain is usually localized over the affected area. May rapidly progress to an epidural abscess where the patient may present with motor or sensory loss, fever and chills in addition to pain over the affected area	Plain x-rays may not show early osteomyelitis. If evident will show disk narrowing and end plate erosion. May need to get radionuclide bone scan. MRI also shows early disease. Blood cultures, CBC, ESR	Orthopedic referral for treatment. Often patients will receive 4-8 weeks of antibiotics and may require debridement of necrotic bone.

Text continued from page 255.

Low back pain is often caused by acute muscle strain. Muscle strain is brought about when acute injury or mechanical stress causes the stretching or ripping of muscle fibers or distal ligamentous attachments of the paraspinal muscles (Kelley, 1997). Often there is spasm, swelling, minor bleeding, and inflammation at the site of injury, causing localized tenderness to the lower back. The discomfort may also occur across the lower back or in the buttock or upper thigh area.

Sciatica or radicular symptoms occur when there is irritation of the lumbar or sacral nerve root, indicating possible disk herniation. The patient experiences sharp or excruciating pain that radiates down the lateral or posterior aspect of the ankle or leg. With disk herniation the patient may experience numbness or tingling, weakness in the distribution of the affected nerve root, and increased discomfort with coughing, sneezing, or a Valsalva maneuver. Disk herniation most commonly (95%) occurs in the lower back at L4-L5 or L5-S1. Figure 14-1 shows the most common sciatica patterns.

When evaluating a patient with a back injury, instruct the patient to perform range of motion of the back and document the degrees that the joints can move up to the point of pain. This includes having the patient bend forward (flexion; 90 degrees), bend backward (extension; 30 degrees), bend to either side (lateral flexion; 35 degrees), and turn one way and then the other (rotation; 30 degrees) (Jarvis, 1996). Palpate for any paraspinal muscle spasms or discomfort over the spinous processes. Evaluate the patient's gait for coordination and the ability to move effectively. The patient should be instructed to walk on the toes (L5-S1 disk; S1 root) and then on the heels (L4-L5 disk; L5 root). Note the quadriceps strength. Conduct the straight leg raising (SLR) test. In the SLR, the examiner lifts the patient's leg to 60 degrees while the patient is in the supine position. Any radicular pain in either leg is noted. Then, the other leg is raised passively to 60 degrees. A positive tests occurs when radicular pain occurs (nerve root irritation) as the sciatica nerve is stretched. Figure 14-2 illustrates the proper technique of performing a SLR.

When conducting a thorough assessment for lower back pain, assess the most common nerve disorders (L4, L5, and S1) and evaluate their motor, reflex, and sensory components. To evaluate L4, test the knee reflex, have the patient dorsiflex the feet, and test sensation over the medial calf. To evaluate L5, have the patient dorsiflex the great toes and test sensation over the medial forefoot. To evaluate S1, test the ankle jerk, have the patient evert both feet, and test sensation over the lateral foot.

To rule out cauda equina syndrome it is important to assess the patient for urinary retention, rectal incontinence, and perineal anesthesia. This syndrome is rare, but requires prompt treatment to restore sacral nerve root function. It signifies extensive midline disk herniation. Patients with cauda equina syndrome may also experience notable bilateral motor and sensory deficits.

Diagnostic Tests   Rarely do lumbosacral x-rays modify treatment or enhance diagnostic judgments. These x-rays cause substantial exposure to radiation. Lumbosacral x-rays cause 20 times the exposure of a chest x-ray. When x-rays show normal disk spaces, you cannot rule out disk herniation, and changes in a disk space do not indicate whether there are degenerative changes or disk narrowing. If patients are over 40 years of age, degenerative changes are common and do not indicate the presence of clinically significant disease. Therefore, x-rays are not indicated unless there has been trauma, lifting (by a patient who is osteoporotic), constitutional symptoms with low back pain, major neurological deficit(s), or history of or suspected malignancy. Pain localized in the thoracic or upper lumbar area is associated with compression fractures and metastatic tumors. MRI is often used to detect osteomyelitis, tumors, abscess, and disk herniation or cord compression. CT may also be used to detect nerve root compression problems, but an MRI is more sensitive in determining the extent of soft tissue involvement.

Diagnostic Impression   W.M. presents to your office with low back pain that occurred after working on his car. The pain from the acute muscle strain continued with manipulations from a chiropractor and continued with his daily work at the building retail store. There were no signs of neurological deficits.

Therapeutic Plan of Care   W.M. should be prescribed light duty for a 1-week period, after

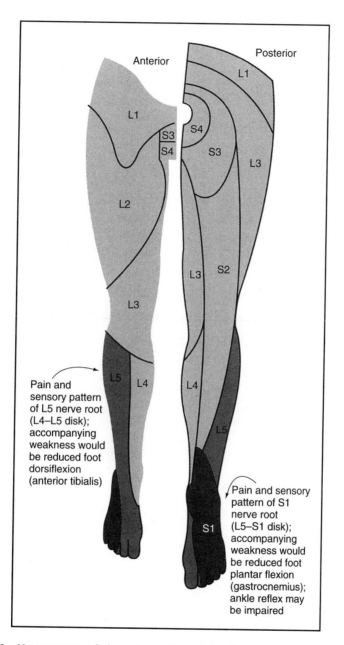

Anterior

Posterior

Pain and sensory pattern of L5 nerve root (L4–L5 disk); accompanying weakness would be reduced foot dorsiflexion (anterior tibialis)

Pain and sensory pattern of S1 nerve root (L5–S1 disk); accompanying weakness would be reduced foot plantar flexion (gastrocnemius); ankle reflex may be impaired

Figure 14-1   Most common sciatica patterns. (From Rubin H, Voss C, Derksen DJ et al: *Medicine: a primary care approach,* Philadelphia, 1996, WB Saunders.)

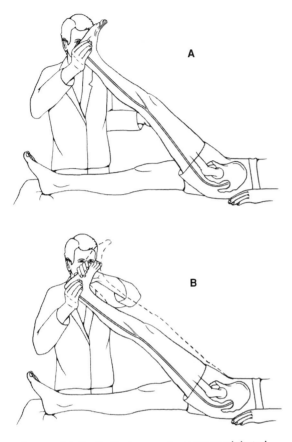

Figure 14-2 Radicular symptoms are precipitated on the left with the straight leg raised (**A**). The leg is lowered slowly until pain is relieved. The foot is then dorsiflexed, causing a return of symptoms (**B**). This indicates a positive test. (Modified from Reilly BM: *Practical strategies in outpatient medicine*, Philadelphia, 1991, WB Saunders.)

which time he should be reevaluated. *Light duty* includes the avoidance of prolonged sitting or standing and limiting the amount of lifting to no more than 20 pounds. Patients should avoid poor posture and bending and twisting motions of the back. Back exercises should be explained and encouraged. Proper back care when lifting should be discussed. Teach proper lifting, maintenance of good posture, and the importance of frequent position changes and lumbar support. An antiinflammatory agent should be prescribed to decrease inflammation and pain. Encouraging the patient to take the

antiinflammatory agent for 5 to 10 days is often effective in treating back pain. A muscle relaxant such as Flexeril may be prescribed for a limited time for the patient who experiences muscle spasms or difficulty sleeping at night from back discomfort. Muscle relaxants tend to cause drowsiness and the patient should be cautioned about this side effect. Their use in the elderly, who are at risk of falling, is not recommended.

Patient Education and/or Community Resources A very important part of patient education is the discussion of back care. Often, patients will ask if spinal manipulation by a chiropractor will improve their low back pain. Patients who have spinal stenosis or disk herniation should avoid spinal manipulation. The guidelines from the Agency for Health Care Policy and Research indicate that spinal manipulation is one physical method for the treatment during the first month of acute back pain without radiculopathy (AHCPR, 1994). If there is not improvement from the spinal manipulation after 4 weeks, the treatment should be stopped and the patient should be reassessed. According to Goroll, May, and Mulley (1995), there are no definitive conclusions regarding the benefits of spinal manipulation, although some trials have shown some benefit.

Teaching the patient proper lifting techniques and providing strengthening exercises for their lower back is a cornerstone of treatment. Teach the patient to keep the back straight and to bend the knees while lifting or picking up items. The leg muscles should be used when lifting, and the items should be kept close to the body and higher than the waist. The patient should not twist, bend, or reach while lifting items. Encourage frequent position changes and the avoidance of prolonged sitting or standing. The patient should rest and sleep on a firm mattress, lying supine with the knees flexed on a small pillow or, if side-lying, with bent knees and hips. To move from a supine to an upright position the patient should turn to the side and push up with the arms to a sitting position; then stand.

Effective prevention techniques to discus include the importance of regular activity on muscle strengthening and maintaining weight control. In addition, discussing the use of antiinflammatory medications, their side effects, and the need to take food with these medications is important. When prescribing physical therapy, discuss its importance so that the patient understand that this treatment is for muscle strengthening and flexibility and that it reduces the chance of reinjury (Goroll, May, and Mulley, 1995).

Rakel (1996) has developed a program for patients experiencing low back pain. Research shows that a systematic approach to back care improves the patient outcomes. The following back program is from the book entitled "Saunders Manual of Medical Practice" and is reprinted from pages 756-758 with permission:

Procedure   Low Back Pain Exercises
Goals in Prescribing Exercises for Low Back Pain Patients

- Decreasing pain, increasing strength, stretching contracted muscles, improving posture, decreasing mechanical stress, improving general fitness, stabilizing hypermobile segments, improving mobility

Types of Exercises Used with Low Back Pain Patients

- Mobility and strengthening exercises
- Lumbar flexion exercises (Williams exercises)
- Hyperextension exercises (McKenzie method)
- There are no good data to favor the utility of one method over another.

Indications

- Acute low back pain after some response to conservative therapy
- Low back pain associated with postural factors
- Fibrositis or fibromyalgia syndrome
- As a part of general rehabilitation and to maintain flexibility
- Chronic low back pain

Contraindications

- Signs and symptoms of systemic illness such as fever, weight loss
- Acute trauma
- The young and elderly who have not had sufficient work-up
- Cauda equina syndrome

- Radiculopathy and muscle atrophy without adequate work-up

Preparation

- Patient's pain should have partially responded to rest, nonsteroidal antiinflammatory drug (NSAID), and/or muscle relaxants
- Patient should be in athletic wear or nonbinding clothes
- Physical therapist or physician should instruct the patient and check progress

Precautions

- Flexion exercises should not be done if:
  There is acute disk prolapse
- Exercise is to begin immediately after prolonged bed rest, because hyperhydrated disk spaces are susceptible to injury
- Back pain is postural due to flexion or lateral trunk list
- Extension exercises may cause an increase in symptoms in patients who:
  - Have acute disk prolapse
  - Have had multiple back operations
  - Have limited flexion due to paraspinous scarring
  - Have spinal stenosis, and have facet syndrome

Technique

A. Mobility and strengthening exercises
  1. Low back stretching
     a. Lie supine on the floor with the legs extended
     b. With the right hand, pull the left leg over the right leg
     c. Shoulders should remain on the floor; turn the head to the left
     d. Pull up the left thigh to stretch the lower back and buttocks
     e. Repeat from the other side
  2. Full spinal stretch (Figure 14-3, *A*)
     a. Lie supine flat on the floor with the knees bent
     b. Place hands on the back of the thighs and bring the thighs on the abdomen
     c. Curl the head up toward the knees; uncurl; repeat

3. Heel cord stretch
   a. Stand facing a solid wall
   b. Place one foot about 18 inches from the wall and the other behind about 8 to 12 inches
   c. Keep the rear foot flat and place hands shoulder high against the wall
   d. Bend the forward leg and move the chest toward the wall and feel the stretch in the calf; change the anterior and posterior feet, and repeat
4. Hamstring stretching
   a. Sit with one leg flexed and one leg straight
   b. Reach toward the toes and stretch gently
   c. Change the position of the legs so that the opposite hamstring is stretched
5. Hip flexor stretching
   a. Lie supine with one leg straight and one flexed
   b. Take the flexed thigh and pull toward the chest
   c. Prevent the extended leg from elevating; repeat by changing legs
6. Back rotation (Figure 14-3, *B*)
   a. Lie supine with both knees flexed
   b. Keep shoulders flat and swing the knees from side to side to tolerance

B. Flexion exercises (Williams exercises): All flexion exercises should begin with the pelvic tilt (Figure 14-3) to decrease lumbar lordosis. The lower back should be flat against the floor.
1. Knee to chest
   a Begin by lying on the back with the knees flexed
   b. Place the hands on the knees and pull to chest
   c. Alternative method: can do one leg at a time
   d. Raising head slightly will stretch neck and other paraspinal muscles
2. Curl up – strengthens the abdominal muscles (Figure 14-3, *C*)
   a. Lie supine with knees flexed and feet on floor
   b. Place hands on chest; pelvic tilt
   c. Bring head and shoulders off the floor and hold for count of three
   d. Relax by uncurling

C. Extension exercises (McKenzie technique)
1. Lying exercises
   a. Lie prone, face to one side, arms to side, and relax. Pain should lessen or move toward the back
   b. Lie prone and then place forearms under shoulders and lift the chest off the floor; hold and then repeat
   c. Lie prone, place hands under shoulders, and push up lifting chest, straighten elbows to tolerance (Figure 14-3, *D*). Eventually get elbows straight and chest and part of the abdomen off the floor
2. Extension in standing (Figure 14-3, *E*)
   a. Stand with feet apart, hands on hips with fingers toward the small of the back or hands clasped in small of the back.
   b. Bend the trunk backward at the waist as far as possible, keeping the knees straight
   c. Repeat after holding a second or two, trying to extend a little farther each time

Follow-Up   When using the McKenzie method exercises, after the acute pain has resolved, flexion exercises should then be followed by extension exercises to prevent recurrence. These exercises also can be used in chronic back pain to maintain flexibility and to strengthen and balance the muscles used in maintaining an erect posture. These exercises are also helpful in the conservative treatment of some herniated disks without neurologic signs.

Follow-Up Plan   Reevaluate the patient in 1 to 2 weeks. If no improvement, or if severe pain or radiculopathy, reevaluate within 24 hours. If the patient is doing well after the second visit, reschedule at 4 to 6 weeks to evaluate and reinforce proper back care. For patients who are improving, but still experience discomfort, reevaluate every 2 weeks until symptoms are resolved. If the back pain is unresolved at 4 weeks and there are no red flags, order lumbosacral x-rays. If pain persists despite conservative treatment, may need to consider further work-up with MRI, bone scan (if diffuse pain), and/or referral for pain management. Possible options for pain management include epidural injection and facet blocks.

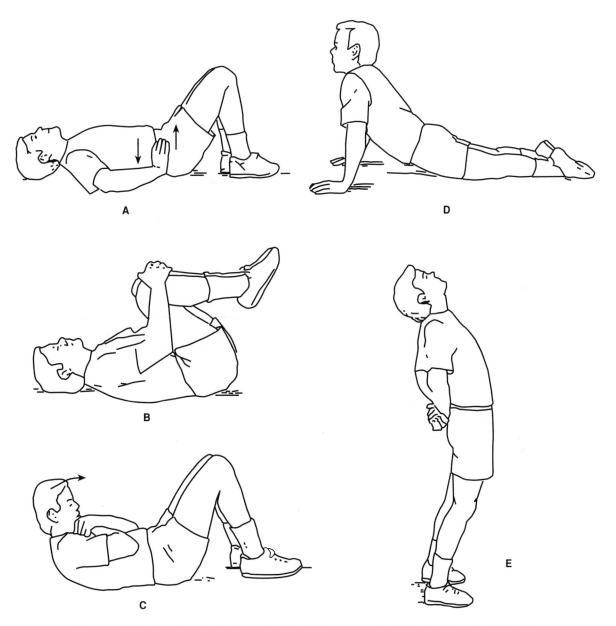

Figure 14-3 Exercises for the lower back. **A,** Full spinal stretch. **B,** Back rotation. **C,** Curl up. **D,** Lying extension exercise. **E,** Standing extension exercise. (From Rakel R: *Saunders manual of medical practice,* Philadelphia, 1996, WB Saunders.)

Case Study 2

CHIEF COMPLAINT: Morning Stiffness in the Fingers and Back

History of Present Illness   S.D. is an 82-year-old Caucasian female who presents with chief complaint of insidious onset of morning stiffness in the fingers of her right hand and in her lower back that is progressively becoming worse over the past 2 years. She reports that when she awakens, her fingers and back feel stiff, but within a half-hour she is able to function fine. S.D. has noticed bumps growing on her fingers, and reports that when she does her daily chores her fingers and back become painful. S.D. states that the more she does, the more she hurts. She takes Tylenol with little relief. Canning season is coming up and she needs to be able to use her hands to can food for the winter. She denies any past or recent trauma.

Past Medical History   HTN, DM, and PUD

Past Surgical History   Hysterectomy 1976; appendectomy 1967

Family History   Mother, DM; father, HTN; brother, glaucoma; sister, HTN

Developmental Stage   Ego Integrity versus Despair

Role-Relationship   S.D. has been a widow for 5 years. She lives in a ranch house with three bedrooms. Her daughter lives 5 miles away and visits almost daily. S.D. enjoys watching her daughter's children. S.D. visits neighbors and is involved in a coffee club at church. She attends a Lutheran church regularly.

Sleep/Rest   S.D. has no set bedtime. She usually falls asleep at 10 PM and arises about 7 AM. Often takes a nap in the afternoon as she reads the newspaper.

Nutrition/Metabolic   S.D. has had upper and lower dentures for 10 years. She fixes three meals per day for herself. Typically, she will have tea and toast for breakfast, a sandwich and piece of fruit for lunch, and a frozen dinner in the evening. Snacks include fruit and crackers.

Activity/Exercise   Performs all activities of daily living without difficulty. Enjoys reading and walking outdoors when the weather permits.

Coping/Stress   Enjoys gardening and growing flowers. Her daughter, neighbors, and friends at church are her support.

Health Management   Does not smoke, drink or use recreational drugs. Td: 1976, Pneumovax 1997. Has signed advanced directive and has durable power of attorney

Self-Perception and Values/Beliefs   Feels like she has had a good life. Is interested in helping others and enjoys her gardening and taking care of her grandchildren.

Medications   Moexipril (Univasc) 7.5 mg qd, glipizide (Glucotrol XL) 10 mg qd, famotidine (Pepcid 20 mg) qd, multivitamin qd, Tylenol Extra Strength 2 tablets tid

Allergies   PCN

Pertinent Physical Findings

Vital Signs   Height 5 feet 2 inches; weight 164 pounds; BMI 30; temperature 98.6° F; heart rate 76; respirations 16; blood pressure 132/88

Skin   Smooth, moist, warm, good turgor, no edema, lesions, exudates. Nail beds pink and smooth, capillary refill less than 3 seconds, no clubbing

Heart   Apical pulse 76 RRR without murmurs, no S_3 or S_4, PMI 5th ICS-LMCL, radial, pedal, femoral pulses 2+ equal bilaterally

Lungs   Clear to auscultation

Musculoskeletal   Extremities pink, warm, without edema, bil negative Homan's sign, joints without evidence of ligamentous laxity, effusions, or erythema. Right hand, Bouchard's nodes on the PIP joints and Heberden's nodes on the DIP joints. Spinal curvature reveals mild kyphosis in thoracic spine and back. No paraspinal tenderness. Active ROM of all joints, but crepitus noted in knees and hips, decreased flexion to 80 degrees bil knees. Mild limitation in internal and external rotation of shoulders bil. Gait stable. Muscle strength upper and lower: able to maintain flexion against resistance with no discomfort

Diagnostics

Diagnostic Tests   X-ray of right hand shows narrowing of the joint spaces and osteophyte formation.

History Data   Questions specific to the chief complaint of morning stiffness include the following:

- Where is the discomfort located? (Determine if it is an articular problem. If it is a joint problem, the pain should be localized to the joint and may involve some degree of functional limitations.)

- Which joints are involved in the discomfort? (Osteoarthritis and psoriatic arthritis commonly occur in the DIP joints.)
- Is it only one joint or is it bilateral and multiple joints? (Monarticular disorders involve gout, Lyme disease, and septic arthritis; whereas polyarticular disorders involve SLE, RA)
- How long does the morning stiffness last? (Less than 15 to 30 minutes, commonly OA; longer periods, RA)
- Do you have redness, swelling, or warmth? (Differentiates between inflammatory and noninflammatory arthritis)
- Have you had any recent or past trauma to the joint(s) involved?
- Are you able to perform all activities of daily living?
- What is your occupation?
- What is your past medical history? (Be sure to cover endocrine, musculoskeletal, and metabolic disorders.)
- Do you have a family history of arthritis?
- What aggravates the discomfort, and are there any associated symptoms? (Determine if there are characteristics of a systemic disease.)
- What medications are you taking, including over-the-counter medications? (Many patients may take aspirin or NSAIDs; often those with RA will experience some relief and take these medications routinely.)
- Have you traveled to an area endemic for Lyme disease? (Determine possibility of tick bite)

Physical Examination Data The focused examination for the chief complaint of morning stiffness and back discomfort includes vital signs, heart, lungs, and musculoskeletal.

Differential Diagnoses Osteoarthritis, rheumatoid arthritis, systemic lupus erythematosus, fibromyalgia, polymyalgia rheumatica, osteoporosis (Table 14-2).

Probable Causes of the Presenting Symptoms
Osteoarthritis affects 20 million Americans. It is the most common form of joint disease. In fact, by the age of 40, a majority of people (90%) will have radiographic evidence of joint disease in their weight-bearing joints. Most individuals, however, do not experience symptoms until after 60 years of age. *Risk factors for osteoarthritis* include obesity, trauma, age, and occupational overuse. Other factors associated with osteoarthritis include congenital musculoskeletal disorders, diabetes mellitus, and metabolic disorders.

Osteoarthritis is a noninflammatory degenerative joint disease characterized by pain that abates with rest, morning stiffness lasting less than 15 to 30 minutes, and minimal inflammation. Osteoarthritis occurs as the articular cartilage is worn down and spur formation begins to develop at the edge of joint surfaces. The synovial membrane lining the joint becomes thickened. Common joint sites are the distal and proximal interphalangeal joints, first metacarpophalangeal joint, knees, hip, and cervical and lumbar spine. The joints feel hard and cool and do not show signs of inflammation. The patient experiences pain that is worse with activity or prolonged standing whereas rest relieves these symptoms. Crepitus may sometimes be felt in the affected joints. In later stages of osteoarthritis the patient may experience the development of hard, nontender nodules over the distal interphalangeal joints (called Heberden's nodes) or over the proximal interphalangeal joints (called Bouchard's nodes).

When determining the cause of the patient's presenting symptom, it is important to review the associated symptoms when making the final diagnostic judgment. For example, morning stiffness is often found in rheumatoid arthritis, whereas in osteoarthritis the discomfort heightens with joint use. If a patient reports a rash, the diagnostic possibilities would include Lyme disease, SLE, and vasculitis. When a patient presents with a fever, diagnostic considerations would include infection, hypersensitivity reaction, or low-grade rheumatoid arthritis. Patients who have morning stiffness, but also complain of sleep disturbances and exhaustive fatigue, may have fibromyalgia or chronic fatigue syndrome. Patients who present with dry mouth and eyes may have Sjögren's syndrome, and these symptoms may also be associated with rheumatoid arthritis. A careful review of all of the associated symptoms may assist in formulating your differential diagnoses.

Table 14-2
Morning Stiffness and Back Pain Differential Diagnostic Cues

Diagnosis	Signs and Symptoms	Lab Data	Treatment
Osteoarthritis (Degenerative Joint Disease) Associated with older age, family history, obesity,trauma, joint instability, and diabetes mellitus Heberden's node (DIP) Bouchard's node (proximal interphalangeal [PIP] or first carpometacarpal joint) Noninflammatory Joints most often affected are the DIP, PIP, first metacarpophalangeal (MCP), knees, hips, and cervical and lumbar spine	Morning stiffness that remits within 15-30 minutes, progressive discomfort with joint activity; late stages develop Heberden's and Bouchard's nodes	Collect history and physical data. Based on these results, order the appropriate tests. If osteoarthritis is suspected (noninflammatory arthritis), may only elect to order an x-ray of the affected area to confirm hypertrophic osteoarthropathy. Some clinicians will make the diagnosis based on clinical data.	Treatment consists of weight reduction to help prevent further degeneration. Acetaminophen (Tylenol) 325 mg (2 tablets) every 4-8 hours should be tried. Other medications include NSAIDs (e.g., ibuprofen [Motrin] 400-800 mg tid prn **OR** oxaprozin [Daypro] 600 mg 2 tablets qd **OR** arthrotec [Diclofenac 50 mg and Misoprostol 200mcg] 50 mg tid **OR** Celebrex 100 mg bid). Topical treatment may be initiated (e.g., capsaicin [Zostiox] cream, a thin layer over painful joints tid-qid). Aerobic exercises routinely are useful to maintain full joint functioning. Warm moist heat or cold treatments prn. Some clinicians will do intraarticular injections with corticosteroids if medications do not provide an adequate response, but they can only be done every 3-6 months. Another option is synvisc (Hylan G-F 20) intra-articular injections each week × 3 for OA patients who fail to respond to conservative therapy. Surgical interventions may be needed for severe cases.
Rheumatoid Arthritis Women affected more often than men (3:1) Rheumatoid factor found in 3/4 of patients Symmetrical distribution Late stages have deformities (e.g., swan-neck flexion of DIP with extension	Insidious onset of symmetrical polyarthritis. Prolonged morning stiffness that decreases during the day. Often presents with fatigue, malaise, weight loss. Have inflammatory signs such as warmth, joint swelling, tenderness, and pain. Commonly affects the wrists, PIP joints, MCP joints, and may affect elbows, hips, knees, ankles, neck, and	Serum protein, rheumatoid factor (present 75% time), erythrocyte sedimentation rate, gamma globulins (specifically IgM and IgG), CBC, platelet count. May decide to selectively order x-ray(s). X-rays are the most specific diagnostic test for RA.	A program plan should be instituted to preserve function, decrease inflammation, and prevent deformities. A rest and exercise program should be instituted. PT and OT can design a home program for patients to implement with periodic evaluations. Rest each day (approximately 2 hours with mild disease) should be followed and support for any inflamed joints should be

Table 14-2
Morning Stiffness and Back Pain Differential Diagnostic Cues—cont'd

Diagnosis	Signs and Symptoms	Lab Data	Treatment
Rheumatoid Arthritis—cont'd			
of PIP), ulnar deviations, boutonniere deformity (i.e., hyperextension of DIP and flexion of PIP) One quarter of patients will exhibit subcutaneous nodules over bony prominences.	back. Extraarticular manifestations are common and multiple (e.g., vasculitis, Sjögren's syndrome, and Felty's syndrome [thrombocytopenia, anemia, splenomegaly]	Early x-ray changes show soft tissue swelling. Late changes show joint space narrowing and erosions. May consider synovial fluid analysis to rule out septic arthritis	maintained. Splints and assistive devices can be used effectively. NSAIDs are first line treatment (e.g., ibuprofen [Motrin] 400-800 mg tid, nabumetone [Relafen] I gram qd). Gastrointestinal side effects with NSAIDs are common with prolonged use. Take with food. If NSAIDs do not control symptoms, add a disease-modifying antirheumatic drug (DMARD). It is important to add a DMARD soon if needed to prevent joint damage. DMARDs include methotrexate, hydroxychloroquine, sulfasalazine, gold, d-penicillamine, azathioprine, cyclophosphamide, and corticosteroids.
Systemic Lupus Erythematosus Incidence is predominately women at age 30 (10:1), but in juvenile or elderly the male to female ratio is 2:1	Multisystem presentation (e.g., oral ulcers, rash over malar eminences, photosensitivity, arthritis, pleuritis, pericarditis, renal involvement [proteinuria >500 mg/d], neurological symptoms [seizures and psychosis], hematological disorders [hemolytic anemia, leukopenia <4,000/ml; lymphopenia <1500/ml; thrombocytopenia <100,000/ml])	Antinuclear antibody titer, urinalysis, anti-dsDNA, anti-Smith antigen, false-positive VDRL, SLE preparation	Important to discuss with the family that this is a chronic disease and describe the pathophysiology, course, and treatment options. Medications used in the treatment of SLE include NSAIDs, hydroxychloroquine, quinacrine, corticosteroids, methotrexate, dapsone, azathioprine, cyclophosphamide, and cyclosporin A. Care should be taken to monitor for side effects of these medications and to draw appropriate lab work.
Polymyalgia Rheumatica Often co-exists with giant cell arteritis Age over 50 Women experience more frequently (2:1) Septic arthritis may be	Pain and morning stiffness of the pelvic area and shoulders of 6 weeks or longer. Fever, malaise, anemia, and weight loss. May have joint swelling of the knees, wrists, and sternoclavicular. May experience H/As, amaurosis	Erythrocyte sedimentation rate (elevated), CBC (may have mild anemia)	Low dose steroids (prednisone 10-20 mg/day) good response within 48 hours. Prednisone is usually given for a period of at least 6 months time and then gradually tapered. Some clinicians add a NSAID when tapering. Occasional relapses

Continued

Table 14-2		
Morning Stiffness and Back Pain Differential Diagnostic Cues—cont'd		

Diagnosis	Signs and Symptoms	Lab Data	Treatment
Polymyalgia Rheumatica—cont'd			
associated with polymyalgia rheumatica	fugax (visual transient ischemic attacks), or scalp tenderness.		occur and treatment must be continued
Osteoporosis Risk factors include menopause, female gender, older age, physical inactivity, low weight (<58 kg), heredity, and low calcium and vitamin D consumption	Usually asymptomatic until the patient experiences either a compression fracture or fall causing injury. May develop kyphosis of the dorsal spine (dowager's hump)	Order tests to rule out endocrine problems (e.g., TSH, parathyroid function, blood sugar, estrogen). Order test to rule out multiple myeloma (e.g., CBC, ESR, and serum protein electrophoresis). Bone mineral density tests (e.g., dual energy x-ray absorptiometry [DEXA], which measures the density of the proximal femur [predictive of fractures] and the density of the lumbar spine [useful for monitoring treatment response]). Other tests that may be ordered include calcium, phosphate, vitamin D, parathyroid hormone, and alkaline phosphatase.	The key for osteoporosis is prevention. The use of estrogen replacement therapy assists with preventing bone loss. Common regimens include conjugated estrogens (Premarin) 0.625 mg qd and medroxyprogesterone acetate (Provera) 2.5-5 mg qd (Provera is added for women with intact uteri) **OR** estrogen patches (Estraderm) 0.5 mg/day – apply patch twice a week and add medroxyprogesterone acetate (Provera) if the woman has an intact uterus. Calcium intake should be adequate. For patients below 18 years old the recommendation is 1800 mg/day; for those under 50 years old the recommendation is 1000 mg/day; for those over 51 years of age, the recommendation is 1500 mg per day if on estrogen. Adding vitamin D (300 IUs) will enhance calcium absorption and is often useful for those older than 51. Avoid cigarette

Diagnostic Tests X-rays of the affected joints will show narrowing of the joint spaces, osteophyte formation, thickened and dense subchondral bone, bone cysts, and sharpened articular margins. With osteoarthritis, laboratory work such as sedimentation rate (inflammation), CBC (hematological involvement), rheumatoid factor testing (rheumatoid arthritis), ANA (SLE, RA, scleroderma, chronic hepatitis), serum calcium, serum phosphorus, uric acid (gout), alkaline phosphatase, urinalysis (glomerular injury) will all be within normal limits.

Diagnostic Impression S.D. presents with symptoms typical of osteoarthritis. She complains of morning stiffness with low back pain lasting approximately 15 minutes upon arising, but the symptoms become worse with joint usage. The discomfort is in her right hand and low back. She also has Heberden's and Bouchard's nodes. Also, consider coexisting osteoporosis due to her status as an elderly female with mild kyphosis of the thoracic spine.

Therapeutic Plan of Care The treatment plan for S.D. includes weight management and diet

	Table 14-2		
	Morning Stiffness and Back Pain Differential Diagnostic Cues—cont'd		
Diagnosis	**Signs and Symptoms**	**Lab Data**	**Treatment**
Osteoporosis—cont'd			
			smoking and heavy alcohol intake. A fall prevention program should be instituted. Other medications that may be used on select patients for prevention and treatment of osteoporosis are: raloxifene HCl (Evista); alendronate sodium (Fosamax); and salmon calcitonin (Calcimir, Miacalcin), either intranasal or parenteral. If vertebral fracture, may use analgesics, heat/cold therapy, proper positioning and scheduled exercises, calcitonin, and may need back support
Fibromyalgia 90% of patients will be women Usually between the ages of 20-50	Fatigue, stiffness, restless sleep, and widespread musculoskeletal pain for at least 3 months. The patient may experience H/As, cold sensitivity, and difficulties functioning effectively at school, home, and work. Pain in at least 11 of 18 trigger point sites on palpation	All laboratory data will be normal: (e.g., erythrocyte sedimentation rate, CBC, RF)	A coordinated program of aerobic exercises, support, and tricyclic medications (e.g., amitriptyline [Elavil] 25 mg at HS **OR** cyclobenzaprine [Flexaril] 20-30 mg at HS may assist with sleep patterns. Patient may use complementary treatments such as massage or acupuncture for symptom relief. Recommendations based on safety and research have not been established for complementary treatments.

counseling (5 feet 2 inches; 164 pounds; BMI 30) including adequate calcium intake, and a scheduled aerobic exercise program. S.D. should continue with Tylenol Extra Strength, which is the mainstay for treatment of OA. She should add capsaicin cream (Zostrix) topically. This medication inhibits substance P mediated pain transmission and should be used three or four times per day on the affected areas. Do not rub medication in eyes or place hand in mouth. She should experiment with cold and warm treatments qid prn to increase her comfort. S.D. should schedule her activities throughout the day to provide for adequate joint rest. She should receive a Td at this visit to update her immunizations.

For S.D., NSAID therapy would have to be carefully considered because of her age and prior ulcer history. Dyspepsia occurs in 30% to 40% of patients with long-term therapy. Gastric ulcerations, a more serious side effect, occur in 3% of patients. Other options, if the topical cream and the Tylenol do not control S.D.'s symptoms, are to use misoprostol (Cytotec) or a proton pump inhibitor (omeprazole [Prilosec]) concomitantly with a NSAID to help avoid gastrointestinal mucosal breakdown. Another option is the newer COX-2 selective NSAIDs such as Celebrex 100 mg bid and Vioxx. These COX-2 NSAIDs may be less likely to cause ulcers or GI bleeding than other NSAIDs. However, all NSAIDs have similar effects on the kidneys and patients need to report any edema or fluid retention. Celebrex is structurally similar to sulfonamides, so avoid use in patients who are allergic to sulfa. Herbal supplements that have been used include primrose oil 2 capsules bid or chondriotia sulfate and glucosamine. These herbal supplements may help with arthritis pain. However, recommendations based on research on safety and efficacy of these herbal preparations has not been established.

Patient Education and/or Community Resources Patient education is an essential part of the management of osteoarthritis. The clinician should assist the patient in developing a plan of care to maintain joint function, improve comfort, and maximize activities of daily living. The cornerstone of treatment is to manage weight reduction, exercise daily, and control pain through medications and local treatments. The patient should avoid strenuous activities, running, sitting for excessive periods, and climbing stairs. Aerobic exercises such as swimming and walking maintain function and strength. Avoid twisting motions when possible.

Follow-Up Plan S.D. should return to the office in 1 to 2 weeks for reevaluation. If her symptoms are then under control, she should be re-evaluated every 3 to 6 months. An evaluation for osteoporosis by ordering a DEXA scan should be considered. If S.D. proves to have osteoporosis, either Fosomax (alendronate as sodium) or Miacalcin (calcitonin-salmon) should be considered.

*C*ase *S*tudy *3*

CHIEF COMPLAINT: Pain and Numbness in Right Wrist

History of Present Illness T.J. is a 36-year-old Caucasian female who is right hand dominant who presents with chief complaint of pain and numbness in her right wrist for 6 months duration. T.J. states that at night she experiences extreme numbness and tingling of the fingers in her right hand and wrist. Her symptoms began 6 months ago with pain during any activity and numbness and tingling that is relieved by shaking her hands. T.J. reports that the pain now shoots up into her forearm and that her grip isn't as good as it used to be. She has tried over-the-counter Tylenol and Motrin with minimal relief. She works as an apple packer.

Past Medical History Asthma

Past Surgical History Lumbar laminectomy in 1992, T&A in 1970

Family History Mother, A&W; father, allergy problems; brother age 32, asthma; brother age 26, A&W; sister age 30, A&W

Developmental Stage Generativity versus Stagnation

Role-Relationship T.J. is divorced and lives alone in an apartment. She has been dating a man for 9 months. She has two boys, ages 5 and 7, whom she takes for a weekend about every other month.

Sleep/Rest Usually sleeps 7 hours per night

Nutrition/Metabolic T.J. does not enjoy cooking food. She eats out most meals, usually at fast food restaurants. Her breakfast usually consists of coffee and a donut. Lunch is usually a sandwich with chips or fruit. Dinner is usually a frozen dinner or fast food. She keeps raw vegetables and fresh fruit at home for snacks.

Activity/Exercise Enjoys swimming and walking. Exercises almost daily (30 to 60 minutes) either at home or at a local health center

Coping/Stress T.J. has many girlfriends with whom she regularly meets to discuss issues. They are very supportive of her, as is her boyfriend. She handles stress by walking, swimming, or talking with her girlfriends.

Health Management Smokes 1 pack per day for 15 years. Drinks socially. On weekends will "party" with her friends and she may drink 4 to 6 beers per night. Td: 1987

Self-Perception and Values/Beliefs States that she enjoys her life and enjoys her friends. Enjoys the time she spends with her boys, but is content with only seeing them every other month.

Medications Albuterol (Ventolin) inhaler 2 puffs qid prn, fluticasone propionate (Flovent) 44 mcg 2 puffs bid, levonorgesterel 0.10 mg, ethinyl estradiol 20 mcg (Alesse) 1 qd

Allergies Sulfa

Pertinent Physical Findings
Vital Signs   Height 5 feet 9 inches; weight 189 pounds; BMI 28; temperature 98.2° F; heart rate 64; respirations 14; blood pressure 120/84

Heart   Apical pulse 64 and regular, no S_3 or S_4, no murmurs

Lungs   Clear to auscultation

Neuromuscular   Examination of the RUE: Positive Tinel's and Phalen's tests. Full range of motion of the R wrist. There is mild focal tenderness over the pronator teres in the R forearm. Right radial pulse is 2+; gross sensation is intact; two-point sensation is intact in all digits; Capillary refill is <3 seconds. Slight muscle wasting over the thenar eminence. Pincer grasp decreased in right compared to the left hand. No masses or swelling noted

Diagnostics
Diagnostic Tests   Right upper extremity nerve conduction test: increased sensory latency

History Data   Questions specific to the chief complaint of pain and numbness of right wrist include the following:

- Is the pain and numbness in your wrist constant or intermittent?
- Is the pain intense or dull?
- Are the symptoms better, worse, or the same at night? (With carpal tunnel syndrome, nocturnal symptoms are usually present.)
- Have you had a recent injury to your hand?
- Do you engage in activities that require repetitive motions or the use of vibrating tools?
- Do you have any bumps or lumps on your hand?
- Do you have rheumatoid arthritis, hypothyroidism, diabetes mellitus, alcoholism, or acromegaly? (Carpal tunnel syndrome is often present with these disorders.)
- Are you pregnant? (Carpal tunnel syndrome may occur in pregnancy.)

Physical Examination Data   The focused examination for the chief complaint of pain and numbness of the right wrist includes vital signs, heart, lungs, and neuromuscular examination of the RUE.

Differential Diagnoses   Carpal tunnel syndrome, ganglion cyst, de Quervain's tenosynovitis, recent injury* (Table 14-3)

Probable Causes of the Presenting Symptoms
In carpal tunnel syndrome the median nerve in the wrist is trapped and compressed in a narrow compartment under the transverse carpal ligament as it passes through the wrist (Gates and Mooar, 1999). Two tests specific to assess for carpal tunnel syndrome are Tinel's and Phalen's. To perform the Tinel's test, tap the palmar aspect of the wrist where the median nerve is located. A positive test will elicit numbness, tingling, and/or pain. To conduct Phalen's test, the patient puts the dorsal aspect of the hands together with the wrists flexed 90 degrees, holding this position for 60 seconds. In a positive test there will be numbness, tingling, and/or burning discomfort with the sharp bending of the affected wrist.

Diagnostic Tests   A nerve conduction test of the affected upper extremity may be conducted if conservative treatment fails.

Diagnostic Impression   This patient presents with symptoms of carpal tunnel syndrome. She is employed in an occupation where she has repetitive wrist movements, she experiences nocturnal exacerbations, and she presents with a positive Tinel's and Phalen's test, and a decrease in pincer grasp in her dominant hand.

Therapeutic Plan of Care   This patient should have a trial of conservative therapy with wrist splint, NSAIDs such as ibuprofen (Motrin) 600 mg tid with food, and wrist rest. If the conservative treatment fails, the patient should be evaluated surgically because she is beginning to have mild thenar eminence atrophy and some mild strength disruption.

Tetanus should be administered at this visit, because T.J. has not had one for over 10 years. In addi-

---

*Other conditions such as pregnancy, hypothyroidism (altered fluid balance), diabetes mellitus (diabetic peripheral neuropathy), cervical spondylosis, alcoholism (neuropathic), rheumatoid arthritis (inflammatory), and acromegaly (anatomical) are also associated with carpal tunnel syndrome.

Table 14-3
Pain and Numbness Differential Diagnostic Cues

Diagnosis	Signs and Symptoms	Lab Data	Treatment
Carpal Tunnel Often found in middle-aged women Occurs in 1% of the population Commonly found among individuals with repetitious work that uses wrist motion in flexion, extension, and gripping Often presents with overuse of wrist and pain without a history of specific injury	Burning and tingling of the 3rd-5th digits of the affected upper extremity; aching pain that may radiate up into the forearm; pain is usually increased by repetitive activities, especially those involving volar flexion or dorsiflexion of the wrist. May experience muscle weakness of the thenar eminence (base of thumb)	Nerve conduction test of the upper extremity. May show increased muscle and sensory delays	Wrist splinting in the neutral position at night, the use of NSAIDs (e.g., ibuprofen [Motrin] 600 mg q6-8 hours with food), rest the affected joint and avoid repetitive activities. Other options to consider include corticosteroid injections if conservative therapy fails. Patients with severe symptoms may need surgical intervention.
Ganglion Cyst Common on the hand or wrist Contains fluid similar to joint fluid The origin of the cyst is usually the wrist joint	Discomfort with increased use or when cyst is accidentally bumped. At times may experience transient numbness and tingling	None	May aspirate with a large bore needle, but reoccurrence rate is high. Surgical intervention will eliminate, but is not used unless the cyst is problematic problematic or disfiguring
De Quervain's Tenosynovitis The site of the dysfunction is the tendons involved with the first dorsal compartment of the wrist	Positive Finkelstein's test (putting the thumb into the palm while making a fist and then ulnar deviating and palmer flexing the wrist). Pain with use of the thumb	None	Conservative treatment involves the use of a removable thumb spica cast used for 10-14 days (may remove for bathing) and NSAIDs. Also may use a corticosteroid injection. Surgical intervention may be required if other treatments fail.
Injury	Pain and swelling over the affected wrist. Guarding and limited range of motion from discomfort	X-ray of wrist	If no fracture, may splint for comfort and rest for 5 to 7 days and use NSAIDs, and apply ice 20 minutes qid to affected area. Instruct patient to elevate affected extremity when possible. If no x-ray findings of a fracture, but there is pain in the snuff box, a thumb spica should be applied and the patient should be re-examined in 2 weeks or referred to an orthopedic specialist.

tion, a pneumovax should be administered due to her history of asthma. A review of her asthma control and smoking history should begin. A plan of care should be developed to assist T.J. to maximum wellness. Periodic follow-up for her asthma, support for a smoking cessation plan, and discussions of decreasing alcohol consumption are important pieces of the plan of care. Assist T.J. to establish her goals and develop effective strategies for her successful health-care plan.

Patient Education and/or Community Resources T.J. needs to understand why she is having the discomfort and numbness and tingling in her wrists. A clear explanation of carpal tunnel syndrome should be discussed with her. She should understand the aggravation of symptoms with repetitive activities. T.J. should be told the side effects of ibuprofen (Motrin), to take it with food, and the need to take it every day for the next few weeks to help decrease the inflammation. She should also be instructed on resting her wrist (may use wrist splint as needed).

Follow-Up Plan Reevaluate this patient in 3 to 4 weeks to determine the progress with conservative therapy and then establish a follow-up schedule for her asthma and lifestyle modifications.

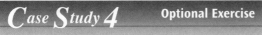

Case Study 4 **Optional Exercise**

CHIEF COMPLAINT: Right Knee Pain

History of Present Illness S.S. is a 17-year-old African-American male who presents with chief complaint of right knee pain and swelling for 1 day. He reports that yesterday he was playing soccer and was hit directly on the lateral side of his knee, causing his knee to bend medially. He fell and had immediate pain. S.S. attempted to play soccer for another half-hour, but the pain increased. He then sat down, took two over-the-counter Motrin, ate, and put ice on his knee to relieve the discomfort. This morning he woke up and found that any twisting motion causes pain. S.S. now notices a slight swelling, and is worried that he "messed up his knee." He reports that he had a left knee injury in soccer when he was in ninth grade, but it resolved

without problems and hasn't had any trouble since. S.S. has played soccer since age 5 and hopes to win an athletic scholarship to a top 10 college.

Past Medical History Unremarkable

Past Surgical History Tubes in ears at age 5, appendectomy at age 16

Family History Father, MI at age 62; mother, HTN and obesity; four sisters, A&W

Developmental Stage Identity versus Role Confusion

Role-Relationship Lives with parents and four sisters in a two-story house in the suburbs. S.S. has many friends with whom he enjoys playing sports, going to movies, and just hanging out. He has been dating a girl in his class for the past 6 months.

Sleep/Rest Falls asleep about 11 PM and awakens at 6 AM

Nutrition/Metabolic Is a vegetarian. Feels he eats healthy foods such as vegetables and fresh fruits. Eats on a regular schedule and eats three meals per day and snacks when he is hungry

Activity/Exercise Very active in soccer. Enjoys competitive games and is always hanging around with his friends, competing with them

Coping/Stress Plays soccer to relieve stress. Talks often to his peers and, at times, with his parents

Health Management Nonsmoker. Does not use alcohol or recreational drugs. Td 7/98

Self-Perception and Values/Beliefs Is excited about attending college by winning a scholarship for collegiate soccer. His goal is to study to be an athletic trainer.

Medications Motrin OTC for pain

Allergies NKMA

Pertinent Physical Findings

Vital Signs Height 6 feet 3 inches; weight 232 pounds; BMI 29; temperature 97.8° F; heart rate 64; respirations 12; blood pressure 124/78

Heart Apical pulse 64 with a regular rate and rhythm, no murmurs, no S_3 or S_4

Lungs Clear to auscultation

Musculoskeletal Extremities: warm, without edema, no varicosities, bil negative Homans sign, dorsalis pedis and radial pulses 2+ bil equal, L knee joint without evidence of ligamentous laxity, effusions, erythema, or swelling, full range of motion. R knee joint with tenderness over the medial joint line to the insertion of the medial collateral ligament, + valgus stress elicits pain, slight laxity of the medial aspect of the knee, and slight swelling over the medial aspect of the knee. Negative varus and valgus laxity; McMurray's, Appley, and anterior cruciate drawer tests; and bulge sign. Able to perform full ROM of R knee, but guards and does slowly. Gait steady, but favors R leg

Diagnostics
Diagnostic Tests   None

Discussion Questions

What type of history data should be collected?

What type of physical data should be collected?

What are the differential diagnoses?

What are the probable causes of the presenting symptoms?

What is your diagnostic impression?

What is the therapeutic plan of care?

What are the patient education and/or community resources?

What is your follow-up plan?

Discussions for optional case study exercises can be found in the accompanying Instructor's Manual.

References

Agency for Health Care Policy and Research: *Understanding acute low back problems* (AHCPR Publication No. 95-0644), Rockville, Md., 1994, U.S. Department of Health and Human Services.

Gates SJ, Mooar PA: *Musculoskeletal primary care,* Philadelphia, 1999, Lippincott.

Goroll A, May L, Mulley A: *Primary care medicine,* ed 3, Philadelphia, 1995, Lippincott-Raven.

Jarvis C: *Physical examination and health assessment,* Philadelphia, 1996, WB Saunders.

Kelley W: *Textbook of internal medicine,* ed 3, Philadelphia, 1997, Lippincott-Raven.

Rakel R: *Saunders manual of medical practice,* Philadelphia, 1996, WB Saunders.

Reilly BM: *Practical strategies in outpatient medicine,* Philadelphia, 1991, WB Saunders.

Richardson J, Iglarsh Z: *Clinical orthopaedic physical therapy,* Philadelphia, 1994, WB Saunders.

Rubin H, Voss C, Derksen DJ et al: *Medicine: a primary care approach,* Philadelphia, 1996, WB Saunders.

Smith BW, Green GA: Acute knee injuries: Part I. History and physical examination, *Am Fam Physician* 51(3):615-621, 1995.)

Tierney L, McPhee SJ, Papadakis MA: *Current medical diagnosis and treatment,* Stamford, Conn., 1999, Appleton & Lange.

Selected Readings

Agency for Health Care Policy and Research: *Acute low back pain in adults: assessment and treatment* (AHCPR Publication No. 95-0643), Rockville, Md., 1994, U.S. Department of Health and Human Services.

Hoppenfeld S: *Physical examination of the spine and extremities,* Norwalk, Conn., 1976, Appleton & Lange.

Mercier LR: *Practical orthopedics,* ed 5, St Louis, 2000, Mosby.

CHAPTER 15

Psychiatric Disorders

Penny Hinkle

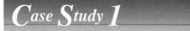

CHIEF COMPLAINT: Acute Epigastric Pain

History of Present Illness J.T. is an 18-year-old Caucasian female college freshman presenting to the student health clinic with complaints of gastric pain and "burning" for 2 days. J.T. recently pledged to a sorority with a reputation for "heavy partying" and attended a sorority party over the weekend. She reports the onset of diarrhea, nausea, and gastric pain the day after the party. The diarrhea and nausea self-resolved within 8 hours, but the gastric discomfort persists. She reports her gastric pain increases when she drinks carbonated beverages and when she has an empty stomach. She denies vomiting with evidence of blood and has not had tarry stools. She admits a similar episode of gastrointestinal disturbance following binge drinking in high school but she did not seek medical treatment. J.T. lives in a co-ed dormitory and likes her suite mates. She is taking a full course load and is majoring in pre-law. J.T. graduated from high school with a B-plus grade average and feels pressured to maintain this average to get into law school.

Past Medical History Unremarkable, regular menses lasting 3 days; LMP 1 week ago

Past Surgical History Tonsillectomy without complications at age 6 years

Family History J.T. has a 20-year-old brother who is living at home with her parents and is working part-time. Her brother left college after the start of his sophomore year secondary to a brief psychiatric hospitalization for treatment of depression with suicidal ideation. He is currently taking an antidepressant and sees a therapist weekly for counseling. J.T. feels her brother's depression is in remission and says he is making plans to return to school next semester. J.T. reports that her father drinks daily, and at times drinks excessively. J.T. does not feel that her father's drinking has interfered with his social or vocational functioning. J.T. is unaware of any other family member having a psychiatric illness.

Developmental Stage Identity versus Role Confusion

Role-Relationship J.T. is the younger of two children. J.T.'s father is a stockbroker and her mother is an interior designer. Both are college educated and live in an upper–middle class neighborhood. Her mother has always had a career and is very active in local politics. J.T. and her mother have a shared interest in tennis but have "never gotten along." J.T. feels that she and her brother have been close, and his hospitalization was very upsetting for her. J.T. has a close female friend who is also in her sorority. J.T. is not currently dating; she ended a long-term relationship with her high school boyfriend during her last visit home. She reports the break-up was a mutual decision.

Sleep/Rest J.T. frequently stays up late to study and socializes on the weekends. In general, she has seen a reduction in the number of hours she sleeps each night since going to college.

Nutrition/Metabolic J.T. eats one full meal a day, generally dinner. She snacks on items out of the vending machine during the day and never eats breakfast. J.T. reports her weight fluctuates 5 to 10 pounds and she has "always had to diet." Her meals are high in carbohydrates and fat.

Activity/Exercise J.T. plays intramural volleyball or tennis 5 days a week.

Coping/Stress J.T. reports feeling "pressure" to meet the social demands of the sorority as well as to maintain her grade point average. She states she regrets taking so many classes this semester, and usually feels overwhelmed by the amount of time needed to study. She admits sadness related to the end of her relationship with her boyfriend.

Health Management J.T. admits binge drinking since high school. She denies other substance use or abuse. She states the frequency and amount of her drinking has increased since joining the sorority. She drinks 1 to 2 six-packs or more of beer on weekends only. She says alcohol increases her appetite and she often binges on fast food after drinking. She reticently admits self-inducing vomiting after food and alcohol binges. She binges and purges two or three times a week. She has seen small fluctuations in her weight and utilizes the purging to keep from gaining. She denies use of over-the-counter diet aids, laxatives, or diuretics. She is a non-smoker by history but admits to smoking recently at parties. She tried "pot" in high school but it made her really hungry and she didn't really like it. J.T.'s last physical examination, which included a baseline Pap smear, was done 3 months ago with no abnormal findings. She denies a history of sexually transmitted diseases or pregnancy. She reports using condoms for contraception when sexually active.

Self-Perception and Values/Beliefs J.T. perceives herself as "fat" and marginally attractive. She has wanted to become an attorney since age 12 but has begun to question whether she is capable of achieving this goal. She attended church when living at home but has not attended since college.

Medications J.T. denies the use of prescribed or over-the-counter medications.

Allergies NKMA

Pertinent Physical Findings
Vital Signs Height 5 feet 6 inches; weight, 135 pounds; BMI 21; temperature 98.6° F; heart rate 90; respirations 16; blood pressure 120/76

General Appearance Pleasant features, well groomed and casually dressed in loose mid-length dress. Appears well-nourished, hair shiny, and nails polished

Heart CVS regular rate and rhythm without audible murmurs

Head/Neck Slight fullness at parotids bilaterally

Lungs Bilaterally clear to auscultation and without adventitious sounds

Abdomen Mild epigastric tenderness increased bowel sounds, without bruits, without rebound, and without palpable organomegaly

Rectum Without palpable lesions or masses, hemocult negative

Skin Right hand with faint abrasion above the third digit

Diagnostics
Diagnostic Tests Chemistry panel with electrolytes and liver enzymes,, serum amylase, CBC with differential, UA, TSH, mental disorder questionnaires for depression and alcohol abuse such as Zung Depression Scale and the CAGE.

The labs will identify underlying medical disorders and the need for further work-up (e.g., ECG, upper GI, or endoscopy). Diagnostic tests must rule out gastric bleed, potential esophageal varices, Mallory-Weiss tear, cardiac dysrhythmia, hypothyroidism, or other endocrine disorder. The Zung Depression Scale and CAGE will screen for co-morbid depression and alcohol abuse.

Lab results obtained for J.T. are listed in Table 15-1.

History Data Questions specific to the presenting complaint of epigastric pain secondary to binge-purge eating and alcohol abuse include the following:

- Describe the severity, character, location, and any factors producing and relieving pain. Is the pain burning, constricting?
- Have you experienced a sharp, severe pain followed by gradually decreasing pain?
- Are you having reflux? If so, is it bitter or acidic?
- Are you having any radiating pain?
- Have you vomited blood or stomach contents with a "coffee ground" presentation?
- Are you having regular bowel movements? Any change in the color or size?
- Have you had any episodes of blacking out or fainting?
- Have you had any episodes of rapid heart rate with irregular beats?
- Have you had prior periods of significant dieting or weight loss?
- When was your last menstrual period? (If patient is a woman) Please describe your full gynecological history including pregnancies and methods of contraception.

Table 15-1
Lab Results for J.T.

Test	J.T.'s results	Normal Range	Test	J.T.'s results	Normal Range
Glucose	87 mg/dl	65-115 mg/dl	**SGOT (AST)**	44μ/l	0-45 μ/l
BUN	6 mg/dl	5-26 mg/dl	**Triglycerides**	189 mg/dl	0-199 mg/dl
Creatinine	0.9 mg/dl	0.6-1.5 mg/dl	**SGPT**	16 μ/l	0-50 μ/l
BUN/Creatinine Ratio	6.7	5.0-25.0	**GGT**	51μ/l	0-70 μ/l
Calcium	9.1 mg/dl	8.5-10.6 mg/dl	**Cholesterol**	191 mg/l	<200 mg/l
Sodium	142 meq/l	135-147 meq/l	**CBC With Differential/Platelets**		
Phosphorus	3.2 meq/l	2.5-4.5 meq/l	WBC	7.1 Thous/μl	4.0-10.5 Thous/μl
			RBC	4.2 Mill/μl	3.8-5.10 Mill/μl
Potassium	3.9 meq/l	3.5-5.3 meq/l	Hemoglobin	13.2 G/dl	11.5-15.2 G/dl
			Hematocrit	37.7%	34%-44%
Chloride	105 meq/l	96-109 meq/l	MCV	90 fL	80-98 fL
			MCH	33.1 PG	27-34 PG
Uric Acid	4.7 mg/dl	2.2-7.7 mg/dl	MCHC	33.0 G/d	32-36 G/dl
			Lymphocytes	27%	14%-46%
Total Protein	6.8 G/dl	6.0-8.5 G/dl	Neutrophils	66%	40%-74%
			Monocytes	6%	4%-13%
Albumin	4.0 G/dl	3.5-5.5 G/dl	Eosinophils	1%	0-7%
			Basophils	0	0-3%
Globulin	2.8 G/dl	2.2-4.1 G/dl	Platelet Count	226 Thous/μl	140-415 Thous/μl
A/G Ratio	1.4	0.9-2.0	**TSH**	3.5 μIU/ml	0.35-5.50 μIU/ml
Total Bilirubin	0.8 mg/dl	0.1-1.2 mg/dl	**UA**	Negative	
Alkaline Phosphatase	67μ/l	25-150 μ/l			

- Please share your history of alcohol or drug use including the age of first use, substances of choice, frequency, and amounts used.
- Are you using any over-the-counter products? Specifically, herbal products, diet aids, Ipecac syrup, laxatives, enemas, or diuretics?
- Please describe the frequency of food binges and the amount of food consumed. How do you induce purging? How often do you purge? Are there any other methods you use to prevent weight gain or expel food?

- Do you feel faint after binge eating and purging?

Questions specific to co-morbid depression and thyroid disorder include the following:

- Are you unusually cold, tired, or having difficulty concentrating?
- Have you gained or lost weight recently? If so, how much?

- Are you having any difficulty sleeping, or finding yourself sleeping more than usual?
- Are you experiencing a loss of interest in your usual activities or a general loss of functioning?
- Have you or anyone in your family been treated for a psychiatric illness? If so, please give specific circumstances.
- Are you having periods of tearfulness or of feeling hopeless?
- Are you having thoughts of "giving up" or harming yourself? Have you ever acted on these feelings? If so, please describe the specific circumstances.

Physical Examination Data   The focused examination for the chief complaint of epigastric pain includes vital signs, general appearance, head, oral cavity, thyroid, heart, abdomen, rectum, and skin.

Differential Diagnoses   Conditions that often present with epigastric pain include eating disorders (e.g., bulimia nervosa, binge-purge type; and anorexia nervosa, binge-purge type), alcohol abuse, acute gastritis/esophagitis, stress, and situational depression/anxiety (Table 15-2).

Probable Causes of the Presenting Symptoms
Binge alcohol abuse and a several-year history of bingeing and purging appear causal for this episode of esophagitis. J.T. meets the diagnostic criteria for an eating disorder, bulimia nervosa. The brief depressive scale administered to J.T. did not indicate symptoms of a depressive disorder meeting the DSM-IV criteria. The etiology of eating disorders is presumed to be complex, with multiple influences from developmental, social, and biological factors (Treasure and Campbell, 1994). Eating disorders are predominantly an illness of young females that present after the initiation of dieting with the dieting becoming a focus of control (Jones, 1997). Eating disorders are chronic, serious diseases with a 15% to 20% rate of mortality from events such as cardiac arrhythmia, gastric hemorrhage, and suicide. When eating disorders present in primary care, it is very important to distinguish among the types to direct treatment and to identify potential serious medical complications. Major depression is the most common co-morbid psychiatric disorder, occurring between 40% and 83% of patients. Obsessive-compulsive disorder and panic disorder follow with 20% to 40% of patients meeting the DSM-IV criteria. Personality disorders are also common, with diagnoses in Clusters B and C of DSM-IV. Personality traits of perfectionism, rigidity, stubbornness, and high expectations of self are seen most commonly (Kaye, 1997).

Anorexia nervosa is defined by DSM-IV as a 20% weight reduction with refusal to maintain a minimally normal weight (i.e., 85% of expected). This occurs in the presence of an intense fear of gaining weight or of becoming fat and a disturbance in self-experience of body weight or shape. Patients present with amenorrhea, at least 20% weight reduction, distortion in body image, overvaluation of thinness, denial of severity of the illness, and treatment refusal.

Prevalence is less than 1% of the general population, with 4% to 6% of those diagnosed being male. Onset is in the early or late teens and is precipitated by stress and initiation of dieting.

Anorexia nervosa subtypes include: (1) the restrictive type, those restricting food intake and excessive exercise; and (2) the binge-purge type, those who restrict caloric intake and weight increase after bingeing with vomiting, laxative, or diuretic abuse. The binge-purge type has the highest incidence of morbidity and mortality, often from metabolic alkalosis initiating cardiac arrhythmia with risk of sudden death.

Bulimia nervosa is defined by DSM-IV criteria as recurrent episodes of binge eating characterized by the consumption of a large amount of food in a short period of time with recurrent inappropriate compensatory behaviors aimed at weight gain prevention. The binge is associated with a feeling of loss of control and ends when no more food is available or when the individual stops eating because of pain. The majority of those with bulimia have irregular patterns of eating, and satiety may be impaired. There are two types of bulimia nervosa: (1) the purging type is classically self-induced vomiting and/or use of laxatives, diuretics, or enemas to prevent weight gain; and (2) the non-purging type, in which the compensatory behaviors are periods of fasting after bingeing and/or excessive exercising. Bulimia is estimated to occur in approximately 5% of teens and young adult women (So-

Table 15-2
Epigastric Pain Differential Diagnostic Cues

Diagnosis	Signs and Symptoms	Lab Data	Treatment
Acute Gastritis Pain in the epigastrium Secondary to alcohol ingestion	Gnawing discomfort in subxiphoid or LUQ May be aggravated by eating or relieved momentarily, then intensifies No radiation, no knife-like pain	CBC, hemoccult	H-2 blocker for 1-2 weeks Diet modification: no caffeine, alcohol, or carbonated beverages
Esophagitis Secondary to alcohol ingestion and irritation from binge-purge pattern	Pressing, constricting pain in substernum may radiate to back	CBC, hemoccult	Same as for gastritis
Anorexia Nervosa Specifiers: restricting type or binge/purge type meets DSM-IV criteria	Extreme loss of appetite and of weight (at least 25% of baseline) Pursuit of weight loss with time spent focusing on weight increasing over time Obsessive thoughts of food and caloric values Dysphoria, depression are common Decreased sexual interest Eating pattern is ritualized Increased exercise, frequency and duration exceeding norms Amenorrhea, absence of at least three consecutive menstrual cycles Low blood pressure, advanced hypotension Low heart rate, advanced bradycardia Skin dry, scaly, often yellow, and more visible in palms, due to carotenemia Emaciation, denial of hunger, fatigue, and thinness Constipation is common Cold intolerance advanced, hypothermia Skeletal prominence is visible, body fat is undetectable Decreased body hair, fine lanugo quality, scalp with diffuse thinning	Anemia, leukopenia Hypokalemic Elevated B-carotene levels Decreased HCT Decreased Hbg Decreased serum albumin Decreased transferrin Decreased IgG, IgM Plasma Fe normal, TIBC decreased Serum amylase $>75l$ U/L Normal T_4, Free T_4, TSH T_3 low, rT_3 elevated Pre-renal azotemia Bun increased 21-25 mmol/L Plasma cholesterol elevated, triglycerides normal Serum glucose decreased <60 LH, FSH decreased with severe weight loss Plasma estrogen normal Plasma testosterone normal in females, decreased in males Prolactin normal ECG prolonged QT interval Hamilton, Beck depression scales confirm dysthymia or major depression, Yale-Brown Obsessive Scale	Hospitalize if the weight reduction has occurred for 6 months or longer. Longer emaciation is more difficult to treat and to restore weight Psychiatric referral, outpatient Therapy types: • Cognitive behavioral • Psychopharmacology SSRI antidepressants are first line pharmacological treatment. Prozac, Paxil, Zoloft, and Celexa are often dosed in the maximum range for eating disorders. Collaborate with psychiatric providers to ensure continuity of care Refer for nutritional counseling in collaboration with psychiatric treatment plan

Continued

Table 15-2
Epigastric Pain Differential Diagnostic Cues—cont'd

Diagnosis	Signs and Symptoms	Lab Data	Treatment
Anorexia Nervosa—cont'd			
	Frank hirsutism Enlarged parotid glands MV prolapse Edema in legs Layering of clothing to mask emaciation	can identify obsessive-compulsive disorder as co-morbidity	
Alcohol Abuse Meets DSM-IV criteria Maladaptive pattern of substance use leading to clinically significant impairment or distress as manifested by: • Evidence of impaired control • Persistent use despite adverse consequences • Positive family history as risk factor	Recurrent esophagitis/gastritis Irritable bowel Injuries related to risk behaviors while intoxicated Easy bruising, poor healing Anemia Hypoglycemia symptoms of dizziness, decreased concentration, sweating, and tremor Pattern of disruption in vocational and interpersonal functioning	Elevated GGT Elevated triglycerides Elevated mean corpuscular volume Positive screening blood alcohol or Breathalyzer Beck Depression Scale (assess co morbid depression) CAGE: Brief screening tool for alcohol abuse/dependence Two positive responses to these questions indicate potential alcoholism: • Have you ever felt you ought to cut down on your drinking? • Have people annoyed you by criticizing your drinking? • Have you ever felt bad or guilty about your drinking? • Have you ever had an eye opener to steady your nerves or to get rid of a hangover?	Develop therapeutic alliance; begin to engage patient in recognizing symptoms of abuse and potential complications Enlist family involvement to aid in reduction of drinking and participation in self-help groups (e.g., Alanon) Establish short-term treatment goals aimed at abstinence if a positive family history of alcohol dependence or uncontrolled use Encourage participation in self-help groups (e.g., Alcoholics Anonymous or Rational Recovery) If psychosocial stresses or evidence of co-morbid psychiatric illness, refer to psychiatric provider Monitor labs for evidence of normalizing values Refer to psychiatric provider if use continues and brief interventions have been ineffective
Depressive Disorder Not Otherwise Specified Includes depressive features that do not meet the criteria for other mood or anxiety disorders in DSM-IV. Depressive	Vary according to other states Subjective anxiety, depression and irritability tends to be time limited in conjunction with catalyst	Work-up should always assess for underlying physiological disorder in addition to anxiety and depression	Patient should be referred for psychiatric evaluation with a specialist if symptoms persist and do not respond to interventions in the primary care setting that are specific to causal factors.

Table 15-2
Epigastric Pain Differential Diagnostic Cues—cont'd

Diagnosis	Signs and Symptoms	Lab Data	Treatment
Depressive Disorder Not Otherwise Specified—cont'd			
symptoms occur in conjunction with other factors such as: • Premenstrual dysphoric disorder • Minor depressive episodes of less than 2 weeks • Post-psychosis or delusional states • General medical conditions or substance induced			
Bulimia Nervosa Meets DSM-IV criteria	Recurrent episodes of binge eating two times a week for 3 months Behavior is compensatory to prevent weight gain Self-induced vomiting or vomiting induced by ipecac Laxative use/abuse in the absence of constipation Diuretic use in absence of edema Binge eating is in response to tension or anxiety Enlargement of parotid glands, submaxillary /mandibular "Chipmunk facies" Skin changes are rare, may see abrasions on hand from self induced vomiting Recurrent gastritis Pedal edema, rare Dental erosion Normal menses Fluctuating weight, weight within 15% of normal range Fatigue, dyspnea, peripheral edema "Holiday heart syndrome," atrial flutter after binge with alcohol Loss of gag reflex over time	Hypokalemic (plasma Kt <3.5 mmol/L) Metabolic alkalosis, arterial pH elevated Thyroid panel is normal Decreased basal prolactin Increased serum amylase 60 IU/L or $>$ with purging ECG may show ventricular arrhythmia, sinus tachycardia CXR may show enlarged cardiac silhouette	Patient should be hospitalized if severe electrolyte disturbances, co-morbid major depression with self-harm ideation, or co-morbid substance abuse requiring withdrawal monitoring Psychiatric referral for therapy types: • Cognitive behavioral • Psychodynamic • Family/marital therapy • Psychopharmacologic SSRIs first line Patient/family education Self-help groups (e.g., Overeaters Anonymous) Referral to cardiologist cardiac symptoms for further evaluation Follow up assessment must include weight, eating behavior, address core eating disorder symptoms, depression/anxiety symptoms, obsessions, and medication evaluation

bel, 1996). A family history of obesity is a risk factor (Knesper, Riba, and Schwenk, 1997). In those with bulimia, 5% will eventually develop anorexia nervosa (Hsu and Sobkiewicz, 1989). There is a high incidence of impulse control problems (Kaye, 1997) and substance abuse in patients with bulimia (Garner, Garfinkel, and O'Shaughnessy, 1985). Patients may binge and purge to regulate intolerable states of anger, tension, and the reduction of guilty feelings associated with weight gain (Kaye, 1997). In bulimic patients with co-morbid depression, anxiety disorder, or severe obsessive features, a combined treatment of psychotherapy, antidepressants, and nutritional counseling is an appropriate initial treatment (Kaye, 1997).

Bulimia nervosa and anorexia have reached epidemic proportions over the past 20 years in female adolescent and young adult populations. This increase appears related to the strong societal demands for thinness and its strong correlates to success (Nagel and Jones, 1992).

Diagnostic Impression   Acute esophagitis with co-morbid alcohol abuse and bulimia nervosa secondary to inappropriate coping mechanisms

Therapeutic Plan of Care   The treatment plan for J.T. includes acute management of esophagitis with OTC or prescription H_2-blockers to decrease acid reflux and allow for reduction of inflammation. If symptoms continue after 2 weeks, and alcohol use has been discontinued, she should be referred to a gastroenterologist to rule out complications and review treatment. Bulimia nervosa can cause complications such as esophageal dilatation/rupture or tear. J.T. should be advised to discontinue alcohol use and avoid caffeine, carbonated beverages, acidic foods, and large food volumes. J.T. should avoid aspirin and NSAIDs, using acetaminophen only when necessary to reduce the risk of GI bleeding. J.T. should be advised that her reported pattern of bingeing and purging and her score on the depression questionnaire indicate that a low-level depression and eating disorder are occurring in conjunction with stress. Referral to a specialist would aid in determining factors underlying her mood and risk behaviors and address alternative coping skills. J.T. should be reassured that treatment at this point could help to better manage

her weight and the demands of school. Advise J.T. that nutritional counseling is available to her and will be coordinated with her referral provider.

Follow-Up   In 2 weeks, check the status of J.T.'s esophagitis and mental health referral. In a non-judgmental manner, reinforce the need to develop alternative coping mechanisms for stress. Emphasize awareness of the social pressure to drink in excess and the tendency to minimize the inherent risks. Schedule a 1-month follow-up if symptoms of esophagitis have abated. At this point the mental health and substance use evaluation should have been completed: determine what treatment has been recommended and support compliance. Address current eating behaviors and nutritional interventions. In 3 months, re-check baseline labs for evidence of continued eating disorder and alcohol abuse. This follow-up reinforces the primary care provider's concern and supports patient treatment compliance.

Patient Education and/or Community Resources
- Anorexia Nervosa and Related Eating Disorders, PO Box 5102, Eugene OR 97405; phone (541) 344-1144; on the Internet at http://www.anred.com
- Eating Disorders Awareness and Prevention, 603 Stewart St., Suite 803, Seattle WA 98101; phone (206) 382-3587; on the Internet at http//members.aol.com/edapinc/
- International Association of Eating Disorders Professionals, 123 NW 13 St. #206, Boca Raton, FL 33432-1618; phone 1-800-800-8126
- National Association of Anorexia and Associated Disorders, PO Box 7, Highland Park IL 60035; phone 1-847-831-3438
- National Self Help Clearing House; phone (212) 354-8525
- Alcoholics Anonymous
- Anorexia Bulimia Nervosa Association, Second Floor-Woodards House, 47-49 Waymouth St., Adelaide South Africa 5000; phone (08) 8212-1644
- 1-800-THERAPIST (a toll-free referral source for therapists specializing in eating disorders)
- Community Mental Health Centers

Case Study 2

CHIEF COMPLAINT: Anxiety, Excessive Worry, and Thoughts of Suicide

History of Present Illness   S.W. is a 45-year-old separated Hispanic female of South American descent referred for evaluation of symptoms of anxiety, excessive worry, difficulty managing activities of daily living, and fleeting thoughts of suicide. S.W. is currently residing in a local shelter for battered women. S.W. initiated a domestic disturbance call to the police and was assisted in obtaining temporary shelter. She reports her current symptoms have been present for many years, but increased in intensity over the past 6 months. She has recently noted additional symptoms of decreased concentration, poor memory, frequent crying spells, and washing her hands unnecessarily. She has not been sleeping well and wakes up at night "soaking wet." She denies intent to act on her suicidal thoughts, stating: "It is a sin in my church to kill yourself." She describes an emotionally abusive relationship with her husband, who is native to this country. Her husband is 10 years her senior and she met him shortly after coming to the United States on a student visa. S.W. planned to obtain a master's degree in English and eventually work in this country. S.W. met her husband at the college campus, where he was employed as a groundskeeper. She married him after a brief courtship and quickly realized she had made "a mistake." S.W. reports her husband became very critical and would often call her "stupid." She became socially isolated and increasingly dependent. She did not continue her graduate studies and began working part-time cleaning office buildings. She reports first feeling severely anxious and depressed after giving birth to her only child. She reports that postpartum she struggled with feelings of excessive fatigue, depression, and overwhelming anxiety that she was incapable of caring for her baby. She reports that fears of contaminating the baby with germs led her to compulsively clean her apartment and her hands with bleach. She rarely left her apartment and had no social contact apart from her husband. She states her fears gradually diminished after a year, but feels she has never returned to the way that she functioned before her son was born. Her 6-year-old son was visiting with her sister

when the domestic disturbance occurred, and he will remain there until she is able to take care of him.

Past Medical History   G1P1, LMP 9 months ago. Her last physical examination was during the immigration process 8 years ago, and had normal results.

Past Surgical History   Denies past surgeries

Family History   Father, deceased at age 59 years from liver cirrhosis secondary to alcohol dependence; mother, 68, without major illness; eight siblings, all A&W

Developmental Stage   Generativity versus Stagnation

Role-Relationship   S.W. is close to her family members, all of whom reside in South America except her sister, who resides in the same city. She maintains weekly telephone contact with her mother. She feels her family is emotionally supportive and they have endorsed her decision to leave her husband. Her son is living with her sister and her family and is attending a local school. S.W. feels she has been a good mother with her only regret being that her son witnessed his father's treatment of her. S.W. has no friends but is becoming acquainted with other women at the shelter.

Sleep/Rest   S.W. sleeps 5 to 6 hours each night with her sleep often disrupted. She doesn't feel rested and usually wakes up early feeling anxious.

Nutrition/Metabolic   S.W. reports a loss of appetite with a recent weight loss of 12 pounds. She eats traditional South American food that is high in fat and carbohydrates.

Activity/Exercise   S.W. denies regular exercise and relates that her activities centered on caring for her child and home.

Coping/Stress   S.W. reports being ashamed to share details of her marital conflicts with her family. She states she feels very stressed and unable to cope. She feels she has lost any sense of personal empowerment over the last several years. She does relate a sense of relief that she is no longer with her husband and is now in a supportive environment at the women's shelter.

Health Management   S.W. denies any alcohol, substance, or tobacco use. Her immunizations were updated during her immigration physical in 1988. Her last well woman examination was 6 years ago following childbirth.

Self-Perception and Values/Beliefs S.W. reports feeling "like a failure" in most aspects of her life. She regrets not finishing her graduate work and having a professional career. She describes herself as having strong religious beliefs and is a member of the Catholic faith. She states her decision to leave her husband was very difficult and is in conflict with her beliefs.

Medications None
Allergies NKMA

Pertinent Physical Findings

Vital Signs Height 5 feet 2 inches; weight 137 pounds; BMI 24; temperature 98.4° F; heart rate 88; respirations 12; B/P 118/72

General Appearance S.W. is a pleasant-featured Hispanic female who is slightly overweight. She is casually dressed in slacks and blouse and is adequately groomed. She is oriented in all spheres, her affect is blunted, and her speech is slightly pressured. She appears anxious as evidenced by her facial expression and by the repetitive twisting of a tissue in her chafed, reddened hands.

Heart RRR and without audible murmurs

Head/Neck Without lymphadenopathy, periorbital edema, or exophthalmos; thyroid, no enlargement or palpable masses or nodules

Lungs Clear to auscultation bilaterally

Abdomen Bowel signs present, no palpable masses, tenderness, organomegaly, renal bruits, or CVA tenderness

Skin Normal temperature, hands erythematous and chafed, nails brittle, hair is thick and shiny

Neurological PERRLA, EOMs normal, normal gait, negative Romberg, and 2+ reflexes in all extremities, equal strength in all extremities, normal muscle tone

Diagnostics

Diagnostic Tests SMAC-24, TSH, FSH, and CBC with differential, UA, TB Tine or PPD, Zung or Beck Depression Scale (Zung available in Spanish), Hamilton or Zung Anxiety Scale

The "Prime MD Today" Patient Health Questionnaire is recommended as a diagnostic tool. It identifies mental disorders in mood, anxiety, alcohol, eating, and somatoform disorders. The questionnaire is available for duplication in English or Spanish at no cost to the provider as a service of Pfizer U.S. Pharmaceuticals.*

S.W. should have laboratory tests including TSH and FSH to rule out subclinical thyroid disease and to confirm menopause. S.W. was negative for thyroid disease with a TSH of 4.5 and her FSH at 47 confirmed menopause. S.W.'s SMAC-24, CBC, and UA were within normal limits. She should have an ECG to rule out co-morbid cardiac disease if her cardiovascular examination was suspect. S.W.'s cardiac symptom presentation and physical examination were negative and she does not warrant further cardiac evaluation. Her neurological examination was negative and further evaluation is not indicated. S.W.'s history indicates a postpartum depression with psychotic features. If S.W. had the onset of a psychotic depression, first episode past the age of 40, a neurology referral would be required. S.W.'s current mental status and her placement in a battered woman's shelter suggest observation for signs of physical abuse or self-mutilation during the physical exam. S.W. should have a well woman examination (i.e., breast, Pap, pelvic, and mammogram). S.W. had a negative TB tine. She scored a 60 on the Zung Anxiety Scale, which warrants a full mental status evaluation. S.W.'s symptom presentation clearly identifies a depressive disorder.

History Data Questions specific to anxiety, excessive worry and suicidal thoughts include the following:

- Have you recently been treated with corticosteroids?
- Have you recently stopped drinking, smoking, or taking a medication?
- Are you taking any over-the-counter medication or herbal product?
- Have you ever been treated for these symptoms before?
- Do you have any other physical complaints?

Prime MD Today, printed in August 1999, was developed by Drs. Robert L. Spitzer, Janet B.W. Williams, Kurt Kroenke, and colleagues with an educational grant from Pfizer Inc. For research information, contact Dr. Spitzer at: rls8@columbia.edu.

- Are you experiencing constipation or diarrhea?
- Have you recently gained or lost weight? If so, how much?
- Have you experienced periods of a rapid or irregular heart rate?
- Have you been having headaches, recent vision changes, unsteady gait, or dizziness?
- Have you ever had a panic attack or a persistent fear that kept you from functioning?
- What do you do to manage your anxiety? Describe the things that are worrying you.
- Have you ever had a head trauma or a time that you have lost consciousness?
- Do your symptoms of anxiety occur after meals?
- Have you ever acted on feelings to harm yourself? If so, please describe the circumstances.
- Describe when your suicidal thoughts occur. Do you feel that you have control over these thoughts? How to you manage not to act on these feelings?

Physical Examination Data   The focused examination for the chief complaint of anxiety, excessive worry, and thoughts of suicide includes vital signs, general appearance, head, neck, heart, lungs, skin, neurological, and abdomen.

Differential Diagnoses   Medical conditions that commonly present with anxiety and depression include cardiovascular (arrhythmias, cardiomyopathies, mitral valve prolapse, congestive heart disease, and coronary artery disease), endocrine (thyroid, adrenal), metabolic (hypoglycemia, vitamin B_{12} deficiency), respiratory (asthma, COPD), secretory tumors (carcinoid, pheochromocytoma), collagen vascular disorders, aspirin intolerance, renal disease, multiple sclerosis, and menopause (Table 15-3). Psychiatric conditions with symptoms of anxiety and depression include bipolar disorders, psychotic disorders, substance abuse, dementia, and adjustment disorders.

Probable Causes of Presenting Symptoms
S.W. is most likely menopausal and experiencing a major mood disorder with anxious and obsessive features. S.W.'s anxiety symptoms do not occur only after meals or fasting, which rules out hypo-

glycemia. S.W.'s thyroid testing was normal and she is without signs and symptoms of other endocrine disorders. S.W. does not complain of heart palpitations and her cardiac examination was normal.

Many patients in primary care exhibit symptoms of both anxiety and depression. Traditionally, depression and anxiety have been viewed as discrete diagnoses. The symptom presentation may not meet DSM-IV criteria for an affective or anxiety disorder, and these patients are often undiagnosed and untreated (Nemeroff, 1997). Patients may deny depressive symptoms due to overwhelming anxiety and the compelling need for symptom relief. Patients with an anxiety disorder without comorbid depression generally do not have anhedonia; the interest in functioning remains despite anxiety symptom barriers. Factors determining symptom presentation include premorbid personality, genetic predisposition, co-morbid medical conditions, and environmental stresses.

Recent research supports viewing these disorders as being one entity, with anxiety at one end of the spectrum and depression at the other. This view can enhance symptom recognition, diagnosis, and treatment in the primary care setting. Approaching treatment from this view would allow adequate treatment for the depression component, which is often missed, and reduce the likelihood of anxiolytic dependence. Patients must be assessed for depression and suicidality. The risk factors for suicide in women are listed in Box 15-1.

Diagnostic Impression   Menopause, anxiety disorder not otherwise specified, mixed anxiety-depressive disorder

Therapeutic Plan of Care   S.W. will be treated with hormone replacement after GYN follow-up. She should experience some symptom reduction from hormone replacement alone but she should be started on a selective serotonin reuptake inhibitor (SSRI) such as Paxil, Prozac, Celexa, or Zoloft (Rubinow, 1996).* S.W. has obsessive symptoms,

---

*Trazodone is a heterocyclic antidepressant with weak serotonin activity that is sedating and has mild anxiolytic effects. Trazodone can be used in subtherapeutic doses with SSRIs without risk of serotonin syndrome to assist with sleep and to reduce anxiety.

Table 15-3
Anxiety and Depression Differential Diagnostic Cues

Diagnosis	Signs and Symptoms	Lab Tests	Treatment
Endocrine Disorders *Thyroid/ Hyperthyroid* Most common Presents with anxiety and depression (Hutto, 1999)	Fatigue Nervousness with irritability Inability to concentrate Restlessness, insomnia, psychosis Overt emotional lability Weight loss without anorexia Palpitations Enlarging neck mass Thyroid bruits Change in appearance of eyes Skeletal wasting Exertional dyspnea Heat intolerance "Silky skin" or hair, onycholysis Hair loss, thinning Hyperpigmentation of bony prominence Postural tremor Sinus tachycardia Systolic flow murmurs Wide pulse pressure Lid lag, stare, or extraocular movement weakness	TSH suppressed < 0.1, $T_4 > 12$, free $T_4 > 2.0$ ECG: arrhythmia, sinus tachycardia	Graves: self-limiting Anti-thyroid drugs may be indicated: Propylthiouracil 100-150 mg q 8 hours Methimazole 5-10 mg bid Check T_4 in 1 month, then every 2-3 months When T_4 is normal, maintain dose with thyroxine
Cushing's Syndrome Glucocorticoid excess, most commonly due to hypersecretion of ACTH from the pituitary with resultant hyperplasia	Deposition of fat in face and upper body producing truncal obesity, "moon facies" and "buffalo hump" Skin changes: • Acne • Generalized hirsutism • Telangiectasia over face • Atrophy/thinning skin • Easy bruising/ecchymosis • Development of purplish abdominal striae • Hyperpigmentation Muscle wasting in the extremities • Virilization in females: • Male pattern baldness • Oligomenorrhea • Increase in upper body muscle mass • Enlarged clitoris	Abnormal suppression with dexamethasone 1 mg at 11-12 AM, plasma cortisol measured at 8-9 AM: normal subjects have cortisol <5 ug/dl	Endocrinology referral

Table 15-3
· Anxiety and Depression Differential Diagnostic Cues—cont'd

Diagnosis	Signs and Symptoms	Lab Tests	Treatment
Mixed Anxiety and Depression *Mixed Symptom State* Has features of anxiety and depressive disorders Meets DSM-IV criteria One of the most common disorders seen in primary care settings	Appetite change Weight loss with anorexia Weight gain secondary to "anxious" eating Feeling of impending doom Irritability Sleep disturbance Palpitations Sweating Tension headaches Inappropriate guilt Poor concentration Anhedonia, depressed mood May report inability to cope, feeling overwhelmed, too anxious to function, and anxious self-doubt	Rule out underlying medical problem; in the absence of physical findings must do basic lab work-up including TSH, FSH if female and irregular menses	Acknowledge to the patient that a medical disorder of anxiety with depressive features has been diagnosed Must assess for suicide, refer immediately if risk present Refer to psychiatric provider if psychosocial stresses and or suicidal ideation are present Document referral and follow-up with a call to the patient to make sure treatment has been obtained If no risk factors are present, the following psychopharmacologic treatment plan should be considered
Hypoglycemia Symptoms present during or after an overnight fast or after meals Types: • Fasting • Postprandial	Sweating, tremor Tachycardia, anxiety Hunger, dizziness Headache, clouding vision Blunted mental activity Decreased fine motor skills Confusion, abnormal behavior	Plasma glucose decreased Postprandial <60 Elevated liver functions	Nutritional counseling, high protein and low carbohydrate diet
Menopause Final episode of menstrual bleeding with progressive loss of ovarian function. Occurs spontaneously between ages 45-55 with median age 50-51 years. Suspect peri-menopause when menses are irregular	Vasomotor instability "hot flashes" Nervousness, anxiety, irritability Depression Sleep disturbance Decreased bone density Osteoporosis Atrophy of urogenital epithelium and skin Short term memory loss Laboratory evaluation Elevated FSH >35 Gradual elevation of LH Gradual reduction of serum estrogen Gradual reduction of androgens Low HDL	Rule out underlying disease Must have well woman examination including PAP, mammogram, and breast self-examination education	Hormone replacement therapy Unopposed estrogen with hysterectomy Estrogen/progesterone combination with intact uterus

Box 15-1

Risk Factors for Suicide in Women

History of depression or other psychiatric disorders, including substance abuse
Family history of suicide or psychiatric disorders
Disrupted family environment
Disappointment in relationships
Presence of firearms or other means
Living alone
Absence of young children living in the household
Presence of physical illness
History of physical, sexual, or emotional abuse
Unemployment
Previous suicide attempts
Premorbid personality traits:

- Impulsivity
- Low frustration tolerance
- Externalization of anger/aggression
- Histrionic
- Overvaluation/devaluation

Adapted from Jacobs DG, Deutsch NL: Screening women for suicidal intent, *Medicine and Behavior Special Report: Women's Health* 2(4):32-33, 1999.

as evidenced by the hand washing, and SSRIs are first line for obsessive disorders as well. Start the SSRI at a low dose, generally half the usual starting dose. If S.W. is fearful of potential side effects, the dose can be started at a quarter of the usual starting dose with the first increase in dose on day 4. Gradually increase the dose of the SSRI each week until achieving a therapeutic dose. Full effects from the SSRI may not be seen until weeks 4 to 6. SSRIs can be activating and have the potential to temporarily increase anxiety and disrupt sleep. S.W. may benefit from trazodone 25 to 50 mg at bedtime to sleep. Trazodone is sedating and has mild anxiolytic effects. She should be followed weekly in the primary care setting while a referral for psychiatric evaluation and treatment takes place. S.W. has multiple psychosocial stresses, which necessitate a combined treatment approach of psychopharmacotherapy and cognitive therapy.

Patient Education and/or Community Resources   Community mental health centers and community social services are excellent referral sources for patients.

Educate the patient on the psychobiology of depression and anxiety. Informational handouts, in both English and Spanish, are available at no cost through pharmaceutical companies that manufacture anti-depressants and anxiolytics.

Self-help groups for women in dysfunctional relationships can be located through community mental health centers.*

Follow-Up Plan   Follow-up weekly with a review of each presenting symptom and monitoring for self-harm ideation for the first month in the primary care or psychiatric setting. As S.W.'s psychosocial issues are addressed and target symptoms subside, medication can be monitored monthly. In the absence of symptoms, monitoring the medication every 3 months is sufficient.

When an anxiety disorder has been diagnosed, the patient should be advised that anxiety occurs in the presence of depression and that symptoms related to the anxiety often foreshadow the awareness of depression. To successfully treat an anxiety disorder, the anxiety must be validated and be the targeted symptom for initial treatment. The patient should be educated that the long-term reduction and elimination of the presenting symptoms requires treatment of the depressive component of this disorder.

A non-sedating antidepressant combined with the short-term use of a benzodiazepine or other anxiolytic is often first-line treatment.

ANTI-ANXIETY AGENTS

Benzodiazepines have been in use for 30 years and are remarkably similar in both their therapeutic and side effects. These agents possess sedative, anxiolytic, anticonvulsant, and muscle-relaxant properties and are prescribed commonly for acute anxiety, generalized anxiety, and panic disorders.

*Anxiety Disorders Association of America, 6000 Executive Blvd. Suite 513, Rockville, MD 20852; telephone (301) 231-9350.

Benzodiazepines are effective in relieving anxiety but should be reserved as monotherapy only in the management of situational anxiety. Benzodiazepines as monotherapy in the treatment of anxiety disorders do not address the underlying cause and can place the patient at risk for drug tolerance and potential dependence. The short half-life benzodiazepines have a greater risk for dependence, and the rapid onset of tranquilization can dissuade a patient from taking additional agents. Benzodiazepine use in the treatment of anxiety disorders should be short-term, with first line use of mid to long half-life agents. The benzodiazepine should be prescribed in conjunction with long-term antidepressant treatment. As the antidepressant becomes effective, the benzodiazepine should be slowly discontinued. Commonly prescribed benzodiazepines are listed in Table 15-4.

Azaperones are novel agents that are chemically unrelated to other anxiolytics and do not have the sedative-hypnotic properties of benzodiazepines. Buspirone is the only azaperone currently available and is indicated for treatment of mild to moderate anxiety. Buspirone does not cause dependence, is non-sedating, and can be abruptly discontinued without risk of withdrawal.

Antidepressant activity has been observed using buspirone in higher doses (60 to 80 mg). Patients with recent benzodiazepine use often reject buspirone (BuSpar) because it does not have rapid tranquilization or the muscle relaxing effects that give patients a sense of immediate relief. Maximum anxiolytic effect from buspirone can take up to 2 to 4 weeks.

Antihistamines such as diphenhydramine and hydroxyzine have anxiolytics effects but are sedating and can cause dry mouth. They can be used for situational anxiety but are not effective in treating anxiety disorders.

Beta-blockers such as long-acting propranolol can assist with situational anxiety and can be used during desensitization with simple phobias.

Antidepressants with anxiolytic properties include the tricyclics, heterocyclics, selective serotonin re-uptake inhibitors, and atypicals.

- *Selective serotonin reuptake inhibitors* (SSRIs, Table 15-5) are the first line treatment for co-morbid anxiety and depression because of their efficacy, few adverse effects, and safety in overdose. When treating depressed patients with symptoms of anxiety, treatment

Table 15-4
Commonly Prescribed Benzodiazepines

Drug	Dose Range (mg/d)	Usual Dose Range	Half-Life	Potency	Comments
Alprazolam	0.75-10	0.25-0.5 tid	4-6 hours	High	High risk for dependence Not recommended for use in treatment of anxiety disorder
Lorazepam	1-10	0.5-1.0 tid	6-8 hours	High	Used for short-term treatment Prescribed concurrently with antidepressant
Clonazepam	1.5-20	0.5-2.0 bid	10-12 hours	Low	Least likely to develop dependence, can be used long term in severe cases of anxiety disorders Should be prescribed with an antidepressant and gradually withdrawn when symptoms of anxiety or no longer prominent

of emergent anxiety and agitation must be avoided. A transient increase in anxiety may occur with SSRIs and may discourage treatment compliance. Patients will generally be more treatment compliant if they experience rapid onset of anxiety symptom reduction from combining a low dose long-acting benzodiazepine with an SSRI. The initial dosing of an SSRI should be increased gradually to minimize side effects. The benzodiazepine should be titrated down and discontinued when the SSRI is in therapeutic range. In the primary care setting, if response is inadequate at the average dose, the patient should be referred to a psychiatric specialist.

Tricyclics are effective for the management of anxiety and depression, but the side effects often contribute to patient medication noncompliance. Patients often complain of sedation, weight gain, constipation, and dry mouth. Current usage of tricyclics is limited to patients who do not respond to non-sedating antidepressants; or tricyclics are given in small doses at bedtime along with other agents. Tricyclics should be avoided due to the risk of lethality in overdose.

Heterocyclics such as trazodone and Serzone are mildly sedating and are excellent choices for patients experiencing mild to moderate depression with prominent anxious features. Trazodone can be administered at bedtime in conjunction with an SSRI to manage sleep disturbance; or administered in very small doses during the day for anxiety instead of a benzodiazepine.

Atypical antidepressants such as bupropion and mirtazapine are often selected for the management of weight or sexual side effects. Bupropion is not known to cause weight gain and in some patients can cause slight weight loss. Mirtazapine causes significant weight gain in most patients. Bupropion and mirtazapine are not known to cause sexual side effects. Bupropion is generally not used as monotherapy for patients with anxiety but is often combined with an SSRI to reduce sexual side effects.

Case Study 3

CHIEF COMPLAINT: Social Isolation, Poor School Performance, and Impulsivity

History of Present Illness S.A. is a 13-year-old Caucasian male presenting for a school physical examination and an immunization update. He is accompanied by his mother who relates increasing worry that S.A. will have "another bad year at school." His mother reports that over the summer break, S.A. spent most of his time in the house playing video games and watching television. S.A. has very few friends and has little or no contact with peers outside of school. He has had poor grades and conduct disturbance since starting school. His relationships in the past have been brief due to his "aggressiveness." S.A. is fidgeting noticeably and he picks up the reflex hammer from the examination room table and begins tapping on the counter. He is avoidant of eye contact, and appears disinterested.

Table 15-5
Selective Serotonin Reuptake Inhibitors

Drug	Starting Dose*	Therapeutic Dose Range	Average Dose
Paroxetine	10 mg	20-60 mg	20 mg
Sertraline	25 mg	50-200 mg	100 mg
Fluoxetine	10 mg	20-80 mg	20 mg
Fluvoxamine	25 mg	100-300 mg	150 mg
Citalopram	10 mg	20-60 mg	40 mg

*Doses for elderly are one-half starting and usual doses; interval for increase 1-2 weeks, 2-6 weeks for full response.

Past Medical History S.A. has a history of seasonal allergies, with fall the most symptomatic. He denies history of major injury or head trauma. Peri-prenatal history: pregnancy planned, uncomplicated, normal delivery. S.A. had a vision and hearing screening last year in school with normal findings.

Past Surgical History None

Family History S.A.'s mother is 39 years old and has been divorced from his father for 6 years. She is a non-smoker, non-drinker with no pertinent medical history. S.A.'s father is 41 years old and recently remarried. He is a non-smoker, social drinker with no pertinent medical history. S.A. is the second of two children born to his parents. His brother is 3 years older and has no pertinent medical history.

Social Family History S.A.'s parents began having marital difficulty when S.A. was 6 years old. His mother reported the divorce was particularly difficult for S.A. He would often cry and be openly angry with his mother. When S.A.'s father remarried, he moved to a nearby town with his wife and her three children. S.A.'s father is a certified public accountant for a large accounting firm. S.A.'s mother reports that his father has not participated in school conferences and often misses his visitations. S.A.'s mother works full time as a receptionist in a dental office.

Developmental Stage Identity versus Role Confusion

Role-Relationship S.A. admires his older brother, who has been a constant in his life. S.A.'s mother reports that his peers often tease him and his brother is very protective.

Sleep/Rest S.A. has difficulty getting to sleep, has a great deal of difficulty getting up in the morning, and is often late for school. He sleeps from around 11:30 PM to 7 AM. He is irritable upon awakening and reports never feeling rested.

Nutrition/Metabolic S.A. is mildly overweight and he eats a lot of sweetened cereal and junk food. His mother reports that he is always in the kitchen snacking and leaves the kitchen in a state of disarray.

Activity/Exercise S.A. plays video games and watches cartoons during his leisure time. He gets no physical exercise outside of physical education class during school.

Coping/Stress S.A. admits being easily frustrated and has been known to quickly give up on tasks requiring prolonged concentration. His mother states that school conduct reports indicate that S.A. is impulsive and distracts other students in class.

Developmental History S.A.'s postnatal developmental milestones, including speech and motor, were within normal limits.

School History S.A. was enrolled in preschool and kindergarten programs before grade school. His mother reports S.A. has had difficulty sitting still since the first grade, and a school counselor in the fourth grade recommended that he be evaluated for learning problems. S.A.'s mother tearfully admits the evaluation was not done because she was overwhelmed with work and with being a single mother. She states she feels "very guilty about this."

Academic History S.A. has a poor academic performance. He has made Cs and some Ds with multiple notations of "not paying attention," "not turning in homework," "not being prepared for tests" and "disruptive behavior."

Self-Perception and Values/Beliefs S.A. relates that he is "stupid" and does not believe he can succeed in school because "the teachers pick on me."

Medications S.A. uses acetaminophen when ill with a cold or flu. He takes over-the-counter allergy and sinus medication on an as-needed basis.

Allergies NKMA

Pertinent Physical Findings

Vital Signs Height 5 feet 4 inches; weight 147 pounds; BMI 25; temperature 98.4° F; pulse 88; respirations 16; B/P 118/72

General Appearance S.A. is short in stature, mildly overweight, has curly dark brown hair, and is casually dressed in a wrinkled shirt and jeans. His eye contact is poor but he becomes animated when defending his poor academic performance.

HEENT PERRLA, extraocular movements are normal, nasal mucosa is pale and boggy, nasal turbinates are enlarged with clear nasal discharge; neck is supple; thyroid is without enlargement and without palpable nodules or masses, neck is without lymphadenopathy, and pharynx without injection or exudate.

Heart CVSRR, without audible gallops or murmurs, and radial pulses are 2+ and equal

Lungs Clear to auscultation bilaterally

Abdomen Soft, nontender, without rebound, without organomegaly, and bowel sounds are within normal limits

History Data Questions specific to the chief complaint of social isolation, poor school performance, and impulsivity include the following:

- Does he or she engage in dangerous activities or criminal behavior?
- Does he or she show any evidence of chronic illness such as hypo- or hyperthyroidism, sensory deficits (e.g., hearing loss), or allergies to medications, food, or environmental agents?
- Is there any family history of psychiatric illness such as bipolar disorder, depression, or schizophrenia?
- Has he or she displayed verbal or physical outbursts?
- At what age were symptoms first noted?
- Are the symptoms interfering with school or peer functioning?
- Is there any evidence of substance use?
- Have teachers ever noted periods when he appears to be asleep or "zones out" in class?
- Any history of seizures or loss of consciousness?

Differential Diagnoses Differential diagnoses for the client complaint of social isolation, poor school performance, and impulsivity include Tourette's syndrome and attention deficit disorder (Table 15-6).

Probable Causes of the Presenting Symptoms S.A.'s presenting symptoms of social isolation, poor academic performance, low frustration tolerance, and inattention are a common constellation of symptoms present in children with an attention disorder. S.A.'s problems were identified during his early school years and were untreated. S.A.'s difficulty in obtaining and sustaining peer relationships may be due to social inattention and low self-esteem.

Diagnostic Tests SMA 24, TSH, CBC. Labs will rule out underlying medical disorders, particularly endocrine, which can influence behavior.

S.A.'s labs were within normal limits; pertinent values were: TSH 3.5, glucose 91, HGB 14.6, HCT 42.9, cholesterol 169, and triglycerides 116.

Diagnostic Impression Attention deficit hyperactivity disorder combined type (inattentive-impulsive)

The physical examination was positive only for signs and symptoms of allergic rhinitis. S.A. is not taking medication that would impair cognitive functioning or stimulate hyperactivity (e.g., sedating antihistamines or sympathomimetics). His laboratory studies are within normal limits. A neurological examination was not warranted in the absence of abnormal movements or vocalizations. S.A. has had symptoms of impulsivity and inattention since his pre-school years with no overt evidence of a learning disability. S.A. has poor peer relationships and school underachievement. S.A. was overactive as a child and is underactive as an adolescent. He does not meet the DSM-IV criteria for an affective disorder but does present with dysphoria and low self-esteem, which are common complications of ADHD (Greenhill, 1998). S.A. has not experimented with drugs or alcohol and is not engaging in antisocial behavior. S.A.'s family history is negative for psychiatric illness but he has psychosocial problems related to abandonment by his father.

PHARMACOLOGICAL TREATMENT

The effective treatment of ADHD with co-morbid psychiatric disturbances requires referral to a specialist who can determine the neurochemical basis of each disorder and apply the appropriate pharmacological tools (Horning, 1998). In a primary care setting, after appropriate psychiatric evaluation, maintenance pharmacological treatment of the ADHD patient without psychiatric co-morbidity may consist of the following (Castellanos, 1996):

Stimulants

- The first line treatment because of well-established safety and efficacy; often requires frequent dosing

Diagnosis	Signs and Symptoms	Lab Data	Treatment
Tourette's Multiple motor and one or more vocal tics have been present at some time during the illness A tic is a sudden, rapid, recurrent non-rhythmic, stereotyped motor movement or vocalization The tics occur many times a day, usually in bouts nearly every day for more than 1 year, never a tic-free period lasting more than 3 consecutive months Onset before age 18 years, usually between ages 2-13 years	Begins with a single tic in 50% of patients Motor tics present initially with progression over time from head to trunk to limbs Average age of onset of motor tics is 7 years Vocal tics may start as single syllable, progress to longer exclamations, and occasionally to complex gestures Average age of onset is 11 years Prior to the appearance of tics many children show impulsivity, hyperactivity, and inattention similar to ADHD ADHD may be seen in 60% of boys with Tourette's (Talbott, Hales, and Yudofsky, 1988)	SMA 24, TSH, UA Elevated LFTs necessitate hepatitis panel to rule out Wilson's disease Neurology exam Rule out other movement disorders EEG Rule out seizure disorders School reports (academic and general behavior) Tic observation	Neuro/psychiatric referral is required Pharmacotherapy may include antipsychotics, and/or antidepressants and clonidine (alpha-2 agonist) Behavioral therapy to assist with social skills training Anxiety disorder: • 25% of children with ADHD meet the criteria for an anxiety disorder • School difficulties reported were greater for ADHD/anxious children than ADHD alone • May occur in 50% of children with ADHD Conduct disorder: • May occur in 30%-50% of children with ADHD • Show more rule breaking, aggression, and impulsivity than seen with ADHD • Medical and perinatal history does not distinguish between conduct disorder and ADHD • Have stronger family history for antisocial behavior in first-degree relatives (Pliszka, 1998) Bipolar disorder: • Positive family history • Cyclical rather than continuous course • 15% of ADHD with co-morbidity for bipolar illness • Suspect in a child with severe ADHD, aggressive outbursts, and chronic irritability Overactivity: • 15% of boys meet criteria for hyperactivity without other ADHD signs • Increased gross motor activity in response to stress but not persistent for 6 months required for ADHD • Not stimulus driven, poorly organized quality of ADHD children • May be seen in mental retardation, activity must be disproportionate to mental age

Continued

Diagnosis	Signs and Symptoms	Lab Data	Treatment
Attention Deficit Disorder The etiology of ADHD is unknown but emerging neuropsychological and neuroimaging literature suggests abnormalities in fronto-striatel dysfunction and catecholamine dysregulation. Genetic and adoption studies suggest a genetic origin for some form of the disorder along with psychological and physiological adversities such as prenatal insult. Up to two thirds of clinically referred school age children with ADHD may have a co-morbid Axis I Disorder. Retrospective research and follow up studies indicate that children with attention disorders are at high risk for developing co-morbid psychiatric disturbances in childhood, adolescence and adulthood (Biederman, 1998). The most common co-morbid psychiatric disturbances in childhood include those of conduct, learning, mood and anxiety (Pliszka, 1998).	At least six of the following symptoms of inattention-hyperactivity must be present Inattention: • Lack of attention to details or careless mistakes in school tasks, or other activities • Difficulty in sustaining attention in tasks recreational activities • Gives impression of not listening when spoken to directly • Failure to follow through on instructions or finish schoolwork • Difficulty in organizing tasks and activities • Avoidance or dislike of tasks that require sustained mental effort • Tendency to lose things necessary for tasks or activities • Distraction by extraneous stimuli • Forgetfulness in daily activities Hyperactivity: • Fidgeting with hands or feet or squirming in seat	Clarify parent's chief complaint related to functioning Obtain the results of any developmental screening, achievement or IQ test that has already been conducted Obtain parent and teacher rating scales Observe parent and child to evaluate symptoms of ADHD or co-morbid condition Obtain family history Observe child's attention and activity level with the parent present and alone Observe the child's level of compliance during an interaction with the parent Assess the child's physical and neurological status Collaborate with teachers to determine if there is a need for psycho-educational, speech, or language tests Diagnosis of ADHD is made exclusively by history: teacher and parent rating scales can support diagnosis. • Child Attention Problems Scale	Treatment criteria: • ADHD symptoms must be persistent and cause functional impairment in school, home, or with peers • No medical contraindication to treatment • Must be 6 years or older • An adult must supervise pill taking • Parents and school staff must be educated that stimulants are drugs of abuse and identify behaviors that reflect abuse • Prescriber must ascertain that no family member in the household is abusing stimulants • School personnel must supervise medication administration during school hours

Diagnosis	Signs and Symptoms	Lab Data	Treatment

Attention Deficit Disorder—cont'd

Diagnosis	Signs and Symptoms	Lab Data	Treatment
Children with multiple co-morbid disturbances are more likely to have antisocial behavior, substance abuse and anxiety/depression spectrum disorders in adulthood (Biederman, 1998). Like their child counterparts, ADHD adults have impulsive, inattentive, and restless behaviors. ADHD adults with co-morbid psychiatric disturbances are at high risk for occupational and interpersonal failures. Awareness of ADHD as a heterogeneous disorder in children can improve the detection, diagnosis, and treatment, thereby reducing adult morbidity and disability (Khouzam, 1997). There are three types of ADHD identified in DSM-IV and are differentiated by predominant symptoms; the subtypes include: • Predominantly inattentive • Predominantly hyperactive-impulsive • Combined type	• Not remaining seated when expected • Subjective feelings of restlessness • Difficulty in engaging in leisure activities quietly • Often "on the go" or "driven" • Excessive talking Impulsivity: • Tendency to blurt out answers before questions have been completed • Difficulty in awaiting turn • Tendency to interrupt or intrude on others	• Conners Parent and Teacher Rating Scales • IQ Test • WISC III (Wechsler Intelligence Scale III) • Wide Range Achievement Test–Revised (can estimate grade level) • Achievement Woodcock Johnson Psycho Educational Battery Rule out medical disorders with concurrent symptoms: • Thyroid (hypo/hyperthyroid) • Sensory deficits (hearing loss) • Seizure disorders • Medication reactions • Fragile X syndrome (characteristic faces and gaze avoidance)	

- Adequate trial of one psychostimulant at a time should be given before changing treatment regimen
- Clinical effects start within 2 days
- Effects persist and show little to no tolerance over years
- 20% to 25% of patients show significant improvement in symptom reduction
- Mechanism of action is not clear

Commonly prescribed stimulants, in order of frequency of use, are listed in Table 15-7.

Antidepressants

- First alternative treatment
- Noradrenergic/dopaminergic are most commonly used
- Treat co-morbid mood and anxiety disorders
- Do not accentuate tics and compulsive phenomena
- Not addictive and will not provide risk for abuse
- Commonly prescribed antidepressants are listed in Table 15-8.

Table 15-7
Commonly Prescribed Psychostimulants for the Treatment of ADHD in Children and Adolescents

Medication	Tablet Strength	Starting Dose	Interval Between Doses (hr)	Titration Rate (mg/wk)	Usual Therapeutic Doses
Methylphenidate	5, 10, 20	5 mg bid	3-4	5-10	0.3-0.8 mg/kg/dose[a]
Dextroamphetamine	5, 10, 15	5 mg d or bid	4-6	5	0.2-0.5 mg/kg/dose[b]
Adderall[c]	10, 20	5 mg qd or bid	4-6	5	0.15-0.4 mg/kg/dose[b]
Pemoline	18.75, 37.5, 75	37.5 mg qam		18.75	1-2 mg/kg/day[d]

Note: Adolescents may require lower mg/kg dosing than school-age patients.
[a]Total daily dose or more than 60 mg is not recommended.
[b]Only rarely should more than 40 mg/day be considered.
[c]Consists of equal parts of amphetamine aspartate, dextroamphetamine sulfate, dextroamphetamine saccharate, and amphetamine sulfate.
[d]Maximum daily dose=112.5 mg/day.

Table 15-8
Commonly Prescribed Antidepressants

Drug	Available Forms	Comments
Venlafaxine	Short-acting 25, 37.5, 50, 75, 100 mg	Inhibits reuptake of serotonin and norepinephrine
	Long-acting 37.5, 75, 150 mg	Nausea and somnolence, most common adverse reaction
		No cardiac conduction problems noted
Bupropion	Short-acting 75, 100 mg	Inhibits neuronal uptake of norepinephrine, dopamine and serotonin
	Long-acting 100, 150 mg	Agitation is common side effect but can be reduced if titrated slowly
Tricyclics	Nortriptyline: 10, 25, 50, 75 mg	Anticholinergic side effects are prominent
	Desipramine: 10, 25, 50, 75, 100, 150 mg	
	Imipramine: 10, 25, 50 mg	

NONPHARMACOLOGICAL TREATMENT

A combination of therapies may result in the best outcome.

- Individual supportive therapy utilizes techniques to structure daily tasks.
- Group therapy provides support from peers while learning techniques to manage symptoms.
- Family therapy is used to improve interpersonal communication and problem-solving skills.
- Cognitive therapy teaches techniques for managing stress and reducing situational conflicts.
- Behavior therapy is used to reward behaviors that lead to diminished hyperactivity and increased attention, the learning of new tasks, and the strengthening of short-term memory.

Therapeutic Plan of Care   S.A. should be referred for a psychiatric evaluation with a provider who has expertise in treating ADHD. S.A. should be referred to an adolescent group that builds social skills and addresses related problems of low self-esteem. S.A.'s mother could benefit from a C.H.A.D.D. support group. The primary care provider will collaborate with the psychiatric provider for needed medical follow-up.

The initial physical examination and laboratory studies are necessary before pharmacological treatment, but not routinely necessary for stimulant treatment. Stimulants are first line treatment unless there is evidence of co-morbid psychiatric illness. Patients prescribed pemoline need liver function tests prior to treatment and every 3 months for the first 6 months and then every 6 months.

Common side effects for stimulants include an initial weight loss that rarely jeopardizes health and reduced growth velocity. Children who are treated year-round have more evidence of reduced growth than do those with drug holidays.

Because S.A. has allergies, special attention should be paid to his diet. S.A. should avoid food products with MSG or other preservatives. Many ADHD children benefit from martial arts such as Tai Chi, which helps build self-control and improve attentiveness.

Patient Education and/or Community Resources
- C.H.A.D.D. (Children and Adults with ADHD), 499 NW 70th Ave., Plantation, FL 33317

- National Attention Deficit Disorder Association, PO Box 972, Mentor, OH 44061; telephone toll-free 1-800-487-2282; fax (216) 350-0223
- Books on ADD: *Why Johnny Can't Concentrate: Coping with Attention Deficit Problems,* by Robert A Moss, 1990, Bantam (ISBN: 0-553-34968-6)

Follow-Up Plan   Primary care provider should place outreach call to mother to determine if she has obtained an appointment for S.A. to be evaluated by a specialist. Mother should be advised to have the specialist submit a consultant report for his medical record.

Mother should be advised that periodic laboratory and medial follow-up is required if S.A. is treated with medication. S.A.'s mother should be supported and encouraged to continue follow-up treatment for him and obtain peer support for herself.

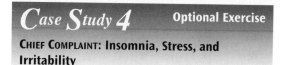

Case Study 4   **Optional Exercise**

CHIEF COMPLAINT: Insomnia, Stress, and Irritability

History of Present Illness   R.H. is a 34-year-old, separated, African-American male presenting with complaints of insomnia and irritability. R.H. was told by his boss to seek medical follow-up because his work performance has declined significantly in the past year. R.H. has been employed by the U.S. Post Office since high school and has been in a managerial position for the last 5 years. R.H. relates feeling overwhelmed at work and in his personal life. R.H. was separated from his wife last year and has been living with his parents to save money. R.H. states that his wife left him when he used their savings to start a franchise business that never got off the ground. R.H. is heavily in debt and is working a second job on the weekends to make extra money.

Past Medical History   R.H. has had elevated blood pressure, as noted on previous annual physicals, but did not follow up as requested by his previous physician.

Past Surgical History   R.H. had a right inguinal hernia repair in junior high and a vasectomy 3 years ago.

Family History   R.H.'s father has hypertension and is taking medication.

Developmental Stage Generativity versus Stagnation

Role-Relationship R.H. is the oldest of three children. He has two sisters who are married and live in the area. R.H. has always been a good provider and his parents are proud of his rapid advancement in the post office. R.H. has two small children residing with their mother. He reports that keeping his family together has "always been important" to him.

Sleep/Rest R.H. relates having trouble sleeping: "I can't get my mind to shut down." He has always been able to get by with very little sleep, 5 or 6 hours a night. In recent months R.H. has been sleeping 3 or 4 hours each night. R.H. was able to work double shifts early in his career while attending the local college part-time.

Nutrition/Metabolic R.H. has maintained his weight within 5 pounds until the past several months. He has lost 10 pounds and says he has "lost his appetite." He reports eating well-balanced meals until recently. He does admit liking salty foods.

Activity/Exercise R.H. has always been involved in softball and bowling leagues through work and exercises two or three times a week at the gym. He often volunteers to raise funds for charities sponsored at work.

Coping/Stress R.H. states he has managed stress in past years but he has been having trouble coping since his separation from his wife.

Health Management Alcohol, R.H. reports that for the past 6 months he has been drinking 3 or 4 beers a night to help him get to sleep. When bowling on his weekly league he drinks excessively. On a few occasion he has needed to have friends take him home because he has had too much to drink. His immunizations are current; last tetanus 1993 after cutting his ankle on chain link fence. He doesn't smoke tobacco or "pot." He denies other drug use, stating he tried "crack" once after high school. He had a "bad reaction" recalling feelings of restlessness and paranoia.

Self-Perception and Values/Beliefs R.H. reports a positive self-image and strong spiritual beliefs. He reports that his family and job are very important to him.

Medications No prescribed medication, will take acetaminophen on occasion

Allergies NKMA

Pertinent Physical Findings

Vital Signs Height 6 feet 1 inch; weight 193 pounds; BMI 27; temperature 98.6° F; heart rate 94; respirations 20; B/P 146/90

General Appearance R.H. is a pleasant-featured African-American male who is well-groomed and dressed in sports coat and slacks. He is articulate and his speech is mildly pressured. He maintains eye contact when responding to questions, but appears restless and is easily distracted by environmental stimuli.

Head/Neck Thyroid without enlargement, without palpable masses/nodules,

PERRLA, EOMS WNL, funduscopic examination without papilledema, AV nicking, hemorrhages or exudates, without lymphadenopathy

Heart CVS RRR without audible murmurs, gallops, without carotid bruits

Lungs Clear to auscultation

Extremities 2+ reflexes, without edema, without muscle weakness or atrophy

Skin Warm dry, without lesions, without bruising

Abdomen Soft, non-tender, without palpable masses, without organomegaly, without renal bruits, hemoccult negative

---

Discussion Questions

What type of history data should be collected?

What type of physical data should be collected?

What are the differential diagnoses?

What are the probable causes of the presenting symptoms?

What is your diagnostic impression?

What is the therapeutic plan of care?

What are the patient education and/or community resources?

What is your follow-up plan?

Discussions for optional case study exercises can be found in the accompanying Instructor's Manual.

References

American Psychiatric Association: *Diagnostic and statistical manual of mental disorders,* ed 4, Washington, DC, 1994, APA.

Biederman J: Attention-deficit/hyperactivity disorder: a life-span perspective, *J Clin Psychiatry* 59(Suppl 7):4-16, 1998.

Castellanos FX: An overview of pediatric psychopharmacology, *Psychopharmacology in Practice: Clinical and Research Update,* 1996.

Garner DH, Garfinkel PE, O'Shaughnessy M: The validity of the distinction between bulimia with and without anorexia nervosa, *Am J Psychiatry* 142(5):581-587, 1985.

Greenhill LL: Diagnosing attention-deficit/hyperactivity disorder in children, *J Clin Psychiatry* 59(Suppl 7):31-41, 1998.

Horning M: Addressing co-morbidity in adults with attention-deficit/hyperactivity disorder, *J Clin Psychiatry* 59(Suppl 17):42-47, 1998.

Hsu LK, Sobkiewicz TA: Bulimia nervosa: a four- to six-year follow-up study, *Psychol Med* 19(4):1035-1038, 1989.

Hutto B: The symptoms of depression in endocrine disorders, *CNS Spectrums* 4(4):51-61, 1999.

Jacobs DG, Deutsch NL: Screening women for suicidal intent, *Medicine and Behavior.* 2(4):32-33, 1999.

Jones K: History and prevention of eating disorders, *The Prevention Researcher* 4(3):1-4, 1997.

Kaye W: A biological basis for treating eating disorders, *Psychopharmacology in Practice: Clinical and Research Update,* 323-396, 1997.

Khouzam HR: Attention deficit hyperactivity disorder in adults: guidelines for treatment, *Consultant* August: 2159-2163, 1997.

Knesper D, Riba MB, Schwenk TL: *Primary care psychiatry,* Philadelphia, 1997, WB Saunders.

Nagel KL, Jones KH: Sociological factors in the development of eating disorders, *Adolescence* 27:107-113, 1992.

Pliszka SR: Comorbidity of attention-deficit/hyperactivity disorder with psychiatric disorder: an overview, *J Clin Psychiatry* 59(Suppl 7):50-58, 1998.

Rubinow D: Psychiatric disorders during peri-menopause, *Psychopharmacology in Practice: Clinical and Research Update* 67-122, 1996.

Sobel S: What's new in the treatment of anorexia nervosa and bulimia? *Medscape Womens Health* 1(9):5, 1996.

Talbott JA, Hales RE, Yudofsky SC: *Textbook of psychiatry,* Washington, DC, 1988, American Psychiatric Press.

Treasure J, Campbell I: The case for biology in the etiology of anorexia nervosa, *Psychological Medicine* 24:3-8, 1994.

Selected Readings

Leibenluft E: Questions and controversies in the treatment of rapid cycling mood disorder, *Psychopharmacology in Practice: Clinical and Research Update* 195-207, 1996.

Medical outlook for psychiatry Vol. 2 No.1 (audiotape), 1998.

Nagel KL, Jones KH: Eating disorders: prevention through education, *Journal of Home Economics* 85(1):53-56, 1993.

Owley T, Sharma R: Drug-induced mania: a critical review, *Psychiatric Annals* 26:659-663, 1996.

"Prime MD Today," Pfizer Pharmaceuticals, 1999.

Reiger DA, Narrow WE, Rae DS et al: The de facto U.S. mental and addictive disorders service system: Epidemiological Catchment Area prospective one-year prevalence rates of disorders and services, *Archive of General Psychiatry* 50:85-94, 1993.

Sheehan DV, Lecrubier Y: Mini international neuropsychiatric interview, *Journal of Clinical Psychiatry* 59 (Suppl 20), 22-33, 1998.

CHAPTER 16

Endocrine Disorders

Jean Nagelkerk, Ruth Ann Brintnall, and Wendy Muma

Case Study 1

CHIEF COMPLAINT: Blurred Vision, Increased Thirst, and Fatigue

History of Present Illness D.S. is a 47-year-old Hispanic male who presents with a chief complaint of blurred vision, increased thirst, and fatigue of 6 months duration. He states that his vision has declined. He reports double vision. D.S. states that he works in a marina and often runs errands. For the past 6 to 8 months his energy has decreased and he is sleepier. Denies weight loss, frequent infections, numbness or tingling in extremities, and sexual dysfunction. Does not experience early satiety. D.S. has not seen a health-care provider for 8 years. The last time he was at his health-care provider's office he was told that he had a mild form of high blood pressure, but was told he did not need any medication at that time.

Past Medical History He fractured his right wrist in 1988 after a fall, no sequelae

Past Surgical History Non-contributory

Family History Mother, age 66, has insulin dependent diabetes since age 42; father, age 70, has hypertension; brother, age 45, has diabetes controlled by oral agents

Developmental Stage Generativity versus Stagnation

Role-Relationship Lives alone in an apartment in the city. Has a close group of friends and family that are supportive

Sleep/Rest Sleeps 7 hours per night. Awakes feeling fatigued

Nutrition/Metabolic Breakfast, coffee (3 or 4 cups with sugar and cream) and a donut or sweet roll; lunch, fast food; dinner, eats frozen dinners or dines out with friends. Snacks consist of chips, candy, and soda

Activity/Exercise Keeps fit by doing physical jobs at his work. Does not feel he needs to exercise when he returns home

Coping/Stress Is very close with his family and visits them often. Also, has a small group of close friends that he meets regularly for dining and recreational activities.

Health Management Td: Unsure, but feels it was over 10 years ago. Nonsmoker. Alcohol, drinks 1 or 2 beers at night. Does not seek preventative health care

Medications None

Allergies NKMA

Pertinent Physical Findings

Vital Signs Height 5 feet 11 inches; weight 207 pounds; BMI 29; temperature 98.2° F; heart rate 78; respirations 12; blood pressure 150/92

General Appearance Alert and oriented to time, place, person; overweight, well groomed, speech clear, coordinated movements, in no apparent physical distress.

Eyes PERRLA, unable to perform Snellen eye chart because of double vision; EOMs intact. Funduscopic: Optic disc cream colored, dot hemorrhages and exudates noted

Neck Supple without JVD, carotid bruits, thyromegaly, or cervical lymphadenopathy; trachea midline

Heart Apical pulse 78 regular rate and rhythm, no S_3 or S_4, PMI 5th ICS-MCL, radial, and femoral pulses 2+ and equal bilaterally

Lungs Clear to auscultation bilaterally, no adventitious breath sounds, resonant throughout lung fields

Abdomen Rounded, active bowel sounds, no abdominal bruits, soft, no masses or organomegaly, nontender, no inguinal lymphadenopathy, no CVA tenderness

Extremities Pink, warm, without edema, no varicosities, joints without evidence of ligamentous laxity, effusions, erythema or swelling; feet, gross sensation intact, capillary refill <3 seconds, pedal pulses 2+, no lesions or open areas, callouses on heels bilaterally

Neurological CN II-XII grossly intact, DTR 2+ bilaterally symmetrical, muscular strength 5+/5, no atrophy or tremors, Romberg neg, sensation intact to light touch and pinprick; sensation with fine filament intact; able to heel-to-toe walk

Diagnostics

Diagnostic Tests Urine dip: + moderate glucose, otherwise negative; fasting blood sugar 259; BUN and creatinine WNL; fasting lipid and liver profile WNL; ECG, NSR; microalbumin 30 mg; TSH, WNL

History Data Questions specific to the chief complaint of blurred vision, increased thirst, and fatigue include the following:

- Do you have a family history of diabetes?
- Has anyone ever told you that you had high blood sugar?
- Have you experienced a change in weight (persons with type 2 diabetes will sometimes experience a gradual weight gain) or experienced hunger or increased urination?
- Do you have frequent infections (if female, inquire about frequent vaginal yeast infections and gestational diabetes), numbness or tingling in extremities, or sexual dysfunction (less likely with females)?

Also, inquire about risk factors for diabetes, such as the following:

- Is the patient >45?
- Does the patient have a family history of diabetes?
- Is the patient Hispanic, African-American, or Native American? (These populations have a higher incidence of diabetes.)

- Is the patient overweight?
- Does the patient have a history of impaired glucose tolerance or delivered a baby with a birth weight of more than 9 pounds?

Physical Examination Data The focused examination for the chief complaint of blurred vision, increased thirst, and fatigue includes vital signs, general appearance, eyes, neck, heart, lungs, abdomen, extremities, and neurological.

Differential Diagnoses Diabetes mellitus type 1 and type 2 (given the patient's age, type 1 DM is highly unlikely), diabetes insipidus, nondiabetic glycosuria, stress from trauma or from glucocorticoids (may cause transient hyperglycemia) (Table 16-1)

Probable Causes of the Presenting Symptoms The symptoms of polyuria, polyphagia, and polydipsia occur because of high glucose levels (hyperglycemia). Individuals with diabetes have a higher than normal serum glucose level from food intake because of altered use, storage, and uptake of glucose by tissues caused by a relative or absolute lack of insulin in the body (Young and Koda-Kimble, 1995). When enough glucose accumulates in the blood, it will exceed the renal threshold and glucose will be excreted in the urine. Water will be excreted along with the glucose through osmotic diuresis. As patients experience polyuria and loss of glucose in the urine, they begin to experience fatigue and polydipsia. Blurred vision and diabetic retinopathy is also a result of the hyperosmolar state. Blurred vision results from a fluctuation in the water balance in the eye from high blood sugar (McCance and Huether, 1995).

There are approximately 16 million Americans with diabetes, half of whom are undiagnosed (Harris, 1995). More than 90% of people with diabetes have type 2 diabetes. In 1997, the Expert Committee on Diagnosis and Classification of Diabetes Mellitus updated the diagnostic and classification criteria for diabetes. Diabetes mellitus is diagnosed using any one of the following three methods and must be confirmed on a subsequent day. The diagnosis of diabetes can be made with (1) a FBS of >126 (fasting is defined as no intake for 8 hours); (2) a random plasma glucose of >200 with

> ### Table 16-1
> Blurred Vision, Thirst, and Fatigue Differential Diagnostic Cues

Diagnosis	Signs and Symptoms	Lab Data	Treatment
Diabetes Mellitus			
Type 1 Old term = insulin-dependent DM or juvenile onset DM Less than 10% of those with diabetes Typically occurs at a young age Sudden onset Often normal weight or below normal weight, especially at the time of diagnosis Destruction of islet cells of the pancreas may be caused by autoimmune response Requires exogenous insulin C-peptide level approximates endogenous insulin level Characterized by honeymoon period	Polyuria, polydipsia, polyphagia, weight loss, blurred vision Ketoacidosis symptoms include N/V, abdominal pain, CNS depression, Kussmaul respirations, dehydration Frequent infections are common Children may have nocturnal enuresis and fail to grow and gain weight	FBS, HgbA1c, lipid profile, urinalysis, random urine for microalbumin, BUN, creatinine, ECG, CBC, TSH, lytes, ABGs if has diabetic ketoacidosis	Consult with physician for treatment or refer to endocrinologist or diabetic specialist. Hospitalization if has ketoacidosis. Insulin therapy: start with total dose of 0.5-1.0 units per kg. Give two-thirds of total insulin dose in AM and one-third of total insulin dose in PM. The AM dose should be two-thirds intermediate insulin and one-third regular insulin. The PM dose should be half intermediate and half regular insulin. During the honeymoon phase the insulin dose may need to be decreased to 0.2-0.5 U/kg/day. With select patients may elect intensive insulin therapy using continuous insulin pump therapy
Type 2 Old term = non-insulin–dependent DM or adult onset DM 90% of those with diabetes Typically occurs >40 years Many are overweight Characterized by insulin resistance Nonketotic hyperosmolar coma if uncontrolled will need hospitalization Strong genetic component 50% will eventually require insulin Many have complications when diagnosed	May be asymptomatic or fatigue, nocturia, frequent infections, polydipsia, polyuria, blurred vision, numbness and tingling in extremities, and frequent infections	FBS, lipid profile, urinalysis, random urine for microalbumin, BUN, creatinine, ECG, CBC, TSH, baseline HgbA1c	If FBS <250 mg/dl may try exercise and weight loss for 3 months. If FBS >250 mg/dl and <400 mg/dl, trial exercise, weight loss, and oral antidiabetic agent. Treatment options include sulfonylurea, biguanide, thiazolidinedione, alpha glucosidase inhibitor, meglitinide, insulin, combination or triple therapy. If the first antidiabetic agent is not effective, add a second agent from a different class. If combination antidiabetic therapy is not effective, consult a physician. May consider triple therapy with oral agents, combination of oral agents with insulin, or initiation of insulin. If a

▢	**Table 16-1**
	Blurred Vision, Thirst, and Fatigue Differential Diagnostic Cues—cont'd

Diagnosis	Signs and Symptoms	Lab Data	Treatment
Diabetes Mellitus—cont'd			
Type 2—cont'd			combination oral antidiabetic regimen fails replace one agent with insulin. Starting dose of insulin is based upon clinical judgment of insulin deficiency, suspected insulin resistance, and patient preference. One approach is to trial 10 units of intermediate acting at HS or 0.25 mg/kg. Adjust q 3-5 days based on fasting blood sugars
Cushing's Syndrome	Central obesity, moon face, buffalo hump, protuberant abdomen and thin extremities, hyperglycemia, polyuria, thin skin, striae, glycosuria, hypertension, weakness, hirsutism, poor wound healing, leukocytosis	Screen for hypercortisolism Give dexamethasone 1 mg at 11 PM and collect cortisol level at 8 AM if >5 ug/dl excludes Cushing's. 24-hour urine collection for cortisol and creatinine. If still uncertain, may do a suppression test by giving dexamethasone 0.5 mg p.o. q 6 hours × 48 hours then collect urine on the 2nd day. Or may do midnight serum cortisol level. May do MRI pituitary or CT of chest and abdomen depending on suspected cause	Refer to endocrinologist. Treatment depends on the cause. If pituitary adenoma may do selective transsphenoidal resection of the pituitary adenoma with hydrocortisone replacement therapy. Adrenal neoplasms or any ectopic tumors should be resected may need hydrocortisone replacement. If unresectable, may be given mitotane, ketoconazole, or metyrapone
Nondiabetic Glycosuria (Renal Glycosuria)	Glucose spills in urine. Serum blood sugar is normal	Urine dip and urinalysis. FBS and glucose tolerance test. BUN and serum creatinine	No treatment, monitor patient annually

Continued

	Table 16-1		
	Blurred Vision, Thirst, and Fatigue Differential Diagnostic Cues—cont'd		
Diagnosis	**Signs and Symptoms**	**Lab Data**	**Treatment**
Diabetes Insipidus (DI)	Polyuria, polydipsia, urine specific gravity <1.006	24-hour urine collection for volume, glucose, creatinine. Serum glucose, urea nitrogen, calcium, K, Na. If central diabetes insipidus is suspected, conduct a vasopressin challenge test. If nephrogenic diabetes insipidus is suspected, measure serum vasopressin during fluid restriction. If nonfamilial central diabetes insipidus is suspected, order MRI of the pituitary and hypothalamus	Refer to endocrinologist. Treatment depends on the cause. Desmopressin acetate may be used for central DI. With central and nephrogenic diabetes insipidus, may consider hydrochlorothiazide. With nephrogenic diabetes insipidus, combined drug therapies are sometimes used. Avoid thioridazine and lithium if drug therapy is needed because they cause polyuria. Avoid aggravators such as glucocorticoids that increase renal free water clearance

acute symptoms of diabetes; or (3) an oral glucose tolerance test using a 75-gram glucose load with a 2-hour plasma glucose >200. The American Diabetes Association (1998) established screening criteria to help identify asymptomatic individuals with diabetes. The criteria included individuals:

- Who are 45 years of age and above (If FBS is normal, it should be repeated every 3 years.)
- Who are obese (i.e., >120% of desirable body weight or a BMI >27)
- Who have a first degree relative with diabetes
- Who have hypertension >140/90
- Who are members of a high-risk ethnic population (e.g., African-American, Hispanic, Native American, Asian, or Pacific Islander)

- Who have gestational diabetes or have delivered a baby with a birth weight of more than 9 pounds
- Who have HDL levels <35 mg/dl and/or triglycerides >250 mg/dl
- Who have a history of impaired glucose tolerance or impaired fasting glucose

The Diabetes Control and Complications Trial (DCCT) in type 1 diabetic patients was completed and reported in September 1993. The study is a milestone in the field of diabetes management. The results of this long term, prospective, longitudinal, multi-center study conclusively demonstrate that glycemic control is a major determinant in the development and progression of diabetic microvascular and neuropathic disease (Lebovitz, 1994). These results were repeated in type 2 diabetics on insulin in the Kumamoto Study (Olefsky, 1997). Tight control is contraindicated in children under 2 years of age; and used with caution with children under 7 years of age, in persons with advanced renal disease, and in the elderly (Tierney, McPhee, and Papadakis, 1999).

Chronic complications of diabetes mellitus types 1 and 2 are microvascular, neuropathic, and macrovascular diseases. Microvascular disease includes retinopathy and nephropathy. Macrovascular disease includes stroke, coronary artery disease, and peripheral vascular disease. Neuropathic diseases include peripheral neuropathies, autonomic neuropathies, and mononeuropathies. Other associated long-term health problems that commonly occur in people with diabetes include cataracts, glaucoma, depression, hypothyroidism, and increased susceptibility to infections.

Macrovascular disease, and particularly atherosclerosis, is the most common of all chronic diabetic complications and accounts for about 80% of total mortality (Garber, 1997). Seventy-five percent of mortality occurs as the result of markedly accelerated coronary artery disease (Garber, 1997). Although diabetes itself can accelerate atherosclerosis by 200% to 400%, diabetic patients often have multiple risk factors for coronary disease (Garber, 1997). Although many of these risk factors are covariants of type 2 diabetes, including hypertension, hyperlipidemia, and smoking, type 2 diabetes is an independent risk factor for cardiovascular disease and is in proportion to the duration of diabetes (Sobel, 1997). The cornerstone of prevention of macrovascular disease is aggressive intervention to modify well-established risk factors. Target blood pressure with treatment should be <130/85 mm Hg, and the NCEP-ATP II guidelines for hyperlipidemia should be followed and aggressive treatment instituted in persons with diabetes.

Peripheral vascular disease (PVD) occurs approximately four times more often in diabetics than in the general public. PVD results in an inadequate blood supply to the lower limbs, depriving the tissues of oxygen and nutrients. The impaired removal of waste products plays a major role in the development of foot ulcerations. Symptoms of PVD include intermittent claudication, cold feet, and pain at rest that is relieved by dependency (Ahron and Hunt, 1998). The single most important treatment in PVD is smoking cessation (Bell,

1991). Daily foot care and monitoring is important in prevention of foot disease.

Neuropathy may lead to a peripheral sensory deficit, autonomic dysfunction, or a mononeuritis. The peripheral neuropathy is predominantly sensory, reducing sensation in the extremities, and may progress to cause pain and dysesthesias (Nussbaum, 1995). Autonomic neuropathy most commonly presents as impotence, orthostatic blood pressure, or lack of appropriate changes in heart rate. Decreased gastrointestinal motility, orthostatic hypotension, and urinary retention are other potential manifestations. Autonomic neuropathy is almost always seen in association with distal polyneuropathy. Its presence is an important predictor for foot and other infections. Diabetic mononeuropathy (also called mononeuritis multiplex) involves discrete cranial nerves, singly or as a mononeuritis (Nussbaum, 1995). Most commonly affected cranial nerves are III and VI. Best prevention is tight blood glucose management and smoking cessation (Nussbaum, 1995).

Diabetic nephropathy, a major cause of renal failure, accounts for 25% of patients in end stage renal failure (Ernst, 1998). Subclinical and histologic findings for diabetic nephropathy are present long before the stage of clinical proteinuria and rising serum creatinine. Within 5 years after the onset of diabetes, the patient experiences a decreased glomerular filtration rate, a positive microalbuminuria, and hypertension. These are clinical signs of incipient nephropathy. Interventions that are aimed at optimizing health and preventing the progression of diabetic nephropathy include controlling blood glucose and blood pressure, preventing insults to the kidney (infection, trauma), using an angiotensin converting enzyme inhibitor (ACE), and decreasing protein intake (Ernst, 1998).

Diabetes is the leading cause of blindness in the United States for persons between the ages of 20 and 74 years (Bernbaum and Stich, 1998). Diabetic retinopathy is often detectable within 5 to 10 years of diagnosis. Since type 2 diabetes often is undetected for years after the onset, 21% of patients have retinopathy at diagnosis. Diabetic retinopathy occurs when the microvasculature that nourishes the retina is damaged, permitting leakage of blood components through the vessel walls. Retinopathy may vary from a mild, asymptomatic form to a severe, rapidly devastating condition. Retinopathy is staged in the terms nonproliferative (e.g., mild, moderate, severe, and very severe) and proliferative. Nonproliferative retinopathy is characterized by microaneurysms, blot hemorrhages, cotton wool spots, venous changes, intraretinal microvascular abnormalities, and retinal capillary loss and ischemia. Proliferative retinopathy is characterized by neovascular changes, which cause fibrosis; vitreous hemorrhages; and retinal detachment. Ophthalmological evaluation is imperative to diagnosis and to patient follow-up. Treatment with laser photocoagulation may halt progression and decrease vision loss. Surgery (vitrectomy) is necessary when a vitreous hemorrhage will not spontaneously clear or when dense fibrovascular proliferation affects the macula and causes severe vision loss. Prevention of eye diseases include a yearly dilated examination, control of blood glucose and blood pressure levels, and smoking cessation (Bernbaum and Stich, 1998).

Medications that may increase glucose levels include thiazide diuretics, phenytoin, niacin, and large amounts of glucocorticoids. Contraceptive medications may impair glucose tolerance.

Diagnostic Tests   Tests useful in evaluation of diabetes mellitus include a urine dipstick to assess glucose, protein, and ketones; urinalysis to assess infection, glucose, protein, and ketones; random urine microalbumin to assess kidney function; and FBS to assess fasting blood sugar levels. A HgbA1c assesses glycemic control for the previous 2 to 3 months. A HgbA1c of less than 8% demonstrates blood sugars of less than 200 mg/dL and those values between 11% to 12% indicate a blood glucose level of more than 300 mg/dL (Goroll, May and Mulley, 1995). Obtain a TSH to assess thyroid function; BUN and creatinine to assess kidney function; ECG; and fasting lipid and liver profile.

Diagnostic Impression   D.J. presents with increased thirst (polydipsia), blurred vision, and fatigue. These are the classic symptoms characteristic of diabetes mellitus.

Therapeutic Plan of Care   D.J. meets the criteria for a diagnosis of diabetes with his fasting blood sugar = 259. FBS the following day was 289. He is also having symptoms that are interfering with his

normal daily activities (blurred vision). An oral agent should be prescribed to lower glucose levels. See Table 16-2 for a listing of oral agents with action, dosage, and side effects.

D.J. could be started with metformin (Glucophage) 500 mg bid initially. A basic discussion of the pathophysiology and signs and symptoms of hypoglycemia and hyperglycemia should be reviewed. In addition, home glucose monitoring should be taught as well as diet management and exercise (Table 16-3). D.J. should also work on weight reduction for better glycemic control. Due to his stage I hypertension (150/92) and diabetes he should be started on an ACE inhibitor (e.g., moexipril 7.5 mg qd) for documented high blood pressure (Joint National Committee on Prevention, Detection, Evaluation, and Treatment of High Blood Pressure, 1997). D.J. should also be scheduled to see an ophthalmologist for an eye evaluation. The ophthalmic changes noted on the funduscopic examination require further evaluation and treatment by an ophthalmologist. He should also be scheduled for outpatient diabetic management classes as part of a comprehensive educational program.

Patient Education and/or Community Resources   Information can be obtained from the American Diabetes Association (ADA) at: http://www.diabetesnet.com/ada.html. Diabetic patients should be offered the opportunity to attend a diabetic education class in their community. These classes typically review the pathophysiology of diabetes and the signs and symptoms of hypoglycemia and hyperglycemia; discuss the long-term complications of diabetes; review meal planning; and discuss medication therapy and home glucose monitoring. Each patient should be encouraged to purchase and wear a medical alert tag to help identify that they are diabetic.

The *signs and symptoms of hypoglycemia* include sweating, restlessness, shakiness, hunger, headache, confusion, and seizures. Patients should be taught to carry hard candies or glucose tablets to take in case of hypoglycemia. Friends and family should be instructed on injecting glucagon (1 mg for adults and adolescents) or placing glucose packets in the buccal mucosa if the patient is unresponsive. The *signs and symptoms of hyperglycemia* include polyuria, polydipsia, polyphagia, weight loss, fatigue, weakness, and frequent infec-

Table 16-2
Oral Antidiabetic Agents

Drug	Action	Dose	Major Side Effects
Second-Generation Sulfonylureas May increase dosage q 2-4 weeks Glyburide (DiaBeta, Micronase, Glynase PresTabs) Glipizide (Glucotrol/ Glucotrol XL) Glimepiride (Amaryl)	Stimulates insulin production from beta cells and helps with insulin resistance	Glyburide: 1.25-10 mg single or divided dose Glynase 0.75-12 mg Glipizide: 2.5-20 mg single or divided dose. Single dose for extended release (XL) Glimepiride: 1-4 mg single dose	Hypoglycemia Weight gain Skin rash GI upset Do not give with sulfa allergy
Meglitinide May increase dosage q 2-4 weeks Repaglinide (Prandin)	Stimulates insulin release from the pancreas. Insulin release is glucose dependent	Repaglinide: 0.5-16 mg in divided doses	GI upset Upper respiratory infections Headaches Hypoglycemia
Biguanides May increase dosage q 4-6 weeks Metformin (Glucophage)	Decreases hepatic glucose, decreases intestinal production and absorption of glucose, and increases insulin sensitivity	Metformin: 500-850 mg tid	GI upset Headaches Metallic taste Lactic acidosis Diarrhea Don't give with renal impairment, dehydration, serious illness. Hold for 24-48 hours after dye for x-rays
Alpha Glucosidase Inhibitors May increase dosage q 2-4 weeks Acarbose (Precose) Miglitol (Glyset)	Delays digestion of ingested carbohydrates	Acarbose: 25-100 mg tid Miglitol: 75-300 mg in three divided doses	GI upset Diarrhea Flatulence Hypoglycemia: use glucose, not sucrose, to treat Elevated ALT/AST
Thiazolidinediones May increase dosage q 8-12 weeks Pioglitazone HCl (Actos) Rosiglitazone (Avandia)	Improves target cell response to insulin, decreases hepatic glucose production, and increases glucose disposal in the skeletal muscles	Pioglitazone HCL: 15-30 mg Rosiglitazone: 4-8 mg	Elevated liver enzymes: closely monitor liver enzymes during treatment Edema Anemia

tions. Early diagnosis and treatment have limited the number of individuals with type 1 diabetes who are hospitalized for ketoacidosis. The *signs of ketoacidosis* are fruity breath odor, impaired consciousness, dehydration, and Kussmaul respira-

tions. Persons with type 2 diabetes usually do not present with ketoacidosis because they have enough circulating insulin to prevent lipolysis. Rare cases may occur with stress, infection, or illness. Persons with type 2 diabetes may experience

Table 16-3
Insulin Preparations

Insulin	Onset	Peak	Duration
Rapid Acting Insulin Lispro	15 minutes	1 hour	3.5-4.5 hours
Short Acting Insulin Regular	30 minutes	2-4 hours	6-8 hours
Intermediate Acting Insulin NPH, Lente	1-3 hours	6-10 hours	18-24 hours
Long Acting Insulin Ultralente	4-6 hours	18 hours	24-48
Premixed Insulin NPH and Regular 70/30 50/50	 30 minutes 30 minutes	 2-12 hours 3-6 hours	 24 hours 24 hours
Lispro 75/25	15 minutes	2-12 hours	24 hours

hyperglycemic hyperosmolar nonketotic coma. *Signs of hyperosmolar hyperglycemic nonketotic coma* include severe dehydration, blood sugar >600 mg/dl, ketosis (rarely), and serum osmolality of >340. New onset diabetes, noncompliance, steroids and diuretics, surgery, chronic illness, and stress can cause hyperosmolar hyperglycemic nonketotic coma. These patients require emergency treatment and hospitalization. Treatment is aimed at fluid resuscitation to restore electrolyte and improve glucose imbalances. Rapidly lowering the blood glucose to <250 mg/dl increases the risk of cerebral edema.

Home glucose monitoring should be taught to each diabetic patient, with return demonstrations to ensure accuracy and proper technique. If the patient is on intensive insulin therapy, frequent blood sugar monitoring is essential. An intensive program includes checking the blood sugar before meals, at HS, and occasionally in the middle of the night (3 AM). Patients who are not on intensive insulin therapy should monitor their blood sugar before meals, at HS, and in the middle of the night for 7 days in order to evaluate their pattern or when changing medications or dosages. Once stable, they should check their blood sugar before breakfast and dinner and then once a day, alternating times. With good control they may be able to check their blood glucose only twice a week, but this should be individualized and blood glucose should be assessed at varying times.

The patient should review *illness management* during diabetic education. The patient should be instructed to continue to take medications as prescribed, and informed that additional medication may be needed (infection may increase blood glucose) based on intensive home blood glucose monitoring. The patient should be encouraged to stay hydrated and eat normally. Nutrition is a very important aspect of diabetic care. Diabetic patients may be taught carbohydrate counting. They typically have 50% to 60% of their calories as carbohydrates. If they take more carbohydrates than scheduled, they may need to administer additional insulin (based on 1 unit of regular insulin to 10 to 15 g of additional carbohydrates eaten) but may experience weight gain. They should limit their cholesterol to 300 mg per day with no more than 30% fats, and of these, only 10% of saturated fat. The recommendation for protein intake is 10% to 20% of daily calories (American Diabetes Association, 1997). Artificial sweeteners may be used.

Foot care is an essential component of diabetic education. The use of monofilament testing to identify loss of protective sensation and to identify those at risk is very helpful. Proper foot care for the diabetic patient includes daily inspection of each foot for any signs of injury. It also includes gently washing and patting the feet dry (especially between the toes). Lotions with perfume or alcohol should not be used because these can dry out the feet and predispose to injury. Additionally, instruct the patient on the use of clean, white, cotton socks; properly fitted shoes; the avoidance of constricting nylons or hose of any type; and encourage patients not to go barefoot or wear sandals because this will help prevent foot injuries. Smoking cessation is a good measure to enhance circulation. If an ulcer is identified, prompt nursing and medical care is needed to prevent further damage and promote healing. Cultures and an x-ray should always be ordered, as well as coverage of common microorganisms with an antibiotic. Proper nutrition and close follow-up is essential.

Follow-Up Plan To provide support and education, a 1-week visit should be scheduled. If the patient is progressing well and has a good basic understanding of diabetes and hypertension, then recheck in 3 to 4 weeks. Once stable, the patient can be reevaluated every 3 months. During the 3-month visit a *HgbA1c* should be drawn to check glycemic control over the past 3 months. If the level is 2% higher or lower than the lab normal, modifications to the treatment plan should be instituted. A HgbA1c <7.5% indicates good control (Uphold and Graham, 1998). Conditions or substances that can provide a false high reading include alcoholism, high dose aspirin use, and uremia. Any type 2 diabetic patient, type 1 diabetics after 5 years of diagnosis, and anyone who has eye problems should schedule annual eye examinations with an ophthalmologist.

Case Study 2

CHIEF COMPLAINT: Fatigue, Weight Gain, and Hair Loss

History of Present Illness P.R. is a 29-year-old Caucasian female who presents with chief complaint of fatigue and hair loss for 9 months and a 12-pound weight gain over the past year. P.R. states that every time she combs her hair she loses several hairs in her comb. She reports cold intolerance, frequent constipation, and dry skin. She has not had a physical since the birth of her last child and has noted that her menses are heavier than normal. P.R. has a heavy menstrual flow for the first 4 days of her 8-day cycle, changing a soaked super tampon every 2 to 3 hours. She attributes this to the tubal ligation that she had after her last child. P.R. is currently on day 3 of her menses. She denies a personal and family history of thyroid problems, pain and swelling of her neck, and radiation to her head or neck.

Past Medical History Gestational diabetes during her second pregnancy

Past Surgical History D&C for miscarriage after her second child

Family History Mother age 61, diabetes controlled with oral agents; father age 63, hypertension; sisters ages 31 and 35, A&W

Developmental Stage Intimacy versus Isolation

Role-Relationship P.R. lives in the suburbs in a three-bedroom, two-story home. She works full time as a secretary for a law firm. Her husband of 7 years works at a factory 10 hours per day, 6 days per week. They have three children ages 2, 5, and 7.

Sleep/Rest Falls to sleep exhausted at 9 PM and awakens at 6:45 AM feeling tired.

Nutrition/Metabolic A 24-hour recall includes a bowl of Grape Nuts cereal and a glass of milk for breakfast; midmorning snack included peanuts, coke, and candy bar; lunch with her girlfriends at Burger King where she had a Whopper, large order of french fries, and Coke; dinner was at Kentucky Fried Chicken and included two pieces of chicken, mashed potatoes with gravy, and cole slaw. The evening snack with the children included chocolate almond ice cream.

Activity/Exercise States she is too busy to exercise while working full-time, cleaning the house, and caring for their three children

Coping/Stress P.R. states that with her lack of energy, she is feeling overwhelmed with her job and home responsibilities. Her husband is very supportive, but works long hours and cannot help very much. P.R. enjoys her job, but feels that unless her energy returns she will have to request part-time employment. The family enjoys reading, riding bikes, and hiking together. They have no religious affiliation.

Health Management P.R. does not drink alcohol, smoke, or take recreational drugs. Last Td: 1 year ago. She has a smoke detector in her home. Her husband owns three guns for hunting that he keeps locked in the basement.

Medications Multivitamin with iron daily and a herbal preparation Q-10 qd to increase her energy level.

Allergies Penicillin causes a red rash

Pertinent Physical Findings

Vital Signs Height 5 feet 9 inches; weight 209 pounds; BMI 31; temperature 98.2° F; heart rate 68; respirations 12; blood pressure 134/84

General Appearance Alert and oriented to time, place, and person; overweight, well groomed, speech clear, coordinated movements, no apparent distress

Integument Skin smooth, dry, warm, good turgor, no edema, or lesions; hair black, smooth and thin, evenly distributed; slight hair loss over lateral eyebrows

Neck Supple without JVD, carotid bruits, thyromegaly, no cervical lymphadenopathy, trachea is midline

Heart Apical pulse RRR with rate of 68; no S_3 or S_4, PMI at 5th ICS-LMCL, radial, pedal, and femoral pulses 2+ and equal bilaterally

Lungs Clear to auscultation and equal bilaterally, no adventitious breath sounds, resonant to percussion over lung fields

Abdomen Abdomen slightly rounded, hypoactive bowel sounds, no abdominal bruits, soft, no masses or organomegaly, nontender, no inguinal lymphadenopathy, no CVA tenderness.

Neurological CN II-XII grossly intact, DTR 1+ bil symmetrical, muscular strength 5+ bil, no atrophy or tremors, Romberg negative, sensation intact to light touch and pinprick, able to heel-to-toe walk

Diagnostics

Diagnostic Tests TSH, sensitive assay, 10 uU/ml (0.5-5.0 uU/ml); free T_4, 0.6 ng/dl (0.7-1.8 ng/dl). CBC: WBC 7.2; hemoglobin 12.0 g/dl; hematocrit 39.2%; platelet count 440,000 u/L

History Data Questions specific to the chief complaint of fatigue, weight gain, and hair loss include the following:

- When did you first notice your symptoms and have they progressed?
- What medications are you taking? (For example, amiodarone causes hypothyroidism in 8% of patients taking this medication.)
- Have you ever been treated for thyroid problems in the past? If so, what treatments were used?
- Do you have a family history of thyroid disorders?
- Have you had radiation to the head or neck?
- Do you have pain in your neck or any swelling?
- Do you have any of the following: hair loss, constipation, fatigue, heavy menses, cold intolerance, and dry skin, weight gain, depression? (These are common signs and symptoms of hypothyroidism.)
- Do you have a history of alcohol abuse, liver disease, or renal disease?

Physical Examination Data The focused examination for the chief complaint of fatigue, weight gain, and hair loss includes vital signs, general appearance, integument, neck, heart, lung, abdomen, and neurological evaluation.

Differential Diagnoses Hypothyroidism, congestive heart failure, depression, macrocytic anemia (Table 16-4)

Probable Causes of the Presenting Symptoms Hypothyroidism is caused by decreased secretions of T_4 and T_3. T_4 is the major thyroid hormone released into the circulation (Rubin, Voss, Derksen et al, 1996). The thyroid hormones are regulated by

Table 16-4
Fatigue, Weight Gain, and Hair Loss Differential Diagnostic Cues

Diagnosis	Signs and Symptoms	Lab Data	Treatment
Hypothyroidism Women are diagnosed more often than men Increased prevalence with age Affects 5% of the elderly	Early symptoms include fatigue, dry skin, menorrhagia, cold intolerance, weight gain, hair loss, constipation, and decreased reflexes Late symptoms include hoarseness, menstrual abnormalities, goiter, pitting edema, and cardiac enlargement	Sensitive TSH, Free T_4. May order antimicrosomal antibody if suspect Hashimoto's thyroiditis. If suspect secondary hypothyroidism, may need thyroid radioiodine uptake study or other testing. ECG if suspect cardiac irregularities. Consider lipid profile	If an infant or child, refer to a pediatric endocrinologist. For adults give thyroid replacement therapy for hypothyroidism. Usual starting dose for healthy adults under the age of 50 with no heart problems ranges from 0.075-0.125 mg/day (1.0-1.8 μg/kg/day). In the elderly or those with coronary insufficiency, the starting dose is 0.025-0.050 and slowly increase to avoid angina, dysrhythmias, or heart failure. Check TSH at 4-6 weeks and may adjust if needed at 0.025 mg/day then redraw TSH at 4-6 weeks to assess thyroid level
Congestive Heart Failure	SOB, dyspnea, edema of lower extremities, paroxysmal nocturnal dyspnea, orthopnea, 3rd heart sound	ECG, CXR, CBC if suspect infection or anemia. If suspect MI, do cardiac enzymes. If suspect endocarditis, get blood cultures. BUN and creatinine to check renal function. Echocardiogram	Remove cause if possible. Consider a diuretic and an ACE inhibitor. Monitor K if on a diuretic. Preventative care includes annual influenza vaccine and a pneumococcal vaccine. Low sodium and low-fat diet.
Depression	Depressed moods, difficulty concentrating, sleep disturbance, loss of interest in surroundings, fatigue, decreased sexual drive, weight gain, and decreased appetite	Consider TSH, CBC, and random blood sugar (RBS) to rule out organic causes. Urine toxicology to assess for substance abuse. ECG if using TCAs	Psychotherapy and medications are often used. The most common medications prescribed are TCAs, SSRIs, and MAOs (third line treatment with dietary restrictions). TCAs have anticholinergic side effects, overdoses may be lethal, and are contraindicated in patients with cardiac conduction problems and narrow-angle glaucoma. SSRIs are usually first line treatment because they are well tolerated and do not have the cardiovascular and anticholinergic SE.

Continued

Table 16-4
Fatigue, Weight Gain, and Hair Loss Differential Diagnostic Cues—*cont'd*

Diagnosis	Signs and Symptoms	Lab Data	Treatment
Macrocytic Anemia Megaloblastic (Folate or vitamin B_{12} deficiency) MCV >125 fL	Fatigue, peripheral paresthesias (B_{12} deficiency), glossitis, decreased appetite, diarrhea	CBC with differential. Vitamin B_{12} and folate level.	If pernicious anemia, will require lifelong treatment. IM of 100 µg of vitamin B_{12} daily × 1 week, weekly × 1 month, and then monthly. Oral cobalamin may be used instead of IM vitamin B_{12}. For folic acid deficiency give folic acid I mg qd

thyroid stimulating hormone (TSH), which is secreted by the anterior pituitary gland. Thyrotropin releasing hormone (TRH) is produced in the hypothalamus and regulates TSH. Hypothyroidism affects most systems of the body, producing a variety of clinical manifestations. The causes of hypothyroidism may be thyroid, pituitary, or hypothalamic disease (Kelley, 1997). Primary hypothyroidism accounts for approximately 98% of cases. In primary hypothyroidism, laboratory values will show an elevated TSH and a low free T_4. Causes of primary hypothyroidism include chronic autoimmune thyroiditis (Hashimoto's thyroiditis may have goiter), radiation therapy, surgery, or iodide deficiency (in developing countries). Medications that are goitrogens (substances that cause goiters) include lithium, amiodarone, iodide, propylthiouracil or methimazole, phenylbutazone, and sulfonamides. A food goitrogen is turnips (Tierney, McPhee, and Papadakis, 1999).

Hypothyroidism, in advanced cases, is often associated with anemia. It is common for a patient to present with hypothyroidism and have a mild normochromic normocytic anemia. Microcytic anemia is often seen from iron deficiency in women who have heavy menstrual bleeding. Macrocytic anemia may be seen, but may resolve with treatment of hypothyroidism. An autoimmune mechanism is implicated for the 10% of patients with hypothyroidism that have pernicious anemia.

With long-standing or very poorly controlled hypothyroidism, myxedematous symptoms can occur. Symptoms that patients experience with myxedema include thick, coarse, dry skin; depression; bradycardia; impairment in mental activities; pretibial edema; hearing impairment; and cardiac enlargement. In rare cases a patient may lapse into a myxedema coma, which is a medical emergency. Signs and symptoms of myxedema coma include coma or altered mental status, bradycardia, hypothermia, and respiratory or cardiac failure. These patients need hospitalization and aggressive supportive treatment.

Diagnostic Tests Sensitive TSH, Free T_4, CBC, and glucose. The TSH and Free T_4 are ordered to assess for primary hypothyroidism (high TSH and low Free T_4). A free T_4 test is a better measure of thyroid function than total T_4. The total T_4 level is altered by changes in thyroid-binding globulin independent of thyroid function (Goroll, May, and Mulley, 1995). The CBC is ordered to assess the patient for anemia, particularly because of the patients heavy menses (increased blood loss). The glucose is drawn because of the patient's positive family history of diabetes (screening). Lipid screening should also be completed.

Diagnostic Impression P.R. reports cold intolerance, heavy menses, fatigue, hair loss, and weight gain. Clinical and laboratory evaluation support the diagnoses of primary hypothyroidism (elevated TSH and low T_4).

Therapeutic Plan of Care P.R. needs thyroid replacement to achieve an euthyroid state. The typical starting range is 0.075 to 0.125 mg/d (1.0 to 1.8 μg/kg/d) (Kelley, 1997). Based on P.R.'s weight (95 kg × 1.0 μg = 95 μg/kg), starting P.R. at 0.01 mg/day is acceptable.

Patient Education and/or Community Resources P.R. should understand that she will most likely need to take thyroid replacement medication for the rest of her life. She should be cautioned to take the proper dosage, and informed that the drug will be titrated slowly because patients with hypothyroidism are sensitive to the effects of thyroid hormones and may experience tremors, nervousness, and palpitations. Taking large doses or increasing the thyroid replacement rapidly may be dangerous to health because cardiac abnormalities (e.g., angina and dysrhythmias) may be produced. The patient should be told that certain medications might interfere with the absorption of thyroid medication. Common drugs include iron preparations, aluminum hydroxide antacids, sucralfate, phenytoin, and cholestyramine. Often, the thyroid replacement dosage must be adjusted for patients who are taking phenytoin, carbamazepine, or rifampin.

P.R. should understand the signs and symptoms of hypothyroidism and hyperthyroidism. The symptoms of hyperthyroidism include tachycardia, weight loss, sweating, tremor, fatigue, menstrual irregularity, and goiter. In thyrotoxicosis there are high levels of free T_3 and T_4. Graves' disease is the most common form of thyrotoxicosis. It is an autoimmune disorder characterized by thyroid enlargement and antibodies development against the thyroid gland. With Graves disease patients may experience infiltrative ophthalmopathy (exophthalmos).

P.R. should also understand the importance of regular follow-up to assess her thyroid level and evaluate for any signs and symptoms of hypo/hyperthyroidism. It is important for P.R. to use the same brand of thyroid replacement, because there may be variations in the biologic activity and hormonal content of commercial preparations.

Follow-Up Plan P.R. should return in 4 weeks for a TSH level to evaluate thyroid control. If the patient is euthyroid, recheck in 3 months; if she is hypothyroid, the thyroid dosage should be in-

creased by 0.025 mg/d and recheck TSH in 4 to 6 weeks. Once stable, check at 3 months and then every 6 to 12 months.

P.R.'s heavy menstrual flow may improve with thyroid replacement. In the absence of an abnormal pelvic examination and Pap test, a trial of NSAIDs for 3 days before her menses and 3 days into the cycle or hormonal therapy may decrease the amount and length of the menstrual flow.

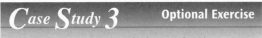

Case Study 3 **Optional Exercise**

CHIEF COMPLAINT: Hypercholesterolemia

History of Present Illness R.W. is a 52-year-old Caucasian female nurse who returns following a complete physical examination to review findings and implications of elevations in total cholesterol, triglycerides, and borderline high density lipoprotein (HDL) noted on her laboratory profile. Her risk factor profile for coronary artery disease (CAD) includes a family history of (1) CAD, (2) diabetes mellitus, and (3) hypercholesterolemia. Negative factors include (1) normal blood pressure, (2) normal blood glucose, and (3) negative smoking history. In general, R.W. feels well and considers herself healthy. She works full time as a charge nurse in surgical critical care at a local medical center.

Past Medical History Broken right wrist at age 12

Past Surgical History Appendectomy at age 40

Family History Father age 75, CAD, DM, hypercholesterolemia; mother age 72, A&W; brother age 50, HTN; sister age 48, DM; sister age 47, A&W

Developmental Stage Generativity versus Stagnation

Role-Relationship R.W. has been married for 27 years and has two children who are married and independent. Children: one son, 25; one daughter, 23

Sleep/Rest Falls asleep at 10 PM and arises at 6 AM feeling rested

Nutrition/Metabolic Breakfast, sausage biscuit or Egg McMuffin at McDonald's with coffee; lunch, sandwich or salad, dessert, and Coke; dinner, meat, potato, vegetable, buttered bread, dessert, and coffee. Snacks on raw vegetables and fruit

Activity/Exercise Walks 1 mile a day with her neighbor

Coping/Stress R.W. and her husband spend 1 hour per night talking, relaxing, and discussing issues. They attend a Catholic church every Sunday and help with religious education classes. They enjoy golfing, swimming, and attending baseball games.

Health Management R.W. routinely has an annual physical examination and mammogram. She has 3 cups of coffee and one or two Cokes per day. Nonsmoker. Drinks a glass of white wine when dining out (about five times a month). Td: 7/6/97; she receives a flu vaccination each fall. Does not own firearms

Medications Multivitamin, daily; Premarin 0.625 mg/daily; Provera 2.5 mg/daily; calcium 500 mg/daily

Allergies Penicillin, causes hives

Pertinent Physical Findings

Vital Signs Height 5 feet 6 inches; weight 150 pounds; BMI 25; temperature 98.4° F; heart rate 64; respirations 12; blood pressure 134/76

General Appearance Appears stated age; alert and spontaneous; good historian

Skin Smooth, moist, warm, good turgor, no edema, or lesions

Eyes PERRLA, optic discs sharp, well defined, cream color, no exudates or hemorrhages, EOMs intact, visual acuity 20/20 OU. No arcus senilis. Xanthomas noted on the eyelids bilaterally

Neck Supple without JVD, carotid bruits, thyromegaly, no cervical lymphadenopathy, trachea is midline

Heart Apical pulse 64 regular rate and rhythm, without murmurs, no S_3 or S_4, PMI 5th ICS-LMCL

Abdomen Round, active bowel sounds in all quadrants, no abdominal bruits, soft, no masses or organomegaly, nontender, no inguinal lymphadenopathy, no CVA tenderness

Extremities Pink, warm, without edema, no varicosities, dorsalis pedis and radial pulses 2+ bilateral, joints without evidence of ligamentous laxity, effusions, erythema or swelling

Neurological Cranial nerves II-XII are intact; no focal deficits are apparent

Diagnostics

Diagnostic Tests CBC is normal; electrolyte profile is unremarkable; total serum cholesterol 245 mg/dl; HDL 34 mg/dl; triglycerides 250 mg/dl. Urine analysis normal. Low-density lipoprotein (LDL) was calculated using the formula: Total cholesterol – HDL – triglycerides/5 = LDL, or 245-34-50=161

Discussion Questions

What type of history data should be collected?

What type of physical data should be collected?

What are the differential diagnoses?

What are the probable causes of the presenting symptoms?

What is your diagnostic impression?

What is the therapeutic plan of care?

What are the patient education and/or community resources?

What is your follow-up plan?

Discussions for optional case study exercises can be found in the accompanying Instructor's Manual.

References

Ahron JN, Hunt C: Management of skin, foot, and dental care. In Funnell MM, Hunt C, Rubin R et al, editors: *A core curriculum for diabetes education,* ed 3, Chicago, 1998, American Association of Diabetes Educators.

American Diabetes Association: Position statement: nutritional recommendations and principles for people with diabetes mellitus, Diabetes Care 20(Suppl 1):S14-S17, 1997.

American Diabetes Association: Report of the Expert Committee on the diagnosis and classification of diabetes mellitus, *Diabetic Care* 21(Suppl 1):S5-S19, 1998.

Bell DS: Lower limb problems in diabetic patients: what are the causes? What are the remedies? *Postgrad Med* 89:237-240, 243-244, 1991.

Bernbaum M, Stich T: Complications: eye disease and adaptive diabetes education for visually impaired persons. In Funnell MM, Hunt C, Rubin R et al, editors: *A core curriculum for diabetes education,* ed 3, Chicago, 1998, American Association of Diabetes Educators.

Ernst KL: Complications: nephropathy. In Funnell MM, Hunt C, Rubin R et al, editors: *A core curriculum for diabetes education,* ed 3, Chicago, 1998, American Association of Diabetes Educators.

Garber AJ: Role of hyperglycemia in the etiology and progression of chronic complications of diabetes mellitus. In Olefoker JM, editor: *Current approaches to the management of type 2 diabetes: a practical monograph,* Secaucus, NJ, 1997, Professional Post Graduate Services.

Goroll AH, May LA, Mulley AG: *Primary care medicine: office evaluation and management of the adult patient,* ed 3, Philadelphia, 1995, Lippincott-Raven.

Harris M: *Diabetes in America,* ed 2, Washington, DC, 1995, National Institutes of Health.

Joint National Committee on Prevention, Detection, Evaluation, and Treatment of High Blood Pressure: The sixth report, *Archives of Internal Medicine* 157:2413-2446, 1997.

Kelley W: *Textbook of internal medicine,* ed 3, Philadelphia, 1997, Lippincott-Raven.

Lebovitz NE: *Therapy for diabetes mellitus and related disorders,* ed 2, Alexandria, VA, 1994, American Diabetes Association.

McCance KL, Huether SE: *Pathophysiology: the biologic basis for disease in adults and children,* ed 2, St Louis, 1995, Mosby.

Nussbaum SR: Approaches to the patient with diabetes mellitus. In Goroll AN, May LA, Mulley AG: *Primary care medicine: office evaluation and management of the adult patient,* ed 3, Philadelphia, 1995, Lippincott.

Olefsky JM: *Current approaches to management of type 2 diabetes; a practical monograph,* Secaucus N.J., 1997, Professional Postgraduate Services.

Rubin H, Voss C, Derksen DJ et al: *Medicine: a primary care approach,* Philadelphia, 1996, WB Saunders.

Sobel BE: Complications of diabetes: macrovascular disease. In Olefsky JE, editor: *Current approaches to the management of type 2 diabetes: a practical monograph,* Secaucus, NJ, 1997, Professional Postgraduate Services.

Tierney L, McPhee SJ, Papadakis MA: *Current medical diagnosis and treatment,* Stamford, Conn., 1999, Appleton & Lange.

Uphold C, Graham M: *Clinical guidelines in family practice,* Gainesville, Fla., 1998, Barmarrae Books.

Young LY, Koda-Kimble MA: *Applied therapeutics: the clinical use of drugs,* Vancouver, 1995, Applied Therapeutics, Inc.

Selected Readings

Singer PA, Cooper DS, Levy EG et al: Treatment guidelines for patients with hyperthyroidism and hypothyroidism, *JAMA* 273(10):808-812, 1995.

U.S. Department of Health and Human Services: *Clinical guidelines on the identification, evaluation, and treatment of overweight and obesity in adults: the evidence report* (NIH Publication No. 4083), Rockville, Md., 1998, Author.

U.S. Department of Health and Human Services: *NCEP report of the expert panel on blood cholesterol levels in children and adolescents* (NIH Publication No. 2732), Rockville, Md., 1991, Author.

COMPLEMENTARY THERAPIES

CHAPTER 17

Integrating Complementary Therapies into Practice

Roxana Huebscher

This chapter presents definitions of Natural/Alternative/Complementary (NAC) care; discusses several NAC practices; describes why NAC therapies are important; and delineates some NAC approaches that the nurse practitioner (NP) can integrate into contemporary practice and thereby increase the repertoire of therapies.

Although most NPs consistently educate and counsel about health concerns, many health-care providers, including NPs, tend to rely on drugs, radiation, and surgery for treatment of symptoms and illnesses. Education on NAC therapies is increasingly important so that both consumer and health-care provider can institute other forms of therapy as complements or as alternatives, thus providing an integrative approach to health care and providing more options for clients. However, health-care providers also need to be knowledgeable about NAC therapies so they may make appropriate decisions about the quality of both the modality and the provider.

Reimbursement is an issue with many NAC therapies. There are a few nursing diagnoses available such as "energy field disturbance" and some CPT codes that may help with payments. NAC therapies are becoming increasingly popular and more health-care organizations are instituting NAC clinic settings, meaning that more plans may pay for the cost of this care. However, clients must often pay for this care out-of-pocket. Costs vary for NAC therapies, and health-care providers would do best to call for the range of prices for a treatment.

DEFINITIONS OF NAC

NAC proponents have defined practices in several ways. These definitions vary from the narrowly defined "interventions neither taught widely in medical schools nor generally available in U.S. hospitals" (Eisenberg, Davis, Ettner et al, 1998; Eisenberg, Kessler, Foster et al, 1993) to Micozzi's (1996) philosophical and comprehensive view:

> Complementary medical systems are characterized by a developed body of intellectual work that underlies the conceptualization of health and its precepts; that has been sustained over many generations by many practitioners in many communities; that represents an orderly, rational, conscious system of knowledge and thought about health and medicine; that relates more broadly to a way of life (or "lifestyle"); and that has been widely observed to have definable results as practiced (p 7).

Eisenberg et al (1993, 1998) documented the percentage of persons in the United States who were using alternative therapies. Their 1997 study showed that 42% of the nation used at least one of 16 therapies surveyed. In addition, the Office of Alternative Medicine (a part of NIH now known as the National Center for Complementary and Alternative Medicine or NCCAM) states that complementary and alternative medicine:

> . . . encompasses all health systems, modalities, and practices other than those intrinsic to the politically dominant health system of a particular society or culture. CAM includes all practices and ideas self-defined by their users as preventing or treating illness or promoting health and well-being (Hufford, 1995, p 94).

Holistic nursing authors have defined alternative therapies this way:

> Interventions that focus on body-mind-spirit integration and evoke healing by an individual, between two individuals, or healing at a distance (e.g., relaxation, imagery, biofeedback, prayer, psychic healing); may be used as complements to conventional medical treatments (Dossey, Keegan, Guzzetta et al, 1995, p 6).

This holistic definition goes beyond the medical definitions and uses terminology that includes body-mind-spirit and healing. Holistic nursing is not synonymous with NAC therapies because holistic nursing encompasses nursing in all areas, whether they be conventional or alternative/complementary. However, NAC practices fit especially well into a holistic perspective.

Another important concept to clarify is the difference between the terms *alternative medicine* and *alternative health care.* Most alternative practices do not require a medical degree in order to practice. When the therapy is termed medical, practitioners run the risk of being accused of practicing medicine without a license. Because treatments such as acupuncture and traditional oriental medicine, Ayurvedic and Tibetan medicine, homeopathy, naturopathy, chiropractic, shamanism, and nutritional and herbal therapy have been practiced for many years by persons other than physicians, to call these practices medical is inaccurate and risky in a legal sense. In other words, these NAC therapies are health-care practices, rather than medical practices.

IMPORTANCE OF NAC AND RATIONALE FOR ITS USE

There are many reasons why practitioners suggest, and clients use, NAC therapies. These reasons include comfort; client control; client confidence/faith in themselves, their health-care providers (HCPs), and the treatment of their conditions; and the "naturalness" of many NAC therapies. In a recent study, Astin (1998) found that:

> . . . the majority of alternative medicine users appear to be doing so not so much as a re-

sult of being dissatisfied with conventional medicine but largely because they find these health care alternatives to be more congruent with their own values, beliefs, and philosophical orientations toward health and life (p 1548).

In addition, use of NAC therapies allows for extension of the client's personal research base to find out "what works" for them. NAC therapies also present a cultural opportunity for both the HCP and client because many therapies are from cultures different than conventional Western health care.

Comfort refers to a person's sense of relief, transcendence, and ease (Kolcaba, 1991). Relief means having a need met; transcendence refers to rising above a concern; and ease refers to a feeling of calm or contentment. Even though comfort is a difficult concept to measure, clients use NAC therapies in order to feel comfortable and often to ease pain.

Control is concerned with the sense that one has some power or direction over a situation and on the outcome of a situation. Many NAC practices are self-care practices, and clients may feel a sense of control when they are able to provide part of their own care. The NP's health care responsibilities include providing as many options as applicable to clients, thus these alternatives should be considered as a part of the treatment plan.

Confidence and faith refer to a knowing that things will work out. Even if Western nursing and medicine tell a person "there's nothing else we can do," NAC options are available. Such options offer hope and faith that something more can be done.

Naturalness means that therapies are less invasive and often non-drug oriented. Herbs, however, often considered as alternatives, are substances just as any medication and thus need to be considered with the same cautions as other drug therapies. (Chapter 18 provides information on herbal therapies.) When pharmaceuticals are offered as the only treatment for a condition, some clients will seek other treatments, not wanting to rely on drugs as the only solution.

In the United States today, there is a compelling drug problem, not just with illicit drugs but also with prescription drugs. This can lead to overdrugging and undertreatment of our clients (Huebscher, 1997). The consequences of this include iatrogenesis (including increased bacterial resistance), drug interactions, and other adverse effects. Lazarou, Pomeranz, and Corey (1998) reported, after an electronic database search from 1966 to 1996, that the overall serious adverse drug reaction (ADR) incidence in hospitalized patients was 6.7% and the percentage of fatal ADRs was 0.32%. They estimated that in 1994, 106,000 hospitalized patients had fatal ADRs, "making these reactions between the fourth and sixth leading cause of death" (1998, p 1200). Thus providing more naturalness and options other than drug therapy, whenever possible, could benefit clients and the health-care system.

NAC THERAPIES MANAGEMENT FOR THE NP

Authors categorize NAC care in many ways. The NCCAM classifies practices into the following: (1) alternative medical systems; (2) mind-body interventions; (3) biological-based therapies; (4) manipulative and body-based therapies; and (5) energy therapies. Box 17-1 delineates each category of the NCCAM classification.

Several concerns could be raised with the classification. For example, the "medical systems" include modalities that would not be considered "medical" by some health-care providers. This category could be problematic for practitioners in the United States, since only physicians can "practice medicine" and other professionals could possibly face legal implications if these modalities are thought of as medical in the Western sense of the word. For current treatment categorizations by NCCAM, access the NIH website at http://nccam.nih.gov/nccam/fcp/classify/index.html

Engebretson and Wardell (1993) classify therapies as physical manipulation, ingested or applied substances, uses of energy, and mental/spiritual modalities. They further divide these into orthodox, marginal, and alternative classifications. These last three terms depend somewhat on the region of the country and the personal point of view. For reasons of clarity, this chapter categorizes NAC care into self-care practices, provider-assisted practices, and traditional healing methods.

Box 17-1

NCCAM Classifications of Alternative Medicine Practices 2000*

I Alternative Medical Systems
Traditional oriental medicine
Native American
Aboriginal
African
Middle-Eastern
Tibetan
Central and South American
Homeopathy
Naturopathy

II Mind-Body Interventions
Meditation
Hypnosis
Dance
Music
Art therapy
Prayer
Mental healing

III Biologically-Based Therapies
Herbal
Special dietary
Orthomolecular
Individual biological therapies

IV Manipulative and Body-Based Methods
Chiropractic
Osteopathic
Massage

V Energy Therapies
Energy fields (biofields, e.g., qigong, reiki, therapeutic touch)
Electromagnetic fields (e.g., pulsed fields, magnetic fields, alternating or direct current)

*These are the categories within which NCCAM has chosen to group the numerous CAM practices; others employ different, broad groupings. (Source: NCCAM website, accessed 8/14/00 at http://nccam.nih.gov/nccam/fcp/classify/index.html)

Self-Care Practices

Self-care practices include those things that persons can do for themselves, including therapies where clients need some provider assistance, training, or education in order to begin maintaining the therapy on their own. Box 17-2 lists some self-care practices.

These practices include modalities that NPs can teach, or for which they can refer clients. This means NPs and other health-care providers must become knowledgeable about these modalities. Having a referral list of reputable practitioners is useful. Ensuring quality is more difficult with NAC therapies because the standards for NAC treatments may not be mandated as they are for nursing care. NPs need to know about the specific NAC practice and about the NAC provider, if the modality has a provider involved. This entails finding the research base as well as regulation and standards for the NAC practice and practitioner.

NPs may teach and/or recommend some appropriate self-care along with routine conventional care; or may initiate the NAC therapy. For example, affirmations are a helpful modality to teach clients who tend to be negative, persons needing demanding procedures or frightening therapies, persons with confidence problems, or those who are making changes in their lives. Affirmations are strong positive, personal, present-tense statements that express a desirable outcome as if it already has occurred. Only positive words are in affirmations. Affirmations are thoughts that clients say to themselves numerous times daily to help immerse the consciousness and produce the desired result. Some examples of affirmations include:

> Every day in every way, I am healthy, happy, and prospering.
> I am strong and full of energy.
> I have a meaningful job that I love.
> I say what I need to say effortlessly, honestly, and tactfully.

This modality operates on the concept that we are what we say we are. Affirmations can be easily used with many other therapies.

In addition, a health-care provider lending library of self-care resources is also helpful. The

---

Box 17-2
Self-Care Practices

Affirmations
Aromatherapy
Art and/or art therapy
Assertiveness/attitude
Bibliotherapy
Biofeedback
Caring for something:
  person, plant, pet
Centering
Color therapy
Deep breathing
Focusing
Hobbies
Imagery/visualization
Journaling
Light therapy
Meditation

Movement: dance, exercise, tai chi, yoga
Music: listening and/or playing/singing
Nutrition/nutritives (e.g., supplements, herbs)
Prayer
Presence
Relaxation
Religious and/or spiritual practices
Ritual
Self-hypnosis
Sleep hygiene
Spiritual practices
Stress management
Values clarification
Volunteer work
Water therapy
Writing

health-care provider can keep audio/video tapes, texts, books, booklets, articles, and handouts for clients to use. Other references may include self-help books and how-to books on topics such as drawing/painting, how to do visualization, stress management, assertiveness, and nutrition. Even appropriate novels and short stories or poetry may have some healing significance.

Movement, whether conventional exercise or NAC modalities, is a self-health care practice available for every client. For example, yoga is a movement therapy that helps with balance, relaxation, and stress management. In a randomized trial of interventions for carpal tunnel syndrome, clients had more effective results with a yoga-based approach than with wrist splinting (Garfinkel, Singhal, Katz et al, 1998). Likewise, T'ai Chi has been used to

improve strength, balance, concentration, and coordination (Spencer and Jacobs, 1999). T'ai Chi and yoga may be useful for cardiorespiratory, neurological, and arthritic conditions.

Another way to view NAC self-care therapies is from the perspective of the symptoms or disease entity the client presents. For example, with a sleep problem, rather than routinely prescribing a sedative or benzodiazepine, consider all the natural sleep hygiene processes plus add the NAC therapies. Box 17-3 lists suggestions that may be given to a client for healthy sleep promotion from a self-care perspective (Huebscher, 1997).

These are just a few examples of self-care practices. There are numerous texts, tapes, and other guides for the health-care provider to use or recommend.

Box 17-3

Sleep Hygiene

Identify any known specific reason for not sleeping and correct this as much as possible (e.g., substances, sleep apnea, noise, unsafe or stressful situation)

Keep a sleep diary for 2 weeks to recognize individual patterns

Maintain consistent sleep and wake times

Provide a comfortable, cool, safe, quiet sleep room

Avoid daytime naps or take short "power naps" of approximately 15 minutes only

Participate in walking or other form of exercise during the day (but not within 3 hours of bedtime)

Benefit from sunlight exposure (or use a light box)

Make sure the bed is used only for sleep, intimacy, or "sleepytime" reading (e.g., no work, paying bills, or eating)

Maintain a bedtime ritual/presleep routine (e.g., brushing teeth, devotional reading, prayer/meditation)

Take a warm shower or bath. Essential oils such as lavender can be used for relaxation

Address pain/discomfort concerns (e.g., with warm bath, liniment rub, medication)

Avoid alcohol, nicotine, caffeine, and other stimulants (even early AM caffeine can affect sleep)

Eat a small, easily digestible protein snack about 1 hour before bed (may need to vary this if GERD is present; for example, may need to eat 2 to 3 hours prior to sleep); tryptophan-containing snacks (e.g., milk, turkey, tofu, nut butters) may be helpful because this amino acid is needed along with the neurotransmitter serotonin for melatonin synthesis

Practice deep breathing: Take 10 deep, SLOW breaths (in for a count of 5; hold for a count of 5; out for a count of 5). This technique may be used to get to sleep or if a person awakens in the night.

Use relaxation tapes such as Emmett Miller's "Healing Journey"* or other comforting sound or music tapes

Keep paper and pencil at bedside. Make a "worry list" (a list of things that need to be done tomorrow or worries that can be "picked up" tomorrow after a good night's rest)

Take herbal preparations such as chamomile tea, 1 teaspoon in boiling water (**Note:** Query for allergies; chamomile is in the Composite family that includes chrysanthemums, black-eyed susans, and ragweed); or valerian, hops, or kava kava

*Healing Journey tapes may be ordered from Source Casettes at 1-800-52-TAPES.

Provider-Assisted Care

Provider-assisted care refers to those health-care practices that require a therapist or a specific practice modality. A few common categories of care include chiropractic, homeopathy, naturopathy, altered states of consciousness (ASOC), bodywork, and energywork. There are many others, including numerous nutritional categories. Chiropractic was founded in the late 1800s and is concerned with spinal bio-mechanical balance. Most clients have treatment for neuromusculoskeletal problems (e.g., back pain, neck pain, headaches) and chiropractic has been found useful for acute low back pain (Shekelle, Adams, Chassin et al, 1992).

Homeopathy was brought to the United States in the early 1800s. This treatment is based on the "law of similars," the principle that "any substance that can cause symptoms when given to healthy people can help to heal those who are experiencing similar symptoms" (Cummings and Ullman, 1997). In other words, homeopathy treatment aims to "let likes be cured with likes." Homeopathic remedies are highly diluted by a process called potentization. Homeopathy is not to be confused with herbal therapy, although herbs may be used in a homeopathic way. Homeopathy is used for many signs and symptoms although emphasis is on the whole person. Respiratory, allergic, dermatologic, digestive, neurologic, musculoskeletal, women's and men's health problems, first-aid, emotional, and sleep problems may be treated homeopathically (Cummings and Ullman, 1997). A meta-analysis of 185 homeopathic trials (Linde, Clausius, and Ramirez et al, 1997), with 89 studies meeting study criteria, found that the combined odds ratio was 2.45 in support of homeopathy, although more systematic research is needed. Spencer and Jacobs (1999) reviewed these findings in their text on CAM.

Naturopathy was brought to the United States in the late 1800s. These therapies include nutrition, botanicals, fasting, homeopathy, medications, biofeedback, acupuncture, hydrotherapy, physical therapy, exercise, counseling, and lifestyle modification. Naturopathy is licensed in several states; some practitioners have limited prescriptive privileges. Some states allow practitioners to aid in natural childbirth.

Altered states of consciousness (ASOC) refers to therapies that work with a level of consciousness other than that used in the workaday mode. Box 17-4 gives examples of ASOC in which health-care providers may become trained or for which they may refer clients or provide reading materials, tapes, or other information. As an example, self-management training (SMT) refers to interventions and integrative functions of the brain that help manage the body. People who know SMT strategies including biofeedback (only one part of SMT) may be able to reduce their need for pharmaceutics. Nakagawa-Kogan (1994) believes that the principles of SMT apply to all chronic conditions, including chronic pain, headaches, temporomandibular joint syndrome, hypertension, chronic arthritis, depression, anxiety reactions, insomnia, and somatic complaints. The SMT program begins by "defining the behaviors, cognition, emotional responses, and physical signs that are to be the targets for self-regulation . . . anger management, anxiety management, and depression management are the basic skills of SMT" (Nakagawa-Kogan, 1994, p 81). Biofeedback uses instruments to feed back psychophysiological information and, as part of SMT, allows clients to become "consciously aware of the interface between bodily status, environmental events, and internal cognitive information" (Nakagawa-Kogan, 1994, p 81).

Hypnosis "relates to an induced, sleeplike state involving motivation, relaxation, concentration and application" (Halo Shames, 1996, p 38). With hypnosis, the inductee, (person being hypnotized) has a

---

Box 17-4

Examples of Altered States of Consciousness

Biofeedback
Hypnosis
Meditation
Relaxation
Dreams
Imagery/Visualization
Prayer
Self-management training

focus or some "work" to do. Several schools of thought exist on hypnosis. One of the most popular is Ericksonian hypnosis. Hypnosis is used in psychotherapy, dentistry, surgery, pediatrics, obstetrics and gynecology, oncology, and in outpatient medical areas such as for procedures, pain management, and smoking cessation programs (Temes, 1999).

Likewise, imagery, visualization, and relaxation have a broad range of uses in the health-care setting. Prayer and meditation may also be suggested for patients receptive to these practices.

Massage, often called bodywork, generally refers to therapies that have direct contact with the body. Energywork refers to a provider working with the subtle energies of the body. There are therapies that combine both energywork and bodywork. Box 17-5 lists forms of bodywork and energywork. Massage is becoming more popular as a treatment for musculoskeletal problems, headache,

and stress relief. The energy therapies include healing touch, therapeutic touch (TT), and reiki. These practices originated in the ancient practice of laying-on-of-hands. Delores Krieger brought TT into nursing through her work at New York University. TT can promote relaxation, reduce pain, accelerate the healing process, and alleviate psychosomatic illness (Krieger, 1993). Healing touch provides TT and other hands-on processes and may work with the chakras. Reiki also has hands-on placement in specific areas. All these therapies include working with energy or energy fields, but have differing philosophies.

Traditional Health Care Practices

Ayurveda, traditional Chinese medicine, Tibetan medicine, shamanism, and curanderismo are considered traditional health-care practices in many parts of the world. For example, ayurveda is the nat-

---

Box 17-5

Bodywork and Energywork

Acupressure	Movement integration
Alexander	Myofascial release
Amma	Myotherapy
Aromatherapy	Neuromuscular
Aston patterning	Polarity
Ayurveda	Prenatal massage
Bindegewebmassage	Reflexology
Bonnie Pruden myotherapy	Reiki
Bowen	Rolfing
Chair/seated massage	Rosen method
Deep tissue	Rubenfeld synergy
Esalen	Russian medical massage
Feldenkrais	Shiatsu
Functional integration	Sports massage
Healing touch	St. John method
Hellerwork	Structural integration
Infant massage	Swedish massage
Jin shin do	Therapeutic touch
Jin shin jyutsu	Trager work
Lomi lomi	Tui na
Lymphatic drainage	Watsu
"M" technique	Zero balancing
Mariel	

ural healing system of India and is the subject of one of the oldest known written histories of health care. Ayurveda encompasses science, religion, and philosophy. It is based on the concept of five elements (ether [space], air, fire, water, and earth) made manifest in the body as the tridosha or biological humors: vata (movement, ether and air), pitta (energy, metabolism, fire and water); kapha (strength, resistance, earth and water) (Lad, 1985). Treatments include pancha karma, therapies that are "cleansing to the body, mind, and emotions" (Lad, 1985, p 70). These processes include vomiting, purgatives, medicated enemas, nasal medication, and purification of the blood. Dietary measures, yoga, breathing and meditation, massage, medicinals, gems, astrology, and colors and other lifestyle modification also are part of treatment. (Lad, 1985).

Traditional Chinese medicine also works with five elements: earth, water, metal, wood, and fire. These elements correspond to organs, colors, seasons, and many other characteristics. For example, the organs that correspond to wood are liver and gallbladder; the color, green; the season, spring; the direction, east; the taste, sour; the sense organ, eyes (Connelly, 1975). Treatments may include herbs, diet, acupuncture, tui na (massage), qi gong (meditation), Tai Chi (movement), astrology, feng shui (harmony of energy in the environment), and other lifestyle modifications. The importance of balance and movement of chi or vital energy through the meridians is stressed. Acupuncturists work with the meridians to help the flow of chi. Recently, the National Institutes of Health concluded that:

> There is "clear evidence" for acupuncture's efficacy for treating postoperative and chemotherapy nausea and vomiting, the nausea of pregnancy, and postoperative dental pain. The panel also concluded that, for a number of pain conditions, acupuncture may be an effective adjunctive therapy. These conditions include, but are not limited to addiction, stroke rehabilitation, headache, menstrual cramps, epicondylitis (tennis elbow), fibromyalgia, low-back pain, carpal tunnel syndrome, and asthma (Villaire, 1998, p 21).

Diagnosis in both ayurveda and traditional Chinese medicine includes assessing tongue and pulse as well as determining specific patterns of the individual. In ayurveda, for example, the vata, pita, kapha constitutions each have different aspects such as body frame, type of emotional temperament, sleep patterns, and numerous other characteristics. In traditional Chinese medicine, there also are qualifiers for conditions including: exterior or interior (relating to the depth of disease); cold and heat (relating to the nature of the disease); deficiency and excess (relating to the "opposing forces in the struggle"); and yin and yang (relating to the category of disease) (Beijing, Shanghai, Nanjing Colleges of Traditional Chinese Medicine and the Acupuncture Institute, 1980). This is an extremely brief introduction to health care practices that span thousands of years, and does not begin to explain the complexity of these two prominent systems and philosophies. In addition, Tibetan medicine, curanderismo, and Native American practices tell wise healing stories. Health-care providers need to be aware of these practices because more clients are using traditional medicine and because these ancient healing modalities have something important to teach us.

Combination of Self-Care and Provider-Assisted Care

Realistically speaking, many clients probably use a combination of self-care and provider-assisted care (with both conventional and/or NAC therapies) for a disorder. Texts are now providing synopses of care for conditions (Eliopoulos, 1999; Snyder and Lindquist, 1998; Spencer and Jacobs, 1999). Thus the following examples are given to pique the reader's interest. Health-care providers will need further investigation into the numerous alternatives available in order to discern the quality and applicability of the therapies and to decide which NAC treatment may be appropriate for which clients.

An example of a combination of self-care and provider-assisted care are the various NAC treatments for depression. Ernst, Rand, and Stevinson (1998) did database searches for NAC treatments for depression. Their research on these NAC practices concluded that rigorous data is "extremely limited" (p 1026), however, there are numerous therapies that have been tried. The areas with the most evidence for beneficial effects are "exercise, herbal therapy (with *Hypericum perforatum*) and, to a lesser extent, acupuncture and relaxation therapies" (p 1026). Their cited research included case series and uncontrolled and controlled studies, some in English and some in other languages. In addition, a recent small study by Allen, Schnyer and Hitt (1998) suggested that acupuncture significantly improved depressive symptoms in women when compared to a placebo-like nonspecifc acupuncture treatment.

Several herbals have been used for depression. However, St. John's wort (*Hypericum perforatum*) has probably received the most study. Linde, Ramirez, Mulrow et al (1996) completed a meta-analysis of randomized clinical trials using St. John's wort for mild to moderate depression and found significant improvement over placebo, and similar efficacy to standard antidepressants. Other herbs commonly used for depression—but without the base of research—include lemon balm, ginseng, basil, wood betony, wild oats (Ernst, Rand, and Stevinson, 1998), as well as kola, lady's slipper, lavender, lime blossom, rosemary, skullcap, valerian, and vervain (Hoffman, 1996).

Other therapies that have been used for depression include aromatherapy, dance and movement therapy, homeopathy, hypnotherapy, massage therapy, music therapy, relaxation therapy (Ernst, Rand, and Stevinson, 1998), and, of course psychotherapy and counseling. Obviously, numerous treatments other than SSRIs exist for depression. Such treatments may help empower clients and decrease the need for dependency on a drug.

A second example is that of fibromyalgia, a process of unknown etiology. Along with education, drugs, and exercise, NAC therapies that have been used include counseling, acupuncture, biofeedback, tender point injections, ultrasound, heat, massage, and music vibration (Chesky, Russell, Lopez et al, 1997; Hellmann, 1998; Freundlich and Leventhal, 1993; Sunshine, Field, Quintino et al, 1996). Both massage and transcutaneous electrical stimulation (TENS) were found to be beneficial in a small study of 30 fibromyalgia patients (Sunshine, Field, Quintino et al, 1996). Support groups, stress reduction, cognitive restructuring, trigger point therapy are also suggested (Maurizio and Rogers, 1997).

In conclusion, there are numerous NAC therapies available for the health-care provider to inte-grate into current conventional practice. Most are less invasive and provide comfort. Supplements and herbal therapies are substances, however and need to be used with the same precautions as over-the-counter and prescription drugs. Health-care providers need to be open to NAC therapies because large numbers of clients are using NAC treatments. However, health-care providers need to assess the quality and appropriateness of the therapies. Health-care providers need a NAC-provider referral base and may wish to become educated as a provider in a NAC therapy. With this broader knowledge base, more options will be available for holistic client care.

References

Allen J, Schnyer R, Hitt S: The efficacy of acupuncture in the treatment of major depression in women, *Psycholog Science* 9(5):397-401, 1998.

Astin J: Why patients use alternative medicine, *JAMA* 279(19):1548-1553, 1998.

Beijing College of Traditional Chinese Medicine (CTCM), Shanghai CTCM, Nanjing CTCM, and The Acupuncture Institute of the Academy of TCM: *Essentials of Chinese acupuncture*, Beijing, 1980, Foreign Languages Press.

Chesky K, Russell IJ, Lopez Y et al: Fibromyalgia tender point pain: a double-blind, placebo-controlled study of music vibration using the Music Vibration Table™, *Jnl Musculoskeletal Pain* 5(3):33-52, 1997.

Connelly D: *Traditional acupuncture: the law of the five elements.* Columbia, Md., 1975, The Centre for Traditional Acupuncture.

Cummings S, Ullman D: *Everybody's guide to homeopathic medicines,* New York, 1997, Tarcher Putnam.

Dossey B, Keegan L, Guzzetta C et al: *Holistic nursing: a handbook for practice,* Gaithersburg, Md, 1995, Aspen.

Eisenberg D, Davis R, Ettner S et al: Trends in alternative medicine use in the U.S., 1990-1997, *JAMA* 280(18):1569-1575, 1998.

Eisenberg D, Kessler R, Foster C et al: Unconventional medicine in the U.S., *NEJM* 328(4):246-252, 1993.

Eliopoulos C: *Integrating conventional and alternative therapies,* St Louis, 1999, Mosby.

Engebretson J, Wardell D: A contemporary view of alternative healing modalities, *Nurse Pract* 18(9):51-55, 1993.

Ernst E, Rand J, Stevinson C: Complementary therapies for depression, *Arch Gen Psychiatry* 55:1026-1032, 1998.

Freundlich B, Leventhal L: The fibromyalgia syndrome. In Schumacher HR, editor: *Primer on the rheumatic diseases,* ed 10, Atlanta, 1993, Arthritis Foundation.

Garfinkel M, Singhal A, Katz W et al: Yoga-based intervention for carpal tunnel syndrome, *JAMA* 280(18):1601-1603, 1998.

Halo Shames K: *Creative imagery in nursing,* Boston, 1996, Delmar.

Hellmann D: Arthritis and musculoskeletal disorders. In Tierney L, McPhee S, Papadakis M, editors: *Current medical diagnosis and treatment,* Stamford, Conn., 1998, Appleton and Lange.

Hoffman D: *The complete illustrated holistic herbal,* Rockport, Mass., 1996, Element.

Huebscher R: Overdrugging and undertreatment in primary health care, *Nursing Outlook* 45(4):161-166, 1997.

Hufford D: Whose culture, whose body, whose healing? *Alternative therapies in health and medicine* 1(5):94-95, 1995.

Kolcaba, KY: A taxonomic structure for the concept comfort, *Image* 23:237-240, 1991.

Krieger D: *Accepting your power to heal,* Santa Fe, N.M., 1993, Bear and Co.

Lad V: *Ayurveda: the science of self-healing,* Wilmot, Wis., 1985, Lotus.

Lazarou J, Pomeranz B, Corey P: Incidence of adverse drug reactions in hospitalized patients, *JAMA* 279(15):1200-1217, 1998.

Linde K, Clausius N, Ramirez G et al: Are the clinical effects of homeopathy placebo effects? A meta-analysis of placebo-controlled trials, *Lancet* 350(9081):834-843, 1997.

Linde K, Ramirez G, Mulrow CD et al: St. John's Wort for depression: an overview and meta-analysis of randomized clinical trials, *BMJ* 313:253-258, 1996.

Maurizio SJ, Rogers JL: Recognizing and treating fibromyalgia, *Nurs Pract* 22(12):18-31, 1997.

Micozzi M: *Fundamentals of complementary and alternative medicine,* New York City, 1996, Churchill Livingstone.

Nakagawa-Kogan H: Self-management training: potential for primary care, *NP Forum* 5(2):77-84, 1994.

Shekelle PG, Adams AH, Chassin MR et al: Spinal manipulation for low back pain, *Ann Intern Med* 117(7):590-598, 1992.

Snyder M, Lindquist R: *Complementary and alternative therapies in nursing,* New York City, 1998, Springer.

Spencer J, Jacobs J: *Complementary/alternative medicine,* St Louis, 1999, Mosby.

Sunshine W, Field T, Quintino O et al: Fibromyalgia benefits from massage therapy and transcutaneous electrical stimulation, *J Clin Rheumatol* 2(1):18-22, 1996.

Temes M: *Medical hypnosis: an introduction and clinical guide,* New York City, 1999, Churchill Livingstone.

Villaire M: NIH Consensus Conference confirms acupuncture's efficacy, *Alt Therapies* 4(1):21-22, 1998.

Suggested Readings by Topic

General

Beal M: Women's use of complementary and alternative therapies in reproductive health care, *Jnl Nurse Midwifery* 43(3):224-234, 1998.

Dreher H: Immune power personality, *Noetic Sciences Review* 39:13-16, 36-40, 1996.

Dreher H: *The immune power personality: seven traits you can develop to stay healthy,* New York, 1996, Plume.

Eisenberg D: Advising patients who seek alternative medical therapies, *Annals of Int Med* 127(1):61-69, 1997.

Haskell W, Luskin F, Marvasti F: Complementary/alternative therapies in general medicine: cardiovascular disease. In Spencer J, Jacobs J: *Complementary/alternative medicine,* St Louis, 1999, Mosby.

Howell S: Natural/alternative health care practices used by women with chronic pain: findings from a grounded theory research study, *NP Forum* 5(2):98-105, 1994.

Luskin FM, DiNucci EM, Newell KA et al: Complementary/alternative therapies in select populations: elderly persons. In Spencer J, Jacobs J: *Complementary/alternative medicine,* St Louis, 1999, Mosby.

Journals

Alternative Therapies in Health and Medicine: November 1998 issues of *Arch Intern Med, Arch Gen Psychiatry,* and *JAMA;* December 1998 issue *NP Forum*

Holistic Nursing

Alternative and Complementary Therapies

Websites

Center for Complementary and Alternative Medicine UC Davis (asthma and allergies): http://www-camra.ucdavis.edu/

U.S. National Institutes of Health Center for Complementary and Alternative Medicine: http://nccam.nih.gov/nccam/

Columbia University Medical Center (CCAM, Aging, and Women's Health Research Center): http://cpmcnet.columbia.edu/dept/rosenthal

Ask Dr. Weil: http:// www.hotwired.com/drweil/

Healthworld Online: http:// www.healthy.net

Acupuncture and Oriental Medicine

Keuler H: Nurse to acupuncturist: a personal transition, *NP Forum* 9(4):202-208, 1998.

Liu G, Jia Y, Zhan L et al: Electroacupuncture of senile and presenile depressive state, *J Tradit Chin Med* 12:91-94, 1992.

Luo H, Jia Y, Feng X et al: Advances in clinical research on common mental disorders with computer controlled electroacupuncture treatment. In Tang L, Tang S, editors: *Neurochemistry in clinical applications,* New York, 1995, Plenum.

Lou H, Jia Y, Wu X et al: Electro-acupuncture in the treatment of depressive psychosis, *Int J Clin Acupunct* 1:7-13, 1990.

Marwick C: Acceptance of some acupuncture applications, *JAMA* 278(Dec 3):1725-1727, 1997.

National Certification Commission for Acupuncture and Oriental Medicine, phone (202) 232-1404.

Ortega, N: Acupressure: an alternative approach to mental health counseling through bodymind awareness, *NP Forum* 5(2):72-76, 1994.

Plawecki H, Plawecki J: Acupuncture: the same difference, *Jnl Gerontolocial Nsg* 24(7):45-46, 1998.

Shaller K: Tai Chi Chih: an exercise option for older adults, *Jnl of Gerontological Nsg* 22(10):12-17, 1996.

Shaller K: Tai Chi/movement therapy. In Snyder M, Lindquist R: *Complementary and alternative therapies in nursing,* New York City, 1998, Springer.

Tao DJ: Research on the reduction of anxiety and depression with acupuncture, *Am J Acupunct* 21:327-329, 1993.

Yang X: Clinical observations on needling extrachannel points in treating mental depression, *J Tradit Chin Med* 14:14-18, 1994.

Altered States of Consciousness (ASOC)

Achterberg J: *Imagery in healing,* Boston, 1985, Shambhala.

Davis M, Eshelman E, McKay M: *The relaxation and stress reduction workbook,* Oakland, Calif., 1995, New Harbinger.

Gimbel MA: Yoga, meditation, and imagery: clinical applications, *NP Forum* 9(4):243-255, 1998.

Hrezo R: Hypnosis: an alternative in pain management for nurse practitioners, *NP Forum* 9(4):217-226, 1998.

Kornfield J: *The inner art of meditation* (videotape), Boulder, Colo., 1996, Sounds True.

Maguire B: The effects of imagery on attitudes and moods in multiple sclerosis patients, *Alt Therapies* 2(5):75-79, 1996.

Mandle CL, Jacobs SC, Arcari PM et al: The efficacy of relaxation response. Interventions with adult patients: a review of the literature. In *Essential readings in holistic nursing,* Gaithersburg, Md., 1998, Aspen.

National Institutes of Health: Technology Assessment Panel on integration of behavioral and relaxation approaches into the treatment of chronic pain and insomnia, *JAMA* 276(4):313-318, 1996.

Zahourek R: *Relaxation and imagery,* Philadelphia, 1988, WB Saunders.

Educational Programs

AHNA: Nurses Certificate Program in Imagery, PO Box 8177, Foster City, CA 94404; email, NCPII@aol.com

Ayurveda

Chopra D: *Perfect health,* New York, 1990, Harmony.

Chopra D: *Ageless body, timeless mind,* 1998, Three Rivers Press.

Frawley D: *Ayurvedic healing,* Salt Lake City, 1989, Passage.

Lad V: *Ayurveda: the science of self-healing,* Santa Fe, N.M., 1984, Lotus.

Chiropractic

Bove G, Nilsson N: Spinal Manipulation in the treatment of episodic tension-type headache, *JAMA* 280:1576-1579, 1998.

Cherkin D, Deyo R, Battie M et al: A comparison of PT, chiropractic manipulation, and provision of an educational booklet for the treatment of patients with low back pain, *NEJM* 339:1021-1029, 1998.

Federation of Chiropractic Licensing Boards, 901 54th Ave Ste 101, Greeley, CO 80634; phone (970) 356-3500; or access the website at: www.fclb.org/fclb

Herbs

Blumenthal M, editor: *American Botanical Council: the complete German Commission E monographs: therapeutic guide to herbal medicines,* Austin, Texas, 1998, Integrative Communications.

Borins M: The dangers of using herbs, *PGM* 104(1):91-99, 1998.

Fetrow C, Avila J: *Complementary and alternative medicines,* Springhouse, Penn., 1999, Springhouse.

Glisson J, Crawford R, Street S: Review, critique, and guidelines for the use of herbs and homeopathy, *NP* 24(4):44-69, 1999.

McIntyre A: *Woman's herbal,* New York, 1994, Holt.

Murray M, Pizzorno J: *Encyclopedia of natural medicine,* Rocklin, Calif., 1998, Prima Publishing.

Murray M: *Encyclopedia of nutritional supplements,* Rocklin, Calif., 1996, Prima Publishing.

Murray M: *The healing power of herbs,* Rocklin, Calif., 1995, Prima Publishing.

Natural Products Quality Assurance Alliance, *Quality and safety standards* (1995), 16770 NE 79th St. Ste 205, Redmond, WA 98052; phone (206) 861-8408.

Tierra M: *Planetary herbology,* Twin Lakes, Wis., 1992, Lotus.

Weil A: *Eight weeks to optimum health,* 1998, Fawcett.

Weil A: *Spontaneous healing,* 1996, Ballentine.

Weil A: *Natural health, natural medicine,* 1998, Houghton Mifflin.

Wong A, Smith M, Boon H: Herbal remedies in psychiatric practice, *Arch Gen Psychiatry* 55:1033-1044, 1998.

Herb Journals

HerbalGram (Journal of the American Botanical Council and Herb Research Foundation

The Quarterly Review of Natural Medicine (Publication of Natural Products Research Consultants) Seattle, WA; access the website at: www.nprc.com

CD ROM

Blake S: *Alternative remedies,* St Louis, 1999, Mosby.

Facts and Comparisons: *Review of natural products,* CD-Rom, 2000, Lippincott, Williams & Wilkins.

Organizations

American Botanical Council, PO Box 201660, Austin, TX 78720; phone (512) 331-8868; access the website at: www.herbalgram.org

American Herbal Products Association, PO Box 2410, Austin, TX 78768; phone (512) 320-8555.

American Herbalist Guild, PO Box 74655, Arvada, CO 80006; phone (303) 423-8800; access the website at: www.healthy.net/herbalists

Herb Research Foundation, 1007 Pearl St. Ste 200, Boulder, CO 80302; phone (303) 449-2265; access the website at: www.herbs.org

Thorne Research (monographs on vitamins and selected botanicals); access the website at www.thorne.com

Homeopathy

American Institute of Homeopathy; access the website at http://www.healthy.net/pan/pa/aih/about_AIH.htm

Council for Homeopathic Certification; access the website at http://www.homeopathy-council.com/

Editorial Board and ISAM: System of homeopathy, *Alternative Medicine* 1(2):104, 1986.

Huebscher R: Homeopathy part II, *NP Forum* 11(4), December 2000 (in press).

Huebscher R: Homeopathy: let likes be vcured by likes, *NP Forum* 11(3), 2000.

Migodow J: An introduction to homeopathic medicine and the utilization of bioenergies for healing, *Alternative Medicine* 1(2):163-168, 1986.

The National Center for Homeopathy; access the websites at: http://www.homeopathic.org/

The North American Society of Homeopaths; access the website at http://skl.home.mindspring.com/NASH_Page.html

Massage

Beck M: *Milady's theory and practice of therapeutic massage,* Albany, N.Y., 1994, Delmar. Access the website at info@delmar.com

Berneau-Eigen M: Rolfing: a somatic approach to the integration of human structures, *NP Forum* 9(4):235-242, 1998.

Byers D: *Better health with foot reflexology,* St Petersburg, Fla., 1991, Ingham.

Carter M, Weber T: *Body reflexology,* West Nyack, N.Y., 1994, Parker.

Complete review guide for national and state certification examinations in therapeutic massage and bodywork, Oviedo, Fla., 1997, Oviedo Physical Medicine and Rehab Inc.

Cox C: *Maternity massage,* Scottsdale, Ariz., 1994, Stress Less Publishing

DePaoli C: *The healing touch of massage,* New York, 1995, Sterling.

De Domenico G, Wood E: *Beard's massage,* Philadelphia, 1997, WB Saunders.

Fritz S: *Mosby's fundamentals of therapeutic massage,* St Louis, 1995, Mosby.

Greene E: Massage. In Jacobs J: *The encyclopedia of alternative medicine,* Boston, 1996, Journey.

Huebscher R: An overview of massage. Part I: history, types of massage, credentialing and licensure, *NP Forum* 9(4):197-199, 1998.

Huebscher R: An overview of massage. Part II. *NP Forum* 10(1):1-2, 1999.

Juhan D: *Job's body: a handbook for bodywork,* Barrytown, N.Y., 1987, The Talman Co.

Kunz K, Kunz B: *Hand and foot reflexology: a self-help guide,* New York, 1984, Prentice Hall.

Lawrence D: *Massage techniques,* New York, 1986, Putnam.

Long C: Reflexology. In Jacobs J: *The encyclopedia of alternative medicine,* Boston, 1996, Journey.

Maxwell-Hudson C: *Aromatherapy massage,* New York, 1994, Dorling Kindersley.

Meek SS: Effect of slow stroke back massage on relaxation in hospice clients, *Image* 25(1):17-21, 1993.

Oleson T, Flocco W: Randomized controlled study of premenstrual symptoms treated with ear, hand, and foot reflexology, *Obst and Gyn* 82(6):906-911, 1993.

Roberts B: Soft tissue manipulation: neuromuscular and muscle energy techniques, *Jnl of Neuroscience Nsg* 29(2):123-127, 1997.

Russell J: Bodywork: the art of touch, *NP Forum* 5(2):85-90, 1994.

Snyder M, Cheng W: Massage. In Snyder M, Lindquist R: *Complementary and alternative therapies in nursing,* New York City, 1998, Springer.

Snyder M, Egan EC, Burns KR: Efficacy of hand massage in decreasing agitation behaviors associated with care activities in persons with dementia, *Geriatric Nursing* 16(2):60-63, 1995.

Tappan F: *Healing massage techniques,* Norwalk, Conn., 1988, Appleton and Lange.

Music Therapy

Aldridge D: Alzheimer's disease: rhythm, timing and music as therapy, *Biomed Pharmacother* 48:275, 1994.

Campbell D: *The Mozart effect: tapping the power of music to heal the body, strengthen the mind and unlock the creative spirit,* New York, 1997, Avon.

Chlan L: Music therapy. In Snyder M, Lindquist R: *Complementary and alternative therapies in nursing,* New York City, 1998, Springer.

Clark M, Lipe A, Bilbrey M: Use of music to decrease aggressive behavior in people with dementia, *Jnl of Gerontological Nsg* 24(7):10-17, 1998.

Cook J: Music as an intervention in the oncology setting, *Cancer Nursing* 9(1):23-28, 1986.

Fitzgerald-Clouthier ML: The use of music therapy to decrease wandering: an alternative to restraints, *Music Ther Persp* 11(1):32, 1993.

Guzzetta C: Effects of relaxation and music therapy on patients in a coronary care unit with presumptive acute myocardial infarction, *Heart and Lung* 18(6):609-616, 1989.

Schroeder-Sheker T: Music for the dying: a personal account of the new field of music thanatology, *Jnl of Holistic Nsg* 12(1):83-99, 1994.

Native American Medicine

Cohen K: Native American medicine, *AT* 4(6):45-57, 1998.

Naturopathy

American Association of Naturopathic Physicians, 601 Valley St. Ste 105, Seattle, WA 98109; phone (206) 328-8510; access the website at: www.infinite.org/Naturopathic.Physician

McCabe P: Natural therapies in Australia: a nurse naturopath's view, *NP Forum* 5(2):114-117, 1994.

Murray M: *Heart disease and high blood pressure: how you can benefit from diet, vitamins, minerals, herbs, exercise, and other natural methods,* Rocklin, Calif., 1997, Prima.

Also by Murray M: *Natural alternatives to Prozac; Natural alternatives for weight loss, The healing power of foods;*

Chronic fatigue syndrome; Menopause; Male sexual vitality; Arthritis; Diabetes and hypoglycemia; Stress, anxiety and insomnia; Premenstrual syndrome; Stomach ailments and digestive disturbances, Chronic candidiasis.

Nutrition

Behm R: A special recipe to banish constipation, *Geriatric Nursing,* 6(4):216-217, 1985.

Belluzzi A, Brignola C, Campieri M et al: Effects of an enteric-coated fish-oil preparation on relapses in Crohn's disease, *NEJM* 334:1557-1560, 1996.

Bland J: Diet and prostate problems, *Alt Therapies Jnl* 1(4):75-76, 1995.

Gann P, Hennekens C, Sacks F et al: Prospective study of plasma fatty acids and risk of prostate cancer, *J Natl Cancer Inst* 86:281-286, 1994.

Packer L, Fuchs J, editors: *Vitamin C in health and disease,* New York, 1997, Marcel Dekker.

Kushi M: *Standard macrobiotic diet,* Becket, Mass., 1996, One Peaceful World Press.

Marchand L, Hankin J, Kolonel L et al: Vegetable and fruit consumption in relation to prostate cancer risk in Hawaii: a reevaluation of the effect of dietary beta-carotene, *Am J Epidemol* 133:215-219, 1991.

Mossad S, Macknin M, Medendorp S et al: Zinc gluconate lozenges for treating the common cold: a randomized double-blind placebo controlled study, *Ann Intern Med* 125(2):81-88, 1996.

Ross R, Henderson B: Do diet and androgens alter prostate cancer risk via a common etiologic pathway? *J Natl Cancer Inst* 86:252-254, 1994.

Stampfer MJ, Malinow MR, Willett WC et al: A prospective study of plasma homocystine and risk or MI in US physicians, *JAMA* 268(7):877-881, 1992.

Stephens N, Parsons S, Schofield P et al: Randomized controlled trial of vitamin E in patients with coronary disease: Cambridge Heart Antioxidant Study, *Lancet* 347:781-786, 1996.

Tinkle M: Folic acid and food fortification: implications for the primary care practitioner, *NP* 22(3):105-106, 109, 112-114, 1997.

Virtamo J, Huttunen J: Vitamin A and prostatic cancer, *Ann Med* 24:143-144, 1992.

Wilt T, Ishani A, Stark G et al: Saw palmetto extracts for treatment of benign prostatic hypertrophy, *JAMA* 280(18):1604-1609, 1998.

Wood R, Vogen B: Feeding the anorectic client: comfort foods and happy hour, *Geriatric Nursing* 19(4):192-194, 1998.

Pets

Dossey L: The healing power of pets: a look at animal-assisted therapy, *Alt Therapies Jnl* 3(4):8-16, 1997.

Huebscher R: Pets and animal assisted therapy, *NP Forum* 11(1):1-4, 2000.

James K: Animals in health care. In Snyder M, Lindquist R: *Complementary and alternative therapies in nursing,* New York City, 1998, Springer.

Spirituality/Prayer

Amenta M, Bohet N, editors: Spiritual concerns. In *Nursing care of the terminally ill,* Boston, 1986, Little, Brown.

Bearon L, Koening H: Religious cognition and use of prayer in health and illness, *The Gerontologist* 30:249-253, 1990.

Brown-Hunter M, Price LK: The Good Neighbor Project: volunteerism and the elderly African-American patient with cancer, *Geriatric Nursing* 19(3):139-141, 1998.

Burkhardt M, Nagei-Jacobson M: Dealing with spiritual concerns of clients in the community, *Jnl of Community Health Nsg* 2:191-198, 1985.

Byrd R: Positive therapeutic effects of intercessory prayer in a coronary care unit population, *Alt Therapies* 3(6):87-90, 1997.

Carson V: *Spiritual dimensions of nursing practice,* Philadelphia, 1989, WB Saunders.

Dossey L: The return of prayer, *Alt Therapies* 3(6):10-17, 113-120, 1997.

Gustafson M: Prayer. In Snyder M, Lindquist R: *Complementary and alternative therapies in nursing,* New York City, 1998, Springer.

Moore N: Spirituality in medicine, *Alternative Therapies* 2(6):24-26, 103-105, 1996.

Shuler P, Gelberg L, Brown M: The effects of spiritual/religious practices on psychological well-being among inner city homeless women, *NP Forum* 5(2):106-113, 1994.

Soderstrom K, Martinson I: Patient's spiritual coping strategies: a study of nurse and patient perspectives, *Oncology Nursing Forum* 14:41-46, 1987.

Therapeutic Touch/Healing Touch/Reiki

Brennan B: *Light emerging: the journey of personal healing,* New York, 1993, Bantam.

Gordon A, Merenstein J, D'Amico F et al: The effects of therapeutic touch on patients with osteoarthritis of the knee, *J Fam Pract* 47(4):271-277, 1998.

Healing Touch Certificate Program (educational program endorsed by AHNA), Colorado Center for Healing Touch, 12477 W Cedar Drive, Ste 206, Lakewood, CO 80228; e-mail: ccheal@aol.com

Huebscher R: Therapeutic touch; what is the controversy and why does controversy exist? NP Forum 10(2): 43-43, 1999.

Krieger D: *The therapeutic touch,* Englewood Cliffs, NJ, 1979, Prentice-Hall.

Krieger D: *Living the therapeutic touch,* New York, 1987, Dodd, Mead and Co.

Macrae J: *Therapeutic touch: a practical guide,* New York, 1987, Knopf.

Mulloney S, Wells-Federman C: Therapeutic touch: a healing modality, *J Cardiovasc Nurs* 10(3):27-49, 1996.

Peck S: The effectiveness of therapeutic touch for decreasing pain in elders with degenerative arthritis, *Jnl of Holistic Nsg* 15(2):176-198, 1997.

Starn J: The path to becoming an energy healer, *NP Forum* 9(4):209-216, 1998.

Stein D: *Essential reiki,* Freedom, Calif., 1995, Crossing Press.

Wytias C: Therapeutic touch in primary care, *NP Forum* 5(2):91-97, 1994.

CHAPTER 18

Common Herbal Therapies

Kathryn Niemeyer

The use of herbs as medicine is an ancient healing tradition. The present practice of herbal medicine in the United States, part of the ancient healing tradition, is an assimilation of herbal knowledge and practice from Native American, Eastern, European, and American folk traditions (Hall, 1998 Hoffman, 1996).

At present, 80% of the world's population relies on herbs as a primary source of healing (Winslow and Kroll, 1998; Gesler, 1992). In European and Asian countries, herbs play an important role in health care as demonstrated by the education of physicians and pharmacists in the clinical use of herbal medicines. The United States, on the other hand, has tended to reject herbal medicine in favor of pharmaceuticals. Although pharmaceuticals have relevant applications, many healers and health-care practitioners have come to the realization that herbal medicines also have relevant applications. The thoughtful concept is to integrate Eastern and Western herbal medicine with modern clinical practice. To this end, herbalists and pharmacists, allopathic, osteopathic, and naturopathic physicians and nurses, botanists, traditional healers, and other health-care providers are entering into a discourse to expand the collective knowledge about the medicinal use of plants.

While health-care practitioners are attempting to sort out and identify the role medicinal herbs play in health and health care, Americans are forging ahead into the world of herbs. People are choosing, purchasing, and using herbal medicines in unprecedented numbers (Brevoort, 1998). Herbs have hit the mainstream of America for both the consumer and the practitioner.

How can herbal medicine be integrated into today's clinical practice? Is there wisdom in herbal medicine that calls out for change in conventional clinical practice? These are questions which health-care practitioners must seek to answer. This chapter provides introductory information regarding herbal medicine.

THE CLINICAL USE OF HERBS

Herbs are used clinically as alternatives to pharmaceuticals; as complements to pharmaceuticals; and in situations where no appropriate pharmaceutical exists. An herbal regimen may be used as an alternative when the pharmaceutical regimen produces ill effects or undesirable side effects. Herbal medicines may constitute a least harmful, least invasive approach to clinical intervention (Duke, 1997). Herbs are also useful as alternatives to pharmaceuticals when the herb or herbs produce the desired effect at a lower financial cost to the patient. An example of an herb used as an alternative to a pharmaceutical would be the use of the saw palmetto in place of finasteride for benign prostatic hypertrophy. Saw palmetto has been shown to be a comparable herbal alternative to the drug finasteride (McCaleb, 1997; Miller, 1998).

Herbal medicines are also used along with or complementary to pharmaceuticals. An example of complementary herbal use would be when an herb is used to minimize the side effects of a drug. The herb ginger can be used with chemotherapeutic agents to relieve the side effect of nausea. Herbs are also complementary when used along with drugs as a measure to decrease dose requirements. The use of the herb hawthorne for heart disease may result in reduced doses of digitalis or ACE inhibitors (Mashour, Lin, and Frishman, 1998). Herbs also support organs when harsh drugs threaten them. For instance, milk thistle is used to heal and support the liver when hepatotoxic drugs such as anticonvulsants are taken (Brown, 1996). The use of herbs along with pharmaceuticals constitutes an appropriate use of herbs. There are many known and yet to be discovered complementary uses of herbal therapies (Weiss, 1998).

The practice of medicine today is often disease centered. Trauma and disease drive health-care delivery, and medicine is often very good with trauma and disease. However, conventional health care is less successful with protection of health and prevention of disease. Herbs are useful in situations when there are no pharmaceuticals to do the job. An example is the use of echinacea to prevent and treat common colds and influenza. The taking of herbs for prevention, support, and strengthening in times of vulnerability are worthy uses of these medications. Herbs can be exceptional assets when used to support wellness.

Herbs are being used to promote wellness in acute illness and chronic diseases along with and in place of pharmaceuticals. The integration of herbal medicine into health care is rapidly becoming a reality. People are participating in time-honored rituals of self-care and family guardianship by calling on the healing power of plants.

THE SITUATION TODAY

We are in a unique situation with today's use of herbs. The consumer is expected to negotiate his or her own health care. While herbal products seem to be available everywhere, the supporting resources are not. There may not be a medicinal herbalist, phytotherapist, or naturopathic physician to assist with the therapeutic or clinical use of the herbs. The consumer may have no alternative but to rely on the advice of a store clerk or glean what information is available from magazine articles on herbs. In fact, people are self-diagnosing and self-prescribing their own herbal remedies. The problem with this arises when herbs are combined with different herbs and pharmaceuticals without professional guidance. Herb-herb and herb-drug combinations are being used regardless of tradition or research into their clinical application. Herbs have a broad range of effects as well as interactions with other herbs and pharmaceuticals.

It is of the utmost importance for the health-care practitioner to be educated in the alternative and complementary use of herbs as medicine. In 1998, 69% of the population in the United States engaged in some alternative health care practice, and 38.5% to 70% of these persons did not inform their primary care physician of the use of alternative health care (Alles, 1998). As the consumer negotiates his or her own health care with herbal use, the practitioner has an opportunity to enter that negotiation and counsel regarding the validity of common herbs and how they interact with pharmaceuticals. It is important for the practitioner to know what resources are available and when it is time to collaborate with a medical herbalist to ensure consumer safety and provide the best care and advocacy for the client.

HOW HERBS DIFFER FROM PHARMACEUTICALS

It is common to see people approach the use of herbs in the same way they approach the use of pharmaceuticals. In the United States, we have been acculturated to believe in and desire for ourselves the quick cure, the "magic bullet" effect from a pill (Gordon, 1996). Even though it is true that 25% of pharmaceuticals have derived from the plant world, herbal medicines are very different than pharmaceuticals (Brown, 1996; Murray, 1995; Weiss, 1998). The clinical use of herbs has traditionally been within a context of holism. The whole person is treated using a number of personal interventions to promote healing. Herbal therapies often accompany education in nutritional changes; exercise and lifestyle modification; hydrotherapy recommendations; bodywork such as massage and spinal manipulation; and energy work. Each of these interventions encourages personal responsibility, self-healing, and balance in life. If a depressed person goes from the office to the automobile to the couch, eating a diet high in processed and refined foods, then only taking St. John's wort will do little for the problem. To maximize the efficacy of medicinal herbs is to use them in a context that supports healing of the whole person; otherwise, the effect will be likened to a drug outcome where there is symptom relief and the pill becomes the cure.

Herbs work differently than drugs do. They often work at multiple sites in the body, and the actions as well as plant constituents often have a synergistic effect (Brown, 1996). That is why it is difficult to substitute a drug for an herb. For example, licorice can soothe the gut, provide phytoestrogen support, and has antidepressant action (Duke, 1997). There are no clear and direct herbal analogs to drugs. Herbal medicines often work to support the body and have a balancing effect (Brown, 1996). Most pharmaceutical drugs act to overwhelm physiology and suppress the body's own functioning and thus provide symptom relief (Gordon, 1996). Herbal medicines nurture and encourage the body's own abilities to heal and resist.

Many phytotherapists consider herbs to be as safe as salad. Botanist James Duke claims that herbs are "about 10,000 times less lethal than pharmaceuticals" (Duke, 1998). Overall, they are gentle on the body and have few or no side effects. (See the section on Precautions with Herbal Medicines.) Many herbs work slowly, taking time to elicit the desired outcome. St. John's wort may take 8 to 10 weeks of therapy prior to manifestation of effects. Vitex takes approximately 30 days, yet echinacea peaks in a couple of hours (Brown, 1996). Herbal medicines remind us that healing takes time, a concept that may be alien in our fast-paced, stress-filled lives. It is much more convenient to take a pharmaceutical, though in the long run it may be more detrimental to personal well being, the well being of our culture, and the well being of the earth. Engaging with plants as medicine takes a genuine commitment and interest in one's own ability to heal and care for oneself. This is a commitment that takes time, a drive to be educated, and perhaps a willingness to make changes in one's life.

RESEARCH ON HERBAL MEDICINES

Herbs have been the subject of scientific inquiry and methodology for approximately 25 years. Recently, randomized controlled clinical trials have become the research method in vogue for evaluating herbs. Prior to this, herbs have been used as medicine for centuries and no one questioned if they worked. For scientists, it is experimental research and empirical data that is convincing.

Up to this point, most of the research on herbal medicines has been conducted and evaluated in Germany. Many European countries have been using herbs in health care for years. Germany established a group of professionals called the German

Commission E that evaluated research, made recommendations for use of herbal medicines, and published research-based guidelines for the use of herbs as medicines. German Commission E Monographs have recently (1998) been translated into English through the work of Mark Blumenthal and other members of the American Botanical Council (Blumenthal et al, 1998). The German Commission E has disbanded, but research in Europe continues to be evaluated by the European Scientific Cooperative on Phytotherapy.

Research in the United States has not been as forthcoming. Companies are hesitant to invest large sums of money in research when they are unable to have a patented product. Recently, as the demand for herbal medicine increases, so has the research. The research on herbs has resulted in the identification of active ingredients or constituents and effective dose ranges based on the percentages of that active ingredient. The increase in the availability and use of herbs in pill and capsule form is also largely the result of research into the identification and isolation of active ingredients.

When evaluating research on medicinal herbs, as with any research, it is important to look at it critically. Not only are the methodology and conclusions important, but also the variables specific to the herb. These may include the form of delivery, the dose tested, and the processing or preparation of the herb. Most herbal research revolves around outcomes within specific populations and are related to the amount of an active ingredient.

The use of many common herbs is supported by research. Ginkgo biloba is an example of a well-researched herbal medicine. There may well be over 400 published studies on this herb (Brown, 1996). It is also one of the most commonly prescribed herbs in Germany. Echinacea is also well researched, whereas dong quai is an example of an herb that has been researched but still lacks a consensus as to what specifically this herb does. Saw palmetto is an herb that has been studied in clinical trials with the drug finasteride, producing well-defined patient outcomes (Braeckman et al, 1997; Wilt et al, 1998).

In the United States, medicinal herb research is in its infant stages. However, in other parts of the world, the use of herbal medicines is a strong clinical tradition supported by significant scientific research.

MEDICINAL HERB DOSING

Traditionally, herbalists have used the whole plant as medicine. This comes from a belief in the synergy of plant constituents, or the ability of the different plant ingredients to work together to achieve the effects. For example, one constituent of the plant may assist by moving another constituent along in the body to where it needs to go to be effective. Another plant constituent may have a secondary effect that complements the primary action, while yet another ingredient may nullify any negative effects on the body. The whole plant has therapeutic value (Hoffman, 1990).

Traditionally, the dosing of medicinal herbs has been very individualized, rather than a one-size-fits-all intervention. Dosing starts low and is titrated up or increased in increments until the desired effect is achieved. This dosing-to-effect method is and has been used because of the overall safety of herbal medicines. Using this approach, the herbalist's recipes and prescriptions—like the human response to medicine—are individual. This approach optimizes the fit of the herbs to the person.

Research has yielded data that has promoted more uniform dosing and standardization in herb delivery. Standardization refers to a guaranteed percentage of active ingredient present in the herb delivered (Duke, 1997). The higher the percent of active ingredient present, the lower the required dose. Pill and capsule delivery forms have become the method of delivery for standardized herbs with specific dosage recommendations. This has promoted safe use of herbs for both the professional and for the consumer who lacks a broad knowledge base or philosophy of herbalism. It has made herbal medicines more available and more approachable to the user. However, it may not be a better or more effective approach than traditional dosing. In fact, such an approach to herbalism may inhibit the healing power of the herb.

PRECAUTIONS WITH HERBAL MEDICINES

As herbal use increases, so do the concerns regarding its safety. This is especially true when herbs are combined with pharmaceuticals or when they are used with conditions or diseases such as diabetes.

When used appropriately, herbs are safe and have few ill effects. But ill effects of herbs may be seen when herbs are used in situations when they are contraindicated. This is true if large medicinal doses are used for prolonged periods of time (i.e., greater than 1 month). Ill effects may also be seen when a more potent form of the herb (e.g., a tincture) is substituted for a weaker form of delivery of the same herb (e.g., a tea or tablet) that produces no ill effect (Brinker, 1998; Brooks, 1995; Ernst, 1998; Tyler, 1996). Tea, coffee, alcohol, and certain foods, such as grapefruit, have a greater effect on drug activity than most common herbal therapies if used within a normal range of consumption (McQuade-Crawford, 1998). As research continues to explore and illuminate the relationship of herbs to pharmaceuticals, as well as the range of herbal activity, health-care practitioners ought to take steps to ensure consumer/client safety based on known information.

It is beyond the scope of this chapter to discuss all known interactions and precautions. Additional information is included in the section on common herbs.

There are several herbs that have a high potential for ill effects when used at any dosage. These are not commonly used herbs and should only be used under the direction and supervision of a professional. Potentially dangerous herbs include ephedra, foxglove, gelsemium root, life root, lily of the valley, lobelia, mayapple root, mistletoe, poke root, rauwolfia root, and tansy. These herbs are strong cardiotonics, abortifacients, cathartics, or paralytics and should only be used with considerable caution (McGuffin, Hobbs, Upton et al, 1997).

Any herb has the potential to elicit an allergic response. A few herbs are more likely to result in allergies, such as arnica, chamomile, echinacea, and feverfew (Brinker, 1998). Specific herbs that can result in photosensitivity include celery, fennel, parsley, St. John's wort, and yarrow (Brinker, 1998). Herbs that can irritate the gastrointestinal system include cinnamon, cayenne, cola, garlic, goldenseal, and horse chestnut (Brinker, 1998). Celery and coffee are examples of herbs that can irritate the genitourinary system (Brinker, 1998). Herbs that can result in increased diuresis can also facilitate the loss of potassium. Those herbs include coffee, cola, horsetail, mate leaves, and guarana.

Licorice results in decreased potassium due to its aldosterone-like effect with high doses (Brinker, 1998).

The issue of herbal use during pregnancy and lactation is a complex one. The conservative approach is to avoid all herbs while pregnant or lactating. In all instances of pregnancy and lactation, herbal medicines should be considered only with the direction and supervision of a trained professional herbalist or a licensed naturopathic physician. Herbs can be classified as emmenagogues, abortifacients, uterine stimulants, oxytocics, uterina relaxants, hormones, teratogens, fetotoxins, or mutagens. Even though larger doses are usually needed for the ill effects of uterine stimulation, it is advisable to approach the use of herbs during pregnancy and lactation with knowledge and extreme caution (Brinker, 1998). Box 18-1 lists common herbs to avoid with pregnancy and lactation.

Another area of concern is the use of herbs with anticoagulants or in conditions where increased risk of bleeding exists. The problem herbs are from plants that contain coumarin or coumarin-like substances, and herbs that inhibit platelet aggregation (Box 18-2). Unlike broad-spectrum antibiotics and some sulfa-based antibiotics, herbal antiseptics do not alter gut flora that produce vitamin K (Brinker, 1998), so herbal antiseptics do not result in bleeding complications. It is also worth noting that natural sources of salicylates, such as willow bark, lack the platelet inhibition effect that the pharmaceutical salicylates have (Brinker, 1998). Any substance that decreases coagulation or vitamin K has the potential to enhance the effect of warfarin products. To elicit increases in bleeding tendencies, herbs need to be used in larger doses and for prolonged periods of time (Brinker, 1998).

Herbal sedatives, such as those listed in Box 18-3, should be used with extreme caution if used concurrently with alcohol, sedating pharmaceuticals, or other sedating herbs. Sedatives used with other sedatives will compound the sedating effects and so put the person at risk for poor judgment and injury. The sedating effect of herbs is highly individual, so an exaggerated effect may result with lower doses of the herbs (Almeida and Grimsley, 1996).

Herbal use with diabetes is, at present, a yet-to-be-researched area of medicinal herbalism. Many herbs have the effect of increasing or decreasing blood sugar (Box 18-4). Herbal preparations are not recommended for concurrent use with insulin (McQuade-Crawford, 1998; Brinker, 1998).

CHOOSING MEDICINAL HERBS

Herbs are considered dietary supplements. The Food and Drug Administration (FDA), in accordance with the Dietary Supplement Health and Education Act (DSHEA) of 1994, regulates labeling claims. Herb companies may make claims related to the effect of the herb on the body's structure and function. They are prohibited from making claims relating to the treatment or prevention of a disease. For example, it can be said that echinacea enhances the immune system; but the manufacturer of the product is unable to claim the herb can prevent and treat the common cold and flu. This is subject to change in the next few years (Chamberlain, 1998). At this time, there is no regulation of product content. So a potential problem is content reliability. The consumer depends on the integrity of the herbal product manufacturer.

Variability is another problem present in herbal products. Variation in the product may arise not only from processing or delivery form but also from soil conditions, time of harvesting, and the part of the plant used (Murray, 1995). For example, the therapeutic effect may differ depending on if the herb was prepared from the plant's root or its flower. The effect may also differ depending on the age of the plant used. Dried herbs are always more potent than fresh herbs. So a tea made from fresh peppermint will need more herb than if dried peppermint is used.

The natural enemies of herbal potency are air, light, and age. Exposure to any of these elements will decrease the therapeutic potency and longevity of the herbal product, as well as dried or fresh herbs. The longer the herbal product sits on the shelf, the less effective it will be. This is also a factor when purchasing herbs. The consumer should know how old the herb was before it reached the shelf. When choosing herbs, it is of value to be aware of the potential variability and to purchase from a company that follows sound herbal preparation protocols.

When choosing herbs, it may be helpful to

Box 18-1

Herbs to Avoid While Pregnant or Lactating*

Alfalfa
Alder
Aloe vera
Anise
Arnica
Ashwaqandha
Balsam pear
Barberry
Basil
Black cohosh
Blessed thistle
Blue cohosh
Calamus
Calendula
Cascara sagrada
Cayenne
Chamomile
Chjevril
Cottsfoot
Comfrey
Dong quai
Eleuthero
Ephedra (ma huang)
Evening primrose
Fennel
Fenugreek
Feverfew
Flaxseed
Garlic
Ginger
Ginseng
Goldenseal
Gotu kola
Guggul
Hops
Hyssop
Juniper berries
Kava kava

Licorice
Lobelia
Marjoram
May apple
Milk thistle
Motherwort
Mountain mint
Mugwort
Pennyroyal
Peppermint
Periwinkle
Poke root
Rosemary
Rue
Sage
Senna
Southern wood
St. John's wort
Stinging nettle
Tansy
Thuga
Thyme
Uva ursi
Vitex
Wormwood
Yarrow
Yohimbe

Adapted from: Brinker F: *Herb contraindications and drug interactions*, ed 2, Sandy, Ore., 1998, Eclectic Medical Publications; Duke JA: *The green pharmacy*, Emmaus, Penn., 1997, Rodale Press; McQuade-Crawford, A: *Herbal remedies for women*, Rocklin, Calif., 1997, Prima Publishing; and Romm A: Gentle expectations, *Herbs for Health* March/April 1997:25-27.

*This list is not all-inclusive. It does include the common, more familiar herbs. Consult with a herbalist or licensed naturopathic physician before using any herb or plant during pregnancy or lactation.

learn about the company processing the herbs. A telephone number or address for the company should be on the product. Look for companies that have quality assurance programs in place. This is usually indicated by the presence of a batch number on the package. Quality assurance provides for

product consistency and internal testing and evaluation for product control. It is helpful to know which companies are involved in research and education. Product or herbal information packages or flyers are usually provided by the company and often are placed near the product in stores. Some herb

Box 18-2

Herbal Precautions

The following herbs should be used with caution if taken concurrently with coagulopathies, thrombocytopenia, warfarin, or with agents that decrease platelet aggregation:

Coumarin-Containing Plants

Horse chestnut
Sweet clover
Sweet vernal-grass
Vanilla leaf

Platelet Aggregation Inhibitor Plants

Bromelain
Cayenne
Chinese skullcap
Feverfew
Flax
Ginger
Ginkgo
Onion
Turmeric Root

Adapted from: Brinker F: *Herb contraindications and drug interactions,* ed 2, Sandy, Ore., 1998, Eclectic Medical Publications.

Box 18-3

Precautions With Herbal Sedatives

Precaution: Herbal sedatives such as calendula, catnip, chamomile, hops, kava kava, lemon balm, motherwort, skullcap, St. John's wort, and valerian may enhance the sedating action of any drug acting on the central nervous system. This includes antiemetics, analgesics, narcotic, beta-blockers, antidepressants, antianxiety drugs, and neuroleptics.

Box 18-4

Herbal Precautions for Diabetics

Herbs that alter blood sugar include the following:

Hypoglycemic Herbs

Agrimony
Aloe
Barley
Bilberry
Bugleweed
Burdock
Cumin
Damiana
Dandelion
Fenugreek
Garlic
Ginseng
Horse chestnut
Juniper
Jute
Mulberry
Psyllium
Prickly Pear
Reishi mushroom
Siberian ginseng

Hyperglycemic Herbs

Cocoa
Coffee
Cola
Guarana
Ma huang (ephedra)
Mate
Rosemary
Tea leaves

Compiled from McQuade-Crawford A: *Phytomedicines: Their expanding role. Conference proceedings: medicines from earth, interactions between herbal remedies and constituents and conventional drugs,* North Carolina, 1998, Gaia Herbal Research Institute; and Brinker F: *Herb contraindications and drug interactions,* ed 2, Sandy, Ore., 1998, Eclectic Medical Publications.

companies also provide educational conferences for persons in the herbal industry. Most of these utilize the expertise of leaders in the field of herbalism. The consumer may also be interested in choosing organic herbs that are either grown by the herb company or purchased from local growers. Many herb companies are very open and receptive to inquiries about their products.

NON-HERBAL DIETARY SUPPLEMENTS

Vitamins, minerals, amino acids, enzymes, synthetic hormones, and other products considered "natural" are also classified as dietary supplements. They are often misunderstood and considered to be herbal. DHEA, or dehydro-epiandro-sterone, is not an herb. It is produced from the herb wild yam, as are some birth control pills and some progesterone creams. The conversion of the herb to the hormone occurs in the lab, where many pharmaceuticals are produced. DHEA is a hormone precursor for estrogen and/or testosterone found in the body. Melatonin is also not an herb but a hormone. It is naturally produced by the pineal gland and helps regulate sleep-wake cycles. The synthetic form is useful in some situations to help with insomnia. Glucosamine sulfate is a glycosylated amino acid, not an herb. It is normally found in the body and is involved in the formation of tendons, bones and ligaments. The synthetic form is often used to improve the structure of articular cartilage, so it may be useful with arthritis. Co-enzyme Q_{10} is often mistaken for an herb and is commonly recommended along with herbs. It is found naturally in the cells throughout the body. It facilitates energy generation in the mitochondria through contributing to ATP synthesis. It is a non-herbal dietary supplement taken to increase cardiovascular strength and immunity (Balch and Balch, 1997).

Herbal medicines, even though classified as dietary supplements, are quite different from other dietary supplements. Herbal medicines are phytotherapies or plant therapies. They are natural; but not all supplements considered natural are herbal.

WILDCRAFTING AND ORGANIC

Wildcrafting refers to the obtaining of herbs from the wild. Though it may sound like a nice way to obtain herbs, it has some major disadvantages. The first relates to the depletion of natural resources. Herbs can be wildcrafted to extinction. A second disadvantage is the danger in foraging for herbs unless one is an expert at herb and plant identification. This poses the risk of making a false plant or herb identification.

Herbs that are termed organic are herbs grown and preserved without the use of irradiation, herbicides, pesticides, or chemical fertilizers (Brown, 1996). Some states, such as California and Oregon, have put in place legal standards to define what constitutes "organic" products.

SPIRITUAL CONNECTION

Healing with herbs is often approached from a spiritual perspective. Herbs can provide a connection to the natural healing capabilities of the earth. Once again, we are reminded of the sustenance we are given from the earth and the opportunity to honor that gift. Herbs may represent a portion of our existence that is not completely harnessed or controlled. The herbs, as part of nature, become greater than we are and indeed have a sacred power to heal. Herbal medicines are ancient. They connect us to our history and past rituals of healing. We are drawn to healing herbs, as if our cells have memory. We become part of an unbroken tradition:

> . . . I believe rational explanations are destroying medicine today, as well as our society at large. To be healed, we need to believe in the possibility of healing and in a greater world, and in higher powers, than our own (Mehl-Medrona, 1977).

ISSUES RELATING TO HERBAL USE IN CLINICAL PRACTICE

Herbal medicine is an area of growing concern. Herbs can be potent medicines with both the power to heal and the power to harm. If used appropriately, herbs are safe, have few side effects, and few dangers associated with them. Herbs should be used with knowledge and treated with respect. The fact that herbs are widely available and can be used and purchased without prescription points up the need for consumer education in order to prevent harm.

A challenge for the practitioner is what to do about herbal medicines. Should the practitioner provide this information? Should practitioners encourage herbal use, discourage herbal use, or prescribe herbs at all? What assessment data is necessary to ensure client safety when herbs are used as medicine? What level of knowledge or qualification does the practitioner need before entering into the area of herbalism? Or should referral be the precedent? Can herbs be used to complement the usual, accepted practice of health care? These questions touch upon just a few areas that come to the attention of the practitioner faced with medicinal herbal use. As research continues and as the knowledge of herbal medicines expands, our awareness and discussions need to continue to define the boundaries of health care practice.

HERB CATEGORIES

Herbs are categorized according to the actions of the herb and what kinds of problems they traditionally treat. The following categories are not all-inclusive but have been included because they may be new or unfamiliar (Hoffman, 1988).

Adaptogens Herbs that strengthen and support normal physiology, these increase resistance to stress and toxins as well as build endurance. They also act to balance neuro-endocrine-immune functioning (examples: ginseng, astragalus)

Alteratives Herbs that act to gradually restore wellness, these enhance change slowly (examples: black cohosh, garlic, burdock)

Anti-oxidants Herbs that block or interfere with the cellular damage from the oxidation of free radicals (examples: ginkgo biloba, green tea ([Box 18-5])

Astringents Herbs that tighten or tone and are anti-hemorrhagic (examples: witch hazel, horse chestnut)

Bitters Herbs that taste bitter and stimulate digestion via the secretion and flow of digestive enzymes (examples: dandelion leaf and root, yarrow)

Box 18-5

Antioxidants

Free radicals are molecules that are unstable because they have an extra electron. Free radicals cause cellular damage and are the result of tobacco use, pollution, pesticides, alcohol, ultraviolet radiation, excessive exercise, and infection.

Antioxidants, substances found in foods and herbs, provide protection against the damage caused by free radicals. The following are some major sources of antioxidants:

- Grape seed extract—has approximately 50 times more antioxidant properties than vitamins C and E
- Green tea
- Ginkgo biloba
- Astragalus
- Evening primrose
- Coenzyme Q_{10}
- Vitamins C and E

Carminatives Herbs that soothe and tone the digestive system. They also stimulate gas expulsion from gastric-intestinal tract (examples: parsley, peppermint, valerian)

Cholagogues Herbs that stimulate the production and flow of bile. They also improve fat digestion (examples: milk thistle, goldenseal root, artichoke)

Demulcents Herbs that protect and soothe irritated or inflamed mucous membranes (examples: fenugreek, marshmallow root)

Emmenagogues Herbs that promote menstrual flow. They also tone and support the female reproductive system (examples: dong quai, black cohosh, motherwort)

Immune-modulators Herbs that promote strong immune function (example: echinacea)

Nervines Herbs that are restorative to the nervous system. These can be relaxants, stimulants, or tonics (examples: St. John's wort, gotu-kola, skullcap)

Rubefacients   Herbs that increase local circulation with topical application (examples: mustard, horseradish)

Tonics   Herbs that strengthen and stimulate functioning of specific systems (examples: hawthorne, goldenseal, nettles)

Vulneraries   Herbs that promote wound healing (examples: comfrey, yarrow, plantain)

MAJOR PLANT CONSTITUENTS (Hoffman, 1988)

Acids   Antiseptic, anti-pyrogenic properties; may also have laxative or diuretic properties

Alkaloids   Narcotic-like, analgesic, nervine stimulant, and antiseptic properties. Can be poisonous in long term use or extracted (pure) form. Diverse group of constituents

Anthraquinones   Laxative properties

Bitters   Several chemical constituents that are bitter to the taste. Digestive stimulant, antifungal, and antibiotic properties

Carbohydrates   Simple sugars and starches. Gums, mucilages, and antiseptics

Cardioactive Glycosides   Cardiotonics. Act to support the mechanical and electrical activity of the heart

Coumarins   Lactone glycosides. Weak anticoagulation properties. Metabolite di-coumetarol has potent anticoagulation action

Flavones and Flavonoid   Immune tonics, antiinflammatory, antioxidant

Glycosides   Antispasmodic, diuretic, and capillary strengthening properties

Phenols and Phenolic Glycosides   Analgesic, diuretic, antiinflammatory, antipyretic, and disinfectant properties

Saponins   Steroidal, antiinflammatory, diuretic, digestive stimulant, and expectorant properties

Tannins   Astringent, antibacterial, antiviral, antior pro-inflammatory, and antioxidant properties

Volatile Oils   Aromatic herbs, essential oils. Antiseptic, antispasmodic, stimulant properties. External use only

MEDICINAL HERBS AND CHILDREN

Children are unique and have their own set of special needs (Bove, 1996). It is beyond the scope of this chapter to explore the roles that herbs can play in the health and wellness of children. The following guidelines will have to suffice:

- When used appropriately, herbs are safe to use with children and do indeed have many uses with acute and chronic childhood disorders. Care should be taken with the use and dosing of herbs in infants and children.
- Palatability is often a problem with the delivery of herbs to children. The taste and smell of herbs can be improved with the use of honey, lemonade, or peppermint in the herbal preparation.
- There are several herbal preparations for children. These extractions are usually water- or glycerin-based rather than alcohol-based.
- Herbal medicines should not substitute for good nutrition. Diets with adequate proteins, essential fatty acids, and vitamins, and low in refined ·sugar and processed foods should come first.
- Dosage adjustments should be made in relation to the recommended adult dose:
  - Infant – ⅛ of the adult dose
  - Child (2-6 years) – ¼ of the adult dose
  - Child (6-10 years) – ⅓ of the adult dose
  - Child (10-14 years) – ½ of the adult dose
- Or specific dose adjustments can be made using Young's formula:

$$\text{Age}/\text{Age} + 12 = \text{portion of adult dose}$$

or Dilling's formula:

Age /20 = portion of adult dose

- Many people choose herbal medicines for their children due to the relatively low toxicity of common herbs and the reduced risk of side effects.
- Whenever using herbs with infants or children, collaboration with a professional herbalist or licensed naturopathic physician is recommended.

DELIVERY OF HERBS (Hoffman, 1988)

Tea
- An infusion of fresh or dried herb in boiling water
  1. If using dried herb, place 1 tsp in 1 C; or 1 oz per 3 C
  2. If using fresh herb, place 3 tsp in 1 C
  3. Steep 10 to 20 minutes
- Can be taken orally or topically, hot or cold
- Always store in refrigerator for longer periods of time
- For use with leaves, flowers, stems, berries, or seeds
- Examples: chamomile, peppermint

Decoction
- An infusion where plant parts are boiled in water rather than steeped like a tea
- Useful with woody, hard parts of the plant such as roots, bark, or rhizomes
  1. Use same proportion of herb to water as for a tea
  2. Boil and simmer for 10 to 15 minutes
  3. Strain while still hot
- Example: willow bark

Tincture
- Concentrated preparation
- Alcohol-based extract; may also be water-, vinegar-, or glycerin-based.
- Usually in a 1:5 proportion, but may be extracted in a 1:1 proportion (Alcohol is an excellent solvent for most plant ingredients.)
- Can be taken orally or topically

- More potent delivery form than tea or tablet/capsule
- For oral delivery, dilute in small amount of warm water or juice
- Example: echinacea

Capsules or Pills
- Delivery for dried or powdered herbs; palatable delivery form
- May not be as absorbent as other forms
- Become less potent with storage
- Capsule or pills should be standardized – processed to guarantee a known percentage of active ingredients in relation to dry weight. The higher the percentage of active ingredient, the lower the required dose

Topical Preparations
- Liniment – oil, vinegar or alcohol preparation of herbs used for massage of muscles
- Salve – oil and beeswax semi-solid preparations
- Poultice – paste made from fresh herb macerated with water or vinegar and/or flour
- Compress – a poultice applied with heat to surface of body

References

Alles W: National CAM survey results. Presented at Conference on Complementary and Alternative Medicine: Scientific evidence and steps toward integration in Palo Alto, Calif. In Udani, J: Resident forum, *JAMA* 280(18):1620, 1998.

Almeida JC, Grimsley EW: Coma from the health food store: interaction between kava and alprazolam, *Ann Intern Med* 125(11):940, 1996.

Balch JF, Balch PA: *Prescription for nutritional healing,* ed 2, New York City, 1997, Avery Publishing Group.

Blumenthal M et al, editors: *The complete German Commission E monographs, therapeutic guide to herbal medicines,* Boston, 1998, American Botanical Council.

Bove M: *An encyclopedia of natural healing for children and infants,* New Canaan, Conn., 1996, Keats Publishing.

Braeckman J et al: A double blind, placebo-controlled study of the plant extract *Serenoa repens* in the treatment of benign hyperplasia of the prostate, *Eur J Clin Res* (9):247-259, 1997.

Brevoort P: The booming U.S. botanical market, a new overview, *Herbalgram* 44:33-45, 1998.

Brinker F: *Herb contraindications and drug interactions,* ed 2, Sandy, Ore., 1998, Eclectic Medical Publications.

Brooks S, editor: Botanical toxicology, *Protocol J Bot Med* 1(1):147-158, 1995.

Brown DJ: *Herbal prescriptions for better health,* Rocklin, Calif., 1996, Prima Publishing.

Chamberlain L: What the labels won't tell you, *Herbs for health* Nov/Dec.:34-37, 1998.

Duke JA: *The green pharmacy,* Emmaus, Penn., 1997, Rodale Press.

Duke JA: Letters: Herbal medicine, *Time,* Dec. 14, 1998.

Ernst E: Harmless herbs? A review of the recent literature, *Am J Med* 104(2):170-178, 1998.

Gesler WM: Therapeutic landscapes: medical issues in light of the new cultural geography, *Soc Sci Med* 34(7):735-746, 1992.

Gordon JS: *Manifesto for a new medicine,* New York City, 1996, Addison Wesley Publishing Company.

Hall N: *Herbs, hormones and the mind.* Paper presented at Conference on Herbs, Hormones, and the Mind, Grand Rapids, Mich., 1998.

Hoffman D: *The complete illustrated holistic herbal,* London, 1996, Butler & Tanner Ltd.

Hoffman D: *The herbal handbook: a user's guide to medical herbalism,* Rochester, Vt., 1988, Healing Arts Press.

Hoffman D: *The elements of herbalism,* New York City, 1990, Barnes and Noble.

Mashour NH, Lin GI, Frishman WH: Herbal medicine for the treatment of cardiovascular disease, *Arch Intern Med* 158:2225-2233, 1998.

McCaleb R: Phytomedicines outperform synthetics in treating enlarged prostate, *Herbalgram* 40:16, 1997.

McGuffin M, Hobbs C, Upton R et al, editors: *Botanical safety handbook,* New York, NY, 1997, CRC Press.

McQuade-Crawford, A: *Herbal remedies for women,* Rocklin, Calif., 1997, Prima Publishing.

McQuade-Crawford A: *Phytomedicines: Their expanding role. Conference proceedings: medicines from earth, interactions between herbal remedies and constituents and conventional drugs,* North Carolina, 1998, Gaia Herbal Research Institute.

Mehl-Medrona L: *Coyote medicine, lessons from Native American healing,* New York, 1997, Simon and Shuster.

Miller LG: Herbal medicinals, *Arch Intern Med* 158:2200-2211, 1998.

Murray MT: *The healing power of herbs,* ed 2, Rocklin, Calif., 1995, Prima Publishing.

Tyler VE: What pharmacists should know about herbal remedies, *J Am Pharm Assoc* 36(1):29-37, 1996.

Weiss RF: *Herbal medicine,* Beaconsfield, England, 1998, Beaconsfield Publishing Ltd.

Wilt TJ et al: Saw palmetto extracts for treatment of benign prostatic hyperplasia. A systematic review, *JAMA* 280(18): 1604-1609, 1998.

Winslow LC, Kroll DJ: Herbs as medicine, *Arch Intern Med* 158(20):2192-2199, 1998.

Selected Readings

Bove M: *Herbal pediatrics, building and maintaining childhood immunity. Conference proceedings: medicines from the earth, phytomedicines: their expanding role,* North Carolina, 1998, Gaia Herbal Research Institute.

Lowe FC, Ku JC: Phytotherapy in treatment of benign prostatic hyperplasia: a critical revi ew, *Urology* 48:12-20, 1996.

McQuade-Crawford, A: *Understanding phytochemicals.* Conference Proceedings: Medicines from the earth, protocols for botanical healing, North Carolina, 1996, Gaia Herbal Research Institute.

Zink T, Chaffin J: Herbal health products: what family physicians need to know, *Am Fam Physician* 58(5):1133-1140, 1998.

part four

4

APPENDIXES

Common Supportive Herbs

Kathryn Niemeyer

CATEGORIES OF HERBS

Immune System

- Astragalus
- Schisandra
- Echinacea*
- Elderberry/flower*
- Garlic*

Sinuses

- Eyebright
- Bayberry
- Goldenseal
- Calamus
- Stinging nettle*
- Hyssop

Central Nervous System

- Skullcap
- Catnip
- Lemon balm*
- Valerian*
- Kava kava*
- St. Johns wort*
- Ginkgo biloba*
- Gotu kola

Joint and Cartilage Health

- Arnica*

Women's Health

- Black cohosh*
- Vitex*
- Motherwort*
- Dong quai*
- Raspberry leaf
- Evening primrose*
- Licorice*
- Fenugreek*
- Flaxseed*
- Alfalfa
- Soy*

Men's Health

- Saw palmetto*
- Yohimbe

Urinary Tract

- Uva urse*
- Yarrow tea*
- Goldenseal
- Cranberry extract

Cardiovascular Health

- Hawthorn*
- Motherwort*
- Garlic*
- Gugulipid
- Ginkgo biloba*
- Antioxidants

Gastrointestinal Support

- Peppermint*
- Chamomile*

*Herbs approved by German Commission E.

- Ginger*
- Milk thistle*
- Licorice*

Adrenal Support

- Ginseng*
  Siberian
  Korean
  American
  Licorice*

Migraines

- Feverfew
- Capsicum

Pain and Inflammation

- Willow bark*
- Feverfew
- Ginger*
- Capsicum
- Turmeric*

COMMON HERBAL THERAPIES

This section is for reference purposes and represents a synthesis and summary of several expert sources. The authors referenced have successfully evaluated years of research on the clinical use of herbs. The dosing recommendations represent consensus and the recommendations of the referenced experts.

Common Name black cohosh, snakeroot, bugwort, squaw root

Botanical Name   *Cimicifuga racemosa*

Active Ingredients   Triterpenes and flavones

Parts Used   Root

Action   Suppresses luteinizing hormone; binds to estrogen receptors optimizing estrogen levels; uterine tonic; diuretic, astringent, alterative, antispasmodic, vasodilator

*Herbs approved by German Commission E.

Uses   Menopausal symptoms, premenstrual syndrome, dysmenorrhea, infertility

Dosage   Tincture – 2 to 5 mg bid; tablet/capsule – 40 mg per day in 2 divided doses; use for 6 months (no research on long-term use)

Precautions   Do not use with pregnancy or lactation

Side Effects   Large doses can cause headache, nausea, dizziness, or change in heart rate

Additional Information   Reasonable alternative to HRT

Common Name chamomile or German chamomile

Botanical Name   *Matricaria recutita*

Active Ingredients   Volatile oils, flavonoids

Parts Used   Dried flower tops

Action   Mild sedative effects; chamomile soothes and calms; antiinflammatory and antispasmodic or muscle relaxation effects on the gastrointestinal tract; stimulates normal digestion; mild diuretic activity; mild antibacterial effect when used topically on wounds

Uses   Anxiety and/or insomnia; indigestion, cramping with diarrhea due to stress, gastritis, irritable bowel syndrome, or spastic colon (long-term management); gastric ulcers; infant colic; inflammatory skin disorders such as eczema and/or irritation of the gums

Dosage   Tea – 1 to 4 cups per day between meals; tincture – up to 1 tsp *OR* 5 ml tid between meals; tablet/capsule – 2 to 3 gm tid between meals. **Note:** Tea can also be used as a mouthwash, in a poultice, or in a bath.

Precautions   May have allergic reaction if allergic to members of the daisy family (e.g., ragweed, asters, and chrysanthemums)

Side Effects   None known

Herb-Drug Interactions   None known

Common Name   chaste-tree or chasteberry

Botanical Name   Vitex, Agnus-Castus

Active Ingredient   Unknown; whole plant is used

Parts Used   Dried fruit

Action   Acts on pituitary gland to increase luteinizing hormone, resulting in progesterone production during the luteal phase of the menstrual cycle; mildly inhibits follicle stimulating hormone; reduces prolactin levels and decreases excess estrogen; effect is balanced progesterone to estrogen to prolactin ratios

Uses   Premenstrual syndrome, irregular menses or amenorrhea, infertility; peri-menopausal symptoms

Dosage   Tincture – 1 to 5 ml every day 30 minutes before breakfast; tablet/capsule – 1 to 175 mg every day

Precautions   Stop dosing 5 to 7 days during menses; discontinue use following menopause; do not take if pregnant or lactating; use of this herb with hormone replacement therapy is not recommended

Side Effects   Short-term rash with itching; occasional gastric upset

Herb-Drug Interactions   None known

Additional Information   Use continuously until improvement, continue an additional 4 to 6 weeks, then stop; for infertility may need to take 12 to 18 months; effects may not be seen for first 30 days; safe for long-term use for prolactin suppression; vitex does not contain hormones, works in a gentle balancing way; safe for use by women without ovaries

Common Name   dong quai

Botanical Name   Chinese angelica

Active Ingredients   Coumarins, flavonoids, and essential oils

Parts Used   Roots and rhizomes

Action   Phytoestrogen activity; binds to estrogen receptors like natural estrogen; emmenagogue and tones uterus; vasodilation secondary to calcium channel blockage; smooth muscle relaxation; inhibition of IgE antibody production

Use   Dysmenorrhea, amenorrhea, metrorrhagia; premenstrual syndrome, menopausal symptoms; cardiovascular support, allergies

Dosage   Tea – 1 to 4 cups per day; equivalent to 1 to 2 gm dried herb; tincture – ½ to 4 ml up to six times a day

Precautions   Do not use with prescription anticoagulants; avoid with history of bleeding disorders, hypermenorrhea, diarrhea, and pregnancy; avoid if at risk for breast cancer

Side Effects   Rash, photosensitivity of skin seen with large doses

Herb-Drug Interactions   Possible additive bleeding effect if used concurrently with anticoagulants, aspirin, NSAIDs

Common Name   echinacea or purple coneflower

Botanical Names   *Echinacea purpura, E. angustifolia, E. pallida*

Active Ingredients   Polysaccharides

Parts Used   Root of *E. pallida* and *E. angustifolia;* aerial parts of *E. purpura*

Actions   Immune stimulation; increased WBC and interferon production and maturation; facilitation of migration to areas of infection; antibacterial; inhibition of bacterial hyaluronidase secretion so bacteria have less access to cells; antiviral, antipyretic actions and topically antifungal

Uses Prevention and early treatment of colds and flu (echinacea can decrease the incidence of cold and flu symptoms and decrease the severity of symptoms once they appear.); recurrent respiratory and urinary tract infections; chronic yeast infections.; recurrent ear infections; topically to treat cold and canker sores, fungal infections, and wounds

Dosage Tea – 1 to 5 cups per day; tincture – up to 10 ml or 2 tsp tid; tablet/capsule – 300 mg tid; may take as often as every 2 hours for 48 hours if needed for prevention; may take up to 2 weeks continuously; may take low dose up to 8 weeks before stopping

Precautions Should not be taken on a continuous basis for longer than 8 weeks (may have hepatotoxic effects if taken continuously; not to be taken with immunosuppressant drugs such as corticosteroids or cyclosporine; should not be taken with chronic systemic diseases involving the immune system such as autoimmune diseases, lupus, HIV, TB, MS, leukosis; use cautiously with diabetes mellitus; may have allergic reaction if allergic to plants in the daisy family

Side Effects Tincture or lozenge may cause temporary numbness or tingling of the tongue

Herb-Drug Interactions Immunotonic effects of echinacea may counteract the immunosuppression of drugs such as corticosteroids and cyclosporine

Common Name	eleuthera or Siberian ginseng

Botanical Name *Eleutherococcus senticosus, Acanthopanax senticosus*

Active Ingredient Glycosides, specifically eleutherosides B, E, and polysaccharides

Parts Used Root

Action Adaptogen; supports and nurtures the normal functioning of adrenal glands; normalizes the pituitary-hypothalamic-adrenal interaction; inhibits the alarm phase of sympathetic nervous system response, therefore enhances energy levels, reactions to stress and resistance; promotes immune functioning by increasing lymphocytes as well as the number and activity of T cells; supports oxygen usage by muscles during exercise; stimulates RBC production; protects against cellular mutation with exposure to carcinogens; decreases blood sugar levels

Uses To assist in adaptation to stress; mental fatigue and physical exhaustion, exercise endurance, and to increase vitality; cold and flu prevention; chronic fatigue syndrome, HIV, lupus; supportive following chemotherapy, and/or radiation therapy; exposure to chemical toxins; recovery from chronic or long-term illnesses

Dosage Equivalent to 2 to 3 gm per day; tea – 1 to 4 cups per day; tincture – 5 to 20 ml per day in 3 or 4 divided doses; tablet/capsule – 2 to 3 gm per day in 3 or 4 divided doses; take for 6 to 8 weeks followed by a 7-day period without taking the herb, then resume; generally, take for 3 months; may need to repeat later

Precautions Should not be taken with hypertension or a BP greater than 170/90; should not be taken if pregnant or lactating; avoid use if bipolar or psychotic disorders are present

Side Effects Occasional reports of diarrhea; insomnia may occur if taken near bedtime

Herb-Drug Interactions May worsen the effects of caffeine; may falsely elevate digoxin levels; may interact with antipsychotic medications; may augment effects of HRT

Common Name	evening primrose

Botanical Name *Oenothera biennis*

Active Ingredient Gamma-linolenic acid (GLA)

Parts Used Oil of the seed

Action GLA is an essential fatty acid in the useable form for the body. It provides the carrier triglyceride enotherol. GLA is necessary for normal structure and function of cells, regulation of cholesterol levels, skin health, intact myelin sheaths, and prostaglandin production.

Uses   Problems with fatty acid synthesis or abnormal prostaglandin production; premenstrual syndrome (PMS); diabetic neuropathies – delays onset and slows progression; chronic inflammatory conditions, such as eczema – the best outcome is with early treatment; diseases of overactive immune systems or autoimmunity, such as rheumatoid arthritis, multiple sclerosis

Dosage   PMS – 3 to 6 gm per day for 6 months, 14 days before menses; inflammatory conditions – 4 to 8 gm per day for 3 to 4 months; MS – 500 mg per day for 3 weeks during exacerbations; take with meals to increase absorption; take total dosage in divided doses tid to qid

Precautions   Not recommended for those receiving epileptogenic drugs such as phenothiazines; seizure threshold may be lowered

Side Effects   Occasional reports of gastric discomfort, nausea, or headache

Herb-Drug Interactions   Anticonvulsant dosage may need to be adjusted with concurrent use of evening primrose.

Common Name	feverfew

Botanical Name   *Tanacetum parthenium*

Active Ingredients   Sesquiterpene lactones, specifically parthenolide

Parts Used   Leaves and flowering tops

Actions   Inhibition of the release of serotonin from platelets; interference with platelet aggregation; blocks development and action of pro-inflammatory mediators, such as prostaglandins, leukotrienes, and thromboxanes

Uses   Long-term management and prevention of migraine headaches, specifically headaches of the hot-throbbing type accompanied by nausea and/or vomiting and visual disturbances (feverfew decreases the severity, duration, frequency, and associated symptoms of migraine headaches); historically used to treat fevers and inflammation; rheumatoid arthritis

Dosage   Tincture – 1 to 5 ml every day in 2 divided doses; decrease to lowest effective dose if favorable results after 90 days; table/capsule – standardized to at least 2% parthenolide 125 mg per day; may increase to 1 to 2 gm with acute attacks; continuous use is recommended for optimal outcomes; may need to take for several months before effect is seen

Precautions   May have allergic reaction if allergic to plants in daisy family (e.g., chamomile, ragweed, or yarrow); do not use during pregnancy or lactation; do not use with children under 2 years of age; if prescription medication is being used for migraines, consult a health-care practitioner prior to using feverfew

Side Effects   Minor mouth sores or gastric distress may be seen when raw leaves are eaten

Herb-Drug Interactions   Nonsteroidal antiinflammatory drugs (NSAIDs) may reduce the effectiveness of feverfew with concurrent use; feverfew may interfere with the action of selective serotonin reuptake inhibitor antidepressants such as Prozac; inhibits platelet aggregation, so avoid concurrent use with anticoagulants

Additional Information   Feverfew represents a safe herbal alternative to NSAID use for the treatment of headaches, arthritis, and low-grade benign fevers.

Common Name	garlic

Botanical Name   *Allium sativum*

Active Ingredient   Allicin

Parts Used   Bulb

Action   Decreases platelet aggregation and increases fibrinolysis; lowers liver production of cholesterol and triglycerides while increasing high-density lipoproteins; has broad antimicrobial activity – inhibits growth of microbes (antibacterial, antiviral, antifungal, and antiparasitic); may mildly lower blood pressure

Uses   Hypercholesteremia; mild hypertension; colds and flu; chronic localized yeast infection

Dosage   The best source is raw garlic cloves or supplements closely resembling raw garlic, such as powdered garlic preparations; further recommendations are for enteric coated capsules – equivalent dose of 5000 mcg of allicin per day in divided doses or a minimum of 1 fresh garlic clove per day; as an antiviral, oil macerate preparations are effective

Precautions   Blood pressure may decrease 30 minutes following ingestion with a return to baseline in approximately 2 hours

Side Effects   Heartburn, flatulence, gastric irritation

Herb-Drug Interaction   Cautious use with anticoagulants due to action of garlic to decrease platelet aggregation and promote fibrinolysis

Common Name   ginger

Botanical Name   *Zingiber officinale*

Active Ingredient   Volatile oils, specifically gingerols (in fresh ginger) and shogaols (in processed ginger)

Parts Used   Rhizome

Action   Acts on the gastrointestinal (GI) tract; stimulates digestion, improves production and secretion of bile; improves motility and tone of intestinal muscles; antispasmodic; decreases platelet aggregation; mild antiinflammatory action by decreasing leukotriene and prostaglandin production; antioxidant activity; decreases absorption and increases excretion of cholesterol; increases calcium uptake in myocardium (positive inotropic effect)

Uses   Nausea, vomiting from pregnancy (short-term use, small doses only), motion sickness or post-anesthesia; abdominal distension; gastric protection with use of NSAIDs; inflammatory joint disease

Dosage   As needed dosing; motion sickness – start 2 days to 2 hours before travel; tea/tablet/capsule – 2 to 4 gm in 2 or 3 divided doses; for inflammatory joint disease may double this dose; for pregnancy related nausea – 1 gm in divided dose for 1 to 4 days; tincture – 1.5 to 3 ml in 8 oz juice qid as needed; take with food

Precautions   Persons with gallstones should consult a health-care practitioner prior to use; long-term use with pregnancy is not recommended; caution with concurrent use with prescription anticoagulants; do not use with thrombocytopenia

Side Effects   Rarely may cause gastric discomfort if taken on an empty stomach

Herb-Drug Interaction   Additive effect if taken with anticoagulants

Common Name   ginkgo biloba

Botanical Name   *Ginko folium*

Active Ingredients   Bioflavonoids and terpene lactones specifically ginkglides

Parts Used   Leaves

Action   Peripheral vasodilation and normalization of blood flow to brain and central nervous system (CNS); ginkgo has an affinity for the hippocampus and protects cell membranes in areas of ischemia by inhibiting peroxidation; promotes Na-K pump function; antioxidant; improves tone and elasticity of blood vessels; reduces platelet aggregation

Uses   Cerebral vascular insufficiency; recovery from CVA (non-hemorrhagic); memory loss associated with aging; poor peripheral circulation (e.g., Raynaud's disease or intermittent claudication); tinnitus, vertigo; neuropathy; retinopathy; impotence; asthma; multiple sclerosis

Dosage   Tincture – 5 to 10 ml bid to tid; tablet/capsule – standardized to at least 24% ginkgo flavone glycosides and 6% terpene lactones 120 to 240 mg daily in 2 or 3 divided doses; effects should be seen in 2 to 3 weeks; 12 weeks regimen is recommended; up to 6 months of herb dosing for intermittent claudication or vertigo

Precautions   Caution if taken concurrent with prescription anticoagulants; ingestion of ginkgo fruit often results in a severe poison-ivy-like allergic reaction; discontinue use 2 weeks prior to surgery

Side Effects   Initially mild transient headaches – usually stops in 48 hours; occasionally mild gastric distress; toxicity – vomiting, diarrhea, irritability, dermatitis

Herb-Drug Interaction   Additive blood thinning effect if concurrent with anticoagulant aspirin or NSAIDs

---

Common Name   ginseng

Botanical Name   *Panax ginseng* – Asian; *Panax quinquefolius* – American

Active Ingredients   Several; research has placed priority on ginsenosides

Parts Used   Roots

Action   Adaptogen; supports endocrine and adrenal function; enhances pituitary-hypothalamic-adrenal interaction; stimulates the immune system and improves antibody response; the result is improved response to stress, increased resistance, energy, endurance, and vitality; protection against toxins; mental concentration and acuity are improved; muscles utilize oxygen more effectively and the fatty acid transformation to energy is enhanced, thus sparing glycogen stores; overall metabolism is improved through the balancing of insulin to blood sugar; platelet aggregation is decreased; American ginseng has an overall cooling effect, whereas Asian ginseng has a warming effect

Uses   Chronic fatigue, mental and physical debilitation, low endurance; chronic stress and cortico-steroid dependency; recovery from surgery, chemo and radiation therapies; athletic training; menopause; white ginseng refers to the dried or unprocessed root; red ginseng refers to the steamed then dried root (used for its greater antioxidant action)

Dosage   Dose to effect; tea – 1 cup up to tid (equivalent dose to 1 to 2 gm dried root); tincture – 2.5 to 5 ml everyday to tid; tablet/capsule – standardized to 4% to 7% ginsenosides 100 mg every day up to tid; use herb for 2 to 3 weeks then remain off the herb for 1 week then repeat; usual duration is 3 months; may repeat if needed

Precautions   Persons with hypertension or on antihypertensive medications should avoid ginseng; caution if used concurrently with anticoagulants; do not use if pregnant or lactating; caffeine and ginseng may cause overstimulation; avoid if bipolar or psychotic disorders are present

Side Effects   Insomnia, hypertension, anxiety, headache, diarrhea, skin rash

Herb-Drug Interactions   Additive effect if used with anticoagulants, aspirin, or NSAIDs; mild additive effect if used with hormone replacement therapy; may possibly have mild additive effects if used concurrent with corticosteroids; if used with MAO inhibitors may cause insomnia, headache, or tremors

---

Common Name   goldenseal

Botanical Name   *Hydrastis canadensis*

Active Ingredient   Berberis alkaloids, specifically berberine

Parts Used   Root and rhizome

Action   Broad spectrum antibiotic activity through inhibition of microbial adhesion to the host cells; useful against various bacteria, protozoa, and fungi; immune stimulant – increases blood to spleen and stimulates production of macrophages; antipyretic; stimulates bile secretion

Uses Infections of mucus membranes, respiratory, digestive and genitourinary tracts; cholecystitis, cirrhosis

Dosage Tea – 1 to 4 cups per day; equivalent dose of 2 to 4 gm dried herb; tincture – 5 to 15 ml tid; tablet/capsule – standardized to 8% to 12% alkaloid content; equivalent dose of 2 to 4 gm per day in divided doses

Precautions Do not take if pregnant or lactating; higher doses or prolonged periods of dosing (greater than 5 to 7 days) may cause increased liver enzymes or malabsorption of B vitamins; avoid with hypertension; goldenseal is endangered, recommended substitutes are Oregon grape root *(Berberis aquifolium),* barberry *(Berberis vulgaris),* or goldenthread *(Coptis chinensis)*

Side Effects May be liver toxic in high doses

Herb-Drug Interactions May antagonize anticoagulant effect of heparin

Common Name gugulipid

Botanical Name *Commiphora mukul*

Active Ingredient Keytones, specifically Z and E guggulsterone

Parts Used Resin

Action Lowers very low and low-density lipoproteins; elevates high density lipoproteins through stimulation of metabolism in liver; stimulates thyroid function; mildly inhibits platelet aggregation and promotes fibrinolysis; antiinflammatory action

Uses High cholesterol; high triglycerides; rheumatoid arthritis

Dosage Tablet/capsule – standardized to 5% guggulsterone, 500 mg tid

Precautions Cautious use with prescription anticoagulants

Side Effects Seen with crude gum, alcohol, or petroleum extracts—diarrhea, rashes; standardized tablet – nontoxic, no side effects

Herb-Drug Interactions May have mild additive effect with anticoagulants

Additional Information Has history of valued use in Ayurvedic medicine

Common Name hawthorn

Botanical Name *Crataegus laevigata, C. oxycantha, C. monogyna*

Active Ingredients Flavonoids, specifically oligomeric procyanidins and cardiotonic amines

Parts Used Ripe fruit, leaves, and flowers

Action Peripheral vasodilation, increased coronary circulation, decreased systemic vascular resistance. Positive inotropic effect and improved myocardial oxygen utilization; antioxidant

Actions Strengthens capillaries; mild diuretic effects; inhibits release of pro-inflammatory substances; may have beta blocker and ACE inhibitor activity

Uses Early CHF; stable angina pectoris; recovery following an MI; mild hypertension

Dosage Tea – 1 cup tid – equivalent of 4 to 5 gm dried per day; tincture – 2.5 to 5 ml tid; tablet/capsule – standardized to 20% procyanidins; 100 to 900 mg per day in divided doses; average dose 100 to 250 mg tid; effect is slow and steady, should be taken long-term; effectiveness seen after 1 to 2 months of therapy

Precautions May need to adjust doses if used concurrently with beta blockers, ACE inhibitors, or digitalis preparations; high doses are contraindicated for people with chronic atrial fibrillation and for those with hypotension secondary to valve dysfunction

Side Effects None known

Herb-Drug Interactions Potentiation of digitalis effect with concurrent use; potentiation of beta blocker effect with concurrent use; potentiation of ACE inhibitor effect with concurrent use

Common Name   kava kava

Botanical Name   *Piper methysticum*

Active Ingredients   Kavalactones

Parts Used   Rhizome

Actions   Sedative and calming action on central nervous system without loss of mental acuity, concentration ability, and memory; may act as a dopamine antagonist; acts on limbic system in the brain and modifies receptor domains; mild neuromuscular relaxation, anticonvulsant and analgesic activity

Uses   Insomnia; anxiety; skeletal muscle spasm

Dosage   Tincture – 1 to 3 ml tid; tablet/capsule – standardized to 70% kavalactones; anxiety – 50 to 100 mg up to tid; insomnia – 180 to 210 mg hs; dosage greater than 300 gm per week not recommended

Precautions   Do not take if pregnant or lactating; not for young children; do not use concurrently with other sedatives, barbiturates, or antidepressants; avoid use with Parkinson's disease and/or the drug levodopa; fat-soluble, so can accumulate and have delayed effects

Side Effects   Mild gastric discomfort, unstable gait, numb tongue, occasional reports of skin rash or allergic reactions; large dose can cause loss of balance and dry, scaly skin; long-term (greater than 3 months) use can cause the skin to turn yellow — if this occurs, discontinue use

Herb-Drug Interactions   May potentiate CNS sedating drugs, especially benzodiazepines

Additional Information   No risk of tolerance developing; good to use with psychotic disorders; reasonable alternative to benzodiazepines; potential for injury with excessive use

Common Name   licorice

Botanical Name   *Glycyrrhea glabra*

Active Ingredient   Flavonoids, glycyrrhizin, and glycyrrhetinic acid

Parts Used   Root and leaf

Action   Antiinflammatory; binds to glucocorticoid receptors (cortisone-like effect); interferes with pro-inflammatory substances; antiallergenic; aldosterone effect – inhibits breakdown by liver by suppressing 5-beta reductase; increases half-life of cortisol and aldosterone; immunosupportive—antibacterial, antiviral activity; hepato-protective—prevents free radical damage and increases bile secretion; antidepressant—mechanism unknown; gastric protective—deglycyrrhizinated licorice (DGL) stimulates normal gastric defenses that prevent ulcer formation; improves quality of gut lining and supports intestinal cells; estrogenic—antagonizes xenoestrogens and potentiates estrogen in higher doses

Uses   Inflammation, viral infections, Addison's disease or adrenocortical insufficiency, depression, menopause, upper respiratory infections; DGL – gastric/peptic ulcers, irritable bowel syndrome, mouth ulcers; topically – herpes, eczema, psoriasis

Dosage   Tea – 3 cups per day – equivalent to 1 to 2 gm tid; tincture – 2.5 to 5 ml tid; tablet/capsule – 200 to 600 mg glycyrrhizin in 3 divided doses; do not take for more than 4 to 6 weeks; DGL – take in a chewable form 20 minutes before meals 300 to 380 mg up to 1200 mg per dose; may take up to 8 to 16 weeks

Precautions   Do not take with hypertension, kidney or liver insufficiency, or if at risk for hypokalemia; use with caution in diabetes mellitus; the higher the dose and the longer the time (greater than 6 weeks) on licorice, the more aldosterone effect is seen; no aldosterone with DGL

Side Effects   Large doses (5000 mg per day) results in aldosterone-like syndrome: increased blood pressure, increased sodium, hypokalemia, edema—will reverse when herb is discontinued; DGL – no side effects

Herb-Drug Interactions May potentiate corticosteroid treatments; may antagonize antihypertensive medications; antagonizes spirolactone; because of potential for hypokalemia, may potentiate digitalis preparations and hypokalemia from diuretics and thiazides

Additional Information Reasonable alternative to low dose corticosteroids

<h2>Common Name   milk thistle</h2>

Botanical Name *Silybum mariarum*

Active Ingredients Bioflavonoids, specifically silymarin

Parts Used Seeds of dried flowers

Action Binds to the hepatocyte stabilizing the cell membrane and protecting it from toxins; promotes regeneration of liver cells through protein synthesis; neutralizes toxins in or around the liver by increasing levels of glutathione and by inhibition of damaging leukotrienes; increased antioxidant activity in the liver; increases solubility of bile; takes part in normal detoxification process of liver

Uses Liver disease secondary to alcoholism, hepatitis, chemical toxins, or drugs; for liver protection with long-term therapy with antidepressants, anticonvulsants, or chemotherapy; cholecystitis; psoriasis

Dosage Tincture – 1 ml tid (avoid alcohol-based tinctures: large amounts of alcohol are needed to obtain therapeutic dose of silymarin); table/capsule – standardized to 70% to 80% silymarin; initially 500 mg per day in 3 divided doses for 6 to 8 weeks; with improvement, decrease dose to 140 to 240 mg per day in divided doses; effect should start to be seen 1 week to 10 days after initiation of herb therapy; may take longer (4 to 8 weeks) with alcohol-diseased livers

Precautions Cirrhotic liver changes will not reverse with herb, but advancement may be slowed and quality of life may be improved

Side Effects Diarrhea may occur the first few days of therapy

Herb-Drug Interactions None known

Additional Information Anticipated outcome – liver enzymes normalizing and symptom reversal

<h2>Common Name   peppermint</h2>

Botanical Name *Mentha piperito,* variety *officinalis* or *vulgaris*

Active Ingredient Volatile oil – terpenoids

Parts Used Aerial parts

Action Carminative – elimination of intestinal gas and relaxation of esophageal sphincter; antispasmodic – blocks calcium influx into muscle cells; stimulates flow of bile and increases solubility of bile; external analgesic – initially cools, then warms; nasal decongestant

Uses Cholecystitis, irritable bowel syndrome (IBS), indigestion, infant colic; topically – itching, musculo-skeletal pain, colds

Dosage Tea – 2 to 3 cups per day; equivalent of 3 to 6 gm dried herbs; tincture/oil – 6 to 12 drops per day in divided doses and diluted; tablet/capsule – IBS and cholecystitis – 1 to 2 enteric coated tablets tid between meals; precaution—consult health-care practitioner for use with cholecystitis or obstructed bile ducts

Side Effects None known

Herb-Drug Interactions None known

<h2>Common Name   St. John's wort</h2>

Botanical Name *Hypericum perforatum*

Active Ingredients Hypericin and pseudohypericin

Parts Used   Flowers

Action   Antidepressant believed to have slight monoamine oxidase inhibition (MAOI) and selective serotonin reuptake inhibition (SSRI) actions; antiviral activity against influenza A and B, Epstein-Barr, and herpes viruses

Uses   Mild to moderate depression, mood swings, neuritis, anxiety, sleep disorders; topically on wounds and burns; viral infections; use with HIV is under investigation

Dosage   Tincture – 5 to 10 ml (1 to 2 tsp) bid to tid; table/capsule – standardized to at least 0.1% hypericin; equivalent dose of 1 mg/day in divided doses; take with food; effects can be seen after 4 to 8 weeks of use; long-term use is recommended

Precautions   Do not use concurrent with prescription antidepressants; do not use if pregnant or lactating; do not use with children under 2 years of age; high doses may result in increased liver enzymes; no need to avoid foods with tyramine due to minimal to no MAOI action; risk of hypertensive crisis is low (under investigation)

Side Effects   Photosensitivity of skin; occasional reports of headache

Herb-Drug Interaction   Synergistic effect when used with prescription antidepressants; potential for serotonin syndrome characterized by lethargy, apathy, headache, agitation, and decreased libido; added photosensitivity if used with piroxicam or tetracycline; serotonin syndrome might also be seen if beta sympathomimetic drugs are used concurrently

Additional Information   St. John's wort is a gentle and nontoxic alternative to prescription antidepressants such as Prozac; St. John's wort is one of the most widely prescribed antidepressants in Germany

Common Name   **saw palmetto**

Botanical Name   *Serenoa repens, Sabazl serrulata*

Active Ingredient   Free fatty acids and esters

Parts Used   Berries

Actions   Inhibits the conversion of testosterone to dihydrotestosterone by blocking 5-alpha reductase; reduces prostate size; decreases pro-inflammatory agents contributing to benign prostatic hypertrophy (BPH); speeds breakdown of estrogen, progesterone and prolactin; diuretic

Uses   BPH, chronic non-bacterial prostatitis, chronic cystitis

Dosage   Tea – 1 cup tid – equivalent dose of 1 to 2 gm per day; tablet/capsule – standardized to 85% to 95% fatty acids 320 mg daily one time or in 2 divided doses; length of treatment should be 45 to 90 days; effectiveness should be seen after 30 days of treatment; if outcome is favorable, herb can be taken long-term

Precautions   Prophylactic use is not known to be advantageous

Side Effects   Rare gastric disturbance

Herb-Drug Interactions   None known, but should avoid use with other hormonal therapies

Additional Information   Saw palmetto is a reasonable alternative to Proscar; may interfere with PSA serum level; should be off the herb for 1 to 2 weeks prior to test

Common Name   **valerian**

Botanical Name   *Valeriana officinalis*

Active Ingredients   Essential oils, specifically valerianic acid and valepotriates

Parts Used   Root

Action   Sedative/hypnotic; binds weakly to GABA-A receptors in the CNS (weak affinity for same receptors as benzodiazepines); increases deep sleep and dream states

Uses   Mild anxiety, insomnia, stress headaches, muscle tension

Dosage   Tea – 1 to 3 cups per day or at hs equivalent to 2 to 3 gm; tincture – 1 to 3 ml; repeat up to two times over 6 hours; tablet/capsule – standardized to 0.5% essential oils; equivalent dose to 2 to 3 gm up to bid; safe for long-term use; may take a few doses before effect is seen

Precautions   Do not take with prescription sedative/hypnotics; isolated valepotriates act as stimulants

Side Effects   Occasionally gastric disturbance or morning hang-over effect; occasionally paradoxical response – anxiety, headache; large amounts can cause CNS depression

Herb-Drug Interaction   Additive sedating effect with barbiturates

Additional Information   No complications of dependence or tolerance; smell is foul; improves dream recall; combination with other sedating herbs, such as lemon balm, skullcap, or hops has favorable outcomes in cases of insomnia; best source is dried root that has been dried under 40° F; more is not better when it comes to valerian; reasonable alternative for Xanax

   Note: The information in this chapter is intended as a resource and for the education of the health-care provider. It is in no way intended to replace or substitute for medical prescription. This information should be used along with and in collaboration with clinical herbalists or naturopathic physicians.

Suggested Readings

Blumenthal M et al, editors: *The complete German Commission E monographs, therapeutic guide to herbal medicines,* Boston, 1998, American Botanical Council.

Blumenthal M, editor: *Herbalgram* 41, 1997

Blumenthal M, editor: *Herbalgram* 44, 1998.

Brown DJ: *Herbal prescriptions for better health,* Rocklin, Calif., 1996, Prima Publishing.

Cech RA: Balancing conservation with utilization, *Herbalgram* 45:18-60, 1999.

Kinder C, Cupp MJ: Kava: an herbal sedative, *Nurse Pract* 23(6):14, 156, 1998.

Liebmann R et al: Industry and organizations form partnership for goldenseal conservation, *Herbalgram* 44:58-59, 1998.

Mashour NH, Lin GI, Frishman WH: Herbal medicine for the treatment of cardiovascular disease, *Arch Intern Med* 158:2225-2233, 1998.

Miller LG: Herbal medicinals, *Arch Intern Med* 158:2200-2211, 1998.

Murray MT: *The healing power of herbs,* ed 2, Rocklin, Calif., 1995, Prima Publishing.

Tyler VE: *The honest herbal,* ed 3, Binghamton, N.Y., 1993, Haworth Press.

Weiss RF: *Herbal medicine,* Beaconsfield, England, 1998, Beaconsfield Publishing Ltd.

Winslow LC, Kroll DJ: Herbs as medicine, *Arch Intern Med* 158(20):2192-2199, 1998.

Zink T, Chaffin J: Herbal health products: what family physicians need to know, *Am Fam Physician* 58(5):1133-1140, 1998.

APPENDIX B

Assessment Aids

Jean Nagelkerk

The following information is presented to assist in using common grading and numbering systems in your documentation. The use of a standard approach to documentation assists in comunicating data accurately and consistently.

Table B-1
Documentation of Amplitude of Pulses

Amplitude of Pulse	Scale
Bounding	4
Full, increased	3
Expected	2
Diminished, barely palpable	1
Absent, not palpable	0

Table B-2
Documentation of Murmurs by Grade

Murmur Intensity	Grade
Barely audible	I
Soft but clearly audible	II
Moderately loud	III
Loud, accompanied with thrill	IV
Very loud, thrill palpated easily	V
Very loud, heard with stehoscope off chest, thrill visible, palpated easily	VI

Table B-3
Documentation of Size of Tonsils

Location of Tonsils	Grade
Visible	1+
Halfway between tonsillar pillars and uvula	2+
Touching the uvula	3+
Touching each other	4+

Table B-4
Documentation of the Extent of Edema

Appearance of Edema	Grade
Slight pitting, disappears quickly	1+
Slightly deeper pitting, disappears within 15 seconds	2+
Pitting is noticeable and lasts a minute or more, extremity looks swollen	3+
Pitting is very deep, lasts up to 5 minutes, pitting is distorting	4+

Table B-5
Documentation of Deep Tendon Reflexes

Deep Tendon Reflexes	Grade
No response	0
Sluggish or diminished	1+
Expected response, active	2+
Brisk, slightly hyperactive	3+
Hyperactive, intermittent clonus	4+

Table B-6
Muscle Strength Grading

Muscle Strength	Grade
Full ROM, full resistance	5
Full ROM, some resistance	4
Full ROM	3
Passive ROM	2
Slight contraction	1
No contraction	0

Table B-8
Characteristic Sounds of Percussion

Percussion Sounds	Examples
Tympany	Gastric air bubble
Resonance	Normal lung
Hyperresonance	Emphysematous lung
Dullness	Liver
Flatness	Muscle

Table B-7
Documentation of Uterine Prolapse

Uterine Location	Degree
One cm into vaginal canal	I
Within vaginal canal	II
Protrudes outside the vagina	III

Figure B-1   Denver Developmental Tool. (Courtesy Denver Developmental Materials, Inc., Denver, Colo.)

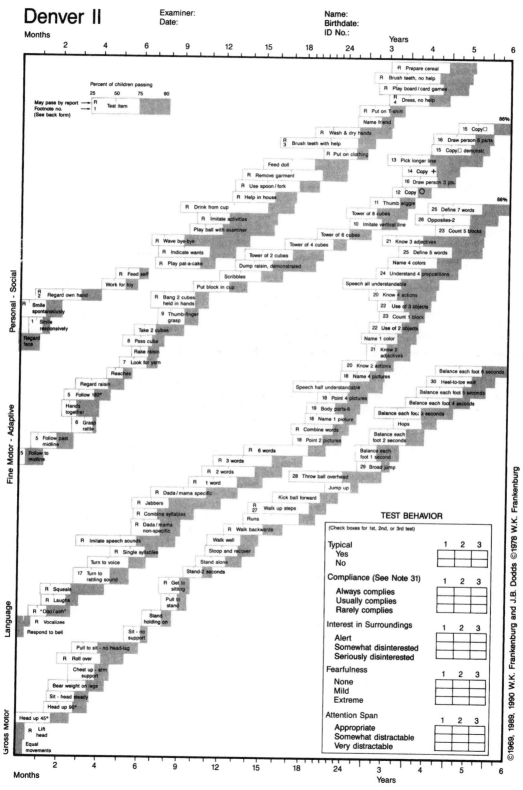

Denver II

APPENDIX B

Continued

DIRECTIONS FOR ADMINISTRATION

1. Try to get child to smile by smiling, talking or waving. Do not touch him/her.
2. Child must stare at hand several seconds.
3. Parent may help guide toothbrush and put toothpaste on brush.
4. Child does not have to be able to tie shoes or button/zip in the back.
5. Move yarn slowly in an arc from one side to the other, about 8" above child's face.
6. Pass if child grasps rattle when it is touched to the backs or tips of fingers.
7. Pass if child tries to see where yarn went. Yarn should be dropped quickly from sight from tester's hand without arm movement.
8. Child must transfer cube from hand to hand without help of body, mouth, or table.
9. Pass if child picks up raisin with any part of thumb and finger.
10. Line can vary only 30 degrees or less from tester's line.⁄
11. Make a fist with thumb pointing upward and wiggle only the thumb. Pass if child imitates and does not move any fingers other than the thumb.

◯	‖	✛	▢
12. Pass any enclosed form. Fail continuous round motions.	13. Which line is longer? (Not bigger.) Turn paper upside down and repeat. (pass 3 of 3 or 5 of 6)	14. Pass any lines crossing near midpoint.	15. Have child copy first. If failed, demonstrate.

When giving items 12, 14, and 15, do not name the forms. Do not demonstrate 12 and 14.

16. When scoring, each pair (2 arms, 2 legs, etc.) counts as one part.
17. Place one cube in cup and shake gently near child's ear, but out of sight. Repeat for other ear.
18. Point to picture and have child name it. (No credit is given for sounds only.)
    If less than 4 pictures are named correctly, have child point to picture as each is named by tester.

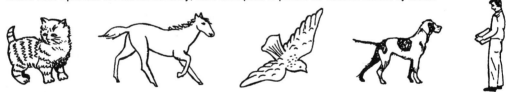

19. Using doll, tell child: Show me the nose, eyes, ears, mouth, hands, feet, tummy, hair. Pass 6 of 8.
20. Using pictures, ask child: Which one flies?... says meow?... talks?... barks?... gallops? Pass 2 of 5, 4 of 5.
21. Ask child: What do you do when you are cold?... tired?... hungry? Pass 2 of 3, 3 of 3.
22. Ask child: What do you do with a cup? What is a chair used for? What is a pencil used for?
    Action words must be included in answers.
23. Pass if child correctly places and says how many blocks are on paper. (1, 5).
24. Tell child: Put block on table; under table; in front of me, behind me. Pass 4 of 4.
    (Do not help child by pointing, moving head or eyes.)
25. Ask child: What is a ball?... lake?... desk?... house?... banana?... curtain?... fence?... ceiling? Pass if defined in terms of use, shape, what it is made of, or general category (such as banana is fruit, not just yellow). Pass 5 of 8, 7 of 8.
26. Ask child: If a horse is big, a mouse is __? If fire is hot, ice is __? If the sun shines during the day, the moon shines during the __? Pass 2 of 3.
27. Child may use wall or rail only, not person. May not crawl.
28. Child must throw ball overhand 3 feet to within arm's reach of tester.
29. Child must perform standing broad jump over width of test sheet (8 1/2 inches).
30. Tell child to walk forward, ⌒⌒⌒⌒➔ heel within 1 inch of toe. Tester may demonstrate.
    Child must walk 4 consecutive steps.
31. In the second year, half of normal children are non-compliant.

OBSERVATIONS:

Figure B-1, cont'd For legend see page 362.

Mini-Mental State Examination

Patient _____ Examiner _____ Date _____

Maximum Score	Score	
		Orientation
5	( )	What is the (year) (season) (date) (day) (month)?
5	( )	Where are we: (state) (county) (town) (hospital) (floor)
		Registration
3	( )	Name three objects: (Apple, Penny, Table) 1 second to say each. Then ask the patient all three after you have said them. Give 1 point for each correct answer. Then repeat them until he or she learns all three. Count trials and record. Trials _____
		Attention and Calculation
5	( )	Serial 7's. 1 point for each correct. Stop after five answers. Alternatively spell "world" backwards.
		Recall
3	( )	Ask for the three objects repeated above. Give 1 point for each correct.
		Language
9	( )	Name a pencil, and watch (2 points)

Repeat the following "No ifs, ands, or buts." (1 point)

Follow a three-stage command:

"Take a paper in your right hand, fold it in half, and put it on the floor." (3 points)

Read and obey the following:

CLOSE YOUR EYES (1 point)

Write a sentence (1 point)

Copy design (overlapping pentagons) (1 point)

Overlapping pentagons

Total score

ASSESS level of consciousness along a continuum _____

Alert   Drowsy   Stupor   Coma

Instructions for Administration of Mini-Mental State Examination

Orientation

(1) Ask for the date. Then ask specifically for parts omitted, e.g., "Can you also tell what season it is?" One point for each correct.
(2) Ask in turn "Can you tell me the name of this hospital?" (town, country, etc.) One point for each correct.

Registration

Ask the patient if you may test his or her memory. Then say the names of three unrelated objects, clearly and slowly, about 1 second for each.

After you have said all three, ask him or her to repeat them. This first repetition determines his or her score (0-3), but keep saying them until he or she can repeat all three, up to six trials. If he or she does not eventually learn all three, recall cannot be meaningfully tested.

Attention and Calculation

Ask the patient to begin with 100 and count backwards by 7. Stop after five subtractions (93, 86, 79, 65). Score the total number of correct answers.

If the patient cannot or will not perform this task, ask him or her to spell the word "world" backwards. The score is the number of letters in correct order, e.g., dlrow = 5, dlorw = 3.

Recall

Ask the patient if he or she can recall the three words you previously asked him or her to remember. Score 0-3.

Language

Naming: Show the patient a wrist watch and ask him or her what it is. Repeat for pencil. Score 0-2.

Repetition: Ask the patient to repeat the sentence after you. Allow only one trial. Score 0 or 1.

Three-stage command: Give the patient a piece of plain blank paper and repeat the command. Score 1 point for each part correctly executed.

Reading: On a blank piece of paper print the sentence "Close your eyes," in letters large enough for the patient to see clearly. Ask him or her to read it and do what it says. Score 1 point only if he or she actually closes his or her eyes.

Writing: Give the patient a blank piece of paper and ask him or her to write a sentence for you. Do not dictate a sentence, it is to be written spontaneously. It must contain a subject and verb and be sensible. Correct grammar and punctuation are not necessary.

Copying: On a clean piece of paper, draw intersecting pentagons, each side about 1 inch, and ask him or her to copy it exactly as it is. All 10 angles must be present, and 2 must intersect to score 1 point. Tremor and rotation are ignored.

Estimate the patient's level of sensorium along a continuum, from alert on the left to coma on the right.

APPENDIX C

Additional Case Studies

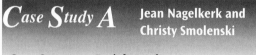

Case Study A — Jean Nagelkerk and Christy Smolenski

CHIEF COMPLAINT: Facial Numbness

History of Present Illness T.J. is a 29-year-old Caucasian male who presents with chief complaint of R sided facial numbness, aching pain behind R ear, increased tearing of his right eye, and loss of taste on the affected side. He felt fine when he went to bed, but when he awoke he became alarmed by the sudden onset of symptoms. T.J. immediately phoned for an appointment with his health-care provider, and is anxious about the possibility of a stroke. He reports that his grandfather died from a stroke 6 months ago. T.J. denies fever, chills, H/A, rash, or decreased hearing. He has not experienced a tick bite and has not experienced any other neurological symptoms.

Past Medical History Treated for bronchitis 2 weeks ago with a Z-Pack at an urgent care center; history of genital herpes

Past Surgical History Negative

Family History Maternal grandfather deceased at age 76 from acute CVA; father age 60, type 2 diabetes; mother age 56, HTN; sister age 28, anxiety disorder

Developmental Stage Intimacy versus Isolation

Role-Relationship T.J. is a single male who works second shift in an automobile factory in Detroit, Mich. He enjoys the second shift because he has time to "party" with his friends after work and sleep late in the morning. T.J. acknowledges several sexual partners in the past year. He resides in a duplex owned by his parents.

Sleep/Rest Typically falls to sleep between 2 and 4 AM and awakens rested between 10 and 11:30 AM.

Activity/Exercise Enjoys lifting weights and uses the bodybuilding equipment daily at a local health club. T.J. owns a motorcycle and a corvette, which he stores in the winter.

Coping/Stress T.J. enjoys his life even though his parents feel he should settle down. Does worry at times about his health because his dad and mother have chronic illnesses and his grandfather recently passed away

Health Management Smokes a half pack per day × 10 years. Drinks at least 3 beers a day, and often more when he "parties" with his friends.

Medications For muscle building, T.J. takes creatine that he gets from a local health food store.

Allergies NKMA

Pertinent Physical Findings

Vital Signs Height 6 feet 1 inch; weight 219 pounds; BMI 29; temperature 98.9° F; heart rate 90; respirations 22; blood pressure 138/88

General Appearance Alert and oriented × 4; casually dressed; speech clear; coordinated movements; fidgeting in chair

HEENT Head normocephalic, atraumatic. Face: mild R facial droop; nasal-labial fold less pronounced; decreased R facial sensation to sharp and dull sensation; skin pink, warm, and dry without lesions. Eyes: PERRL for direct and consensual light reflex and accommodation, EOMs intact; fundoscopic: optic discs sharp, well defined, cream color, no exudates or hemorrhages; inability to fully close R eye. Ears: TMs gray, landmarks intact with distinct cone of light, no vesicular eruptions in ear canal. Nose: Patent bilaterally, septum midline, no discharge, polyps, or sinus tenderness. Throat: Oral mucosa pink, moist, no lesions, tonsils 2+, uvula midline

Neck   Supple without limitation of motion, no cervical lymphadenopathy, trachea midline, no thyromegaly or carotid bruits

Heart   Apical pulse 90 regular rate and rhythm, no S₃ or S₄, PMI 5th ICS-MCL

Lungs   Clear to auscultation

Neurological   CN II-XII grossly intact, DTR 2+ bil symmetrical, muscular strength intact bil, no atrophy or tremors. Cerebellar function intact with rapid alternating hand movements—finger to nose, Romberg negative, sensation intact to light touch and pinprick, able to heel-to-toe walk

---

Discussion Questions

What type of history data should be collected?

What type of physical data should be collected?

What are the differential diagnoses?

What are the probable causes of the presenting symptoms?

What diagnostic tests would you consider?

What is your diagnostic impression?

What is the therapeutic plan of care?

What are the patient education and/or community resources?

What is your follow-up plan?

Discussion, references, and selected readings for this optional case study exercise can be found in the accompanying Instructor's Manual.

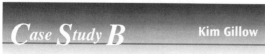

Case Study B   Kim Gillow

CHIEF COMPLAINT: Open Wound

History of Present Illness   C.M. is a 72-year-old Caucasian male who presents with chief complaint of a "sore on my stump." C.M. had bilateral below-the-knee amputations in 1995 secondary to diabetes. He is ambulatory with bilateral prostheses and canes. He received a new pair of prostheses 2 weeks ago, and noticed an open area on the lateral side of his left stump 6 days ago. C.M. states "this new leg is rubbing on it." His wife, who is accompanying him, has been cleaning the area with hydrogen peroxide and states it was draining through several 4×4s for 3 or 4 days, but now has minimal drainage. She has been using Duoderm under a 4×4 the last 3 days. She states, "it had lot of yellow stuff on it, but that all came off." C.M. denies pain at the site; however, he has a history of peripheral neuropathy.

Past Medical History   Type 2 diabetes mellitus, hypertension

Past Surgical History   Bilateral BKA, 1995

Family History   Mother deceased (age 70) diabetes; father deceased (age 72) HTN; sister (age 70) HTN

Developmental Stage   Ego Integrity versus Despair

Role-Relationship   Married 53 years. C.M. and his wife live on the family farm in a two-story house. He is able to climb the stairs with his prostheses. Their daughter and her family live next door and visit almost daily. C.M. and his wife attend a variety of church and social functions and go to Florida for 2 months every winter.

Nutrition/Metabolic   C.M.'s own teeth are in good repair. His wife prepares all of his meals or they go out to eat. He eats three balanced meals a day plus a protein snack at bedtime. He states, "I'm real careful because of my diabetes."

Sleep/Rest   Usually goes to bed around 11:30 PM and is up by 8 AM. He rarely naps during the day.

Activity/Exercise   Performs all activities of daily living without difficulty. Attaches his own prostheses. Still farms part-time and can drive his tractor

Coping/Stress   C.M. has a large circle of support. According to his wife he has always been "easy-going." Wife states, "I'm doing fine. We're in this together. Always have been for 53 years now."

Health Management   Does not smoke, drink, or use recreational drugs. Self-monitors blood sugars bid with usual range of 110 to 120 in the morning and 140 to 160 at 4 PM. Self-monitors B/P weekly with usual reading around 130/60.

Carefully controls his diet. Td 1995; pneumovax 1995. Has signed advanced directives and wife is designated as durable medical power of attorney

Self-Perception and Values/Beliefs C.M. believes he's had a good life and looks forward to the future. He has adjusted to his amputations, stating "I still get around pretty well. Just not as fast. I'm in no hurry." His wife is willing and capable caregiver. There is an obvious bond of affection between them.

Medications Monopril 20 mg qd; Novolin 70/30 insulin 10 units AM and 5 units PM.

Allergies NKMA

Pertinent Physical Findings

Vital Signs Height with prostheses 6 feet 0 inches; weight 165 pounds; BMI 22; temperature: 98.2° F; heart rate 72; respirations 16; blood pressure 134/70

Skin Open area measuring 1.5 cm × 1.4 cm on lateral aspect left leg just below knee. Not directly over incision scar. Wound bed pink. No exudate on dressing. Periwound border dry and scaly, extending 0.5 cm out then pink intact tissue with capillary refill in less than 3 seconds. No erythema, maceration, or induration

Peripheral Vascular Popliteal pulses 2+ bilaterally

Neurological Loss of pinprick sensation midthigh and below bilaterally

---

Discussion Questions

What type of history data should be collected?

What type of physical data should be collected?

What are the differential diagnoses?

What are the probable causes of the presenting symptoms?

What diagnostic tests would you consider?

What is your diagnostic impression?

What is the therapeutic plan of care?

Discussion Questions—cont'd

What are the patient education and/or community resources?

What is your follow up plan?

Discussion, references, and selected readings for this optional case study exercise can be found in the accompanying Instructor's Manual.

Case Study C   Mary Moran Barr

CHIEF COMPLAINT: Abdominal Pain and Tenderness

History of Present Illness C.R. is a 52-year-old Caucasian female executive secretary who presents with a 10-day history of intermittent generalized abdominal pain. She reports episodes of alternating diarrhea and constipation for the past month. She also reports having the flu, diffuse abdominal pain, and a slight fever (99.5° F orally) for a 2-day period 2 weeks ago. Her abdominal pain is now constant and she grades it an "8" on a scale of 1-10, with 10 being most severe. She reports no rectal bleeding and her last stool was hard (constipated) 2 days ago. She has eaten little in the last 48 hours because her appetite has decreased with her increasing pain. Her last menstrual period was 3 years ago and she is menopausal, taking hormone replacement therapy. She is not currently sexually active.

Past Medical History Has a history of HTN for the last 8 years, well controlled with a beta-blocker

Past Surgical History Bladder suspension surgery at age 40, no complications. G-V, Para-II, Ab-III, with 2 uncomplicated deliveries and 3 D&Cs. Appendectomy at age 10

Family History Father 86 A&W; mother, 85, in a nursing home with cerebrovascular dementia; five siblings with HTN; one sibling with CAD and diverticulosis

Developmental Stage Generativity versus Stagnation

Role-Relationship Married for 27 years, living with husband. Two grown daughters live in other cities. C.R. is close with her husband and daughters. She has worked at her present place of employment for 12 years.

Sleep/Rest   Sleeps 8 hours at night and awakens feeling rested. Infrequent insomnia related to occasional increased stress at work

Nutrition/Metabolic   Eats a light breakfast, usually a plain bagel, orange juice, and coffee. Lunch is sporadic – sandwiches or salad and other times yogurt and fruit, but sometimes skips lunch altogether. Snacks in late afternoon on crackers and cheese and a glass of wine. C.R. eats a large dinner consisting of meat, salad, rolls, and dessert. Snacks on crackers, popcorn, and ice cream

Activity/Exercise   Remains active. Does not like to be sedentary. Routine exercise is "spotty." Sometimes walks or swims, but has no pattern or regularity

Coping/Stress   Is occasionally anxious. C.R. feels pressure to do more and is easily overwhelmed when she takes on too much. Feels she needs to budget time, activity, and rest more evenly. Her husband and children are supportive. Does not attend church and does not take time for self-reflection

Health Management   Routinely schedules annual examinations with Pap and mammogram. Non-smoker. Alcohol, has 8 ounces per day (wine). Drinks 3 cups of coffee per day (half of this coffee is decaffeinated)

Self-Perception and Values/Beliefs   General positive feeling, but occasionally discouraged in self-image related to being overweight. Believes she is a good person and well accomplished, but compares herself to others with resulting negative self-image.

Medications   Multivitamin qd, Prempro (0.625 mg estrogen and 2.5 mg progesterone) qd, atenolol qd

Allergies   Renografin-iodine based x-ray dye (anaphylaxis)

Pertinent Physical Findings

Vital Signs   Temperature 100.5° F; BP 152/95; pulse 64; respirations 18; weight 170 pounds; height 5 feet 7 inches; BMI 27

General   Well developed, moderately obese, muscular, large breasted and pear-shaped, in moderate distress

Lungs   CTA without adventitious sounds

Heart   Apical pulse with regular rate and rhythm, no murmurs, heaves, or thrills

Abdomen   Abdomen round, slightly distended with hypoactive bowel sounds. Abdomen is firm and tender in LLQ with both direct and rebound tenderness. No hepatomegaly or splenomegaly. No CVA tenderness

GU/Rectal   Pelvic examination was deferred at this time due to patient's pain level. Rectal examination reveals marked tenderness and fullness. There is no stool present in the rectum. There is a fleck of dark brown stool on gloved examination that tests hemoccult +

Discussion Questions

What type of history data should be collected?

What type of physical data should be collected?

What are the differential diagnoses?

What are the probable causes of the presenting symptoms?

What diagnostic tests would you consider?

What is your diagnostic impression?

What is the therapeutic plan of care?

What are the patient education and/or community resources?

What is your follow-up plan?

Discussion, references, and selected readings for this optional case study exercise can be found in the accompanying Instructor's Manual.

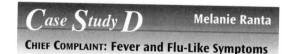

Case Study D   **Melanie Ranta**

CHIEF COMPLAINT: Fever and Flu-Like Symptoms

History of Present Illness   K.R. is a 23-year-old Caucasian female who presents with vague complaints of fever and "not feeling well." Two weeks ago she was seen for a cellulitis of her right hand that had erupted spontaneously, was well demarcated, and had no apparent open areas. She was treated with Keflex 500 mg qid × 10 days with res-olution of symptoms. Since that time, she feels that she has never returned to her usual state of good health. She is running a low-grade temperature (be-low 101° F) and has flu-like symptoms. K.R. re-ports feeling so tired that she could go back to bed in the morning after she has been up for only 3 or 4 hours. Taking her dog for a walk around the block exhausts her. K.R. does not have a good appetite. She denies weight loss, chills, rash, chest pain, dys-pnea, or heart murmur. K.R. has not used appetite suppressants and does not engage in recreational drug use.

Past Medical History Cellulitis of R hand; oth-erwise unremarkable

Past Surgical History Unremarkable

Family History Mother, 50, has type 2 dia-betes well controlled with diet; father, 55, has HTN treated with medication; no siblings

Developmental Stage Intimacy versus Isola-tion

Role-Relationship K.R. is married to a 30-year-old electrical engineer. K.R. works as a med-ical social worker in a hospital setting. She attends a Catholic church with her husband every Sunday.

Nutrition/Metabolic Typically eats a well bal-anced diet and limits red meats. For breakfast has fruit or cereal. Lunch consists of a half sandwich, piece of fruit, and milk. Dinner consists of pasta, vegetables, and meat. Snacks include fruit, crack-ers, or raw vegetables

Sleep/Rest Usually goes to bed at 10:30 PM and awakens at 6:30 AM rested. Now is experienc-ing extreme fatigue and is constantly tired. Fre-quently naps when arrives home from work and falls asleep by 9 PM.

Activity/Exercise K.R. and her husband enjoy outdoor activities such as swimming, biking, and hiking. She usually works out at the local health spa every night, but has not been doing this because of extreme fatigue. Her husband is concerned about her because she is not interested in any recreational activities and prefers to lie around the house.

Coping/Stress K.R. has a very supportive hus-band and parents. She has many girlfriends that she calls, and is active in a golf and basketball league.

Health Management Schedules annual physi-cal examinations ever since age 20 when she be-came sexually active. Schedules dental examina-tions and cleanings every 6 months, last dental visit was 3 weeks ago. Nonsmoker. Alcohol, has a mixed drink at social events. Does not use recreational drugs. Td: 6/5/2000

Self-Perception and Values/Beliefs K.R. is sat-isfied with her life. Enjoys her husband, parents, and friends. Tries to help out with community ac-tivities through her church

Medications Triphasil qd; does not use any herbal preparations

Allergies NKMA

Pertinent Physical Findings

Vital Signs Temperature 100.8° F; pulse 92; respirations 16; BP 98/62; Height 5 feet 2 inches; weight 120 pounds; BMI 20

General Appearance Alert and oriented × 4; well-developed and well-nourished female

Skin No rashes or suspicious moles present. Tender, reddened, raised areas of 1 to 2 mm on tips of fingers. No petechiae

HEENT Head: Normocephalic, nontraumatic, symmetric features and expression. Eyes: Conjunc-tiva not injected, free of lesions, sclera non-icteric. Lids without exudate or lesions, PERRL, EOMs in-tact. Optic discs are flat and of normal sized. Retina free of exudate or hemorrhage. ENT: Ears and nose fee of lesions, scars or masses. TMs pearly gray with landmarks intact. Canals clear with pink mu-cosa, no masses. Hearing is grossly normal to con-versation. Nasal mucosa pink with no lesions, sep-tum midline, turbinates normal with no bogginess. Lips free of lesions, teeth in good repair, gums fee of swelling or redness. Oral mucosa moist and pink, hard and soft palate free of lesions, tongue midline with no lesions, tonsils not enlarged, post pharynx with no erythema. Uvula midline

Neck Supple, symmetrical with no masses, no adenopathy. Trachea midline, no crepitus. Thyroid not enlarged no tenderness present, no masses. No carotid bruit

Lungs Normal diaphragmatic movement without use of accessory muscles. No retractions. Chest clear to percussion and auscultation. Breath-ing even and nonlabored

Heart PMI non-displaced. No thrills, lifts or heaves. S_1 and S_2 audible and regular, grade 3/6 SEM audible with radiation throughout chest and with midsystolic clicks. Nailbeds pink with spontaneous refill, no clubbing, and no splinter hemor-rhages. Femoral, pedal, radial pulses 2+ and even bilateral. No peripheral edema

Abdomen Soft, rounded, no masses or organomegaly, no tenderness. No abdominal or in-guinal hernias

Musculoskeletal Normal gait, no imbalance with movement. Back straight without bony tender-ness. Equal strength of extremities bilaterally, full ROM to joints upper and lower extremities

Neurological CN II-XII grossly intact. DTRs brachial and patellar symmetric, sensation intact to touch

---

Discussion Questions

What type of history data should be collected?

What type of physical data should be collected?

What are the differential diagnoses?

What are the probable causes of the presenting symptoms?

What diagnostic tests would you consider?

What is your diagnostic impression?

What is the therapeutic plan of care?

What are the patient education and/or community resources?

What is your follow-up plan?

Discussion and references for this optional case study exercise can be found in the accompanying Instructor's Manual.

---

*C*ase *S*tudy *E*   **Michelle Elmendorf**

CHIEF COMPLAINT: Pelvic Pain and Dysmenorrhea

History of Present Illness B.P. is a 30-year-old Caucasian female who presents with chief com-plaint of generalized pelvic pain and dysmenorrhea for 6 months. B.P. describes the pain as constant aching pain that begins about 2 to 3 days prior to menses and becomes increasingly severe until her menstrual flow ceases. B.P. reports that her men-strual flow has increased and she is experiencing premenstrual spotting every month. Her menstrual cycle is otherwise normal with 28-day cycles and normal flow lasting 4 or 5 days. B.P. reports painful intercourse 5 to 6 days prior to menses. Denies dy-suria, urgency, hematuria, dyschezia, or rectal bleeding. She denies having similar symptoms in the past. She has tried over-the-counter Ibuprofen and Midol with minimal relief.

Past Medical History Migraine headaches, G3 P3, no complications with pregnancies, NSVD × 3.

Past Surgical History Unremarkable

Family History Mother age 55, breast CA; fa-ther age 57, HTN; sister age 29, A&W

Developmental Stage Intimacy versus Isola-tion

Role-Relationship B.P. is married and lives with her husband and their three children, ages 1, 3, and 5 years old. She is staying home to care for the children and does not work outside of the home.

Nutrition/Metabolic B.P. cooks meals for her family. She eats out once per week with her hus-band. Breakfast usually consists of cereal and juice. Lunch consists of a sandwich with cold cuts, fresh or canned fruit, and milk. Dinner is generally a casserole, or meat, potatoes, vegetables, and milk. She keeps raw vegetables and fresh fruit at home for snacks during the day, and snacks on chips and cheese or popcorn in the evening.

Sleep/Rest Normally sleeps 6 to 7 hours per night and wakes feeling rested

Activity/Exercise Enjoys walking for 45 to 60 minutes every day

Coping/Stress B.P. has many friends in her neighborhood that are supportive and that she reg-ularly talks with. Her husband is also supportive of her. She has been married for 6 years and de-nies any marital problems. She handles stress by talking with her mother or sister and by taking walks alone.

Health Management Non-smoker, does not use alcohol or recreational drugs. Routinely sched-ules annual physical examination and biannual dental examinations. Does not perform self-breast examinations. Last tetanus was in 1994

Self-Perception and Values/Beliefs Enjoys her life, family, and friends. Attends a Methodist church weekly. B.P. has a bachelor's degree and is a certified public accountant. She plans on returning to work when her children are in school.

Medications Ortho Tri-Cyclen one pill every day

Allergies NKMA

Pertinent Physical Findings

Vital Signs Height 5 feet 5 inches; weight 120 pounds; BMI 20; temperature 98.0° F; apical pulse 80; respirations 20; B/P 130/80

General Appearance B.P. is a 30-year-old, well-developed, well-nourished Caucasian female in no acute distress

Lungs Clear to auscultation bilaterally, symmetric chest expansion

Cardiovascular Regular rate and rhythm with normal S_1 and S_2. No murmur, gallop, rub, or thrill

Abdomen Abdomen is soft, without bulges or masses. Mild tenderness to palpation in suprapubic region. Bowel sounds are active in all four quadrants. No organomegaly

Genital Generalized pelvic tenderness during examination; tender adnexa; slightly enlarged, retroflexed uterus, tender indurated nodules in the cul-de-sac; no vaginal or cervical discharge

Rectal No masses, small external hemorrhoids, hemoccult negative stool in anal vault, intact anal tone

---

Discussion Questions

What type of history data should be collected?

What type of physical data should be collected?

What are the differential diagnoses?

What are the probable causes of the presenting symptoms?

What diagnostic tests would you consider?

What is your diagnostic impression?

What is the therapeutic plan of care?

What are the patient education and/or community resources?

What is your follow-up plan?

Discussion and references for this optional case study exercise can be found in the accompanying Instructor's Manual.

APPENDIX D

Key to Abbreviations

Jean Nagelkerk

ACD	Anemia of chronic disease	**CEA**	Carcinoembryonic antigen
ACE	Angiotensin converting enzyme	**CHD**	Coronary heart disease
ACP	American College of Physicians	**CHF**	Congestive heart failure
ACR	American College of Radiology	**CIS**	Carcinoma in situ
AD	Alzheimer's disease	**CMT**	Cervical motion tenderness
ADHD	Attention deficit/hyperactivity disorder	**CNS**	Central nervous system
		CPT	Physicians' current procedural terminology
ADR	Adverse drug reaction		
ALT	Alanine aminotransferase	**CRP**	C-reactive protein
ANA	Antinuclear antibody	**C&S**	Culture and sensitivity
AOM	Acute otitis media	**CT**	Computed tomography
AP	Alkaline phosphatase	**CTA**	Clear to auscultation
A&P	Anterior and posterior	**CVA**	Costovertebral angle
ASA	Aspirin sensitive asthma	**CXR**	Chest x-ray
ASCUS	Atypical squamous cells of undetermined significance	**D&C**	Dilation and curettage
		DCCT	The diabetes control and complications trial
ASO	Antistreptolysin O		
ASOC	Altered states of consciousness	**DENVER II**	Denver developmental screening tool
AST	Aspartate aminotransferase		
AV	Arteriol/vein ratio	**DEXA**	Dual energy x-ray absorptiometry
AVN	Avascular necrosis	**DHEAS**	Dehydroepiandrosterone sulfate
A&W	Alive and well	**DM**	Diabetes mellitus
B_{12}	Vitamin B_{12} (cyanocobalamin, extrinsic factor)	**DMARD**	Disease-modifying antirheumatic drug
BCC	Basal cell carcinoma	**DRSP**	Drug resistant streptococcus pneumonia
BCP	Birth control pills		
BKA	Below-the-knee amputation	**DtaP**	Diptheria and tetanus toxoid acellular pertussis vaccine
BMI	Body mass index		
BP	Blood pressure	**DTR**	Deep tendon reflexes
BPH	Benign prostatic hypertrophy	**DUB**	Dysfunctional uterine bleeding
BSE	Breast self examination	**DVT**	Deep vein thrombosis
BUN	Blood urea nitrogen	**ECF**	Extracellular fluid
BV	Bacterial vaginosis	**ECG**	Electrocardiogram
CAD	Coronary artery disease	**ED**	Emergency department
CAM	Complementary and Alternative medicine	**EOM**	External otitis media
		EOMI	Extraocular muscles intact
CBC	Complete blood count	**EPS**	Expressed prostatic secretions

ESR	Erythrocyte sedimentation rate	**MCL**	Midclavicular line
ESWL	Extracorporeal shock wave litho-	**MCP**	Metacarpophalangeal
	tripsy	**MCV**	Mean corpuscular volume
FB	Foreign body	**MM**	Malignant melanoma
FBS	Fasting blood glucose	**MMR**	Measles, mumps, and rubella vac-
FDA	Food and drug administration		cine
FNA	Fine needle aspiration	**MRI**	Magnetic resonance Imaging
FVC	Forced vital capacity	**MVA**	Motor-vehicle accident
GABHS	Group A beta-hemolytic strepto-	**NAC**	Natural alternative complemen-
	coccal pharyngitis		tary
GERD	Gastroesophageal reflux disease	**NAD**	No apparent distress
HBIG	Hepatitis B immunoglobulin	**NCCAM**	National Center for Complemen-
HBV	Hepatitis B virus		tary and Alternative Medicine
H&H	Hemoglobin and hematocrit	**NCEP**	National Cholesterol Education
H&P	History and physical examination		Program
HbsAg	Hepatitis B surface antigen	**NKMA**	No known medication allergies
HCG	Human chorionic gonadotropin	**NP**	Nurse practitioner
HDL	High density lipoprotein	**NSR**	Normal sinus rhythm
HIB	H. influenza type B conjugated	**NSAID**	Nonsteroidal antiinflammatory drug
	vaccine	**NSVD**	Normal spontaneous vaginal de-
HPV	Human papillomavirus		livery
HRT	Hormone replacement therapy	**N/V**	Nausea and vomiting
HSIL	High-grade squamous intraepithe-	**OA**	Osteoarthritis
	lial lesion	**OB**	Obstetrics
HSV	Herpes simplex virus	**OCP**	Oral contraceptive pills
HTN	Hypertension	**OM**	Otitis media
IBS	Irritable bowel syndrome	**O&P**	Ova and parasites
ICF	Intracellular fluid	**PCN**	Penicillin
ICS	Intercostal space	**PERRLA**	Pupils equal, round, react to light
IDA	Iron deficiency anemia		and accommodation
IgM	Immunoglobulin M	**PET**	Positron emission tomography
INR	International normalized ratio	**PID**	Pelvic inflammatory disease
IUD	Intrauterine device	**PIP**	Proximal interphalangeal
IVP	Intravenous pyelogram	**PMI**	Point of maximal impulse
JVD	Jugular venous distention	**PMH**	Past medical history
KUB	Kidney, ureter, and bladder	**PMN**	Polymorphonuclear neutrophil
LBP	Lower back pain	**PROM**	Premature rupture of membranes
LMCL	Left midclavicular line	**PSA**	Prostate-specific antigen
LDL	Low density lipoprotein	**PT**	Prothrombin time
LES	Lower esophageal sphincter	**PTT**	Partial thromboplastin time
LMP	Last menstrual period	**PUD**	Peptic ulcer disease
LMW	Low molecular weight	**PV**	Polycythemia vera
LSB	Left scapular border	**PVD**	Peripheral vascular disease
LSIL	Low-grade squamous intraepithe-	**PVR**	Post voiding residual
	lial lesion	**RA**	Rheumatoid arthritis
LVH	Left ventricular hypertrophy	**RAST**	Radioallergosorbent testing
MCH	Mean corpuscular hemoglobin	**RBC**	Red blood cells
MCHC	Mean corpuscular hemoglobin	**RBS**	Random blood sugar
	concentrate	**RDW**	Red blood cell distribution width

RF	Rheumatoid factor	**TIA**	Transient ischemic attacks
ROS	Review of systems	**TIBC**	Total iron-binding capacity
RRR	Regular rate and rhythm	**TMJ**	Temporomandibular joint
RSV	Respiratory syncytial virus	**TRH**	Thyrotropin releasing hormone
RUE	Right upper extremity	**TSH**	Thyroid stimulating hormone
SBFT	Small bowel follow-through	**TT**	Therapeutic touch
SCC	Squamous cell carcinoma	**U/A**	Urinalysis
SE	Side effect	**UGI**	Upper gastrointestinal infection
SIL	Squamous intraepithelial lesion	**URI**	Upper respiratory infection
SLE	Systemic lupus erythematosus	**UTD**	Up to date
SLR	Straight leg raising	**UTI**	Urinary tract infection
SOB	Shortness of breath	**VDRL**	Venereal Disease Research Laboratory
SPECT	Single photon emission computed tomography	**VLDL**	Very low density lipoprotein
SPT	Skin phototype	**VPPM**	Voiding post prostatic massage
SSRI	Selective serotonin reuptake inhibitor	**WBC**	White blood count
T&A	Tonsillectomy and adenoidectomy	**WNL**	Within normal limits
TCT	Thrombin clotting time	**XL**	Extended release
TENS	Transcutaneous electrical nerve stimulation		

Index

Page references with "t" denote tables: page references in italics denote figures.